Neocortical Dynamics and Human EEG Rhythms

Neocortical Dynamics and Human EEG Rhythms

Paul L. Nunez
Tulane University

With Contributions by

Brian A. Cutillo
EEG Systems Lab

Alan S. Gevins
EEG Systems Lab

Lester Ingber
Lester Ingber Research

Fernando H. Lopes da Silva
University of Amsterdam

Kenneth L. Pilgreen
Tulane University

Richard B. Silberstein
Swinburne Centre for Applied Neurosciences

New York Oxford
OXFORD UNIVERSITY PRESS
1995

Oxford University Press

Oxford New York Toronto
Delhi Bombay Calcutta Madras Karachi
Kuala Lumpur Singapore Hong Kong Tokyo
Nairobi Dar es Salaam Cape Town
Melbourne Auckland Madrid

and associated companies in
Berlin Ibadan

Published by Oxford University Press, Inc.,
200 Madison Avenue, New York, New York 10016

Oxford is a registered trademark of Oxford University Press

Library of Congress Cataloging-in-Publication Data
Neocortical dynamics and human EEG rhythms /
edited by Paul L. Nunez.
p. cm. Includes bibliographical references and index.
ISBN 0-19-505728-7
1. Neocortex--Electric properties. 2. Electroencephalography.
3. Visual evoked response. I. Nunez, Paul L.
[DNLM: 1. Cerebral Cortex--physiology.
2. Electrophysiology. 3. Electroencephalography.
WL 307 N438 1995] QP383.12.N46 1995 612.8'25--dc20
DNLM/DLC for Library of Congress 94-5465

9 8 7 6 5 4 3 2 1

Printed in the United States of America
on acid-free paper

Preface

Electroencephalography (EEG) is a genuine global measure of neocortical dynamic function with sufficient temporal resolution to follow the millisecond time changes associated with information processing. However, this "window on the mind" is often opaque, revealing only shadows of mental activity. Progress has been slow because good experimental design and data analysis depend on prior knowledge of both passive current flow in the head volume conductor and dynamic properties of neocortical current sources. But such knowledge requires data so substantial trial and error in the design of experiments is required. Another obstacle is the highly interdisciplinary nature of EEG; each scientist can be competent only in a few of the relevant fields. Thus EEG is currently dominated by experimental studies having minimal theoretical basis in the underlying dynamics.

This book has two major aims. (1) To facilitate communication between anatomical, physiological, behavioral, neuropharmacological, engineering, physics and other fields related to EEG. (2) To provide a conceptual framework based on these disparate data that is sufficiently general to embrace brain theories applied to different experimental designs, scales, and brain states. This framework can guide future experimental design and data analysis, and should lead to new or modified theories.

Because of the critical need to communicate between fields, I have avoided the typical edited book with isolated chapters. However, the subject matter demands experts in different fields. This dilemma was addressed by choosing chapter authors with unusual backgrounds in both physical science and neuroscience and experience with EEG data. Since the chapter authors have long experience with interdisciplinary research, many connections between disparate fields were provided; more may be discovered by the reader. We tried to avoid the superficial views of neuroscience or physical science often adopted by practitioners too firmly entrenched in either camp.

We assaulted the usual communication barriers associated with lack of mathematics and physical science training by extensive use of brain metaphors. Such metaphors are distinguished from genuine theory based on physiological data which both suggest and limit metaphors. The mathematics was chosen selectively to supplement words and figures. The density of equations is 0.5 per page compared, for example, to about 3 equations per page in advanced physics texts.

While written words often allow different interpretations, mathematics has more universal meanings. For example, concepts like spatial-temporal scale, pacemaker, wave, top-down interactions, phase transitions, and self organization take on deeper meanings when verbal descriptions are supplemented with matching mathematics. To use a modern metaphor, these concepts have a fractal character not fully revealed in written text. We tried to include just enough mathematics to keep the presentation honest. That is, our inclusion of minimal mathematics makes it far less likely that readers will misinterpret complex ideas or that we have fudged agreement between theory and experiment.

Another communication barrier is spatial or temporal scale chauvinism in which the inherent limitations of any experimental measure are fully appreciated only in the context of other persons' data. But we treat all hierarchal levels with respect in this book. The first three chapters provide both an introduction and overview of later chapters in order to counter parochial views of neuroscience.

Chapter 1 introduces some general characteristics of EEG and magnetoelectroencephalographic (MEG) data in relation to neocortical current sources. The issues of spatial and temporal scale are considered in connection with different measures of brain function. The spatial filtering of fields by the head volume conductor and new high resolution EEG methods are discussed. Volume conduction was treated more extensively in my earlier book *Electric Fields of the Brain: The Neurophysics of EEG* (Oxford University Press, 1981).

Chapter 2 takes a physical science view of neocortex. That is, we propose a model cortex having interactions between functional units ranging from neuron to neural masses at columnar scales. Top-down and bottom-up interactions are discussed. Neocortex is considered a global system in which the dynamic interactions between different parts is its essential feature (in a manner analogous to dynamic interactions of persons, nations, and so on in social systems).

In Chapter 3 a metaphorical link between (mind, brain, scientific method) and (music, violin, physics) is offered to illuminate connections between the issues of scale interactions, neural plasticity, pacemakers, local circuits, standing waves, external control of conscious states, and EEG frequencies. New EEG data that exhibit quasi-stable, coherent spatial structure are provided in support of these ideas. A long time scale (several seconds) is identified which may be related to the short term memory mechanisms discussed in Chapter 14.

Chapter 4 by Ken Pilgreen gives an overview of clinical aspects of EEG with emphasis on dynamic properties. EEG correlates of altered brain state are described. For example, Altzheimer's disease, which has dramatic socioeconomic implications, may be caused by neuromodulatory defects which alter neocortical control parameters. Dr. Pilgreen is a practicing neurologist with a master's degree in physics and experience in both operational and theoretical aspects of EEG.

Chapter 5 by Fernando Lopes da Silva considers the kinds of EEG rhythmic behavior exhibited at scales ranging from single neurons to neural networks. The emergence of novel properties in networks under the control of modulating systems is described. Methods to estimate chaotic attractors of EEG are also discussed. Dr. Lopes da Silva has a medical degree, post graduate study in engineering and physics, and a Ph.D. in neurophysiology. He has long experience with EEG studies in animals and humans in his laboratory at the University of Amsterdam.

Chapter 6 by Richard Silberstein describes relations between cognitive processes and steady-state visual evoked potentials. The visual stimulus is used during both task and control states to allow study of spatial-temporal patterns in narrow frequency bands which are relatively artifact free. The data also suggest that evoked potentials are partly a mixture of traveling and standing neocortical waves. Dr. Silberstein has an honors degree in physics and a Ph.D. in neurophysiology. The EEG data discussed in Chapters 3, 6, 12, and 13 were recorded at the Swinburne Centre for Applied Neurosciences in Melbourne, headed by Dr. Silberstein.

Chapter 7 by Alan Gevins and Brian Cutillo describes relations between cognitive processes and transient evoked potentials. The chapter reviews traditional evoked potentials as well as modern studies of task-related shifting patterns of statistical interdependency between electrode sites carried out at EEG Systems Laboratory in San Francisco (The famous "shadows of thought" that also provide experimental support for the regional and local circuits discussed in Chapter 13). Dr. Gevins has a background in engineering and psychology and has been director of EEG Systems Lab since 1974. Dr. Cutillo is a psychophysiologist who also has long EEG experience.

Chapter 8 reviews discrete linear systems in which physical or physiological variables exhibit time dependence. It provides a background for local neural circuit models and spectral and coherence measures of EEG dynamics.

Chapter 9 reviews continuous linear systems in which variables are functions of both time and location in physical or neural media. Topics include physical and neural wave propagation and membrane diffusion. Background required for more advanced study of complex global systems is provided.

Chapter 10 introduces nonlinear systems using simple examples of electric circuits, mechanical oscillators, and ecologic systems. Jump phenomena, limit cycles, and temporal chaos are included. More advanced topics associated with continuous nonlinear systems include stable spatial structures with temporal chaos and statistical measures of dynamic properties. A critique of correlation dimension estimates of EEG data is provided.

Chapter 11 suggests that global dynamic behavior is expected in a cortex-like system. In certain limiting cases coherent spatial modes governed by linear or quasi-linear differential equations are predicted. It is argued that local circuit and global dynamic behavior coexist naturally, and changes from more local to more global brain states occur due to selective changes in local and global control parameters. Part of the motivation for this theory is to explain aspects of EEG in terms of the underlying physiology. However, the quantitative description of distinctions between local and global dynamic behavior has broader implications. The mathematical developments are presented in the Appendix.

Chapter 12 provides data on the dynamic properties of EEG that appear to support the theory of Chapter 11 for states in which global properties are dominant. Multichannel data on alpha rhythm, steady-state evoked potentials, and EEG under halothane anesthesia are included. These EEG exhibit coherent, stable spatial structure that can apparently coexist with complex temporal behavior including limit cycle and chaotic modes. Apparent nodal lines of standing waves appear consistently in the data.

Chapter 13 by Richard Silberstein considers the selective action of several neuromodulators in different cortical layers. Since different layers are predominately associated with intracortical or corticocortical fibers, neuromodulators may selectively alter local and global control parameters to change brain states. Local resonances (typically in the 40 Hz range) are contrasted with global and regional resonances (below 20 Hz). Brain diseases including Parkinson's disease, Tourette Syndrome, and schizophrenia are viewed as pathologically hypercoupled or hypocoupled states resulting from faulty control parameters. These ideas can be tested with new EEG experiments. If even partly correct, they should have an impact on neuropsychiatry.

Chapter 14 reviews the statistical mechanics of neocortical interactions at multiple scales as developed over the past 20 years by Lester Ingber. The theory describes macroscopic neocortical variables such as EEG with a chain of arguments involving overlapping microscopic and mesoscopic scales. The general methods originate in quantum and gravitational field theory. This approach of nonlinear nonequilibrium statistical mechanics has a complementary relationship to the strictly macroscopic theory of Chapter 11, similar to the relationship between classical kinetic theory of gasses and fluid mechanics. An important prediction of the statistical theory is that the number of neural firing patterns that can simultaneously persist for several seconds is in the range of 5 to 10. Theses patterns may store short-term memories that are known to be limited to 7 ± 2 items. This work may also provide a quantitative theoretical foundation for the local and regional circuits suggested earlier, which produce spatial temporal patterns of EEG associated with particular brain states. Dr. Ingber holds a Ph.D. in theoretical physics and has developed theoretical approaches to nuclear physics, social systems, optimization, and financial markets.

Several colleagues provided papers describing their original work. However, the imposing volume of this material forced many omissions, often because I was unable to place material within our central focus. I tried to avoid long lists of unrelated citations (admittedly with only partial success). Historical perspectives, mathematical derivations, and experimental design were mostly omitted. A number of familiar brain metaphors also were not described. For example, the brain-hologram analogy may have some limited use in describing interference phenomena and global memory storage. However, these processes occur in simple mechanical and electrical systems (Chapters 2, 3, 9 and 10) so the brain-hologram analogy was not used. There is a more compelling similarity between localized-extended wave function states in disordered solids (such as superconductors) and local-global brain states. However, this metaphor is of minimal use to readers lacking background in quantum mechanics so it was not discussed. Esoteric metaphors may allow so much room for reader interpetation that their communication function is eclipsed, thus we have mostly avoided them.

This book provides connections between fields that may benefit electroencephalographers, neurologists, neuropsychiatrists, neuropharmacologists, cognitive neuroscientists, artificial neural networkers, and physicists or engineers interested in complex systems. It suggests new directions for interdisciplinary research. It can also serve as a textbook in interdisciplinary graduate courses if properly supplemented. For example, the material in Chapters 1 through 3 and 8 through 11 was used in several advanced biomedical engineering math courses at Tulane University to provide both an introduction to neuroscience and motivation to work math problems in supplementary notes and texts. We made implicit agreements with students reluctant to take advanced math to limit mathematics to about half the course.

Helpful comments on individual chapters were provided by Valentino Braitenberg, Ted Bullock, Peter Cadusch, Walter Freeman, Evelyn Hogan, John Kounios, Helmuth Petsche, Sam Ridgway, Dirk Roekaerts, James Theiler, and Jim Wright. The EEG research described in my chapters was carried out by the Brain Physics Group in the Department of Biomedical Engineering at Tulane University in New Orleans, including contributions by Guangchang Cao, Richard Hart, Denny Nelson, Sam Law, Ken Pilgreen, Ramesh Srinivasan, Andrew Westdorp, Ranjith Wijesinghe, and Yuchen Yan. Dr. Wijesinghe and Mr. Cao created many high resolution EEG plots, including the Laplacian phase plot of one-second of my alpha rhythm on the book cover (which suggests standing waves). We were supported by grants from the National Science foundation (ECE 8521101) and National Institutes of Health (1R01NS243314); other support is cited by chapter authors. My wife Kirsty typed most of the manuscript and cheerfully provided editorial and other amoral support. My children Lisa (born about the time Chapter 11 was completed), Michael, Michelle, Shari, and Cindy also contributed to a happy (if sometimes hectic) work environment.

New Orleans Paul L. Nunez
December, 1994

Contents

Contributors

Brian A. Cutillo, Ph.D.
Psychophysiologist, EEG Systems Lab
San Francisco, California

Alan S. Gevins, Ph.D.
Director, EEG Systems Lab
San Francisco, California

Lester Ingber, Ph.D.
Director, Lester Ingber Research
McLean, Virginia

Fernando H. Lopes da Silva, M.D., Ph.D.
Professor, Institute of Neurobiology
University of Amsterdam
Amsterdam, The Netherlands

Paul L. Nunez, Ph.D.
Director, Brain Physics Group and Professor, Biomedical Engineering
Tulane University
New Orleans, Louisiana

Kenneth L. Pilgreen, M.D.
Neurologist, Neurological Services
Anniston, Alabama
Adjunct Professor
Tulane University
New Orleans, Lousiana

Richard B. Silberstein, Ph.D.
Professor of Physics and Director, Swinburne Centre for Applied Neurosciences
Swinburne University of Technology
Melbourne, Australia

Neocortical Dynamics and Human EEG Rhythms

1

Quantitative States of Neocortex

PAUL L. NUNEZ

Communication Between the Appropriate Subfields

This book is about communication at many spatial and temporal scales, that is, communication between neurons, between cortical macrocolumns containing hundreds of thousands of neurons, and between human brains containing roughly 10^{11} neurons. I emphasize the plural "brains" to indicate that all brains are not the same, neither in their fundamental approaches to research nor in the electroencephalographic (EEG) patterns they exhibit. The study of brains, or more specifically, neocortical dynamic function and its electrical signals, is highly interdisciplinary. Thus, this book draws important bits of information from neurophysiology, neuroanatomy, neuropharmacology, cognitive neuroscience, EEG, physics, and engineering. Other fields, such as neural networks, chaos theory, information science, traditional cognitive psychology, mathematics, clinical neurology, and membrane biophysics contribute to a lesser degree to the particular description chosen here.

Perhaps one way to indicate the approach of this book is to contrast it with typical neural network studies. The field of "neural networks" may be concerned with how a neural system (typically a relatively simple system) works, but often the emphasis is on a computer design. The field is strongly influenced by computer scientists and others with mathematical, but not necessarily physical or neuroscience, backgrounds. By contrast, realistic descriptions of neocortical dynamics must include theoretical issues of spatial and temporal scale, and the relation of genuine EEG data to neural activity recorded at distinct scales. Studies of complex systems, often at multiple scales, in which successful connections between theory and experiment have been achieved are mostly the province of certain branches of physics and engineering, fields emphasized here that are usually neglected in neural network research.

Another important distinction is between mathematics (as practiced by mathematicians) and mathematical engineering or mathematical physics. In the former case, mathematics is an end in itself; in the latter case, it is used as a tool to reveal nature's secrets. All equations presented in this book belong to the latter category. Still another distinction is made between traditional cognitive psychology, which often has minimal connection to known brain structure and function, and cognitive neuroscience, in which the importance of the brain in cognition is explicitly acknowledged. In the words of Alan Gevins and Brian Cutillo (see Chapter 7), "The language of brain processes is not the language of cognitive psychology." Here we are explicitly concerned with brain function.

An important goal of this book is to provide a common pool of knowledge, despite the diversity of language and approaches, to researchers interested in neocortical dynamics who may have different backgrounds and expertise. But this goal has considerable obstacles. For example, the engineer or physicist may strongly resist the study of cortical anatomy, especially at the fine level of qualitative detail that interests the neuro-anatomist. Furthermore, the physical scientist will probably be frustrated by the lack of quantitative information easily available from any superficial study of anatomy. The problems faced by the typical neuroscientist in obtaining relevant information from the physical sciences are likely to be even more severe, if only because of high barriers associated with lack of physical science and mathematical training. Thus, the neuroscientist may find more quantitative information than he or she could ever want but no clear idea of how to apply it to the nervous system. In either case, road maps could help scientists to not waste time and intellectual energy in areas that have little apparent connection to their research. This book and its references is intended as such a map.

Another obstacle to establishing good communication across fields has to do with level of presentation. The usual serial approach of a typical textbook, a detailed progression from simple to complex issues, will not work here. If, for example, we tried to give a comprehensive treatment of physics or systems engineering, we would quickly lose most readers with medical and biological backgrounds. Furthermore, we would create a large set of books with little space devoted to neuroscience applications. On the other hand, neither will strictly introductory treatments of the relevant fields suffice. The neocortex is a complex system; ideally the full arsenal of advanced theoretical/experimental methods should be available to the neuroscientist. Obviously, this ideal cannot be fully satisfied in a single book. Rather, we tried to approach the ideal with parallel rather than serial treatments of various fields relevant to neocortical dynamics. We emphasize apparent connections between fields rather than their isolated developments, and thus many important details must be omitted. But this limited information can be supplemented by consulting the references as needed.

The need for a parallel approach to the study of neocortical dynamics may be further illustrated using Table 1-1, which is a basic, semiquantitative description of various levels of expertise attained in particular fields of knowledge. We imagine a logarithmic scale, similar to that used to quantify earthquakes, such that the attainment of each level requires roughly an order of magnitude more time and effort than that of the next lower level. Of course, not everyone reaches these levels in the same time. However, even the most capable persons are unlikely to reach level 4 in more than a few fields. Becoming an expert in the seven major

Table 1-1 Levels of Scientific Expertise

Level 1	Familiar with the terminology and some of the major issues in the field. A level that can be obtained by studying literature aimed at the intelligent layman.
Level 2	Ability to reproduce some of the major results in the field and to work simple problems. Some understanding of deeper issues. Typical level of the first-year graduate student.
Level 3	Understanding of most of the central issues. Ability to work complex problems. Ability to carry out a significant research project and produce original results. Typical level of new Ph.D.
Level 4	Recognized experts in the field.

Minimum hours of required study is estimated to be proportional to $10^{(\text{level number})}$.

fields cited in the first paragraph of this section appears impossible. Furthermore, even if this monumental effort were, in fact, accomplished, the critical task of integrating knowledge from these disparate fields would still remain.

Dynamic Neocortical Processes

The main goal of this book is to offer a preliminary framework for both experimental and theoretical studies of neocortical dynamic function, the process by which many neurons collectively interact to produce human consciousness. Perhaps the most direct measure of this dynamic process, especially over the short time scales on which the brain processes information, is the EEG, which is typically recorded in humans using scalp electrodes. Thus, the EEG provides an important window, albeit an often clouded one, to the operations of certain parts of the brain, especially the upper portion of neocortex that lies close to scalp electrodes, as indicated in Figure 1-1. The information provided by the routine scalp EEG may be supplemented by intracranial data obtained in patients who have electrodes implanted for medical reason, and by intracranial recordings in animals.

In addition to scalp potentials, neural current sources also produce weak magnetic fields that may be recorded with special superconducting equipment. This relatively new technology (available since the late 1960s) is called magnetoencephalography (MEG). With MEG, the magnetic field component perpendicular to the scalp surface is recorded. Such recordings provide somewhat different information than does the EEG, although there is considerable overlap. Much of what is described here for EEG also applies to MEG, so we will mostly avoid cumbersome labels such as "EEG and MEG." Further complication of the terminology occurs because of the distinction between spontaneous and evoked activity, such as scalp potentials produced as a result of visual, auditory, or somatosensory stimuli. There are, for example, evoked potentials, event-related potentials, evoked fields, and event-related fields, the latter two referring, by convention, to magnetic fields but not to electric fields. We use "EEG" as a general term to describe all these processes, except when distinctions are important.

This book emphasizes "neocortical" rather than "brain" dynamics for the following reasons:

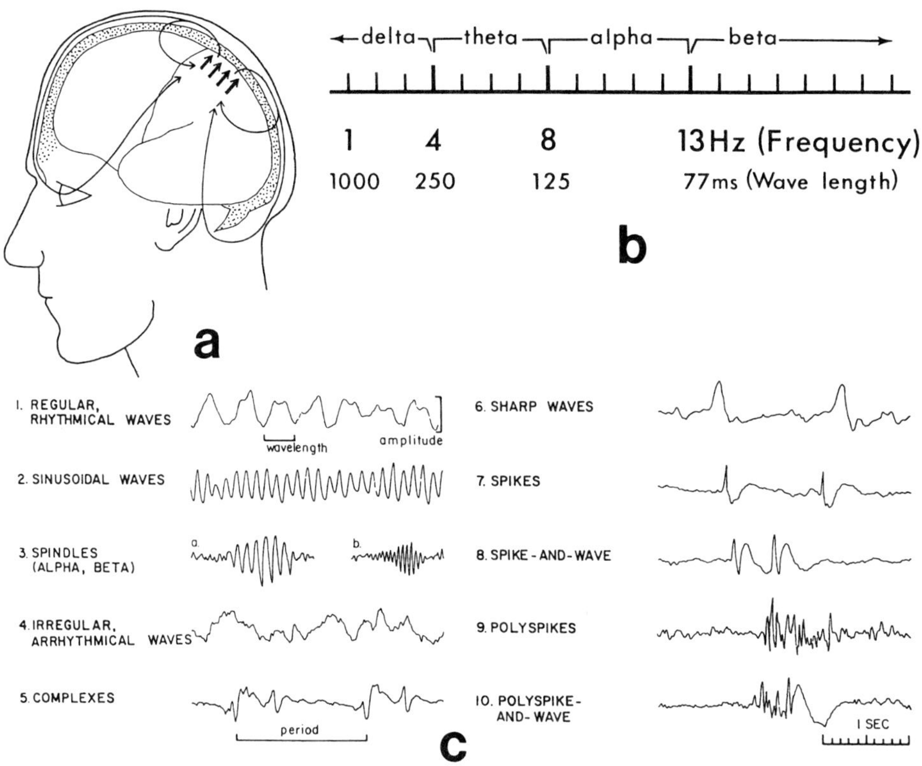

Figure 1-1. **a.** Current sources forming a neocortical dipole layer (heavy arrows) result in a distribution of scalp currents determined by the location of the dipole layer and the volume conductive properties of the head. The relatively high resistivity of skull causes substantial smearing (that is, space averaging) of neocortical sources. (Reproduced with permission from Nunez, 1990a.) **b.** Standard EEG terminology for various frequency ranges of importance in both clinical and research work. The terminology is, however, often used very loosely. For example, records containing substantial high-frequency content are often labeled "beta" based on visual inspection of raw data, even though Fourier analysis may reveal either a dominant alpha peak or broad spectral content, as in the case of 1/f noise. **c.** A few characteristic EEG waveforms and corresponding medical terminology. (Reproduced with permission from Spehlman, 1981.)

1. Most of the available EEG data in humans is believed to be generated by sources in neocortex. The contribution from subcortical structures is usually only important for some averaged evoked potentials that are time locked to the stimulus.

2. Sensory and especially cognitive processing of information is critically involved with neocortical dynamic function. In fact, conscious experience is probably not possible in humans without neocortex.

3. Mammalian neocortex exhibits a relatively high degree of macroscopic homogeneity and isotropy in directions tangent to its surface, thereby making it more accessible to theoretical description.

4. Much, if not most of what makes us individuals is apparently due to differences in neocortex and its system of long-range interconnections, the corticocortical fibers (that is, association fibers) that form most of the white matter located just below the neocortical layer.

5. The human neocortex is very densely interconnected by both short-range (typically less than 1 mm) intracortical fibers and by about 10^{10} long (as long as 20 cm) corticocortical fibers. The human neocortex is much more densely connected to itself than to other brain structures, which partly justifies treating it as a separate system in which input from the midbrain may be considered as external control. The high density of corticocortical fibers in humans compared with lower mammals has been suggested as an important factor in making the human brain "human" (Braitenberg, 1978; reviewed by Katznelson, 1981).

This book focuses on the relation of EEG to neocortical dynamics. Although this connection is complex, we present evidence from several disparate studies that suggests that the approach will be rewarding. We view neocortex as we would a complex physical system, with EEG as its measured output and sensory or other information as its input. In this manner, we can hope to at least pose questions about brain operation in a scientific context. Perhaps we can even gain some modest insights into what many view as the most profound issue for our age—the relation between mind and brain.

As a practical, operational strategy, neocortex can be viewed as a distinct state of matter like solid, liquid, gas, or plasma, with its properties at various spatial and temporal scales subject to theoretical description and measurement with EEG. This optimistic view may, to some, appear inconsistent with observations of the complexity of even a single neuron. A system containing 10^{10} or so strongly interacting neurons might then appear hopelessly complex. One reason for optimism is that ample EEG data are available in humans at the regional level of cortex (typically involving tens to hundreds square centimeters of surface area). Thus reasonable descriptions of neocortical dynamics at large scales, involving the interaction of neural masses (cortical columns, for example), are believed possible.

Many examples from the physical sciences have been studied in which macroscopic descriptions (often of very complex and poorly understood processes at microscopic scales) have predictive value. Thus, in our relative ignorance of brain function, it is natural to search for analogies from the physical sciences. However, we must be aware of the dangers of analysis by analogy. Grossberg (1988) noted in a historical survey:

> While most mind and brain experimentalists ignored theory and most theorists looked for more hospitable frontiers, there arose the widespread tendency to interpret brain function in terms of whatever technological development happened to be current. The ever expanding list of technological metaphors to which the brain has been compared includes telegraph circuits, digital computers, linear control systems, catastrophes, holograms, and spin glasses. All of these metaphors have been unable to explain a substantial data base about brain and behavior, as well they might, since none of them arose from a sustained analysis of behavioral or brain data.

To that list we might add analogies to quantum mechanics (for example, in the case of the uncertainty principle supposedly providing a basis for free will) and more recently, chaos theory. Although this warning about brain metaphors is appropriate, it is perhaps overstated. For example, electric cable theory provided a basis for understanding the subthreshold behavior of neurons. The extension of this description into the highly nonlinear region (that is, nonlinear conductive properties of the membrane) suggested experimental designs and ultimately provided a theoretical basis for action potential propagation along axons (Cole, 1968).

Of course, there are many other examples in science in which analogy to a familiar system is used to obtain a preliminary understanding of an unfamiliar system. A famous case is the behavior of an electron. In some experiments, the electron behaves like a wave; in others, it appears to be a particle. This observation has been called "wave-particle duality." However, the electron is neither wave nor particle, as these terms are defined in the macroscopic world. It is an entirely new entity whose behavior follows the Schrodinger equation of quantum mechanics. However, historically, it was the wave and particle analogies that led to (that is, provided the paradigm for) the development of Schrodinger's equation and quantum mechanics. We use apparent analogies between neocortex and physical systems extensively in this book without apology. The reader may judge, in each case, if the analogy is convincing.

In the case of neocortical dynamics, we can derive plausible equations from anatomy and physiology that may be partially predictive, at least in certain limiting cases. Typically, these equations contain several parameters that in theory are measurable but whose magnitudes are poorly known. These equations may not look like any known equation from the physical sciences. However, in certain limiting cases (for example, when certain parameters are small), the equations may reduce to a known set, one whose physical consequences have been at least partly worked out. In this case, analogy can be very useful. We can then say, for example, this is what happens with spin glasses, hot plasmas, or some other physical system. Perhaps something similar may occur in the brain during a physiologic state that matches this case. Or perhaps such brain states never occur. But at least we have a set of testable hypotheses that have theoretical bases in the underlying physiology and anatomy. We will return to this issue often in this book.

An important goal in brain research and clinical applications, which can be pursued to some degree in the absence of any theoretical description of cortical function, is associating dynamic patterns of EEG with the physiologic or clinical state of the brain. Here we define "pattern" in the broad sense to indicate temporal and spatial properties. The former are likely to include spectral content but may also include new dimensionality measures proposed for nonlinear and chaotic systems. The spatial information is likely to include amplitude distribution over the scalp but may also include patterns of coherency (as with spontaneous EEG) or correlation (as with evoked potentials). However, pattern recognition may be much more effective if based, at least partly, on theoretical descriptions of neocortex so that the parameters of the theory are fitted to the EEG data. This kind of approach has been successful in engineering and the physical sciences.

With these arguments in mind, it is perhaps appropriate to note specific analogies between neocortical dynamics (as measured with EEG) and several physical systems—for example, atmospheric turbulence (measured with velocity, pressure, or temperature sensors) or ocean wave height. Some evident similarities include the following.

1. Measurable quantities may be viewed as stochastic (that is, random) variables, dependent on time and spatial coordinates over a closed surface.
2. Some important rules (often expressed as equations) governing each system's dynamic behavior may be known; however, the system is generally far too complicated for long-range predictions. Of course, far more is known about atmospheric or water wave rules than about neocortical rules, but nonlinear effects are clearly important in both systems.
3. Each system is affected by external input (for example, sensory information, chemical activation by the brainstem, solar energy, wind) that is only partly known.
4. Important phenomena occur at multiple spatial and temporal scales, and important interactions apparently take place across these scales.

For an example of the scaling issue (4), note that inertial fluid forces produce a transfer of energy from large- to small-scale components of motion, thereby assisting in the formation in the flow of sharp, small-scale phenomena (whorls) that characterize turbulence (Monin and Yaglom, 1975). The formation of tornados is a practical example. This is an example of a top-down influence across hierarchical scales in the physical sciences. In later chapters we address possible counterparts in neocortical function.

Certainly we are not suggesting that turbulent fluid phenomena are especially similar to neocortical dynamics. Rather, we can perhaps exploit some fundamental similarities in EEG. There are, of course, also obvious fundamental differences. For example, atmospheric turbulence and water waves can apparently be described by local rules of interaction (for example, differential equations). Thus a disturbance in Moscow can affect the weather in New York only by its transfer through the intervening atmosphere. By contrast, neocortical interactions are both local and nonlocal, the later occurring when corticocortical fibers connect distant regions of cortex. Later, we will draw some analogies to ionized atmospheres (plasma) that also involve nonlocal interactions.

Scaled Windows to Brain Function

The human brain can be studied in many ways. One is to study its structure. Anatomists have discovered hundreds of distinct structures that are evident at macroscopic and submacrosopic scales. The modern methods of computed tomography (CT) and magnetic resonance imaging (MRI) allow us to view normal and abnormal tissue in living humans. Although they provide no direct measure of brain function, anatomic studies are, of course, critical to the development of theories of the brain, which must be consistent with these data.

Another important field is brain chemistry. Neuropharmacology encompasses the psychotropic drugs that alter mood and behavior. For example, general anesthetics, anticonvulsants, hypnotics, and narcotics act on the central nervous system. Although many drugs exert their influence by interacting with neurotransmitters, others are known to modulate pre- and postsynaptic transmission. The electrical and chemical states of the brain are strongly coupled by many subtle mechanisms that are largely unknown. Thus current models of brain electrical activity typically contain parameters that partly reflect the chemical background state of the brain with, for example, dynamic coupling between synaptic action and chemistry either ignored or treated superficially. Such approximations may be justified if chemical parameters change over much longer time scales than the EEG, which is often the case.

One way to study brain function directly is with positron emission tomography (PET), a technique that estimates local cerebral blood flow, oxygen and glucose consumption, and other regional metabolic changes with typical spatial resolution of about 6 mm. That is, PET provides space-averaged data over cortical regions typically containing 10^6 to 10^7 neurons, that is, 10 to 100 cortical macrocolumns. Thus many metabolically active and inactive cortical columns contribute to the smallest volume of detection (the voxel). Furthermore, considerable white matter (with a metabolic rate of about 25% of gray matter) may be present in the volume element, thereby reducing the estimate to less than its actual value (Roland and Widen, 1988). Because of the inaccuracy of absolute measures, PET plots are presented as differences in metabolic activity between brain states.

With cortical activity, the spatial resolution of PET is better than the best scalp EEG methods by perhaps a factor of five. With deep sources, PET has even more advantage for spatial resolution. However, the temporal resolution of PET is in the range of minutes to hours, whereas EEG is sensitive to changes that occur in milliseconds. Thus EEG has an advantage of about five orders of magnitude in temporal resolution. Magnetic resonance imaging is another approach to observe brain function. Recently the new methods of functional MRI have improved temporal resolution substantially. However, temporal resolution of metabolic variables is fundamentally limited by metabolic inertia (diffusion processes, for example) to about 1 second.

The purpose of such comparisons is, of course, not to suggest that any one method is necessarily better than another. Rather it is to emphasize that each technique has its own region of applicability, determined partly by the spatial and temporal scale of interest and partly by the dependent variable to be measured. For example, an increase in metabolic activity may parallel increases in excitatory and inhibitory synaptic action, but the EEG may or may not change substantially during the same period. Each measure (that is, dependent variable) may or may not be closely correlated to the specific brain state observed in a particular study.

Spatial and temporal scales are emphasized repeatedly throughout this book. By contrast to descriptive mathematical or verbal models, a scientific theory must make direct connections to experiments. With electrophysiology, experimental results depend critically on the size and location of electrodes and on the period over which signals are averaged. Thus any theory of brain function or EEG must address the question of scale directly if it will be seriously considered a realistic description. Many, if not most "theories" of neocortical dynamics do not meet this simple test. It is far more difficult to devise a genuine theory that makes predictions (especially quantitative predictions) that can be tested experimentally (that is, have the potential to be proved wrong) than to derive a set of equations and solve them, with the implication that perhaps someone with stronger theoretical skills can determine how to relate dependent variables to actual experiments. This ability typically separates theoreticians from mathematicians, a point not always appreciated by neuroscientists.

The importance of spatial and temporal scales (terminology normally used in the study of complex physical systems such as turbulent fluids, magnetic materials, or spin glasses), or hierarchical level (a less quantitative term often used in brain sciences) has long been recognized in general studies of the brain. One view of this issue is given by Rose (1976):

> Confusion may arise either if one regards these hierarchical levels (ranging from the sociological and psychological at upper levels to chemical and ultimately physical at lower levels) as rigid—made by nature rather than by man—or if attempts are made to cross the levels of the hierarchies of explanation. If, for instance, one says "being in love" is "*caused* by changes of such-and-such in molecular structure in the brain" one is attributing a *causal* relationship between the point-set on one level and that on another, where it is not always legitimate to attribute more than a *correlative* relationship. A causal explanation means that we are saying, for instance, that "being in love" is a *result* of such and such changes in molecular structure. But we could also say such and such changes in molecular structure are a *result* of "being in love." Such causal statements imply both a temporal sequence—one event always precedes the other—and a non-reversibility: *Either* A causes B *or* B causes A. A correlative relationship, on the other hand, does not imply that one event is the result of the other, merely that when one event occurs, the second also invariably takes place: When the state "being in love" occurs, then such-and-such changes in molecular structure also always occur.
>
> Describing the properties of the brain in molecular terms is not the same—as seems sometimes feared—as explaining away these properties, reducing their significance at higher hierarchical levels. In my view, much of the confusion over the relationship of mind to brain has arisen because of attempts to cross hierarchical levels of discourse. . . . The "mind" may be defined as equivalent to "the sum total of brain activity" for discussions within the universe of discourse at a hierarchical level above that of the physiological description of the interaction of cells and below that of social analysis.

A more quantitative (if less romantic) description of the spatial and temporal scales of experimental brain studies, offered by Churchland and Sejnowski (1988), is shown in Figure 1-2. The boundaries indicate approximate regions where several

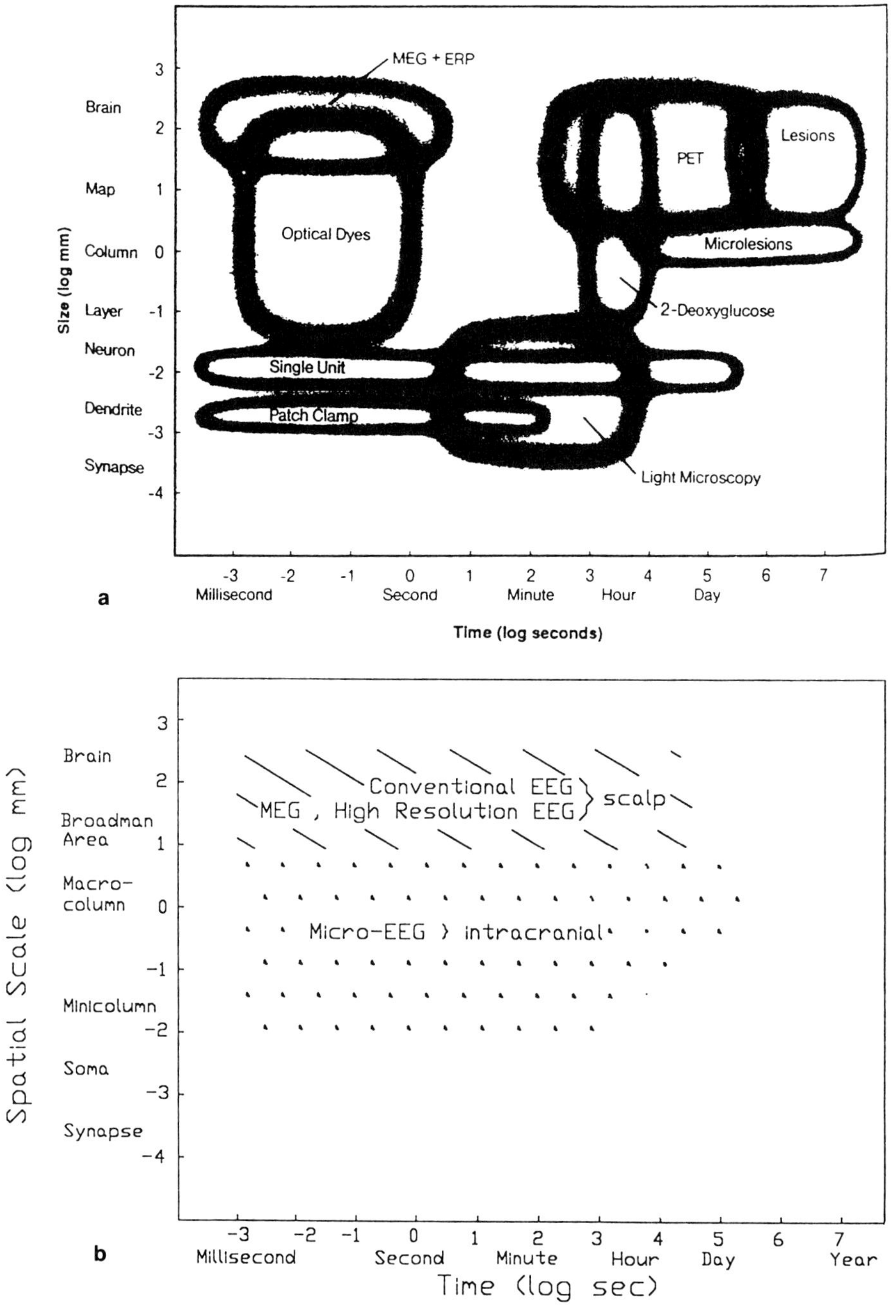

Figure 1-2. **a.** Schematic illustration of the ranges of spatial and temporal resolution obtained with several methods to study the brain. (Reproduced with permission from Churchland and Sejnowski, 1988.) **b.** Similar plot showing more accurate representation of EEG studies. Normal operating ranges are shown rather than fundamental limits.

techniques are commonly used; they do not necessarily indicate fundamental limitations. The interrelation between the observables (or dependent variables in brain theories) in these studies can be shown quantitatively in the following manner.

Suppose we imagine that some quantity $\Phi(\mathbf{r}, t)$ can, in principle, be measured at location r and time t in the brain, at small scales. By "location r and time t," of course, we refer to a space average over an even smaller volume and a time average over an even shorter time than our "descriptive scale," which is chosen to match experiments performed at that scale. For example, $\Phi(\mathbf{r}, t)$ might represent the electric potential in the extracurricular fluid measured with an electrode with a tip diameter of approximately 10^{-4} cm and a digitization rate of 10 KHz. Alternately $\Phi(\mathbf{r}, t)$ might be the potential difference across a cortical minicolumn of diameter 5×10^{-3} cm, with an electrode of the same diameter and digitization rate that could be either the same or different than in the previous example.

A simple, spatial and temporal average of $\Phi(\mathbf{r}, t)$ is obtained from the relation

$$\hat{\Phi}(\mathbf{r}, t) = \frac{1}{T\Delta V} \int_{t}^{t+T} dt' \int_{\Delta V(r)} \Phi(\mathbf{r}', t')\, d^3\mathbf{r}' \tag{1.1}$$

where T is the time over which the time average is obtained and ΔV is the volume over which the space average is taken. For example, if $\Phi(\mathbf{r}, t)$ is potential defined at the minicolumn scale, then a new variable, the potential at the macrocolumn scale, may be defined by (1.1), simply by summing the contribution of the approximately 10^4 minicolumns that form a macrocolumn. Our volume element ΔV is, in this case, not a cube. We want ΔV to enclose only cortical tissue because $\hat{\Phi}$ is defined as the transcortical potential, a quantity subject to direct measurement. Thus we might, for example, record a transcortical evoked potential (perhaps due to electrical stimulation of a nerve) at the macrocolumn scale. However, evoked potentials are often masked by much larger spontaneous EEG so that they can only be observed by time averaging. Thus our measured $\hat{\Phi}$ may be the time average of Φ over a T of several minutes and a space average over several square millimeters of cortical surface. In the case of scalp evoked potentials, the space average probably involves several square centimeters with good experimental techniques and perhaps several tens of square centimeters when no special method is used to improve spatial resolution. Thus scalp-recorded potentials typically involve space averages over cortical regions containing about 10^7 to 10^9 neurons. Some examples of this large-scale activity are shown in Figure 1-3.

Consider now a new observable at small scales $\eta(\mathbf{r}, t)$—for example, metabolic activity at some sub-millimeter and sub-millisecond scale. With PET, one measures $\hat{\eta}$, which involves both time and space averages analogous to (1.1). Such averaging tends to filter out higher frequency components in the signal. A similar effect occurs in the spatial domain; that is, higher spatial frequencies (in each of three directions) tend to be removed by volume averaging. The variables η and $\hat{\eta}$ may exhibit a much different character, especially if they are separated in scale by several orders of magnitude. Thus use of the same letter symbol for each may be misleading. Variables could actually be more closely linked by scale than by

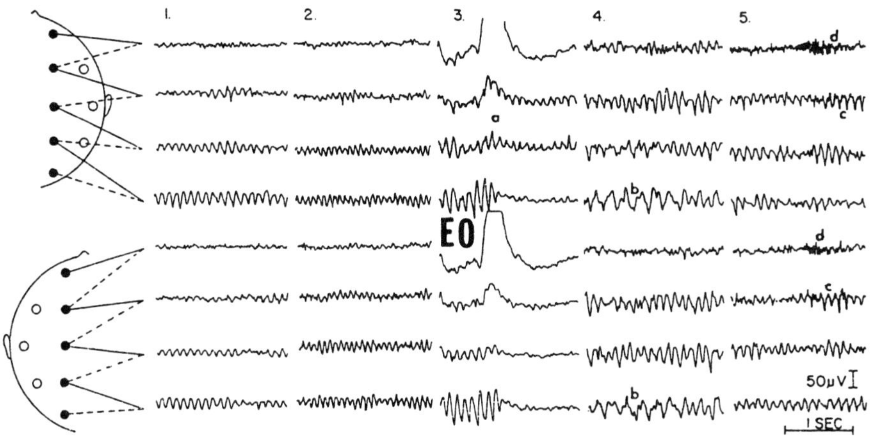

Figure 1-3. Several normal patterns of resting EEG in adults. 1. Alpha rhythm of 9 Hz in the posterior head regions and mixture of alpha and beta activity in the frontal regions. 2. Alpha rhythm of 12 to 13 Hz extending from the posterior to the central regions. 3. Alpha rhythm of 9 to 10 Hz in the posterior head regions is present at the beginning of this part and is blocked by eye opening (EO); a central mu rhythm on the right side persists after eye opening (a). 4. Slow alpha variant of 4 to 5 Hz, maximal in the occipital regions (b), alternates with alpha rhythm of about 9 Hz in a wider distribution in the posterior head regions; beta rhythm is present in the frontal regions. 5. Alpha rhythm of 8 to 9 Hz posteriorly, mu rhythm of similar frequency frontocentrally (c), and beta rhythm frontally (d). Since visual inspection of waveforms emphasizes faster frequencies, the term "beta" may be used to describe frontal rhythms, even though the dominant spectral peak is in the alpha band. The alpha peak is typically observed over the entire scalp in healthy relaxed subjects with eyes closed. (Reproduced with permission from Spehlmann, 1981.)

physical quantity; for example, $\hat{\eta}$ may behave more like $\hat{\Phi}$ than η. Furthermore, use of the hat symbol to indicate averages may not be sufficiently precise, because neocortical dynamics apparently involve interaction at several (or more) scales. We could replace $\hat{\Phi}$ by $\Phi(\mathbf{r}, t; \Delta V, T)$ to show explicitly the dependence of potential on both spatial and temporal scales.

A further point is that (1.1) represents only a special case of the different ways in which averages are obtained. More generally, the variable $\Phi(\mathbf{r}, t)$ may be considered as part of a statistical ensemble of all similar variables, created by a fixed set of external conditions on the system. The averaging integral, in this case, is similar to (1.1), but includes a probability density function that may weight ranges of the integral differently. This kind of mathematical operation is important for making theoretical connections between variables measured at different spatial and temporal scales. It is the province of stochastic field theory. Some applications of this theory are discussed in Chapters 10 and 14.

Selective Sensitivity of EEG and MEG

The extracranial recording of EEG and MEG due to cortical sources is illustrated in Figure 1-4. The arrows represent current dipole moments per unit volume at

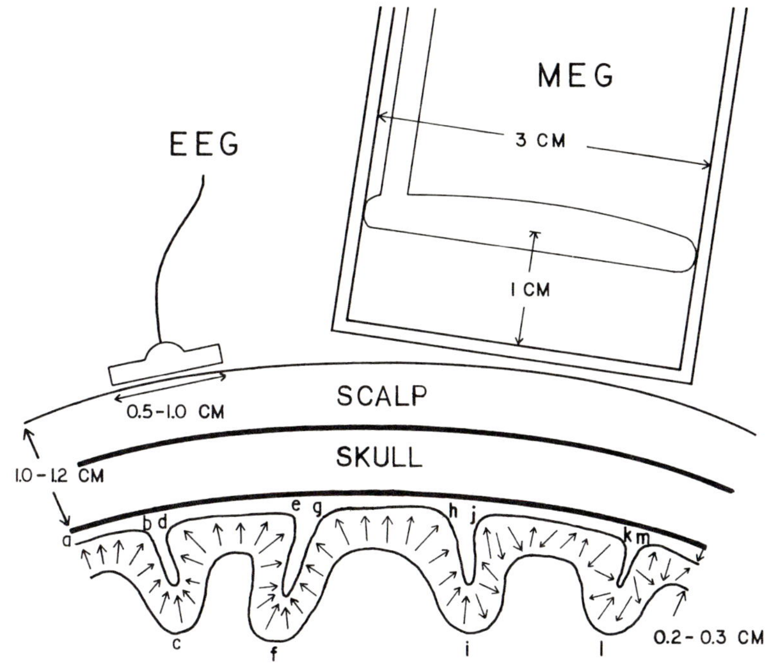

Figure 1-4. Extracranial recording of electroencephalographic (EEG) and magnetoencephalographic (MEG) data. EEG is most sensitive to correlated dipole layer in gyri (ab, de, gh), less sensitive to correlated dipole layer in sulcus (hi), and insensitive to opposing dipole layer in sulci (bcd, efg) and random dipole layer (ijklm). MEG is most sensitive to correlated dipole layer in sulcus (hi) and much less sensitive to all other sources shown because of opposing dipoles, randomly oriented dipoles, or radial dipoles. (The external magnetic field due to a radial dipole in a medium of spherically symmetric conductive layers is zero.) MEG is measured with a superconducting quantum interference device, typically consisting of several coils used to cancel spatially constant magnetic fields. Only the coil closest to the head is shown here. (Reproduced with permission from Nunez, 1990b.)

the scale of a few millimeters, often called in the literature, simply "sources" or "generators." Each "macrosource" (that is, source at the macrocolumn scale) represents space-averaged synaptic and action potential currents in a macrocolumn containing approximately 10^6 neurons and 10^{10} synapses. Several general points are illustrated in Figure 1-4. The first is that both EEG and MEG are limited to a spatial resolution of order of 1 cm. Although the MEG has an important advantage in that it avoids field spreading by the skull, this advantage is partly canceled by the fact that the closest MEG sensing coil must be further from the sources than the EEG electrode (at least with current technology). The general issue of spatial resolution is not the same thing as accuracy of dipole localization. With spatial resolution, we imagine two dipoles moved closer and closer together. When they are separated by some characteristic distance, which is typically of the order of their depth below the sensor, we can no longer tell that there are two separate sources. It is this distance, the "spatial resolution," that is normally limited to a few centimeters (Nunez, 1981; Wikswo and Roth, 1988). The accuracy with which a single dipole can be located with extracranial sensors is perhaps a little better than 1 cm (at least for MEG), but probably no better than a few millimeters (Cohen et al, 1990; Cuffin et al, 1991). Because the cortical macrocolumn of 3-mm diameter lies just below the apparent limit of spatial resolution of extracranial recordings, it is convenient to choose this scale of sources for descriptive purposes in the context of scalp-recorded EEG.

Figure 1-4 also shows that EEG, and especially MEG, are selectively sensitive to particular subsets of brain sources. They obviously tend to be more sensitive to neocortical sources than other sources farther from the sensors. In addition, cortical anatomy further amplifies this preference for recording cortical sources because the large cortical pyramidal cells are lined up perpendicular to the cortical surface, thereby allowing for large, correlated cortical dipole layer sources. In this case, the measured fields are large because of the superposition of coherent sources. Of course, deep sources can be recorded if they are time-locked to some stimulus. In such cases, scalp fields may be recorded by averaging over as many as several thousand stimuli to increase the signal-to-noise ratio (noise in this case is mostly spontaneous EEG generated in the cortex). An example is the brainstem auditory evoked response, elicited in patients by a rapid series of clicks from headphones, which has become a standard clinical test. Because brainstem responses to stimuli (unlike cortical responses) do not have much "personality" (that is, they tend to be very similar in healthy persons), abnormal responses are indicators of multiple sclerosis, brainstem tumors, structural lesions causing coma, and other disorders.

There is additional important selectivity of EEG and MEG recordings that must be remembered in any physiologic interpretation of data. For example, the EEG due to the sources in Figure 1-4 is most sensitive to the correlated dipole layer in gyri (ab, de, gh), where dipoles are lined up. The EEG is insensitive to opposing parts of the dipole layer in sulci (bcd, efg) because the tangential dipoles tend to cancel. The EEG is also insensitive to the random dipole layer (ijklm) because of canceling of both radial and tangential dipoles.

The MEG is most sensitive to the correlated dipole layer in the sulcus (hi) and apparently much less sensitive to all other sources shown because of opposing dipoles, randomly oriented dipoles, or radial dipoles. The latter tend to be excluded because the external magnetic field caused by a radial dipole in a medium of spherically symmetric conductive layers is zero. Although this symmetry condition is not fully satisfied in actual heads, it is close enough so that measured magnetic fields caused by radial dipoles are typically much smaller than fields caused by tangential dipoles of the same strength and depth.

Selective sensitivity is also predicted by time-domain influences. Consider the issue of coherency among individual dipole sources. Coherency is similar to the common EEG concept of synchrony, which, in the EEG field, is typically a loosely defined qualitative measure. By contrast, coherency is a precise technical term defined by (8.12). It is a correlation coefficient, expressed as a function of frequency, which measures the phase consistency between two signals. For example, if two sources are out of phase (at a fixed frequency), but the phase difference remains constant over time, the coherency is equal to one. This would be the case of the coherency between potentials measured at two different nodes of a linear, noise-free electric circuit, for example. In general, the coherency between two signals lies between zero and one because of external influences, nonlinearity, or noise.

Suppose some EEG phenomenon is due to source generation in cortical pyramidal cells that form a dipole layer. For purposes of discussion, imagine that the dipole layer is composed of a mixture of M coherent sources (coherency = 1) and N incoherent sources (that is, uncorrelated; coherency = 0) located within roughly the same distance of a scalp electrode. The potentials due to individual coherent sources combine by linear superposition to produce the summed contribution to scalp potential. In contrast, the contribution of the incoherent sources is due only to statistical fluctuation. Thus the relative contribution of coherent to incoherent sources is estimated to be $M/\sqrt{N}$. For example, approximately 10^7 pyramidal cells line up in parallel within a 1-cm^2 portion of cortical gyrus. If only 1% are coherent, the relative contribution to scalp potential of these minority neurons would then be approximately $10^5/\sqrt{10^7}$, or about 30 times greater than that of the 99% of neurons that produce incoherent sources (Elul, 1972; Nunez, 1981). These are only crude estimates because the effect of different distances between sources and scalp electrode and the effect of coherencies between zero and one have not been considered. However, the general idea that scalp potentials are due primarily to combined contributions from sources with high coherence is valid.

The relative importance of coherent sources can be much less with micro EEG measurements using small electrodes in the cortex. For example, suppose an electrode with a tip diameter of about 10^{-3} cm is placed reasonably close to a cell body. In this case, typically fewer than 100 neurons are close enough to contribute substantially to the measured potential (Abeles, 1982). If we suppose that about 100 neurons contribute, and 10% are coherent, the relative contributions of coherent and incoherent sources are about equal in this case. Of course, if the electrode is placed very close to the cell body, only the local neuron will make a substantial contribution to the measurements. Other equivalent estimates can be obtained for different sizes and locations of electrodes to illustrate the relative importance of coherent and incoherent sources. These examples show the critical importance of spatial scale in the study of EEG. That is, they suggest one important cause for misunderstandings that occur between electroencephalographers, who are concerned with potentials generated in populations of perhaps 10^7 to 10^9 neurons, and physiologists, who typically record potentials due to anything between one and perhaps 10^5 neurons.

Further selectivity in scalp-recorded data occurs when time averages are used. That is, when a field is due to a combination of both stationary (stimulus-to-stimulus) and nonstationary sources, the former may be expected to make the greater contribution to the averaged field. Several researchers have apparently not fully appreciated the importance of the selectivity of their measuring devices and experimental techniques. As a result, studies have been published in the EEG and MEG literature that suggest very localized sources, although good evidence exists that such sources are actually distributed over large regions of the brain. For example, when the source distribution is a large, correlated dipole layer, the EEG pattern may suggest a single deep dipole below the middle of the layer. Also, the MEG tends to be largest at certain parts of the edge of the layer, where only one side of a fissure or sulcus produces coherent sources.

The selective sensitivity of EEG and MEG is illustrated by the simulation shown in Figure 1-5. In this case, a three concentric sphere model representing brain, skull, and scalp (Nunez, 1981) was used to model volume conduction in the head. That is, given a certain set of sources, this model allows estimation of surface potential or magnetic field distribution over the scalp. In this case, the model cortex is divided into regions of macrocolumn size, and each one may produce a dipole source. Positive and negative radial dipoles are indicated by dots and open circles, respectively (a). Arrows and x's indicate tangential dipoles, and the latter differ by having random magnitude and direction. The surface potential distribution (b) mainly reflects the "source clumps" at A and B and the unopposed tangential dipoles at C. The radial component of the magnetic field (d) mainly indicates the unopposed tangential dipoles at C. This plot is very similar to (c), the radial magnetic field due only to dipoles at C, thereby illustrating how easy it is to be confused into thinking that distributed sources are local.

EEG and Cognitive Processing

With all the limitations of extracranial recordings, we might at first wonder if anything of value can be extracted from these signals. However, it has long been appreciated (almost since the first human scalp recordings in 1928) that EEG is a genuine measure, albeit a crude one, of conscious experience. For example, the human alpha rhythm is a 10-Hz, near-sinusoidal oscillation that occurs in about 95% of healthy persons when sitting quietly and relaxed with eyes closed. In some persons, mental calculations cause "blocking" of the alpha rhythm. That is, the 10-Hz rhythm with a typical apparent bandwidth of 1 or 2 Hz is replaced by low-amplitude potentials that may appear in the frequency domain as low-pass noise. A general idea of the gross temporal changes in spontaneous EEG with physiologic state may be obtained from Figure 1-6. More detailed data on spontaneous EEG are provided in Chapters 3 and 4.

An interesting description of alpha blocking is provided in an early study of a well-known experimental subject by Penfield and Jasper (1954):

> Einstein was found to show a fairly continuous alpha rhythm while carrying out rather intricate mathematical operations, which, however, were fairly automatic for him. Suddenly his alpha waves dropped out and he appeared restless. When asked if there was anything wrong, he replied that he had found a mistake in the calculations he had made the day before. He asked to telephone Princeton

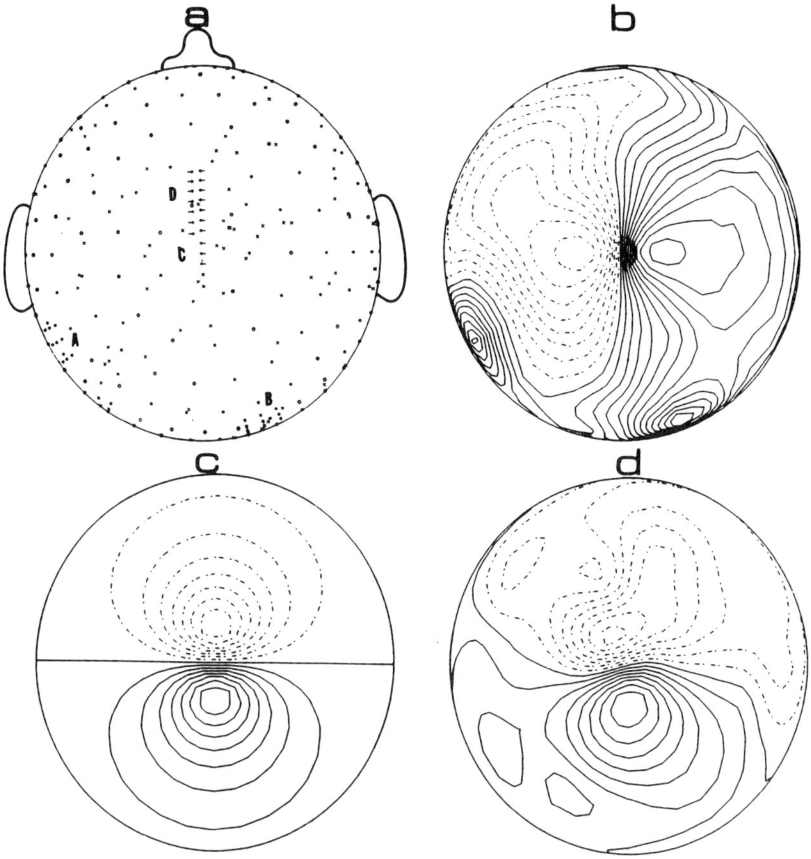

Figure 1-5. **a.** Assumed source distribution consisting of positive radial dipoles (dots), negative radial dipoles (open circles), directed tangential dipoles of fixed magnitude (arrows), and random (in both magnitude and direction) tangential dipoles (crosses). Source strengths of tangential dipoles are made five times larger than those of radial dipoles to simulate dipoles distributed over depths of fissures and sulci. **b.** Surface potential map based on 648 surface samples with no interpolation. Solid lines indicate positive potentials with respect to infinity. The two positive clumps of radial dipoles (A and B) and unapposed dipole layer (C) contribute most to the potential map, with much less contribution from either random or apposed dipoles (D). **c.** Map of radial component of magnetic field (MEG) due only to the unapposed dipole layer (C). **d.** The MEG map due to all sources (similar to map c). (Reproduced with permission from Nunez et al, 1991.)

> immediately. This illustrates how concentration of attention is just a special case of arousal, a local or focused waking response, employing similar neuronal mechanisms.

In some persons, the alpha rhythm continues without obvious time-domain changes during mental calculations but with a sharp decrease in intercortical coherency. This effect is illustrated in Figure 1-7, in which the subject showed a

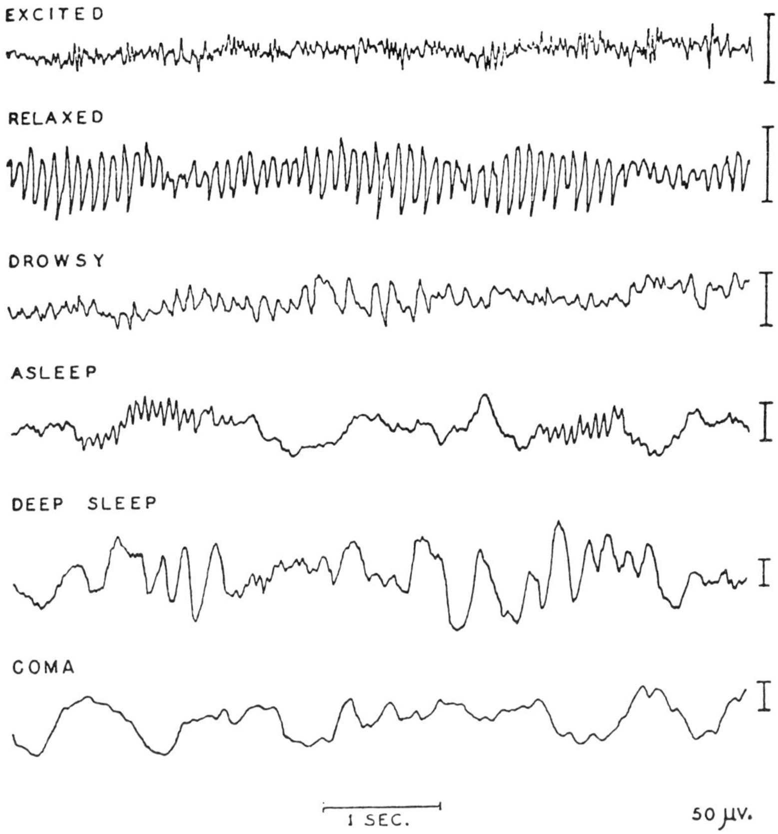

Figure 1-6. Characteristic EEG rhythms during several states of consciousness. Vertical bars denote 50 μV amplitude. Note change of scale; that is, large amplitude slow oscillations are typically associated with sleep and coma. (Reproduced with permission from Penfield and Jasper, 1954.)

coherency decrease during the last 4 minutes of a 6-minute period of mental arithmetic. Another example is the EEG typically recorded during the rapid eye movement (REM) stage of sleep, which is closely related to dreaming. A recent sleep study showed large interhemispheric coherence in the 11- to 15-Hz band in all stages of sleep except REM (Poiseau et al, 1991). During REM, the coherence in this band decreases to a level similar to that shown by the rest of the spectrum. In general, the human spontaneous EEG exhibits the following characteristics: High-amplitude, spatially coherent, sinusoidal potentials distributed over the entire scalp are typically associated with lack of cognitive processing as in the states of deep sleep, anesthesia, and coma. The awake alpha rhythm is somewhat of an intermediate case, being of moderate amplitude and of largest magnitude over the back half of the head. Low-amplitude, broad-spectrum EEG typically occurs in awake persons with their eyes open or perhaps when performing difficult cognitive tasks.

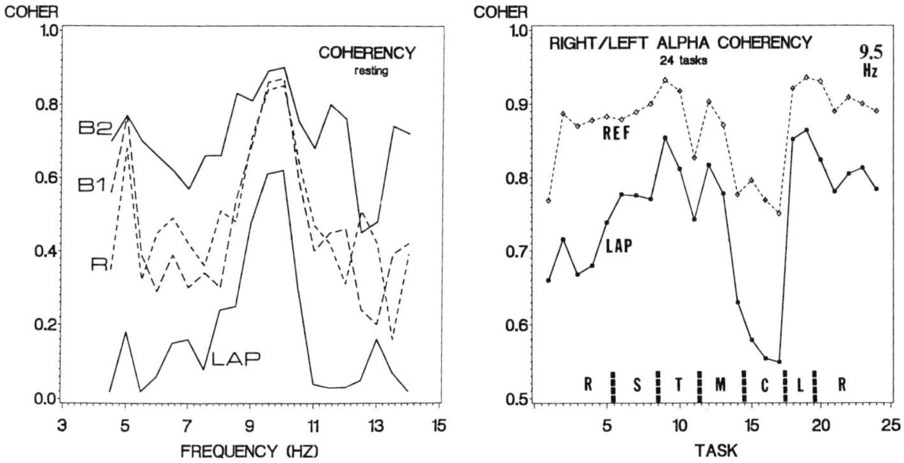

Figure 1-7. **A.** Interhemispheric coherency of 1 minute of eyes-closed, spontaneous EEG (alpha rhythm). (Coherency is a correlation coefficient expressed as a function of frequency.) Data were obtained with two five-electrode Laplacian arrays centered at P3 and P4 (3-cm spacing). Coherency estimates were calculated using four separate homologous derivations: bipolar pair closest to midline (B2), bipolar pair most distant from midline (B1), Fz reference (R), and Hjorth Laplacian (LAP). The Laplacian method removes most of the erroneous high coherency due to volume conduction from opposite hemisphere. (Reproduced with permission from Nunez and Pilgreen, 1991.) **B.** Right-left alpha coherency at 9.5 Hz (frequency peak of both average power and coherency) as a function of tasks performed. Each dot represents 1 minute of data. M and C refer to mental calculations and counting backward, respectively. Other tasks were more passive. The Hjorth Laplacian method shows lower interhemispheric coherency estimates over all tasks. The decrease in coherency during tasks M and C for the reference estimate is only about 10%, whereas the corresponding Laplacian decrease is about 30%. This suggests that Laplacian estimates may provide more robust measures of the interhemispheric coherency of EEG during cognitive processing. (Reproduced with permission from Nunez and Pilgreen, 1991.)

In addition to a history of almost seven decades of spontaneous EEG data, in the past 25 years researchers produced a large body of evoked- (or event-related) potential data. Both transient and steady-state evoked potentials have been recorded (Regan, 1989). The transient response to some stimulus (auditory, visual, or somatosensory) is averaged over many stimuli to remove at least some of the spontaneous EEG, biological noise, and system noise to produce a temporal waveform in the few hundred milliseconds after the stimulus. Transient responses are determined not only by stimulus properties or motor activity (exogenous factors) but also by cognitive processing (endogenous factors). For example, the contingent negative variation refers to a shift in scalp potential as the result of an expected stimulus. Another well-known transient response, P300 (positive potential over the top of the head with respect to ear reference at a latency roughly 300 milliseconds from the stimulus), depends on the perceived significance of the stimulus (see Chapter 7). For example, a series of auditory tones of constant frequency are

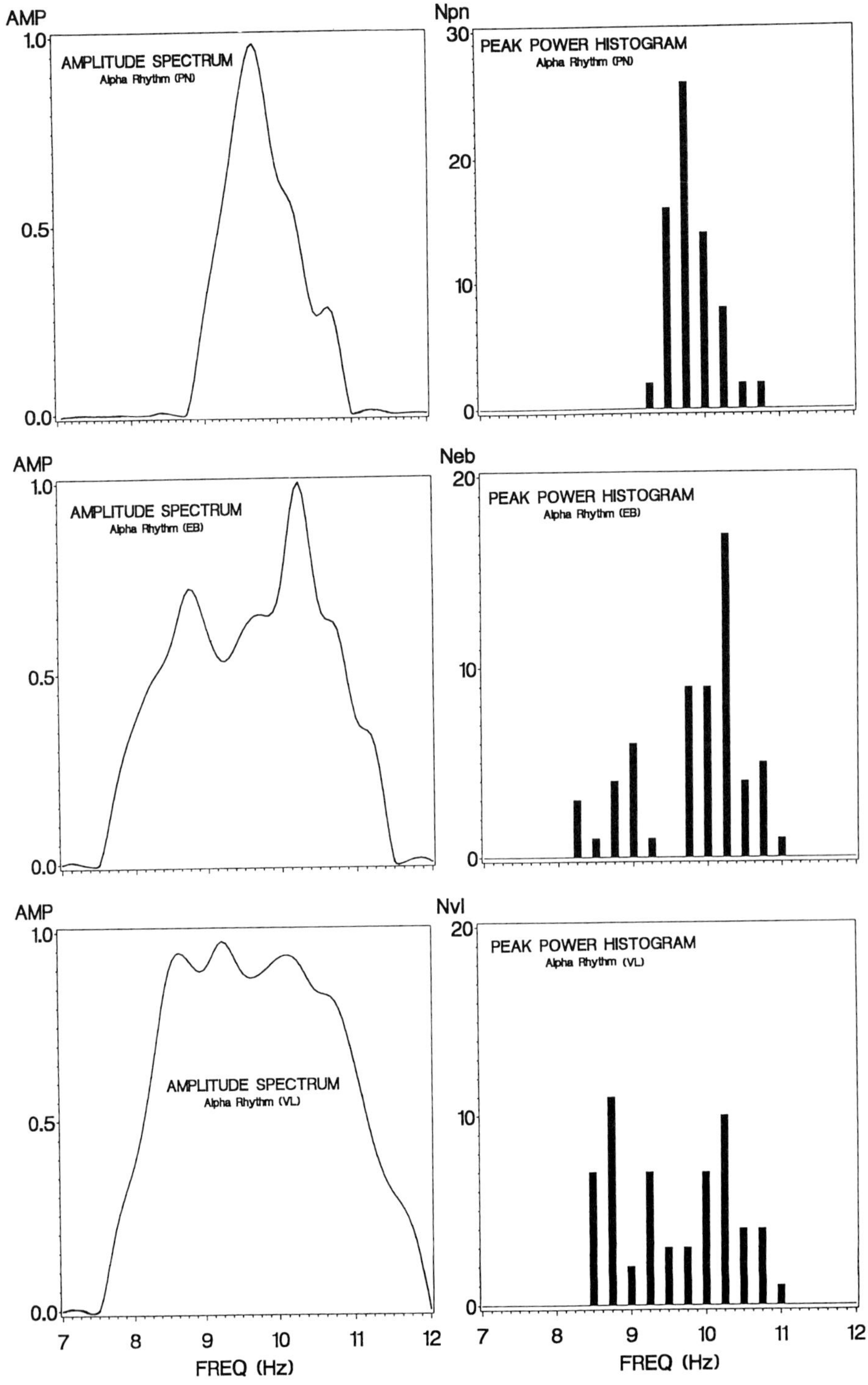
AMP
AMPLITUDE SPECTRUM
Alpha Rhythm (PN)
Npn
PEAK POWER HISTOGRAM
Alpha Rhythm (PN)
AMP
AMPLITUDE SPECTRUM
Alpha Rhythm (EB)
Neb
PEAK POWER HISTOGRAM
Alpha Rhythm (EB)
AMP
AMPLITUDE SPECTRUM
Alpha Rhythm (VL)
Nvl
PEAK POWER HISTOGRAM
Alpha Rhythm (VL)
FREQ (Hz)
FREQ (Hz)

presented, randomly interspersed with a few tones of a different frequency. The person being tested is asked to count the irregular (odd-ball) tones. Whereas the irregular tones evoke a P300 response, regular ones do not.

With multichannel recordings (typically 16 to 64), spatial and temporal properties of EEG and event-related potentials have been studied in relation to cognitive processing (Livanov, 1977). For example, visual imagery can change the location of maximum alpha root-mean-square amplitude on the scalp (Lehmann et al, 1987). Changes in interhemispheric and intrahemispheric coherency patterns of alpha rhythm are associated with mental arithmetic, mental reading, or listening to music (Pockberger et al, 1988; Rappelsberger and Petsche, 1988). Scalp covariance patterns of event-related potentials have been shown to change distinctly in preparation for a cognitive task, and they depend on whether the task was later accurately or inaccurately performed (Gevins et al, 1981, 1983, 1990, 1991). These later data suggest formation of specific functional neural networks (perhaps more appropriately called "cortical columnar or neural mass networks") appropriate for specific types of cognitive processing on time scales in the 10- to 100-millisecond range and spatial scales measured in centimeters. These networks apparently involve neurons in many widely spaced regions in both neocortical hemispheres. The relation of transient evoked potentials to mental activity is considered in greater detail in Chapter 7. Chapter 6 contains an outline of cognitive connections using steady-state evoked potentials with more emphasis on neocortical dynamic theory.

EEG in Medicine

A variety of pathologic conditions occur for which EEG provides an important clinical test. Of course, such tests must account for differences among patients, especially in the case of cortical sources that have their own "personality" or "fingerprint" characteristic of the specific patient. Consider, for example, the spectral contents of the eyes closed, spontaneous EEG recorded from occipital regions in several healthy persons (Figure 1-8). A normal EEG does not necessarily mean normal brain function, at least with the relatively crude technical methods available now. As better methods to improve EEG spatial resolution and pattern

←

Figure 1-8. Amplitude spectra (*left column*) and corresponding peak power histograms (*right column*) for three healthy adults (*three rows*) in the resting, eyes-closed state. Bipolar recordings from occipital region. Each plot represents about 4 to 5 minutes of data (4-second epochs) with suspected artifact removed. Peak-power histograms are determined by choosing the single frequency component (0.25-Hz resolution) of each epoch, which yields the highest spectral power. No contributions to peak-power histograms were found outside the frequency range shown on the plots. The results can be interpreted as a number of closely spaced modes, perhaps both local and global, which are revealed through a small amount of nonstationarity. More details of this idea are described in Chapters 2, 3, 6, and 11. Experimental methods are described in Nunez, 1981 on pages 222 to 229.

recognition are developed, the scope of EEG clinical tests may be expanded substantially (Nunez, 1990a; Nunez and Pilgreen, 1991; Nunez et al, 1994).

Many diseases appear as abnormal spontaneous EEG. However, each abnormal EEG pattern can be caused by more than one disease, and some diseases cause more than one abnormal EEG pattern. Thus the EEG alone usually is not used to make a specific clinical diagnosis but rather to suggest a set of possible diagnoses (Spehlmann, 1981; Niedermeyer and Lopes da Silva, 1993). Abnormalities in the EEG may be either localized or generalized (global); an important case in point is EEG associated with the epilepsies, a set of diseases that afflict approximately 1% of the population.

Localized (that is, focal) epileptiform EEG typically consists of localized, single, or repetitive spikes in the record and sharp waves, perhaps combined with slow waves. These characteristic spatial and temporal patterns may last less than a few seconds, in which case they normally appear between seizures (interictal activity). A sample EEG containing several kinds of interictal temporal behavior is shown in Figure 1-9. Abnormal patterns may persist for a long time and be associated with seizures (ictal or seizure activity). Generally epileptiform EEG has a higher amplitude and is less regular than normal EEG. To a physical scientist, its waveforms may suggest underlying nonlinear interactions.

Generalized epileptiform EEG patterns differ from focal epileptiform activity in that they appear over most or all parts of both cerebral hemispheres and usually have similar shapes, amplitudes, and timing in homologous areas (Spehlmann, 1981). In some cases, epileptiform activity starts locally and spreads over the entire cortex, typically producing a generalized seizure. In the physical sciences, a propagating instability, for example in hot plasma, may have analogous features.

Figure 1-10 also illustrates another way in which unequivocal EEG abnormally shows up (that is, considerable EEG asymmetry between hemispheres). For example, cortical tumors cause an abnormal amount of delta activity (1 to 4 Hz) in the region containing the tumor, perhaps superimposed on the normal alpha rhythm (8 to 13 Hz). Stroke and head injury are other conditions that may cause obvious EEG asymmetry.

Generalized asynchronous slow waves (of relatively low coherence and with frequency less than 8 Hz) during the awake, eyes-closed state are still another indication of possible disease. This kind of EEG pattern may indicate, for example, the presence of infectious disease, Alzheimer's disease, cerebrovascular disease, severe head injuries, or multiple tumor sites. Bilaterally synchronous slow waves have relatively high coherence between homologous locations in each hemisphere or perhaps between all pairs of locations, and have frequencies less than 8 Hz. This type of EEG pattern may be due to diseases impairing deep brain midline structures. Many of the same diseases causing generalized asynchronous slow waves also cause synchronous activity. Another EEG phenomena is alpha coma, sinusoidal activity similar to the normal awake alpha rhythm, except that it typically occurs with high amplitude over the entire scalp. These and other kinds of spatially coherent, global oscillations like the 3 Hz wave of epilepsy are of special interest in connection with the standing wave theory of EEG, described in Chapter 11.

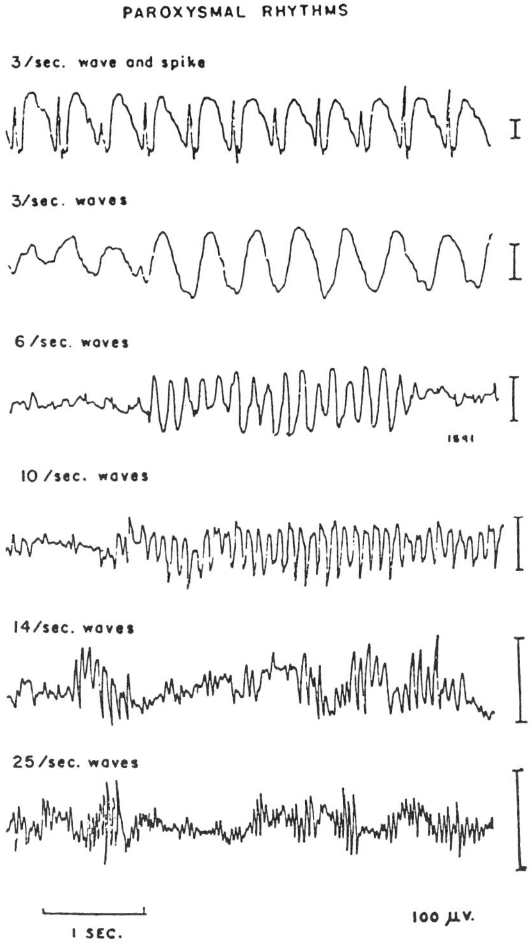

Figure 1-9. Paroxysmal rhythms from the scalp of epileptic patients. Note decrease in amplitude (calibration at right) with the increase in frequency. The 10- and 25-per-second waves occurred in the normal waking EEG and the 14-per-second waves in normal sleep. In epileptic patients they appeared in bursts of relatively large amplitude waves, that is "paroxysmal hypersynchrony without dysrhythmia." (Reproduced with permission from Penfield and Jasper, 1954.)

Evoked potentials are also used in clinical diagnosis, primarily to test conduction in the visual, auditory, or somatosensory systems. Typically the transient response to a sensory stimulus is recorded at the scalp. The latency of some standard waveform in the response has a certain normal range. In patients with lesions along a sensory pathway, abnormally long latency is often observed. With some diseases, this technique can detect lesions not found with other tests. Abnormal evoked potentials also occur in other disorders that are more conveniently diagnosed using other means.

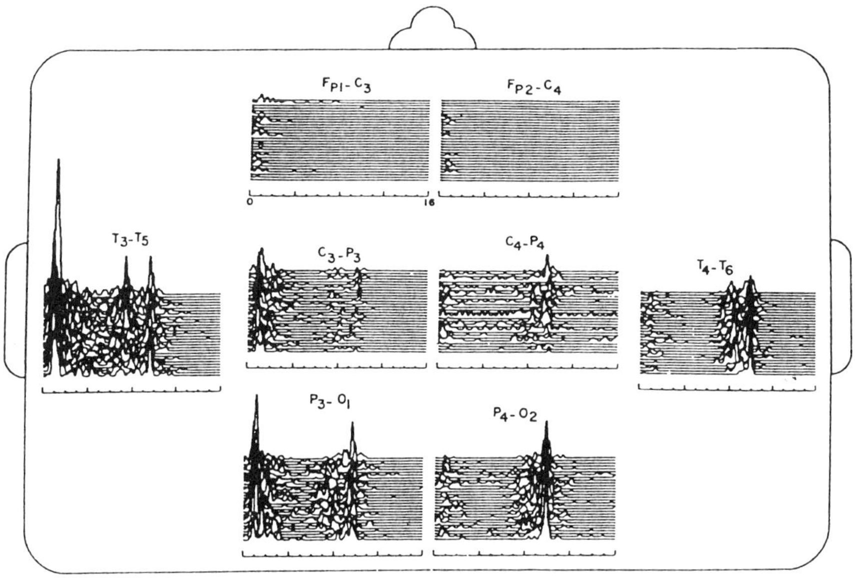

Figure 1-10. Compressed spectral arrays of EEG recorded simultaneously from four homologous locations on each side of the head. The horizontal frequency scale shown is 0 to 16 Hz. Time progresses along the vertical scale. The right side shows normal alpha rhythm; the left side shows abnormal delta activity, indicating temporal lobe tumor. Note that the introduction of a region of inhomogeneous tissue results in the introduction of new EEG modes. (Reproduced with permission from Bickford, 1973.)

Use of evoked potentials in studies of cognitive and psychiatric disorders is suggested by work on the endogenous evoked potentials, that is, those related to cognitive processing. Patients with cognitive and psychiatric disorders occupy a large portion of the hospital beds in western countries. These patients have cognitive disorders that range from those with relatively limited disabilities such as agnosia, apraxia, and amnesia to those with extensive dysfunction such as dementia. The psychiatric disorders include depression and schizophrenia (Yudofsky and Hales, 1992). Use of spontaneous EEG and evoked potentials to diagnose specific disorders and perhaps follow the course of drug treatment are active areas of research. The development of pattern recognition methods that are sufficiently sophisticated to deal effectively with the complexities of neocortical dynamics will probably have major clinical importance. This consideration provides strong motivation for the efforts outlined in this book, beyond that of pure scientific interest. Medical applications of EEG are discussed in more detail in Chapters 4 and 13.

Macrocolumn Sources of EEG

Specific theories of neocortical dynamics are considered later in this book in detail. At this stage of our very limited understanding, any such theory must be preliminary and controversial. However, several quantitative issues must be addressed in any attempt to connect neocortical function with EEG and behavioral observations. Several of these are considered in Chapters 1 to 3.

Consider the following general ways to define the physiologic state of neocortex. One way is by the behavior of the person being studied. An awake subject clearly is in a different state than one who is asleep. Of course, subtle changes of state are likely to be difficult or impossible to quantify with only behavioral observations. A much more quantitative way to define state is with the EEG, either by itself or combined with other physiologic measures. For example, the different sleep stages are distinguished by a combination of EEG, muscle, and eye movement recordings. Of course, these specific measures are of special interest primarily because they are closely correlated with behavioral and cognitive measures.

Neural source activity is, of course, not generally accessible to direct measurement. Some data are available in patients with electrodes implanted for medical reasons (candidates for epilepsy surgery, for example). Other data are available in nonhuman mammalian cortex and other neural structures, but extrapolation to humans presents a separate problem, especially with cognitively related data. However, even if ethical considerations did not prohibit most intracranial recordings in humans, the information obtained in such experiments would still be severely limited by practical considerations, for example by the number of recording sites possible in a living brain whose function must not be substantially affected if data are to reflect normal operation.

Further practical limitations are apparent. For example, suppose we imagine some experiment of the distant future, in which the limitations due to a small number of recording sites is somehow removed. That is, in this thought experiment, data from a large fraction of the 10^{11} neurons of the human brain are recorded separately. Or, perhaps more realistically, a large fraction of the 10^4 cortical macrocolumns is monitored. How do we make sense of this incredible volume of data? That is, we may fail to appreciate the forest if we get lost in the big trees, let alone the bushes, branches, and leaves. Perhaps one of the first ideas would be to reduce the data based on some transformation, for example, a Fourier transform in time and three spatial dimensions. A special case of such transformation (for zero time and spatial frequencies) is the simple time and space average defined by (1.1).

The point of this thought exercise is that both scalp and cortical EEG involve space averages of neural source activity, but at different spatial scales. The averaged EEG is one of the variables that would certainly be examined closely in our idealized thought experiment. Fortuitously, the head volume conductor provides a data reduction approach that might well be used in this thought experiment. Of course, averaging at such large scales may "wash out" so much neural source information that no correlation between behavior and EEG remains. But we know this is not so. Even with the very crude EEG methods used commonly, there is a strong correlation between the spatial-temporal pattern of EEG and "coarse grained" behavior (that is gross cognitive state). In addition, we have good reason to believe that new EEG methods, which increase spatial resolution by a factor of perhaps three to five over conventional methods and use much more effective pattern recognition, will be able to detect more subtle changes in clinical, behavioral, or cognitive state. Such development will have profound implications in medicine, cognitive science, and several related fields, and is, of course, a primary motivation for writing this book.

It is convenient to first define state variables that are easily connected to experimental EEG data. Later we must relate the dependent variables of neocortical dynamic theories to these EEG-related state variables. To begin we note that the cortical macrocolumn (diameter of about 3 mm) lies near the apparent theoretical limit of spatial resolution available in scalp recordings. Furthermore, the macrocolumn apparently constitutes a distinct unit of neocortical dynamic function, an issue considered in detail in Chapter 2. Thus one way to imagine neocortical dynamics is in terms of the interaction of macrocolumns. Of course, simultaneous interactions can also be expected to take place at other spatial scales (for example, between neurons, minicolumns, corticocortical columns, cytoarchitecture regions, and so on).

A cortical macrocolumn contains approximately 10^5 to 10^6 neurons and 10^{10} synapses. These synapses cause microsources at the postsynaptic membrane and at more remote membrane surfaces, as required for current conservation. Electrophysiologic studies span a spatial scale of about five orders of magnitude, including microelectrode studies of transmembrane potential with electrodes having a tip diameter of about 10^{-4} cm, micro-EEG studies with a tip diameter of 10^{-3} to 10^{-1} cm, and studies with a scalp electrode of about 1 cm diameter (Petsche et al, 1984, 1988). However, because the scalp electrode is separated from neural sources by both distance and the poorly conducting skull, the spatial resolution of scalp recordings of EEG is typically closer to 5 or 10 cm than to 1 cm (Nunez, 1981, 1988a). That is, surface potentials recorded by a scalp electrode are due to neural sources averaged over a surface of cortical tissue that is typically at least ten square centimeters and often much larger.

To be more precise about neural sources defined at multiple spatial scales, it is convenient to define the current polarization or simply polarization of a volume ΔV of tissue as the current dipole moment per unit volume. That is

$$\mathbf{P}(\mathbf{r}, t) = \frac{1}{\Delta V} \int_{\Delta V} \mathbf{r}' s(\mathbf{r}', t)\, d^3\mathbf{r}' \tag{1.2}$$

where the polarization $\mathbf{P}$ can be expressed in $\mu A/mm^2$ (microamperes per square millimeter), the microcurrent sources, $s(\mathbf{r}, t)$ have units of $\mu A/mm^3$ (microamperes per cubic millimeter), and the vector $\mathbf{r}'$ locates each source within the volume of tissue. By changing the size of the volume over which the integral is taken, sources can be defined at different spatial scales. This definition of current polarization is analogous to the usual charge polarization used in the physical sciences to characterize the state of dielectric material. That is, in the case of a dielectric, $s(\mathbf{r}', t)$ is the local charge density and (1.2) yields charge polarization. In Figure 1-11, the volume of tissue ΔV is understood to be that of a macrocolumn. The micro-

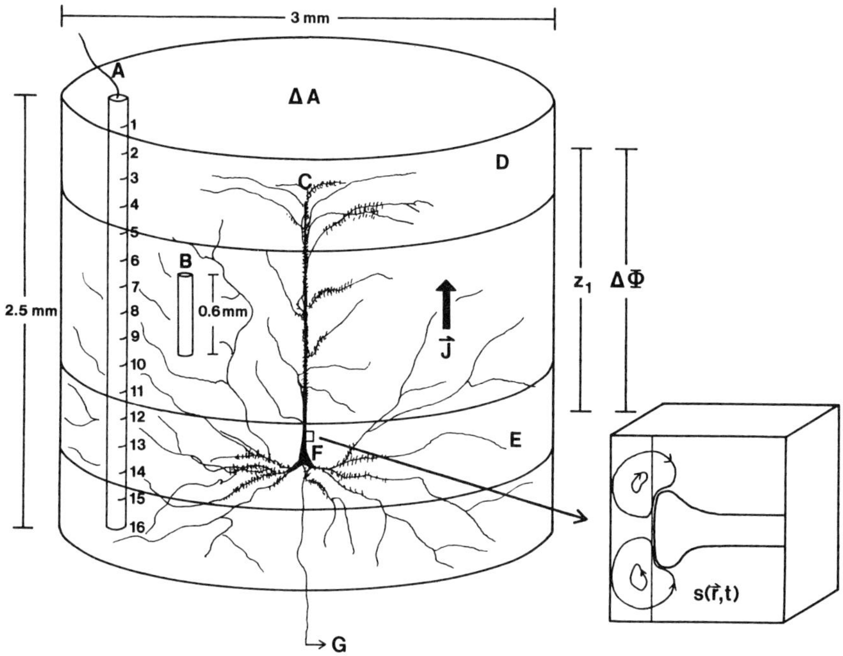

Figure 1-11. A macrocolumn of neocortex, defined by the spatial extent of axon branches (E) that remain within the cortex (recurrent collaterals). The large pyramidal cell (C) shown here is one of about 10^5 to 10^6 neurons in the macrocolumn. Approximately 80% cortical cells are pyramidal cells, and nearly all pyramidal cells send an axon into the white matter (G), which re-enters the cortex at some distant location. Each large pyramidal cell has about 10^4 to 10^5 synaptic inputs (F), which cause microcurrent sources and sinks s(**r**, t) along membrane surfaces. Space-averaged source activity may be measured with a probe (A), shown here with 16 electrode contacts within the cortex. Estimates of current source density typically refer to space averages over volumes represented by small columns (B), which contain many synaptic microsources. In applications involving scalp potentials, it is often convenient to idealize this complicated current source distribution by a small dipole layer (D and E). At some fixed instant in time, a slight imbalance in sources over sinks in region E and/or imbalance in sinks over sources in region D cause a net outward macroscopic current density **J** and macroscopic potential difference ΔΦ across the cortex. (Reproduced with permission from Nunez, 1990a.)

sources s(**r**, t) are related to extracellular micropotentials Φ(**r**, t) by Poisson's equation (Plonsey, 1969; Nunez, 1981)

$$\nabla \cdot \sigma(\mathbf{r}) \nabla \Phi = s(\mathbf{r}, t) \tag{1.3}$$

where σ(**r**) is tissue conductivity, defined at the same scale as the sources and potential.

Source estimates in three dimensions generally require measurement of field potentials at nine or more closely spaced points for each source estimate, a difficult, if not impossible task in living tissue. However, in a laminated structure such as neocortex, with a neuronal population relatively homogeneous and isotropic in directions parallel to the surface and many active synapses over a continuous cortical area, equipotential surfaces may reasonably be assumed to be approximately parallel to the surface (Petsche et al, 1984, 1988). Under these conditions, the probe (A) shown in Figure 1-11 may be used with (1.3) to estimate source activity averaged over a spatial scale depicted by the cylindrical region (B). That is

$$s(z, t) \sim \sigma \frac{\partial^2 \Phi}{\partial z^2} \sim \frac{\sigma}{\Delta z^2} (\Phi_{n+1} - 2\Phi_n + \Phi_{n-1}) \tag{1.4}$$

Where z is the coordinate normal to the surface, Δz is the spacing between electrodes, Φ_n refers to potentials recorded at various depths, and conductivity is assumed to be constant. In other experiments, only cortical surface potentials or perhaps potentials at a few depth locations are obtained. In this case, direct estimates of source distributions are not possible; however, crude estimates of the macroscopic current source density **J** normal to the surface can be obtained. In Figure 1-11, the complex source distribution in the cortex is idealized so that the superficial level (D) produces an excess of sinks (at some instant in time) and the deeper layer (E) produces an excess of sources, which is qualitatively consistent with several studies of evoked (Humphrey, 1968) and spontaneous EEG (Lopes da Silva and Storm van Leeuwen, 1978). In this ideal case, polarization of the macrocolumn is roughly the macroscopic current source density, space averaged across the cortex (Nunez, 1990)

$$P_z \sim J_z \tag{1.5}$$

Of course, current sources are actually distributed across the cortex, so that (1.5) may be only a crude approximation; however, it does provide an intuitively appealing physical interpretation of the polarization **P**, which is more precisely defined by (1.2). As shown in Table 1-2, microsources s(**r**, t) space averaged over volumes comparable to the cylindrical volume B of Figure 1-11 are about 0.1 to 1 $\mu A/mm^3$ for spontaneous EEG and perhaps 20 times larger for penicillin-induced epileptic spikes (Petsche et al, 1984, 1988), with an assumed cortical resistivity of 3500 Ω-mm. In other experiments, the electrode spacing used to estimate vertical Laplacians may be larger, so direct comparison of source magnitudes may not be warranted. That is, for some range of scales, the larger the scale over which either potentials or source densities are averaged, the smaller the expected magnitudes of these variables due to more canceling of positive and negative source contributions at smaller scales. This prediction is partly supported by the data summarized in Table 1-2.

The potential difference across the macrocolumn is approximately related to the macroscopic current density by (Nunez, 1990)

$$\Delta\Phi \approx \frac{J_z z_1}{\sigma} \tag{1.6}$$

where z_1 is the effective pole separation in the dipole layer. Note that current

Table 1-2 Neocortical Potentials and Sources*

Authors	Animal	Experimental Conditions	L (mm)	Δz (mm)	Φ (μV)	$\partial^2\Phi/\partial z^2$ μV/mm²
Cooper et al, 1965	Human	Alpha rhythm, cortex	4	†	100	†
		Alpha rhythm, scalp	10		30	
Humphrey, 1968	Cat	Electrical stimulation of pyramidal tract	0.3	0.2	300	5000–10,000
Mitzdorf and Singer, 1978, 1979	Cat	Electrical stimulation of optic nerve tract	0.003	0.05	2000	50,000–100,000
Lopes da Silva and Storm van Leeuwen, 1978	Dog	Alpha rhythm	0.1	0.35	100	‡
Abeles, 1982	Cat	Spontaneous EEG, 1	3	†	20	†
		Spontaneous EEG, 3	2		30	
		Spontaneous EEG, 7	1		40	
Petsche et al, 1984, 1988	Rabbit	Spontaneous EEG	0.01	0.15	200	2000
		Penicillin-induced spikes	0.01	0.15	6000	50,000

Reproduced with permission from Nunez, 1989.

*L = characteristic size of electrode recording surface, Δz = separation of electrodes tips in depth. Φ is the typical magnitude of recorded potential. $\partial^2\Phi/\partial z^2$ is the estimate of Laplacian value in the direction perpendicular to the cortical surface obtained with finite difference formula (1.4).

†Depth recordings were not obtained.

‡No estimate of source magnitudes was made.

source density and volume (return) current density have opposite signs. ΔΦ is about 200 microvolts for spontaneous EEG (Lopes da Silva and Storm van Leeuwen, 1978; Petsche et al, 1984, 1988) and is typically about several millivolts for cortical potentials induced by electrical stimulation of nerve fibers or penicillin-induced spikes (Humphrey, 1968). Equation (1.6) yields macroscopic current densities across the cortex for spontaneous EEG of approximately 0.03 μA/mm² or 3 μA/cm², with current densities associated with epileptic spikes typically 10 to 100 times larger. For comparison, diffuse current densities due to stimulating electrodes of about 1 mA/cm² (approximately 300 times larger than that of spontaneous EEG) are apparently required to excite nervous tissue (Myklebust et al, 1985).

Broad Classification of Macrocolumn Sources

The neocortex consists of about 10^4 macrocolumns, for which we may define polarization vectors **P** by (1.2). The choice of macrocolumns (rather than some other scale) for this discussion is mostly arbitrary; however, with scalp EEG recordings, smaller scales are not of direct interest because resolution of the polarization vector, even at the macrocolumn scale, is not possible with current technology. The macrocolumns may then be pictured as forming a dipole layer covering the entire cortical surface. Polarization vectors of the dipole layer may be random, highly correlated, or anything in between. Furthermore, the nature of the dipole layer can depend on the period T of time averaging. For convenience, EEG macrosources (that is, the polarization vector **P** at the macrocolumn scale) may be separated into several idealized categories (Nunez, 1988b; Nunez and Pilgreen, 1991).

Type I. Localized and Stationary

Cortical sources are sufficiently localized so that scalp potentials may be approximated by a single transcortical dipole. In practice, this means that the polarization is large over a few square centimeters or less of cortical surface. That is

$$P_z(x, y, t) \sim f(t)\delta(x - x_1)\delta(y - y_1) \tag{1.7}$$

where x_1 and y_1 locate the dipole in directions tangent to the cortical surface and are time independent with respect to the time scale T used in the experiment. Somatosensory evoked potentials over some latency range appear to fit this definition for sources in primary sensory cortex at location x_1, y_1.

Type II. Localized and Nonstationary

These sources differ from type I by allowing a few (M) dipoles to move around. That is

$$P_z(x, y, t) \approx \sum_{m=1}^{M} f_m(t)\delta[x - x_m(t)]\delta[(y - y_m(t)] \tag{1.8}$$

and epileptic spike activity with multiple foci might fit this idealized case to some degree.

Type III. Distributed and Stationary

Current sources are distributed over a relatively large area of neocortex, so that neither of the approximations (1.7) and (1.8) apply. However, characteristic spatial patterns (of amplitude, coherence, and so on) are relatively constant in time, when one time average is compared with the next. That is,

$$\hat{\mathbf{P}}(\mathbf{r}, t, T) \approx \hat{\mathbf{P}}(\mathbf{r}, T) \tag{1.9}$$

where the averaging period T is sufficiently long to produce a constant characteristic spatial pattern. For example, if T is approximately 1 minute, a characteristic alpha average scalp potential distribution is obtained, which may be repeated in subsequent averages as long as the person's physiologic state is not changed. However, (1.9) may not accurately represent the alpha rhythm if the averaging period T is shortened to the one second range (Remond et al, 1969; Lehmann 1971, 1988; Lehmann et al, 1987; Nunez, 1981; refer also to Chapter 3). There are probably many EEG and evoked phenomena for which the averaging period is critical to source characterization. The steady-state evoked potentials at fixed frequency described in Chapter 6 fit this category during the resting state (that is, no cognitive task).

Type IV. Distributed and Nonstationary

None of the approximations applied to source types I to III are valid. Fundamental anatomic and physiologic data (Nunez, 1981, 1988a, 1988b), a variety of human EEGs recorded with depth electrodes (Sem-Jacobsen et al, 1953) and from the scalp (Lehmann, 1971, 1987; Nunez, 1981), and several evoked potential studies (Gevins et al, 1981, 1983, 1991) suggest that type IV sources in the brain are the rule rather than the exception. A prudent viewpoint for the experimentalist is then one of treating any new EEG phenomena as being due to type IV sources until proved otherwise. Obviously experimental protocols should not depend on a priori assumptions (either implicit or explicit) about sources. However failure to appreciate this point fully has apparently led to the publication of several incorrect conclusions about brain function in the EEG and related literature.

Some EEG researchers have emphasized the inverse problem, that is finding the source distribution associated with a given scalp potential map. In practice, these studies have often assumed the character of "brain statics" rather than brain dynamics. The inverse problem in EEG or MEG has no unique solution. That is, for any given potential (or magnetic field) distribution over the scalp surface, a variety of possible neural source distributions exists that can produce the same surface map. This limitation applies even in the idealized case of perfect surface information. But in actual practice, surface data are recorded only at discrete locations, over only the upper region of the surface; noise is present; models of the head are imperfect; and so forth. Thus inverse solutions involving practical questions in EEG or MEG are typically much less unique than idealized solutions. That is, the number of possible current source distributions that may match (within the limits of experimental error) a given set of surface data may be large.

Because of the nonuniqueness of the inverse problem, actual solutions involve the constrained inverse problem in which information about neurophysiology and anatomy is used to limit possible source distributions. The three most common constraints are the following.

1. The sources consist of a single or small number of dipoles (type I), typically at linear scales of about 1 cm or larger. The word dipole is used to indicate the current polarization or dipole moment per unit volume in this context. This subfield of the inverse problem, called "dipole localization," has been developed in both EEG (Henderson et al. 1975; Kavanaugh et al, 1978; Nunez, 1981; Wood, 1982; Fender, 1987; Cuffin et al, 1991) and MEG (Cuffin and Cohen, 1979; Hari and Kaukoranta, 1985; Weinberg et al, 1987; Williamson and Kaufman, 1987; Romani and Rossini, 1988; Cohen et al, 1990).

2. Sources, for example dipoles, may change strength but not location or orientation during a specified time interval (type I). This spatial–temporal constraint was recently added to dipole localization algorithms (Scherg and von Cramon, 1985, 1989; Scherg, 1989). Also refer to review by Nunez (1990a, 1990b).

3. Sources are all located at the same depth, for example in neocortex. This subfield of the inverse problem in EEG has been called "spatial deconvolution" (Nicholas and Deloche, 1976), "software lens" (Freeman, 1980), "de-blurring" (Gevins, 1990), or "cortical imaging" (Kearfott et al, 1991; Sidman, 1991). It is based on the unique relation between surface potentials and sources at a fixed depth (Katznelson, 1981; Nunez, 1981, 1987). This approach is applicable to all four general source types but cannot locate subcortical sources. Often cortical imaging refers only to estimates of cortical surface potential, in which case no assumptions about sources are required (Nunez et al. 1994).

An important issue in EEG is the appropriateness of these constraints for specific applications. For example, a single dipole may be assumed to be the source of a visual evoked potential due to half visual field stimulation and the dipole then located at the correct location in the contralateral hemisphere (Wood, 1982). In studies of patients with known, implanted dipole sources, localization accuracy with EEG is typically about 1 cm, with MEG accuracy possibly a little better for sources with large tangential dipole moments (Cohen et al, 1990; Cuffin et al, 1991).

Although the approach of dipole localization has several apparent applications (such as location of epileptic foci), its general extension to cases of unknown sources that may be distributed over large regions of the brain has little apparent justification. Of course, when confronted, dipole localizers of distributed sources may emphasize that these are only "equivalent dipoles," a purely descriptive concept used to quantify the observed spatial distribution of potential or magnetic field. However, it is suggested here that there are many other (and better) ways to quantify EEG data that do far less damage to realistic views of neurophysiology and neuroanatomy. Our emphasis on brain dynamics over brain statics is suggested by Sherrington's often quoted poetic description:

> It is as if the Milky Way entered upon some cosmic dance. Swiftly the brain becomes an enchanted loom where millions of flashing shuttles weave a dissolving pattern, always a meaningful pattern though never an abiding one; a shifting harmony of subpatterns.

As implied by the enchanted loom allegory, a proper study of cognitive processing would appear to involve a study of brain dynamics, that is, a study of changing spatiotemporal patterns of neuronal firing (Freeman and Skarda, 1985; Gevins et al, 1983, 1986; Nunez, 1981, 1989a, 1989b). The problem of improving spatial resolution remains paramount, but the goal is not localization per se, because at any instant sources can be anywhere and everywhere. Rather we require methods to better characterize dynamic spatial and temporal patterns of both cortical sources and scalp potentials.

Sources as Stochastic Field Variables

Many physical and biological phenomena produce data that are not deterministic. We need not be concerned now whether some fundamental randomness exists in the process or whether the apparent randomness is due only to our ignorance of underlying mechanisms. For example, the height of waves in a rough sea, the acoustic pressures generated by turbulent air flow through a pipe, the voltage output of a noise generator, and most of EEG are data that cannot be described accurately by deterministic mathematics. Rather they may be described by probability statements and statistical averages. A single time history X(t), representing data created by some phenomenon that cannot be described easily by an explicit mathematical relation, may be considered a sample record. The collection of all possible sample records (that is, the ensemble of all records) is called a stochastic (random) process (Bendat and Piersol, 1986).

With EEG, the idea of temporal stochastic processes must be extended to include the spatial domain. These ideas can be applied at any spatial scale, but it is convenient to limit this introductory discussion primarily to macrocolumn sources $\mathbf{P}(\mathbf{r}, t)$ and their corresponding scalp potentials $\Phi(\mathbf{r}, t)$, both of which may be considered stochastic fields (Yaglom, 1987; Monin and Yaglom, 1975). The application of stochastic field theory specifically to EEG is considered by Katznelson (1982). Thus, in general, both sources and potentials exhibit statistical connections between several points in space-time; for example, source activity at one cortical location at one time may be highly correlated to activity at another location at some later time because of the delay inherent in signal propagation. Examples of this are provided in Chapter 7. Or, activity at two locations may be highly correlated (i.e., high coherency) only over a narrow frequency band. Ex-

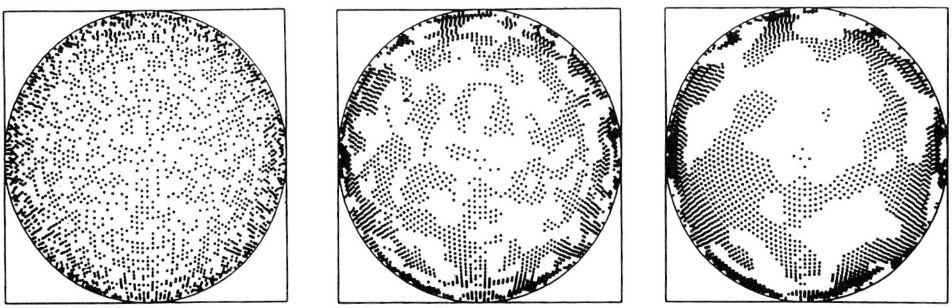

Figure 1-12. A simple simulation of cortical source dynamics at the macrocolumn scale based on (1.10). Each of the 4200 macrocolumns on the surface of the sphere contributes a source $P_{i,k}$, where the index i denotes source location and k is the iteration number. In the far left plot ($k = 0$), sources were determined by a random number generator. Substantial clumping occurred in the middle plot ($k = 3$) due to the dynamic rule (1.10), and still more clumping (long effective correlation length) occurred after $k = 9$ iterations, as shown in the far right plot. (Reproduced with permission from Nunez et al, 1991, which also shows corresponding scalp potentials and Laplacians.)

amples of the later case are shown for alpha rhythm in Figure 1-7 and in Chapter 3. Of course, space-time statistical correlations in complex systems can generally be expected to be more subtle and complex than these simple examples.

To convey visually some of the general properties that may characterize a stochastic neocortical field, we return to our model cortex containing approximately 10^4 macrocolumns, as indicated in Figure 1-12. We imagine some rule that governs the evolution of spatial pattern with time. In this example, the magnitude of each macrosource $P_{i,k}$ at some particular "time" (that is iteration number k) is assumed to be a linear combination of its own source magnitude plus that of its eight nearest neighbors at an earlier time. That is

$$P_{i,k} = AP_{i,k-1} + B \sum_{j \neq i} P_{j,k-1} \tag{1.10}$$

where the sum is over the eight nearest neighbors in the grid. The constant parameters A and B may be normalized such that $A + 8B = 1$ to indicate the relative contributions of surrounding sources at earlier times $(k - 1)$ to source i at time k. As the magnitude of B increases relative to A, macrosources evolve more rapidly into clumps (that is, in fewer iterations).

The initial field $P_{i,k}$ in Figure 1-12 is chosen by a random-number generator. At each successive iteration k, the macrosources become more clumped as a result of the successive operation of the simple rule (1.10). This example does not constitute a theory; rather it is essentially a computer game with minimal connection to real physiology and anatomy. However macrocolumns do interact through intracortical connections partly to their nearest neighbors. They also interact through corticocortical fibers (most of the subcortical white matter in humans) to more distant macrocolumns, but this effect is neglected in Figure 1-12. Furthermore a possibly similar clumping effect has been observed in rabbit neocortex during epileptic seizure (Petsche et al, 1984; Petsche, 1992).

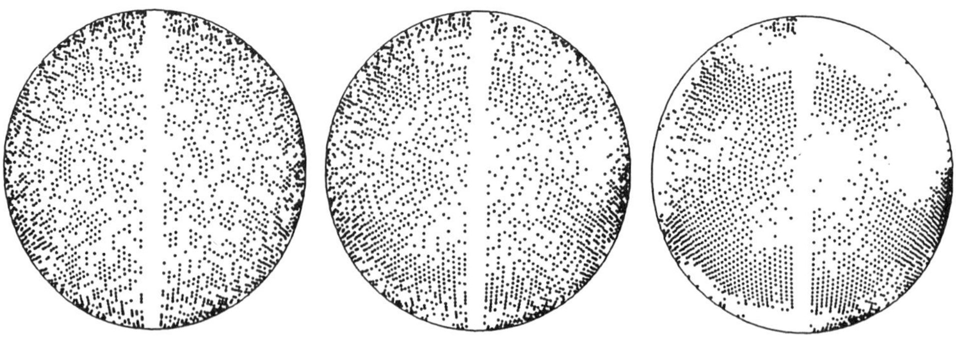

Figure 1-13. A simple simulation similar to that shown in Figure 1-12, except this one includes inhibitory feedback as described by (1.11): far right plot ($k = 0$), middle plot ($k = 3$), far left plot ($k = 5$).

A more complicated algorithm is used to govern the evolution of the field $P_{i,k}$ shown in Figure 1-13. In this instance, sources evolve according to

$$P_{i,k} = AP_{i,k-1} - B \sum_{j \neq i} P_{j,k-1} + C \sum_{j \neq i}{}' P_{j,k-1} \tag{1.11}$$

where the parameters A, B, and C are all positive. The first sum is over all sources located within 5 mm of the i th source, simulating relatively short-range negative feedback. The second sum is over all sources within the radial zone between 5 and 10 mm, simulating positive feedback from more distant sources. For this rule to be more similar to real anatomy and physiology, we would evidently like the range of inhibitory feedback to be shorter by two orders of magnitude (see Table 2-2). However this change would require a large increase in the number of sources in simulations with an enormous increase in required computer time. Alternatively, one could simulate the dynamics in a much smaller region of neocortex. However, in this case, the effects of long-range interactions would be neglected. Possible ways to avoid the complications inherent in systems for which interactions between the basic fundamental units occur at multiple spatial scales are considered in Chapters 2, 10, 11, and 14. More realistic rules for dynamic interaction should include dense connections to homologous regions of opposite cortex and intracortical connection densities that decrease according to

$$B_{ij} \sim e^{-\lambda r_{ij}} \tag{1.12}$$

These particular spatial patterns are shown in part to illustrate the general concept of a stochastic field but also because they appear to have analogous neocortical counterparts. That is, states of minimal cognitive processing such as deep sleep, coma, and anesthesia appear to occur primarily with spatially coherent scalp EEG, apparently more similar to the more clumped patterns of Figures 1-12 and 1-13. Of course, the simple rules of macrocolumn interaction used in these simulations allow patterns to progress only in one general direction, from random fields to more clumped or correlated spatial patterns of macrosources (that is, correlated, dipole layers). However more realistic models (such as those used in neural network studies) allow dynamic changes in either direction. Furthermore the effects of several kinds of subcortical input may be included. These features allow for more complex and realistic theories of neocortical dynamics, as discussed in later chapters.

Quantitative Characterization of Spatial–Temporal Patterns

Spontaneous EEG rhythms are typically displayed by raw traces of amplitude as a function of time. Most clinical electroencephalographers are trained to look only at these time histories, which may involve flipping through many pages of EEG record in each patient. Abnormal EEGs are then discovered through partly subjective pattern recognition methods by the clinician's brain. Like most of medicine, this process involves a combination of art and science. In some research and clinical settings, such methods have been replaced in part by spectral analyses of individual EEG channels to obtain data compression and quantification. Evoked potentials have been characterized primarily by the latency of peaks in the averaged waveform from the stimulus onset. There are, of course, many other ways in which time history can be characterized. Some of these are described in later chapters.

A stochastic field is a function of time and spatial variables. Because quantification of spatial patterns of EEG has received only minimal attention and spatial patterns appear to be correlated to physiologic state, spatial properties are emphasized in this section. The spatial patterns shown here can be thought of as either patterns at fixed instants in time or patterns at fixed frequency (that is characteristic EEG patterns of signals of duration typically lasting a few seconds to a few minutes that have been Fourier transformed in time). When characteristic spatial patterns in a system tend to be associated with specific temporal frequencies, they are called the "eigenfunctions" of the system, a term usually associated with standing wave phenomena. Possible eigenfunctions of spontaneous EEG are shown in Chapter 3. Similar patterns of steady-state evoked potentials are shown in Chapter 6.

With this background, we can, for example, focus on either of the stochastic field variables $\mathbf{P}(\mathbf{r}, t)$ or $\mathbf{P}(\mathbf{r}, \omega)$, corresponding to either of the cases above, representing the dipole moment per unit volume (polarization) at the macrocolumn scale (macrosources). For simplicity, the component of $\mathbf{P}$ perpendicular to the cortical surface may be followed and the time or frequency independent variable of this field can be suppressed with the understanding that the description may apply to either of the two cases above. Furthermore, we will at first apply the description to a two-dimensional medium with surface coordinates x and y, an approach that is accurate when relatively small regions of cortical surface are discussed. Later the treatment can be extended to spherical coordinates to account, in an approximate manner, for the closed cortical surface. With these caveats, we then follow the stochastic field $P(x, y)$.

If important statistical properties of $P(x, y)$ are constant over some surface area, the stochastic field is said to be homogeneous over this area. Homogeneity is the spatial analog of stationarity in the time domain. In practice, we cannot estimate all statistical properties, so the concepts of homogeneity and stationarity can only apply to small (but typically important) subsets of variables. In particular, if the average value of some measured time series P and its autocorrelation function do not vary substantially during some period T, P is said to constitute a stationary sample record. Similarly, if the average measured value of P and its spatial correlation function do not vary substantially over the area, P may constitute an approximately homogeneous sample field (Bendat and Piersol, 1986). The concept of isotropy differs from that of homogeneity; that is, an isotropic stochastic field $P(x, y)$ is one in which statistical properties do not depend on the directions x and y; it has no physical analog in the time domain.

Each field variable has its own statistical properties. For example, the macrosources $P(x, y)$ are independent of volume conductor properties. However scalp potential depends on both the macrosources and volume conductor. Thus, for example, a homogeneous, isotropic stochastic field of macrosources may produce an inhomogeneous, anisotropic stochastic field of scalp potential. We will return to this issue later. In addition, the usual definitions of stationarity and homogeneity involve ensemble averages of sample functions of the stochastic process rather than time and space averages. The statistical property that allows these two basic operations to be equated is ergodicity. However, we leave this and several related theoretical issues to the references because we must address so many more immediate operational issues in neocortical applications.

The concepts of homogeneity and isotropy can be applied to neocortex only with great care. For example, neocortex shows a gross anatomic homogeneity and isotropy in directions parallel to its surface. By contrast, neocortex is easily distinguished in perpendicular directions by distinct layers. There we use these concepts to describe anatomic statistics such as number densities of specific kinds of neurons, synapses, and so on, variables that may also be considered as stochastic fields. This type of quantitative information is limited, but tangential homogeneity and isotropy seem to apply to first approximation, at least at large scales. Important differences occur between some cytoarchitectonic areas of cortex defined by anatomic structure as revealed by several staining techniques (see Figures 1-14 and 2-17). In primary sensory cortex, these anatomic borders coincide with known function, such as visual, auditory, motor, and so on (Jones, 1987). Otherwise their functional importance is unknown.

Gross anatomic homogeneity and isotropy do not, of course, imply that these characteristics are shared by macrosources P(x, y). First, each cortical macrocolumn can be expected to receive continuous input from midbrain structures. Second, each macrocolumn is interconnected to a considerable fraction of all 10^4 cortical macrocolumns by corticocortical (that is, association) fibers. No data strongly suggest that these connections are homogeneous and isotropic, although it is useful to at least assume homogeneity at large scales in approximate theoretical models. This issue is addressed in the context of the global EEG theory in Chapter 11.

One important way to characterize a stochastic field P(x, y) is by its spectral density function $G(k_x, k_y)$, where k_x and k_y are wave numbers (that is, spatial frequencies) in the x and y directions, respectively. The application of spatial spectra to neocortex is valuable because the scalp acts as a low-pass spatial filter and because there are natural connections to theoretical models of neocortical dynamics. The spectral density function or "spatial power spectrum" is the square of the two-dimensional, spatial Fourier transform, defined mathematically by (9.22). Consider, for example, the two-dimensional grids and corresponding spectral density function shown in Figure 1-15. The spectral density function is sharply peaked at the spatial frequencies corresponding to spatial patterns given by

$$P(x, y) \sim \sin k_x x \sin k_y y + \text{small amount of noise} \tag{1.13}$$

Without the addition of noise to (1.13), the peak in Figure 1-15 has zero width.

Let us imagine a patch of neocortex, as in Figure 1-16. For this general discussion, it is not important whether the cortical patch lies in a plane or partly in

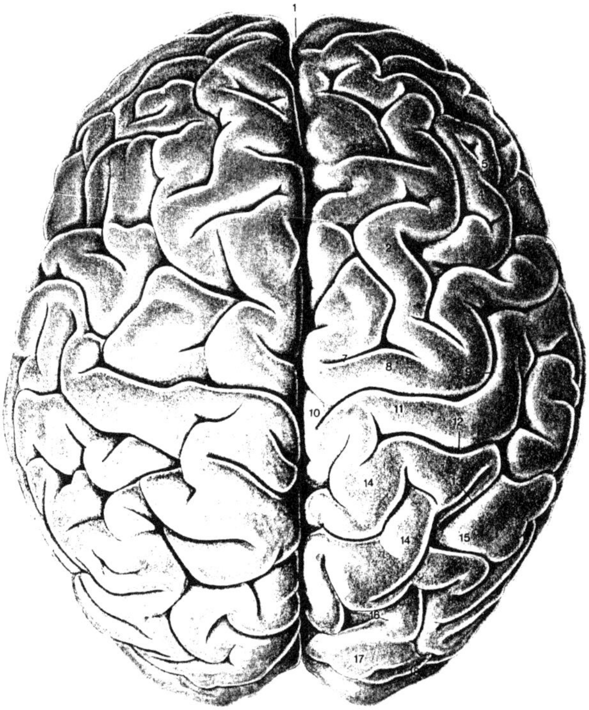
1
5
6
2
7
8
9
10
11
12
14
14
15
16
17

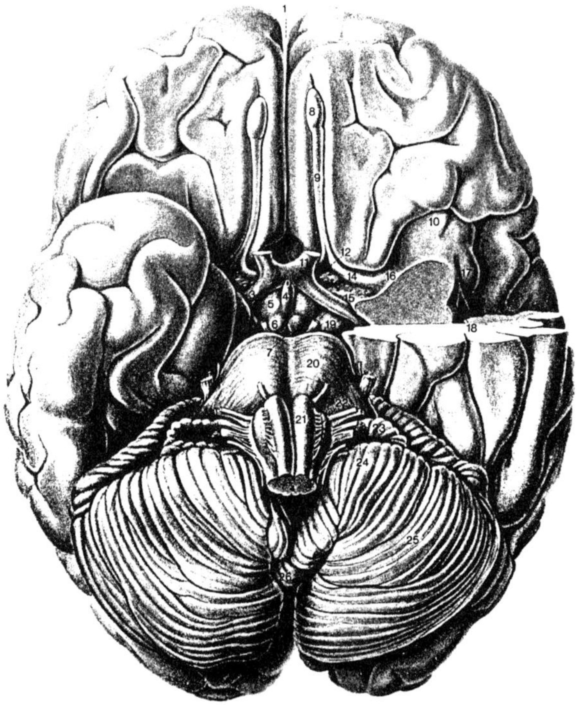
1
8
9
10
12
14
16
17
15
5
4
6
19
18
7
20
21
23
24
25

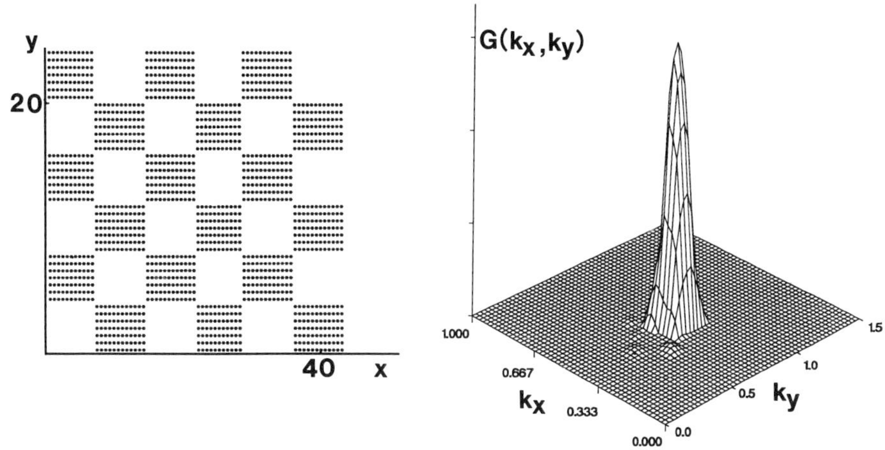

Figure 1-15. Sinusoidal spatial pattern (left side) given by (1.13) and corresponding spatial spectra $G(k_x, k_y)$ on the right. Spatial wavelengths $= 2\pi/k$ in the x and y directions. Thus spectral peak occurs at spatial frequencies $k_x = 2\pi/15$, $k_y = 2\pi/8$. The broadening of the spectral peak occurred because of the addition of noise to the spatial pattern. If x and y are measured in centimeters, the units of k_x are cm^{-1}. Spatial frequencies in cycles/cm are obtained by dividing k_x and k_y by the factor 2π.

fissures or sulci. In the later case, the x and y coordinates follow the cortical surface. The cortical patch shown in Figure 1-17 consists of a grid of 70×42 points. Thus, if we choose the large cortical patch of Figure 1-16, each grid point is the size of a macrocolumn. Alternately the grids might represent a patch of 2 $\times$ 1.2 mm, in which grid points are the size of minicolumns. Minicolumns are defined by the spatial extent of inhibitory connections (2 to 5×10^{-2} mm); they contain approximately 100 neurons. These general ideas also apply to other spatial scales.

The sources $\Delta\Phi$ in Figures 1-17 and 1-18 are distributed between -200 μV and $+200$ μV, with root-mean-square source potentials fixed at 116 μV. This is the same general range of transcortical potentials of spontaneous EEG recorded using intracortical "micro-EEG" electrodes (Lopes da Silva and Storm van Leeuwen, 1978). In Figure 1-17, the number of positive macrocolumn sources (filled spaces) is close to the number of negative sources (empty spaces). By contrast, the percentage of positive sources is progressively higher in parts A and B of Figure 1-18. The predicted surface potentials of Figure 1-18 are in the general

←

Figure 1-14. The human brain as seen from above and below. The upper end of the brainstem, hemispheres of the cerebellum, and underside of the cerebrum are shown in the lower figure. Each hemisphere of the cerebrum is covered by the cerebral cortex. (Reproduced with permission from R. Nieuwenhuys, J. Voogd, and C. van Huijzen. *The Human Central Nervous System*, second revised edition, Berlin: Springer-Verlag, 1981.)

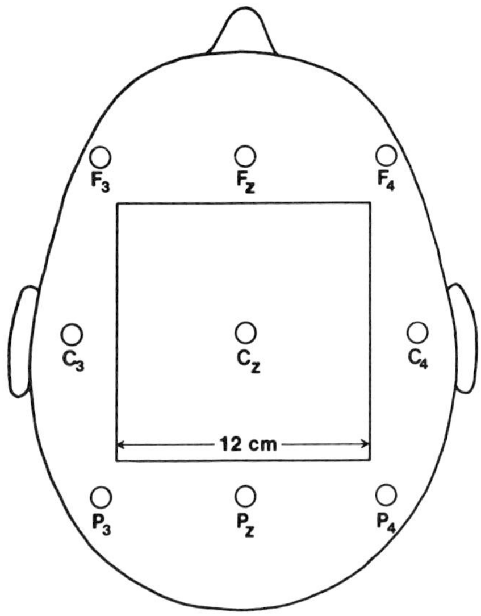

Figure 1-16. Square indicating assumed region of active cortex for several computer simulations using the three concentric sphere model. Refer also to Figures 1-17 and 1-18.

range of scalp-recorded spontaneous EEG in humans. These simulations assume that all sources outside the boxed region of Figure 1-16 are zero. However the potential contours of Figures 1-17 and 1-18 remain unaltered if the entire cortex outside the boxed region produces random sources similar to those shown in Figure 1-18A. Each pattern shown might represent a fixed instant in time. Alternatively the spatial patterns might refer to a narrow frequency range, obtained from perhaps several minutes of EEG data.

The patterns of Figures 1-17 and 1-18 show different degrees of "clumpiness." Clumped patterns are, of course, reflected by spatial patterns with more relative power at low spatial frequencies. The more random spatial patterns cause random or noisy spectral density functions. Band-limited white noise may be defined spatially in a manner analogous to noise in the time domain, such as when $G(k_x, k_y)$ is relatively constant up to maximum cut-off spatial frequencies in each of the x and y directions.

To help imagine spectral density functions, consider a familiar physical phenomena, ocean waves. A typical spectral density function for ocean wave height might look something like Figure 1-19 (Bascom, 1964), indicating that energy in ocean waves is distributed over several kinds of waves, each with a characteristic range of spatial wavelength (or wave number k). With an isotropic ocean wave field, energy can be expressed in terms of wave number magnitude $k = (k_x^2 + k_y^2)^{1/2}$ rather than its separate x and y components. Because the ocean surface is composed of waves, rather than some more general spatial–temporal field, spatial and temporal properties are not independent; rather they are related through a dispersion relation. The rules governing water dynamics force wave frequency to obey the dispersion relation,

$$\omega = k(g/k + bk)^{1/2} \tanh(kh) \tag{1.14}$$

where g is the acceleration of gravity, b is a parameter proportional to surface

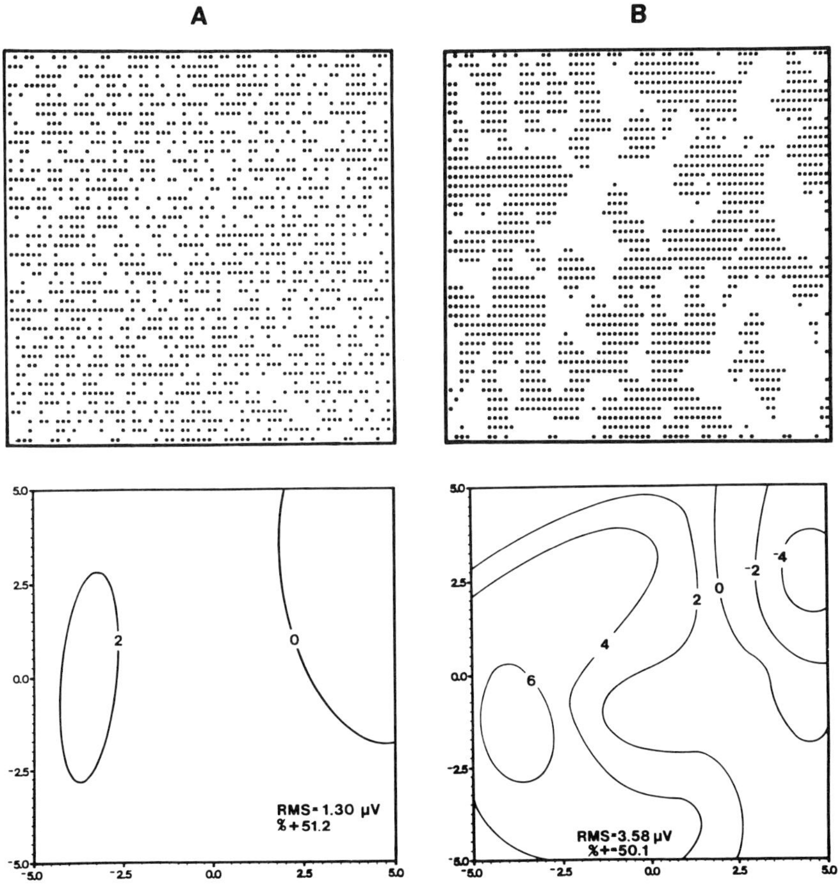

Figure 1-17. Assumed distribution of neocortical macrosource activity ΔΦ (Figure 1-11) in columns of area 3.5 mm^2 (*upper row*) and corresponding theoretical scalp potential distribution (*lower row*) over the same total area indicated by Figure 1-16. Surface potentials at 121 locations were calculated using the three-concentric sphere model with an assumed skull-to-brain resistivity ratio of 80. The contour plots of scalp potential were obtained from the 121 discrete scalp potentials; each value of scalp potential was then due to 2940 cortical sources. Plots were constructed using a spline interpolation. All contour labels are microvolts. The sources ΔΦ were assumed to be distributed between −200 μV and +200 μV, with root-square-mean source potentials held fixed at 116 μV. A filled space indicates a positive potential (surface with respect to depth), whereas an empty space represents a negative potential. The percentages of positive sources are indicated in the lower row and remain close to 50% for both source distributions. In **A**, the sources are completely random (between −200 μV and +200 μV). The resulting root-mean-square scalp potential of the 121 scalp surface locations is 1.30 μV. In **B**, the sources are determined by both random input and the magnitudes of the eight nearest-neighbor sources so that the effective correlation length of macrosources increases from 1 grid space in A to 8 grid spaces in B, with corresponding increases in predicted root-mean-square scalp potentials. (Reproduced with permission from Nunez, 1990a.)

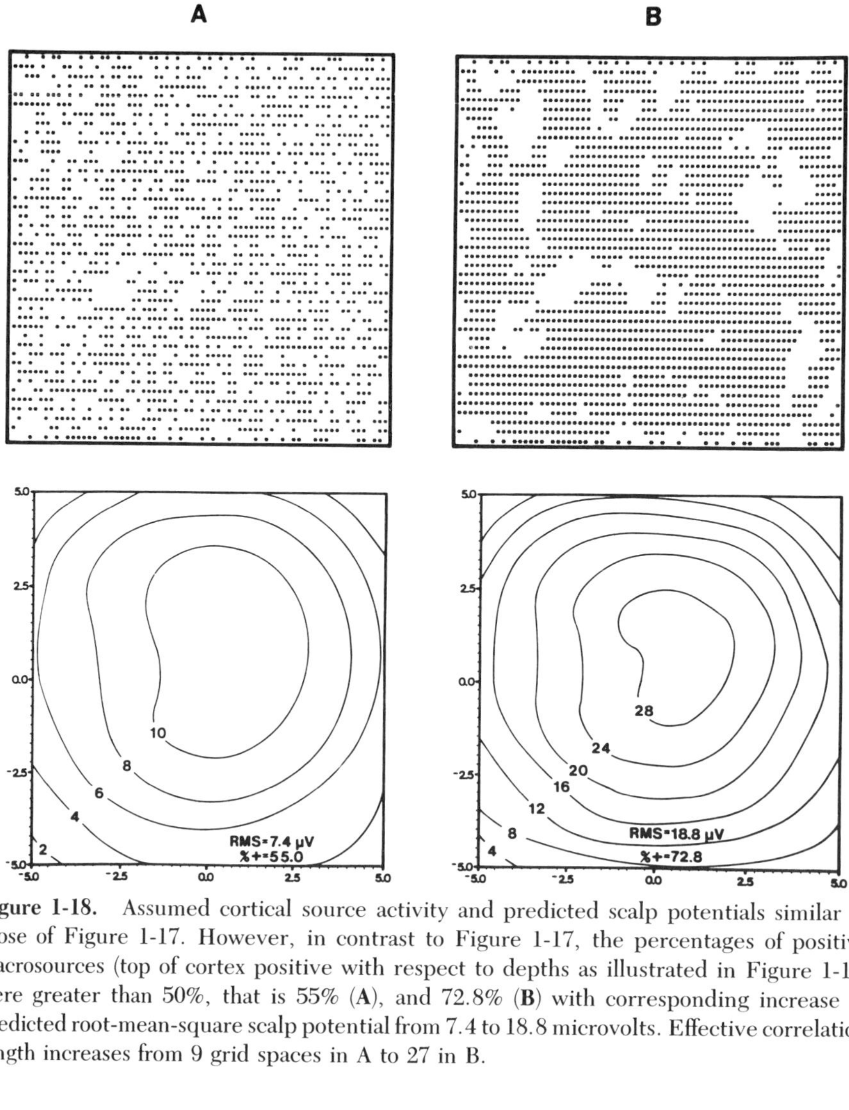

Figure 1-18. Assumed cortical source activity and predicted scalp potentials similar to those of Figure 1-17. However, in contrast to Figure 1-17, the percentages of positive macrosources (top of cortex positive with respect to depths as illustrated in Figure 1-11) were greater than 50%, that is 55% (**A**), and 72.8% (**B**) with corresponding increase in predicted root-mean-square scalp potential from 7.4 to 18.8 microvolts. Effective correlation length increases from 9 grid spaces in A to 27 in B.

tension, and h is ocean depth. Thus (1.14) shows that ocean waves with long wavelengths (small k) are dominated by gravitational forces, whereas ripples are governed mainly by surface tension. Knowledge of a wave's spatial wavelength ($2\pi/k$) implies knowledge of its period ($2\pi/\omega$).

The ocean wave metaphor has some advantages in addition to being easy to visualize. We can illustrate several fairly general properties of linear waves with a simple water wave example. Suppose someone dives into the ocean. There is a region close to the entry point of the diver called the near field, where surface disturbance depends strongly on details such as the diver's speed, angle, arm extension, and so forth. This disturbance is not a wave, but rather a more general

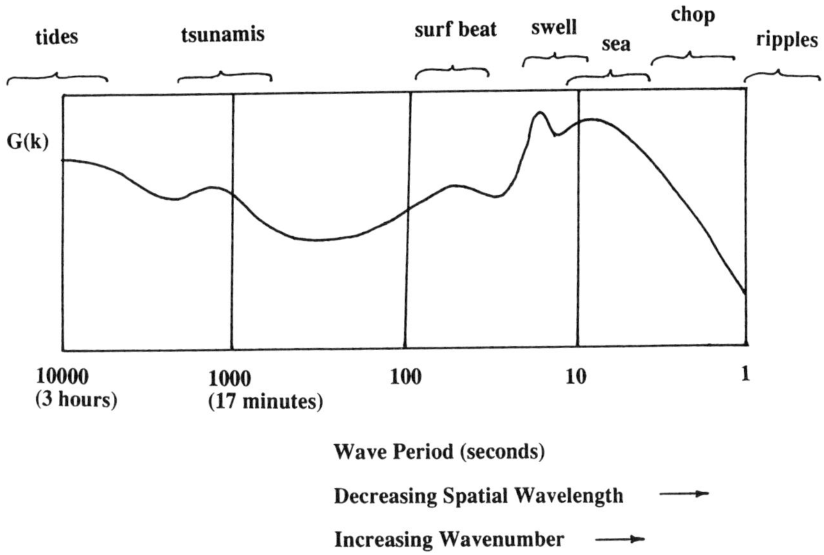

Figure 1-19. An estimate of the ocean wave spectral density function G(k), expressed in terms of wave period = $2\pi/\omega(k)$, where $\omega(k)$ is given by the dispersion relation (1.14). (Modified with permission from W. Munk in Bascom, 1964.)

spatial–temporal pattern. However, as the disturbance moves out from the entry point, the nonwave parts of the disturbance are removed according to the rules of water dynamics, leaving only the wave packet. The region located somewhat away from the entry point is called the far field or wave field, in which the wave packet (composed of a mixture of waves with different wavelengths) travels with group velocity characteristic of the water medium. The same general ideas and terminology apply to other waves, such as electromagnetic waves generated by a transmitter.

Consider the case of a water wave packet, produced by a diver, consisting of a mixture of waves of different wavelengths but distributed over a narrow wave number range near k_0 (Jackson, 1975). The details of the diver's entry into the water determine the actual wave number distribution and its peak near k_0. However, once this disturbance is forced on the water, the wave packet travels in a radial direction away from the central disturbance with the group velocity $d\omega/dk$, which may be obtained as the first derivative of (1.14). With relatively long wavelengths ($k^2 << g/b$) and deep water ($kh >> 1$), the dispersion relation (1.14) reduces to

$$\omega \sim (gk)^{1/2} \tag{1.15}$$

Group (v_G) and phase (v_p) velocities are defined by

$$v_G = d\omega/dk = 1/2(g/k)^{1/2} \tag{1.16}$$

$$v_p = \omega/k = (g/k)^{1/2} \tag{1.17}$$

so that water wave group velocity is about one half of phase velocity, in this limiting case. Phase velocity is the velocity of a single wave component; group velocity is the net velocity of a mixture of wave components. This mixture of wave components forms the wave pulse, which is a disturbance of the medium with finite spatial extent which propagates at the group velocity.

By contrast to water waves, waves with dispersion relation

$$\omega = ck \tag{1.18}$$

are called nondispersive. These are the usual low-amplitude sound waves, electromagnetic radiation in a vacuum, waves in a linear stretched string, and so on. Nondispersive waves have phase and group velocities equal to c, for example, the velocity of light, sound, string deflection, and so on. A wave packet (pulse) of particular shape and spatial extent will propagate undistorted through the medium. By contrast, in a dispersive medium (water, for example), (1.18) does not hold. In this case, different components of the wave packet travel with different speeds and tend to change phase with respect to one another. This leads to a change of shape of the wave packet as it travels, hence the name "dispersion relation," which applies to different kinds of physical and putative brain waves (1.14), (1.15), (1.18), (2.3), (2.10), (9.8), (9.9), (9.53), (9.57), (11.10), (11.14), (11.27), (11.33), (11.47), (14.42). In the example of water waves satisfying (1.15), new wave components form continually at the rear of the advancing wave packet, pass through it, and disappear from the front, as required by the fact that phase velocity is twice that of group velocity. By contrast, the very short waves, for example ripples with $k^2 >> g/b$ in (1.14), have phase velocity that is only about two thirds that of group velocity. In Chapters 11 and 12, certain kinds of putative macroscopic brain waves are described that have group velocity greater than phase velocity.

Despite the variety of behavior possible because of different dispersion relations and different boundary and initial conditions, the deep water waves discussed in this section are linear. As a consequence, two waves can pass through each other with undistorted waveform. For example, several speakers together in a room can talk at the same time without one speaker's sound waves distorting another's waves. Intersecting waves produce linear interference patterns, which disappear after wave packets have completely passed through each other. Waves that are nonlinear but still sufficiently close to linear (that is, quasilinear) are expected to have qualitatively similar behavior, but with distortion. Strongly nonlinear waves (shock waves, action potentials, solitons, for example) involve entirely new phenomena, as discussed in Chapters 10, 11, 12, and 14.

Because a relatively simple relation exists between spatial and temporal frequencies of ocean waves does not imply that the resulting wave field is simple. As Bascom (1964) described it,

> The simultaneous existence of so many kinds and sizes of waves on the surface of the ocean, coming from different sources, moving in many directions, and changing inexplicably from day to day made it difficult for man to learn the ways of waves.

This description could easily apply to many other phenomena, such as electromagnetic or sound waves in the environment or possibly brain waves. The complications of different wave types, directions of travel, and dispersion can apply to both linear and nonlinear waves.

For the analogy between ocean waves and spatial–temporal fluctuations of electric potential on the cortical surface to be plausible, we must imagine a magic ocean that can dramatically change its physical properties, perhaps because of pressure or temperature changes. Although earth's oceans normally do not behave this way, other media, such as plasmas, spin glasses, and magnetic material, can undergo dramatic change of properties (called phase changes in physics), but such phenomena are not as easily visualized, and thus the ocean wave analogy has some limited use. We can imagine the normal ocean as a limiting case of a more general medium, the magic ocean, which would not necessarily support the simple wave phenomena of normal oceans. For example, phase changes in the magic ocean generally lead to new dispersion relations replacing (1.14), or much more general spatial–temporal properties of surface motion in which no dispersion relation exists. Extreme changes in the behavior of dynamic systems which occur as a result of changes in external control mechanisms are termed "bifurcations" in modern dynamic systems theory. The potential complexity of this magic ocean can be appreciated in part by visualizing the turbulent, nonlinear behavior of breakers in the shallow water near a beach. These turbulent phenomena are not waves in the scientific sense. Thus we see that waves, that is, phenomena with dispersion relations, are special cases of stochastic fields. In this context, changes in ocean properties may be analogous to changes in the brain's physiologic state. Chapters 3, 11, and 14 examine the idea that neocortical dispersion relations (that is, relatively simple wave phenomena) may occur as limiting cases of much more complex phenomena in certain physiologic states.

Closely related to the spectral density function is the spatial correlation function, analogous to the autocorrelation function in time series analysis. If P(x, y) is a homogeneous, isotropic field, the spatial correlation function can be defined in terms of a single variable (Katznelson, 1982). The spatial correlation function R(r), in this idealized case, yields a measure of how closely grid points separated by a distance r are related, independent of direction. When spatial patterns are even more idealized so that the correlation function assumes a particular, simple form, a correlation length may be defined. However the usual definition of correlation length is apparently not precise in neocortical applications because the idealizations involved may be physiologically unrealistic. However we may define an effective correlation length applicable to any discrete spatial pattern. The effective correlation length for a random pattern is of the order of one grid spacing, whereas the effective correlation length for a highly clumped pattern is approximately the diameter of a typical clump, as illustrated in Figures 17 and 18.

A discrete spatial pattern **P**(x, y) is precisely defined by its value at every grid point, and the introduction of global concepts such as correlation length are simply attempts to obtain general descriptors to help classify complex patterns, much in the manner that we might try to verbalize a human face, for example. These ideas of pattern also extend naturally into the spatial–temporal domain. For example, spatial patterns that have long effective correlation lengths at fixed instants in time tend to produce large correlation function coefficients in an EEG record between pairs of locations at zero or small lag times. Correlated spatial patterns associated with a narrow frequency band (that is, after Fourier transform in time) tend to exhibit large coherency in this frequency band between pairs of locations separated by distances less than the effective correlation length. Distant regions of the cortex are often strongly connected by corticocortical or callosal fibers, the latter connecting the two cortical hemispheres. For example, homologous locations of the brain hemispheres tend to be densely connected. In such cases, the correlation function or coherency of **P**(x, y) should not necessarily be expected to decrease regularly with distance. In fact, EEG coherency may be larger at specific distant locations than at close locations, as shown in Chapter 3. In such cases, effective correlation length may not be a useful concept.

Another way to represent the spatial–temporal properties of a dynamic pattern of sources is by the probability density function f(**r**, **P**, t), defined such that f is proportional to the probability that a neural mass at location **r** will have polarization **P** at time t, due to sources at some smaller scale. The probability density function can be defined at the macrocolumn scale, in which case **r** represents two surface coordinates. When using "location **r**," we mean the center of a macrocolumn in this case; **P** refers to an average over the sources of the macrocolumn. Alternately f can be defined at smaller scales, for example 0.1 mm^3, a volume containing approximately 10^5 synapses whose microsources collectively produce polarization **P**(x, y, z, t) of elemental volumes at this scale.

This kind of probability density function is a central concept in plasma physics, in which case f(**r**, **v**, t) is proportional to the number of charged particles at location **r** that also have velocities **v** at time t. Of course, other quantitative measures (probability density of neural firings, for example) may be more convenient in theoretical descriptions, but measured EEG fields are directly connected to **P** or f. The connection between probability of neural firings and EEG may not be obvious, although modulation of these variables may be similar. Application of modern statistical methods to neocortex is described in detail in Chapter 14.

Relation of Macrosources to Surface Potentials

Surface potentials Φ(**r**, t) are related to macrocolumn sources **P**(**r**, t) through (1.2) and the macroscopic version of Poisson's equation (1.3), but with sources, potential, and conductivity defined at the macrocolumn scale. The references can provide mathematical details of volume condition (Kavanagh et al, 1978; Nunez, 1981, 1987; Rush and Driscoll, 1968, 1969), but note that the volume conductor (brain, cerebrospinal fluid, skull, and scalp) provides a spatial weighting function relating

P and Φ (Katznelson, 1982), as depicted by the following integral over the cortical surface S:

$$\Phi(\mathbf{r}, t) = \int_S \mathbf{W}(\mathbf{r}, \mathbf{r}') \cdot \mathbf{P}(\mathbf{r}', t)\, d^2\mathbf{r}' \tag{1.19}$$

where $\mathbf{W}(\mathbf{r}, \mathbf{r}')$ is the weighting function that depends on the locations $\mathbf{r}'$ of macrosources and scalp surface location $\mathbf{r}$ and the conductivities and boundaries of various tissues. In the idealized case of a volume conductor composed of spherically symmetric layers of homogeneous, isotropic tissue and sources at equal depths, $\mathbf{W} = \mathbf{W}(|\mathbf{r} - \mathbf{r}'|)$, that is, the weighting function depends only on the distances between macrosources and scalp location. The spatial Fourier transform of the weighting function is, in this case, simply the spatial transfer function of the volume conductor. When subcortical sources contribute substantially to surface potentials, (1.19) must be replaced by a volume integral over the whole brain.

Two qualitative effects of the head volume conductor are well understood. The first is that cortical source effects tend to be "smeared" (that is, space averaged) between cortex and scalp, which is caused mainly by the separation between sources and scalp electrodes and by the poorly conducting skull (Cooper et al, 1965; DeLucchi et al, 1975). The second is that the transfer of signal through tissue is independent of frequency in the range of spontaneous EEG (Plonsey, 1969; Nunez, 1981). Thus, if a dipole is implanted in the cortex and the frequency of oscillation of the current source varied, both the amplitude and spatial distribution of scalp potential are, to excellent approximation, unchanged (Cooper et al, 1965; Nunez, 1981).

The smearing effect of the head volume conductor can be described in a quantitative manner in several ways. Consider, for example, a dipole layer of constant polarization $P_{\tilde{z}}$ over its surface. This may be modeled by a spherical cap of sources occupying the inner surface of the three-sphere volume conductor model of the head, as shown in Figure 1-20. The potential due to this dipole layer is calculated on the inner (cortex) and outer (scalp) surfaces over the center of the dipole layer. The potential ratio is plotted in Figure 1-20 for three skull resistivities that appear to bracket the realistic range. The resulting plots are consistent with the following observations of spontaneous EEG, which have been well known to electroencephalographers for several decades:

1. root-mean-square amplitudes of spontaneous EEG recorded from the cortex are typically two to five times the amplitude of simultaneously recorded scalp potentials (Penfield and Jasper, 1954; Cooper et al, 1965; Nunez, 1981).
2. At least several square centimeters of cortical surface must be "synchronously active" (that is, roughly in phase) for the same potentials to be recorded on the scalp without averaging (Cooper et al, 1965; DeLucchi et al, 1975).
3. The amplitudes of alpha and sleep rhythm potentials recorded from several centimeters deep within the brain are of magnitudes similar to that of potentials recorded on the cortical surface (Sem-Jacobsen et al, 1953).

These experimental observations and the theoretical predictions summarized

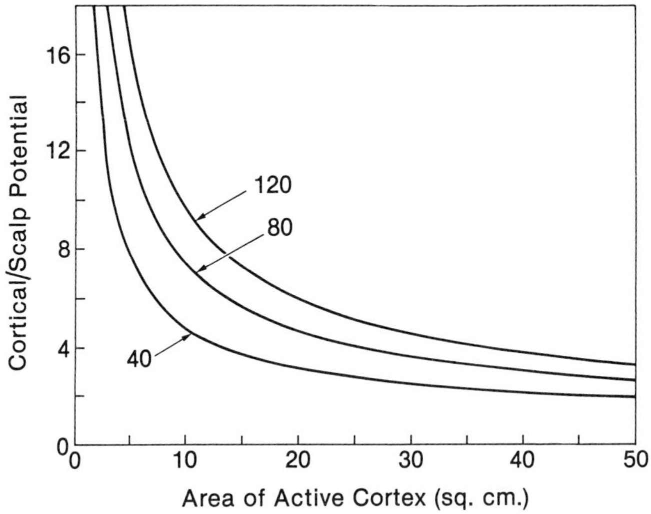

Figure 1-20. Theoretical ratio of cortical-to-scalp potential when a dipole layer formed a spherical cap of depth 1.4 cm below outer sphere of radius of 9 cm. Scalp potential was calculated over the center of the cortical dipole layer. Potential difference across the dipole was assumed to be fixed (similar to Figure 1-18B, with all grid locations filled). Three curves correspond to different ratios of skull-to-brain resistivity. Potentials were calculated with respect to infinity, but ratios shown are qualitatively correct for comparison with either bipolar or reference recordings. The single dipole source is equivalent to a small active surface area, with cortical-to-scalp potential ratio of more than 200. (Reproduced with permission from Nunez, 1990a.)

here are self-consistent if spontaneous EEG is viewed as originating in large neocortical dipole layers (perhaps hundreds of square centimeters) with sources showing relatively long effective correlation lengths to produce cortical potentials of relatively large magnitude. By contrast, some epileptic spikes and evoked potentials (over some latency ranges) apparently can be pictured as due to just a few localized dipole sources.

These general ideas are also supported by an analysis performed by Katznelson (1982), who developed an equation for the root-mean-square amplitude of surface potential in terms of three variables: the magnitude of cortical sources (1.4), the average depth of sources, and the correlation length of the dipole layer. Although this study was very approximate because both an infinite, homogeneous medium and dipole layer sources represented by a single correlation length were assumed, it provides a rough idea of the effect of correlation length on surface magnitudes. When source magnitudes due to direct stimulation of nerve tracts or epilepsy are used in the formula (for example, in Table 1-2), Katznelson's analysis predicts sources of correlation length short compared with depth beneath the scalp (approximately 1 cm). However, when source strengths based on spontaneous EEG are used, predicted correlation lengths are long compared with depth (Nunez, 1986). This later result can be anticipated by the simulations shown in Figures 1-17 and 1-18.

The three-sphere model of the head can also be used to obtain a rough estimate of head transmission dependence of potentials between cortex and scalp on wave number (that is, spatial frequency). For the practical wave number range of $0.1 < k < 1.0\ cm^{-1}$, corresponding to spatial wavelengths of 62 to 6 cm, the three-sphere model predicts a ratio of scalp to cortical spectral power of

$$G_s(k)/G_c(k) \sim k^{-\delta} \qquad (1.20)$$

where the exponent δ is obtained by fitting the actual solution (expressed as an infinite series of Legendre polynomials) to (1.20) for simplicity of presentation (Nunez and Srinivasan, 1993). The exponent $\delta = 2.5 \pm 0.3$ fits the solution for the skull to brain resistivity range of 40 to 160, the range also used in the calculations of Figure 1-20.

Bipolar recordings using close electrodes provide a higher pass spatial filter than is obtained with reference recordings. This method counteracts part of the smearing of cortical potentials, thereby providing a simple and often effective recording strategy. Refer, for example, to Figure 2-14.

A direct experimental check of (1.20) is not available because we know of no data published on the human cortical spectrum $G_c(k)$. However several estimates of the scalp spectrum $G_s(k)$ of spontaneous EEG and evoked potentials have been obtained. The scalp spectral density function for spontaneous EEG has been estimated using a circular array around the circumference of the head to obtain more accurate estimates at long wavelengths (Shaw, 1991). The spatial spectrum was fitted to the function

$$G_s(k) \sim k^{-\alpha} \qquad (1.21)$$

where $\alpha \sim 3.0$ (resting, eyes closed; that is alpha rhythm) and $\alpha \sim 2.3$ (eyes open, fixed position). Comparison of (1.20) and (1.21) suggests that eyes-open spontaneous EEG in the cortex may not be much different from spatial white noise over the wave number range $0.1 < k < 1.0$ because the scalp power decrease with wave number can be explained adequately by volume conductive effects alone. In contrast, the alpha rhythm spectral density function (over a broad temporal frequency range) would decrease more rapidly with increasing wave number. A study of wave number spectra of the visual evoked potential (Gevins, 1990) estimated the decrease of power with wave number in the range of $0.5 < k < 2.8$ for the N170 and P350 peaks. When these data are fit to (1.21), a rough estimate of $\alpha \sim 3$ is also obtained.

These estimates apply to a broad band of temporal frequencies. By contrast, estimates of frequency–wave number spectra (the spectral density function) have been obtained with 0.5 Hz resolution, as shown in Figure 1-21, with spontaneous EEG data recorded using a two-dimensional electrode array over one hemisphere (Nunez, 1981, 1988a). Because of the poor resolution at long and short wavelengths, it is not possible to obtain accurate estimates of the exponent α from these data. However, when these data were fit to (1.21), exponents were found to be in the approximate range $\alpha \sim 3$ to 5 for $0.25 < k < 0.5\ cm^{-1}$, suggesting that cortical power in the (apparent) resonant frequency bands of 8.0 Hz (mu

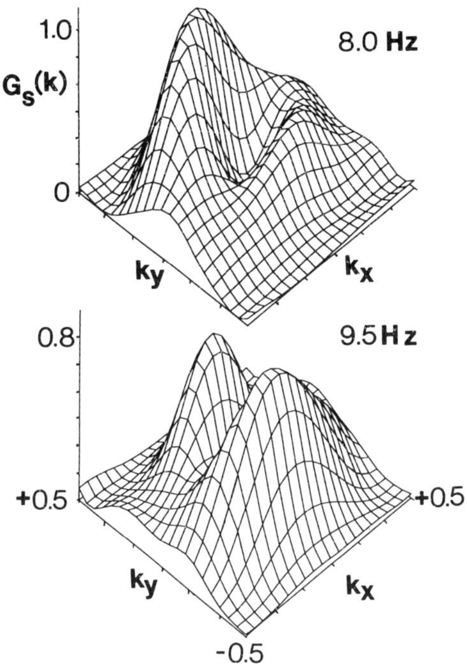

Figure 1-21. Estimates of the scalp spectral density function $G_s(k_x, k_y, \omega)$ in an adult for 1 minute of resting, eyes-closed EEG. Obtained with 16 scalp electrodes covering the right hemisphere; k_y refers to wave propagation in the anterior–posterior direction; k_x is perpendicular. The two plots corresponding to temporal frequency peaks at $\omega_\mu = f_\mu/2\pi =$ 8.0 Hz ("mu rhythm," upper figure) and $\omega_\alpha = f_\alpha/2\pi = 9.5$ Hz ("alpha rhythm," lower figure). An average reference transformation was used to remove power near $k_x = k_y = 0$. The mu rhythm spectrum is consistent with posterior-to-anterior traveling waves. The alpha rhythm spectrum shows symmetric peaks for positive and negative k_y, consistent with standing-wave phenomena. Other interpretations of these data are possible, however. (Reproduced with permission from Nunez, 1981, 1988a.)

rhythm) and 9.5 Hz (alpha rhythm) decrease more rapidly with wave number than that outside the resonant band. That is, within narrow frequency bands, EEG is dominated by relatively long wavelength behavior. This observation is confirmed in part by results obtained in a separate study of four subjects in whom $G_s(k, \omega)$ was fit to $k^{-\alpha(\omega)}$. The frequency dependence of the exponent $\alpha(\omega)$ is shown in Figure 1-22, indicating that $\alpha \sim 4$ near the peak alpha frequency in eyes-closed data.

The independence of tissue resistivities on frequency over the low frequency range of EEG may seem to imply that the time dependence of scalp potentials should be identical to the time dependence of cortical sources. This, however, is not consistent with observation because in some EEG studies high temporal frequencies of the sources $P(x, y, t)$ tend to occur with high spatial frequencies because of the rules of neocortical dynamic interaction. If we accept this property

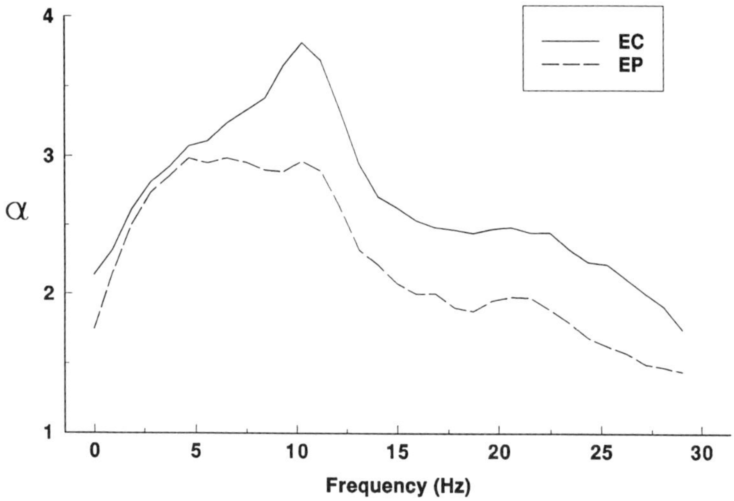

Figure 1-22. The scalp spectral density function $G_s(k, \omega)$ for resting EEG was fit to the function $k^{-\alpha(\omega)}$. The exponent $\alpha(\omega)$ was plotted versus frequency ($\omega/2\pi$) for two cases: EC (eyes-closed, that is, the usual awake alpha rhythm) and EP (eyes opened and positioned). The curves refer to an average over four persons. Data were recorded from a 32-electrode array around the circumference of the head to obtain more accurate estimates of $G_s(k, \omega)$. The maximum exponent $\alpha(f) \sim 4$ occurs in the alpha band $f \sim 10$ Hz for the eyes-closed case, that is, spectral power decreases most rapidly with increasing wave number (short spatial wavelengths) in this frequency range. Plots obtained by private communication from G.R. Shaw to P.L. Nunez. Experimental methods described in G.R. Shaw, 1991.

of the dynamics (evidence presented in Chapters 2 and 12), it clearly follows that less high temporal frequency power occurs on the scalp because the volume conductor acts as a low pass spatial filter, as indicated by the example of spectral density functions for spontaneous EEG shown in Figure 1-21. This plot shows very little relative power at the scalp for spontaneous EEG wave numbers greater than 1 cm^{-1}; that is, wavelengths less than 6 cm. The dynamic behavior of the sources is more difficult to explain, but the occurrence of high temporal frequencies with high spatial frequencies (as described by the dispersion relation) is a nearly universal property of wave phenomena, as this term is used in the physical sciences.

This issue of dispersion relation is addressed several times in this and later chapters. However we can provide some crude reasoning as follows: Suppose a disturbance (for example, modulation of synaptic action) occurs in some local region of neocortex, in a manner somewhat analogous to our imagined diver entering the ocean. The local disturbance may not be described accurately as a wave. However, perhaps neocortical dynamic action filters out the nonwave part of the disturbance as it moves away from its center of origin. We can imagine similar processes at multiple epicenters (the terminology of Lopes da Silva in Chapter 5). In this case, we expect to observe primarily wave field and interference patterns on the cortical surface, which, because of their wave natures, exhibit consistent relations between spatial and temporal frequency. Data that appears consistent with interference patterns in the cortex are shown in Chapters 3 and 12.

Methods To Improve Spatial Resolution

Scalp electrodes measure scalp currents, which are imperfectly related to cortical currents and sources. In conventional EEG practice, scalp spatial resolution is limited by

1. the volume conductor, for example, the smearing effect of the skull and cerebrospinal fluid and the separation distance between electrode and neural sources (Rush and Driscoll, 1968, 1969; Nunez, 1981a; Nunez et al, 1994). Other potentially important issues are current flow through skull holes, and skull resistivity variations over the surface (Yan et al, 1991).
2. the effect of the reference electrode placement; that is, there is no practical place to put the reference electrode that will generally yield the famous "potentials with respect to infinity" adopted by physicists (Katznelson, 1981; Nunez, 1981, 1990a; Nunez et al, 1991).
3. electrode density; that is, spatial sampling.
4. signal-to-noise ratio, which is an important issue in some applications but not critical in others.

With stationary (types I or III) sources, time locked to some stimulus, signal-to-noise ratio of the resulting evoked potential can be improved substantially by increasing the number of stimuli averaged. Increased spatial sampling by itself causes only marginal improvement in spatial resolution because the volume conductor and reference electrode issues remain. Three methods have been used to improve the spatial resolution of scalp signals generated by cortical sources.

1. Magnetoencephalography. The skull is transparent to magnetic fields, which eliminates an important smearing effect. However other problems may be introduced, including the selectivity of the method to specific sources illustrated in Figures 1-4 and 1-5 and smearing due to increased distance of the sensor from neural sources (Romani and Rossini, 1988; Wikswo and Roth, 1988).
2. Spatial deconvolution or cortical imaging. A volume conductor model of the head (for example, concentric spheres analytic model or finite element model) is used to project surface potentials to the cortical surface. This amounts to solving equation (1.19) for the polarization or cortical surface potential in terms of a measured scalp potential Φ, given information about the volume conductor required to determine the weighting function $\mathbf{W}$. This approach is very similar to that used in geophysics, in which the vector geomagnetic field generated by electric current sources in the earth's core is specified near the surface by its scalar potential. If no sources in the superficial layer (the mantle) occur, we can extrapolate surface measurements down to the core–mantle boundary (Lowes, 1974). Accuracy of this approach in either application depends on the accuracy of the volume conductor model used in the extrapolation procedure. Applications

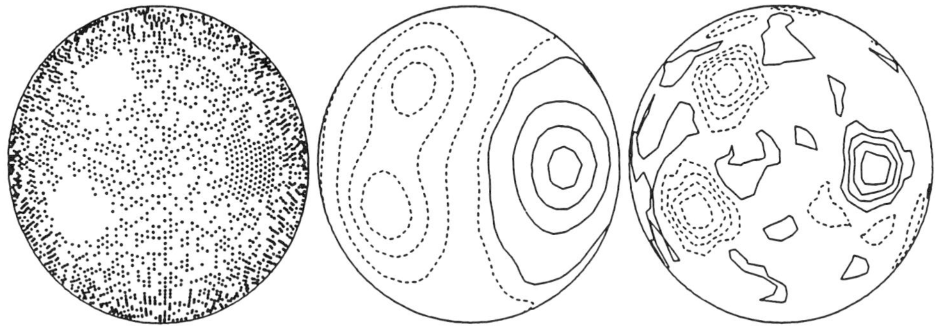

Figure 1-23. (**Left**) An example source distribution at the macrocolumn scale. Dots indicate positive polarization; empty spaces indicate negative polarization (that is, neocortical "dipoles"). Sources $\Delta\Phi$ are randomly distributed between ± 200 μV except in the three clumped regions where sources are either + or -200 μV (refer to Figure 1-11). (**Middle**) Isopotential lines. Plots were obtained using 648 surface samples. Maximum and minimum potentials were $+22$ and -25 μV, respectively (with respect to infinity). Potentials are calculated using the three-concentric spheres model of the head. (**Right**) The corresponding surface Laplacian plot reveals major source clumps. The surface Laplacian plot was also calculated from the three-concentric spheres model. Plots were obtained using 648 surface samples. By convention, the word "Laplacian" was used to indicate the usual surface Laplacian plot with a negative sign so that the sign of the Laplacian matches the sign of local cortical potential. Maximum ($+8.4$ μV/cm^2) occurred over the single positive clump. Two negative regions (-8.1 μV/cm^2) and (-8.4 μV/cm^2) occurred over the two negative source clumps.

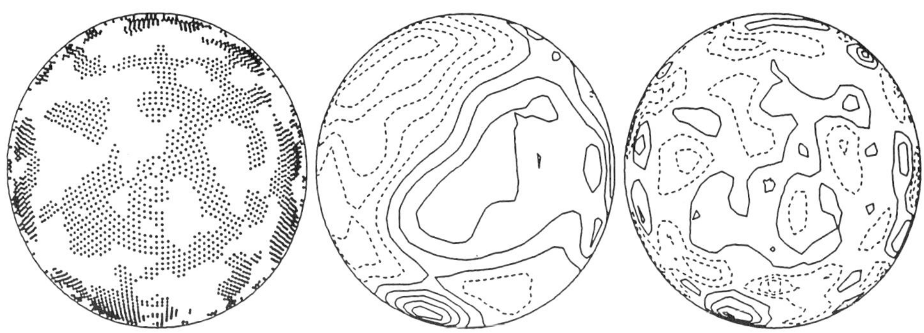

Figure 1-24. (**Left**) This is similar to Figure 1-23 except for a more complicated clumping pattern. Sources are distributed between ± 200 μV. (**Middle**) Isopotentials do not pick out major features of the source pattern even though sampling is very high (648 surface points) and potentials were calculated with respect to infinity (no reference electrode effects). Maximum and minimum potentials were $+11$ and -10 μV respectively. (**Right**) The corresponding surface Laplacian picked out major features at the scale of about 2 cm so that the source pattern (*left*) was very similar to the Laplacian pattern. Maximum and minimum Laplacian values were $+9$ μV/cm^2 and -4 μV/cm^2, respectively.

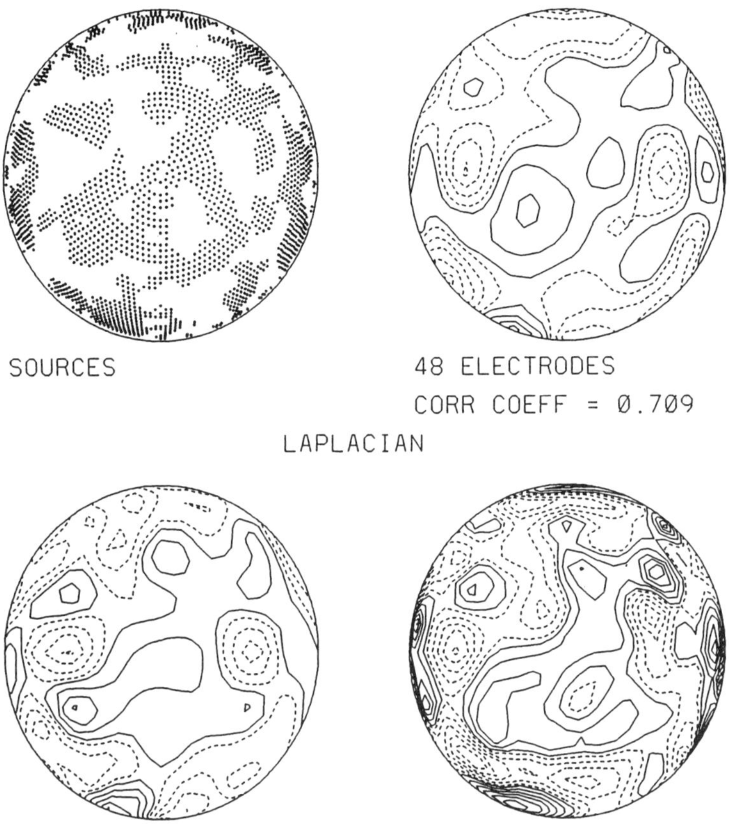

Figure 1-25. The effect of spatial sampling densities on the estimated surface Laplacian map using the three-dimensional spline methods. The plot at upper left shows the same source distribution as that used in Figure 1-24. The number of sampling points (electrodes of 1-cm diameter) and correlation coefficients with actual cortical potential are shown under each plot.

to EEG are considered in Nunez, 1987; Sidman, 1991; Cadusch et al, 1992; Nunez et al, 1994; Le and Gevins, 1993.

3. Laplacian or current source density. In the most modern version, a spline function is used to fit the surface potential distribution at fixed times. The second spatial derivative of the spline function with respect to the two local surface tangent coordinates yields estimates of local current passing perpendicular to the skull surface into the scalp and local cortical potential. This physical interpretation follows directly from the law of current conservation and from the idea that tangential current flow in the skull is small (Nunez, 1981; Katznelson, 1981). Applications of this approach are discussed in Perrin et al, 1987a, 1987b, 1989; Nunez, 1988a, 1990a; Nunez and Pilgreen, 1991; and Nunez et al, 1991, 1994.

The best of the spline–Laplacian and cortical imaging methods appear to be effective in resolving distributed, neocortical sources. These two approaches are shown to yield similar estimates of cortical potential distribution (Nunez et al, 1994). A comparison of the potential and Laplacian surface distribution due to a theoretical pattern of 4200 distributed cortical sources at the macrocolumn scale is shown in Figures 1-23 and 1-24. Source magnitudes vary between +200 and −200 μV, as in Figures 1-18 and 1-19. As source distributions become more clumped, scalp potential magnitudes increase in a manner similar to the simulations of Figures 1-17 and 1-18, except sources are distributed over the entire upper surface of a hemisphere of cortex. These plots were created by calculating potentials and Laplacian values at 648 scalp locations to show that even in the limit of very high spatial sampling, the surface potential distribution does not accurately represent neocortical source clumps at the scale of a few centimeters. This failure occurs even without reference electrode problems, which may be severe. In contrast, the analytic surface Laplacian estimate accurately reflects source distributions at the scale of about 2 cm and is reference independent.

In practice, the effects of spatial sampling and noise must be included in such comparisons. However, the net result of adding these complications is that the Laplacian approach, when combined with a high electrode density (64–128 channels over the entire scalp, for example), can increase spatial resolution over conventional EEG by at least a factor of three (Nunez et al, 1991, 1994). The effect of different spatial sampling is illustrated in Figure 1-25 in which the source pattern of Figure 1-24 is used again.

Spatial Filtering by the Head Volume Conductor

Another way to illustrate the differences between high resolution and conventional EEG is by their different spatial filtering properties. With clinical EEG, different choices of reference electrode emphasize certain sources at the expense of others. Thus the choice of reference electrode (or particular bipolar montage) can be viewed as a spatial filter with respect to source location. An extension of this idea is that of a spatial filter with respect to the size of the correlated source region (Nunez, 1988).

To illustrate the spatial filtering properties of various methods, we use natural functions for spherical surfaces known as the spherical harmonics $Y_{\ell m}(\theta, \phi)$. Here θ and ϕ are the usual spherical coordinates, essentially latitude and longitude in the case of the earth's surface. (Refer to the spherical coordinates shown in the upper left corner of Figure 1-26.) For illustrative purposes, we consider the north pole to be at C_Z. The index ℓ can take on any integer value from 0 to ∞. The index m can take on any value from $-\ell$ to $+\ell$. The $Y_{\ell m}$ functions form an orthogonal set of (many) functions on the surface of a sphere. The larger the index ℓ, the higher the "spatial frequency" in the θ direction. The larger the index m, the higher the "spatial frequency" in the ϕ direction. We place the words "spatial

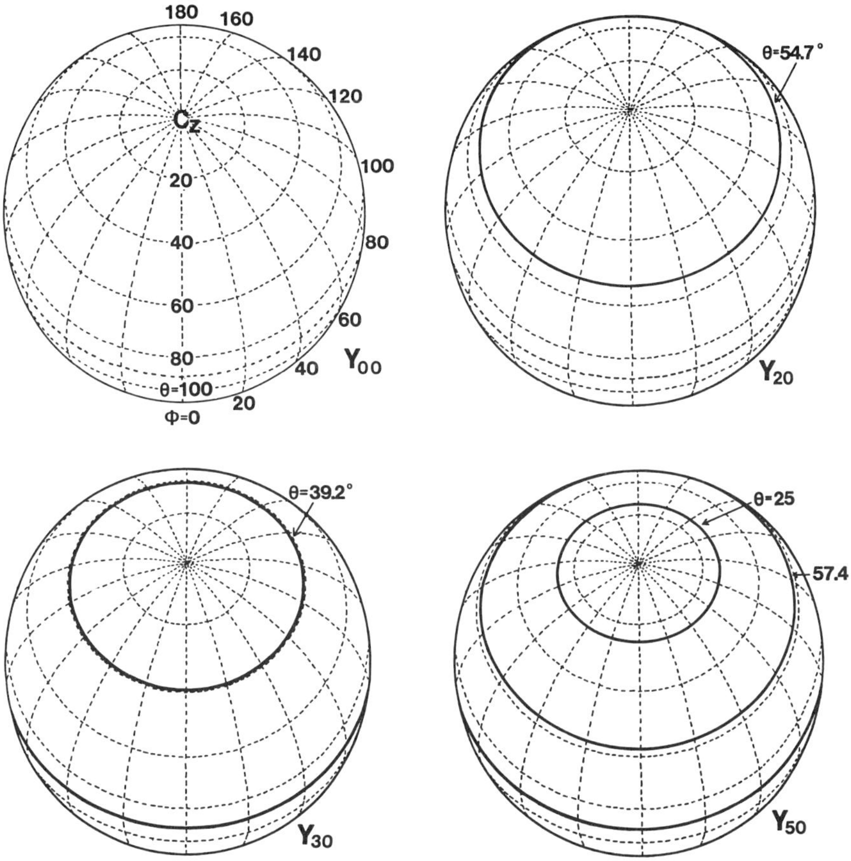

Figure 1-26. The functions $Y_{\ell 0}(\theta)$ with the ℓ index equal to 0, 2, 3 and 5. In electroencephalographic applications, we may choose the coordinate system so that C_Z is the location $\theta = 0°$ (north pole) and the left ear is near $\theta = 90°$ and $\phi = 0°$. The solid (nodal) lines are determined by the angles θ such that $Y_{\ell 0}(\theta)$ equals zero, that is they separate positive and negative regions.

frequency" in quotes because this term is not precisely defined for nonsinusoidal functions. However the general intuitive idea of spatial frequency applies well to these functions, as shown in Figures 1-26 and 1-27 and by the approximate relations

$$k_\theta = \frac{\ell + 1 - |m|}{R} \qquad \ell = 0, \infty$$

$$k_\phi = \frac{|m|}{R \sin\theta} \qquad m = -\ell, +\ell \qquad (1.22)$$

Here R is sphere radius and k_θ and k_ϕ are spatial frequencies (cm^{-1}) in the latitudinal and longitudinal directions, respectively. (Spatial frequencies may be expressed in cycles per centimeter by dividing k_θ and k_ϕ by the factor 2π.) For

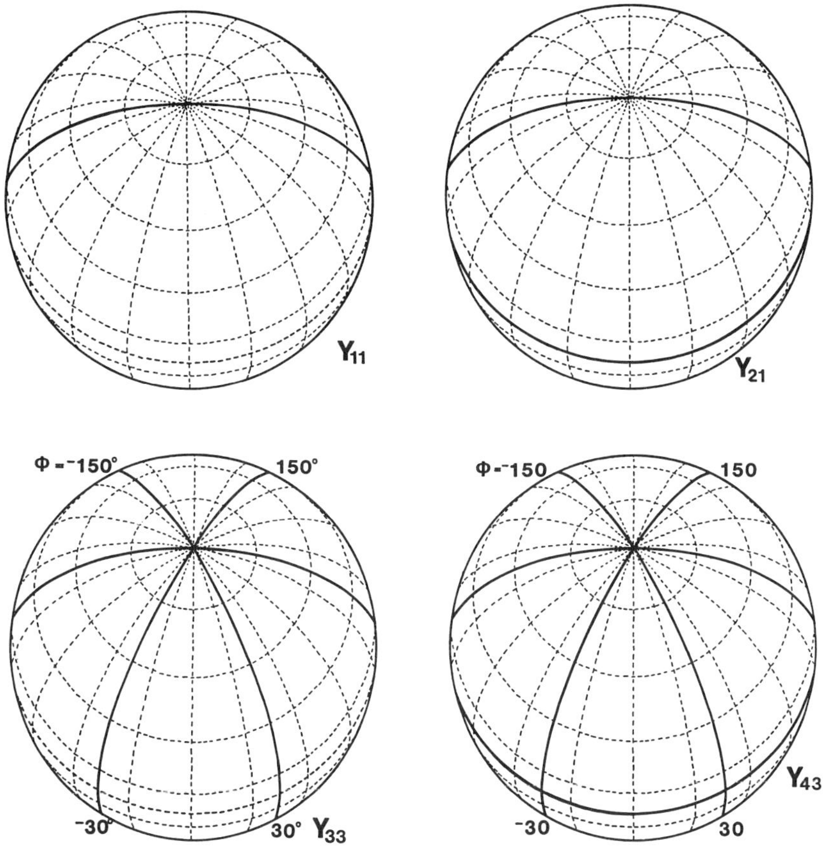

Figure 1-27. The functions $Y_{\ell m}(\theta, \phi)$ for $m \neq 0$ are given by $Y_{\ell m}(\theta, \phi) = Y_{\ell 0}(\theta)e^{im\phi}$, which partition the spherical surface into longitudinal sections in addition to the latitudinal partitions produced by the ℓ index. The real parts of several $Y_{\ell m}(\theta, \phi)$ functions are plotted.

example, with a sphere radius (brain) of $R = 8$ cm, $Y_{10}(\theta)$ has a spatial wavelength in the θ direction of about 25 cm and $Y_{80}(\theta)$ has a wavelength of about 6 cm.

The spatial filtering properties of different methods are illustrated by assuming that cortical source strength is proportional to the functions $Y_{\ell m}(\theta, \phi)$ for different indices ℓ and m. These functions represent different frequencies in the θ and ϕ directions. The predicted scalp potential is calculated using the standard four concentric spheres model of the head (Nunez, 1981). The root-mean-square magnitudes of the potential and Laplacian provide a general idea of the average scalp magnitude of each EEG measure to be expected from each source distribution. That is, an estimate of the sensitivity of each measure is obtained as a function of spatial frequency, k_θ (essentially averaged over the spatial frequencies k_ϕ so estimates are independent of the m index).

Raw scalp potential (Figure 1-28) is most sensitive to very low spatial frequencies. This result (together with reference electrode effects not considered here) indicates why conventional methods provide such poor localization of sources.

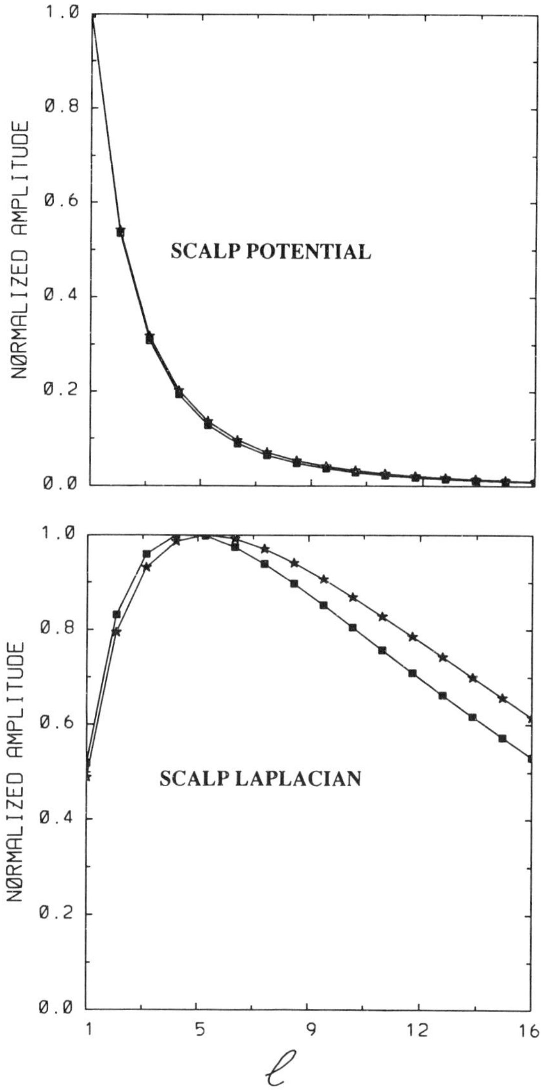

Figure 1-28. The spatial filtering properties of the head volume conductor are estimated using a four concentric spheres model of the head. Radial dipole sources in the cortex are assumed to be distributed such that source strengths are proportional to the $Y_{\ell m}(\theta, \phi)$ functions plus complex conjugates. The resulting scalp potential magnitude (square root of integrated squared potential over the entire surface) is shown in the upper figure. The equivalent plot for the analytic scalp surface Laplacian is shown below. Both measures are independent of the m index. The plots are obtained using an assumed ratio of skull to brain resistivity of 80. Squares refer to a head model with no cerebrospinal fluid layer. Stars are obtained with a cerebrospinal fluid layer of 2 mm, with a brain to cerebrospinal fluid resistivity ratio equal to 5. The relation between spatial frequency and the ℓ index is given by equation (1.22). Scalp potential is a low pass estimate of cortical potential, whereas scalp Laplacian is a band pass estimate of cortical potential. In practice, the high frequency Laplacian cut-off is determined by electrode spacing and the order of the spline function used to estimate the Laplacian.

The Laplacian estimate is sensitive to a relatively broad range of spatial frequencies. As such it is sensitive to the spatial frequency range in which raw potential is insensitive. Thus we can conclude that raw potential and Laplacian estimates provide somewhat complementary but partly overlapping information, with the former mainly valuable to study large-scale (low spatial frequency) sources if reference electrode distortion is not too great. Spline-based cortical imaging methods developed by the Melbourne group provide filtering properties similar to the spline–Laplacian method when scalp potentials are recorded at 64 (or more) surface locations (Nunez et al, 1994).

An approximate idea of the amount of new information potentially available in the EEG can be obtained when spatial resolution is improved. For example, suppose that conventional EEG allows us to monitor the activity of M scalp regions. In the case of standard EEG (that is, a 10/20 system), one might effectively monitor only M = 4 distinct regions with minimal overlap. For example, we might monitor anterior and posterior regions of both hemispheres. Of course, we would like for M to be much larger, perhaps equal to the number of electrodes, but field spreading by volume conduction and reference electrode effects severely limit this procedure when conventional methods are used. A simple approach that minimizes volume conduction spreading is to use 20 EEG channels to obtain Laplacian estimates over four regions, each containing five electrodes with perhaps 3-cm spacing (Nunez and Pilgreen, 1991). If, for convenience, we think of each region as producing S possible neocortical states, the number of different spatial patterns

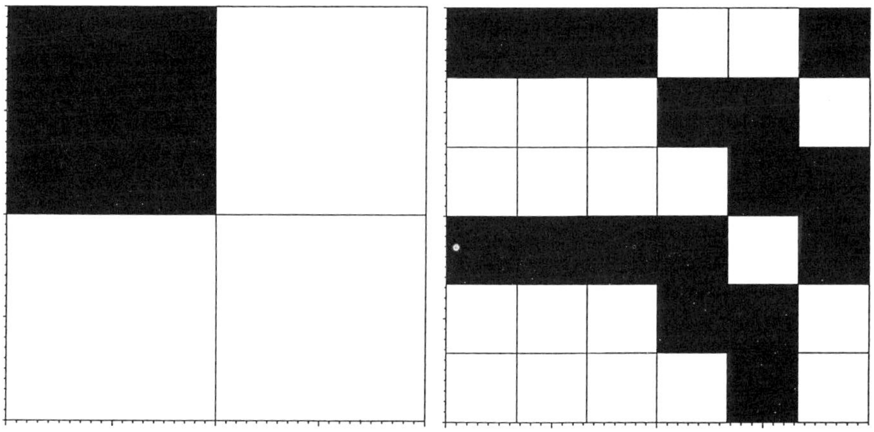

Figure 1-29. Illustration of the number of distinct spatial patterns (states) that may be achieved within a fixed surface area. If each small square can be only black or white, and total area is divided into M squares, the total number of possible patterns is 2^M. EEG spatial resolution using standard 10/20 reference-dependent methods is no better than about 6 to 10 cm. This condition is crudely represented by the plot on the left showing 16 possible spatial states that can be observed with conventional EEG methods. Dense Laplacian arrays (~128 channels over the scalp) can achieve resolution of about 2 cm, as represented very approximately by the right plot, allowing for the observation of 2^{36} = 68,719,000,000 distinct spatial states.

that can be resolved is S^M. When spatial resolution is increased by a linear factor of R, the number of regions that can be monitored separately increases by R^2, and the number of possible spatial patterns is S^{MR^2}. Thus the number of possible spatial patterns is increased by the factor $S^{M(R^2-1)}$.

Suppose we adopt modern methods to increase spatial resolution by a factor of $R = 3$ and conservatively assume that only binary states can be distinguished in each scalp region (for example, polarization vectors either up or down) so that $S = 2$. The arguments proposed above suggest that the number of distinct global states that can be resolved with scalp recordings using high resolution methods is increased by a factor of 2^{32}, that is by about four billion as illustrated in Figure 1-29. Although we have neglected many details, including the fact that we are often interested in spatial–temporal patterns, these estimates emphasize the importance of improved spatial resolution and good pattern recognition algorithms to make sense of potentially complex patterns.

Summary

The EEG is viewed here as a stochastic field variable having spatial–temporal statistical properties that are correlated with the physiologic state of the brain. Thus far in EEG, the study of these correlations has been limited severely by poor spatial resolution of scalp-recorded potentials, misunderstanding of volume conduction, lack of full appreciation of the importance of distinct spatial and temporal scales, and lack of physiologically based quantitative pattern recognition techniques. To overcome these limitations, we adopted several ideas from the physical sciences.

This presentation emphasized building bridges between disparate fields of study rather than rigorous development of isolated fields. Several general approaches can (with suitable modification) be carried over to EEG from the physical sciences to extract much more information from EEG signals. These include methods to improve spatial resolution and the development of effective spatial–temporal pattern recognition methods to be applied in experimental EEG studies. Theoretical models can be of great value in achieving these goals.

The general philosophy of this book may be illustrated by a metaphor of human knowledge represented as a landscape consisting of patterns within patterns within still more patterns at many spatial scales. The knowledge landscape contains many regions with fractal properties. That is, the more we focus narrowly on some field of study, the more we become aware of intricate details whose nature cannot be imagined in any superficial study. This small-scale structure of the knowledge landscape can be appreciated only with substantial intellectual effort. But when such endeavors spurn parallel studies at large (general) scales, formidable barriers to communication between fields may arise. This is illustrated by the old adage about the doctor of philosophy who "learned more and more about less and less until he finally learned everything about nothing," an idea similar to what mathematicians call a "set of measure zero."

Immense communication barriers also exist between the generalists (those who only appreciate the large-scale patterns of our imagined landscape). These barriers occur because many of the connections between disparate fields occur at smaller scales. For example, certain connections between fields may be effectively communicated only between persons who have achieved level two or three of expertise (Table 1-1). This book consists of a series of sample connections between fields taken from different regions of the landscape and from different scales. Although our particular choice of samples is not random, neither is it unique. Thus we may anticipate many alternate sets of samples in other studies of neocortical dynamics.

References

Abeles, M. *Local Cortical Circuits*. New York: Springer-Verlag, 1982.

Bascom, W. *Waves and Beaches*. New York: Ancor Books, 1964.

Bendat, J.S. and Piersol, A.G. *Random Data: Analysis and Measurement Procedures. 2nd Ed.* New York: Wiley, 1986.

Bickford, R.G. *Clinical Electroencephalography*. New York: Medcom, 1973.

Braitenberg, V. Cortical architectonics: general and areal. In: *Architechtonics of the Cerebral Cortex*. (M.A.B. Brazier, Petesche H., Eds.) New York: Raven Press, 1978.

Cadusch, P.J., Breckon, W., and Silberstein, R.B. Spherical splines and the interpolation, deblurring and transformation of topographic EEG. Pan Pacific Workshop on Brain Electric and Magnetic Topography, Melbourne, Australia, February 17–18, 1992.

Churchland, P.S. and Sejnowski, T.J. Prospectives on cognitive neuroscience, *Science*. 242:741–745, 1988.

Cohen, D., Cuffin, B.N., Yunokuchi, K., Maniewski, R., Purcell, C., Cosgrove, G.R., Ives, J., and Kennedy, J. MEG versus EEG localization test using implanted sources in the human brain. *Ann. Neurol*. 28:811–817, 1990.

Cole, K. *Membranes, Ions, and Impulses*. Berkeley, CA: University of California Press, 1968.

Cooper, R., Winter, A.L., Crow, H.J., and Walter, W.G. Comparison of subcortical, cortical and scalp activity using chronically indwelling electrodes in man. *Electroencephalogr. Clin. Neurophysiol*. 18:217–228, 1965.

Cuffin, B.N. and Cohen, D. Comparison of the magnetoencephalogram and electroencephalogram. *Electroencephalogr. Clin. Neurophysiol*. 47:136–146, 1979.

Cuffin, B.N., Cohen, D., Yunokuchi, K., Maniewski, K.R., Purcell, C., Cosgrove, G.R., Ives, J., Kennedy, J., and Schomer, D. Tests of EEG localization accuracy using implanted sources in the human brain. *Ann. Neurol*. 29:132–138, 1991.

Delucchi, M.R., Garoutte, B., and Aird, R.B. The scalp as an electroencephalographic averager. *Electroencephalogr. Clin. Neurophysiol*. 38:191–196, 1975.

Elul, E. The genesis of the EEG. *Int. Rev. Neurobiol*. 15:227–272, 1972.

Fender, D.H. Source localization of brain electrical activity. In: *Handbook of Electroencephalography and Clinical Neurophysiology* (revised series). Vol. 1. (A.S. Gevins, Redmond A., Eds.) New York: Elsevier, pp. 355–403, 1987.

Freeman, W.J. Use of spatial deconvolution to compensate for distortion of EEG by volume conduction. *IEEE Trans. Biomed. Eng*. 27:421–429, 1980.

Freeman, W.J. and Skarda, C.S. Spatial analysis, nonlinear dynamics, and perception: The neo-Sherrington view. *Brain Res. Rev*. 10:147–175, 1985.

Gevins, A.S. Analysis of multiple lead data. In: *Event-Related Brain Potentials*. (J.W.

Rohbraugh, Parasuraman, R., Johnson, J.R., Eds.) New York: Oxford University Press, pp. 44–56, 1990.

Gevins, A.S., Doyle, J., Cutillo, B., Schaffer, R., Tannehil, R., Ghannam, J., Gilcrease, V., and Yeager, C. Electric potentials in human brain during cognition: new method reveals dynamic patterns of correlation of human electrical potentials during cognition. *Science*. 213:918–922, 1981.

Gevins, A.S., Schaffer, R.E., Doyle, J.C., Cutillo, B.A., Tannehill, R.L., and Bressler, S.L. Shadows of thought: Rapidly changing asymmetric brain-potential patterns of a brief visuomotor task. *Science*. 220:97–99, 1983.

Gevins, A.S. and Cutillo, B.A. Signals of cognition: In: *Handbook of Electroencephalography and Clinical Neurophysiology* (revised series). Vol. 2. (F.H. Lopes da Silva, Strom van Leeuwen, W., Remond A., Eds.) New York: Elsevier, pp. 335–381, 1986.

Gevins, A.S., Brickett, P., Costales, B., Le J., and Reutter, B. Beyond topographic mapping: Towards functional-anatomical imaging with 124 channel EEGs and 3-D MRIs. *Brain Topography*. 3:53–64, 1990.

Gevins, A.S., Le, J., Brickett, P., Reutter, B., and Desmond, J. Seeing through the skull: Advanced EEG's accurately measure cortical activity from the scalp. *Brain Topography*. 4:125–132, 1991.

Grossberg, S. Nonlinear neural networks: Principles, mechanisms, and architectures. *Neural Networks*. 1:17–61, 1988.

Hari, R. and Kaukoranta, E. Neuromagnetic study of somatosensory system: Principles and examples. *Prog. Neurobiol.* 24:233–256, 1985.

Henderson, C.J., Butler, S.R., and Glass, A. The localization of equivalent dipoles of EEG sources by the application of electric field theory. *Electroencephalogr. Clin. Neurophysiol*. 39:117–130, 1975.

Humphrey, D.R. Re-analysis of the antidromic cortical response. II. On the contributions of cell discharge and PSPs to the evoked potentials. *Electroencephalogr. Clin. Neurophysiol*. 25:421–442, 1968.

Jackson, J.D. *Classical Electrodynamics. 2nd Ed.* New York: Wiley, pp. 299–303, 1976.

Jones, E.G. Broadmann's areas. In: *Encyclopedia of Neuroscience*. (G. Adelman, Ed.) pp. 180–181, 1987.

Katznelson, R.D. *Deterministic and Stochastic Field Theoretic Models in the Neurophysics of EEG*. Ph.D. Dissertation. LaJolla, CA: University of California at San Diego, 1982.

Katznelson, R.D. Normal modes of the brain: Neuroanatomical basis and a physiological theoretical model. In: *Electric Fields of the Brain: The Neurophysics of EEG*. (P.L. Nunez) New York: Oxford University Press, 1981.

Kavanagh, R.N., Darcey, T.M., Lehmann, D., and Fender, D.H. Evaluation of methods for three-dimensional localization of electrical sources in the human brain. *IEEE Trans. Biomed. Eng*. 24:421–429, 1978.

Kearfott, R.B., Sidmann, R.D., Major, D.J., and Hill, C.D. Numerical tests of a method for simulating electrical potentials on the cortical surface. *IEEE Trans. Biomed. Eng.* 38:294–299, 1991.

Law, S.K., Nunez, P.L., and Wijesinghe, R.S. High resolution EEG using spline generated surface Laplacians on spherical and ellipsoidal surfaces. *IEEE Trans. Biomed. Eng.* 40:145–153, 1993.

Le, J. and Gevins, A.S. Method to reduce blur distortion from EEG's using a realistic head model. *IEEE Trans. Biomed. Eng*. 40:517–528, 1993.

Lehmann, D. EEG maps and map analysis. In: *Statistics and Topography in Quantitative EEG*. Paris: Elsevier, pp. 27–48, 1988.

Lehmann, D. Human scalp EEG fields: Evoked alpha, sleep, and spike-wave patterns. In: *Synchronization of EEG Activity in Epilepsies.* (H. Petsche, Brazier, M.A.B., Eds.) New York: Springer-Verlag, 1971.

Lehmann, D. Principals of spatial analysis. In: *Methods of Analysis of Brain Electrical and Magnetic Signals. Handbook of Electroencephalography and Clinical Neurophysiology.* (revised series). Vol. 1. (A.S. Gevins, Remond A., Eds.) New York: Elsevier, 1987.

Lehmann, D., Ozaki, H., and Pal, I. EEG alpha map series: Brain microstates by space oriented adaptive segmentation. *Electroencephalogr. Clin. Neurophysiol.* 67:271–288, 1987.

Livanov, M.N. *Spatial Organization of Cerebral Processes.* New York: Wiley, 1977.

Lopes da Silva, F.H. and Storm van Leeuwen, W. The cortical alpha rhythm in dog: The depth and surface profile of phase. In: *Architectonics of Cerebral Cortex.* (M.A.B. Brazier, Petsche, H., Eds.) New York: Raven Press, pp. 319–333, 1978.

Lowes, F.J. Spatial power spectrum of the main geomagnetic field and extrapolation to the core. *Geophysic. J. Royal Astron. Soc.* 36:717–730, 1974.

Mitzdorf, U. and Singer, W. Excitatory synaptic ensemble properties in the visual cortex of the macaque monkey: A current source density analysis of electrically evoked potentials. *J. Comp. Neurol.* 187:71–83, 1979.

Mitzdorf, U. and Singer, W. Prominent excitatory pathways in the cat visual cortex (A17 and A18): A current source density analysis of electrically evoked potentials. *Exp. Brain. Res.* 33:371–394, 1978.

Monin, A.S. and Yaglom, A.M. *Statistical Fluid Mechanics. Mechanisms of Turbulence. Vol. 1.* Cambridge: MIT Press, 1975.

Myklebust, J.B., Cusick, J.F., Sances, A. Jr., and Larson, S.T., Eds. *Neural Stimulation, Vols. 1 and 2.* Boca Raton, FL: CRC Press, 1985.

Nicholas, P. and Deloche, G. Convolution computer progressing of the brain electrical image transmission. *Int. J. Biomed. Comput.* 7:143–159, 1976.

Niedermeyer, E. and Lopes da Silva, F. *Electroencephalography: Basic Principles, Clinical Applications, and Related Fields.* 3rd Ed. Baltimore, MD: Urban and Schwarzenberg, 1993.

Nunez, P.L. *Electric Fields of the Brain: The Neurophysics of EEG.* New York: Oxford University Press, 1981.

Nunez, P.L. Unpublished letter to R.D. Katznelson, 1986.

Nunez, P.L. Removal of reference electrode and volume conduction effects by spatial deconvolution of evoked potentials using a three-concentric sphere model of the head. The London Symposium. *Electroencephalogr. Clin. Neurophysiol.* 39 (Suppl): 143–148, 1987.

Nunez, P.L. Spatial filtering and experimental strategies in EEG. In: *Statistics and Topography in Quantitative EEG.* Paris: (D. Samson-Dollfus, Ed.) Paris: Elsevier, pp. 196–209, 1988a.

Nunez, P.L. Methods to estimate spatial properties of the dynamic cortical source activity. In: *Functional Brain Imaging.* (G. Pfurtscheller, Lopes da Silva, F., Eds.) Berlin: Springer-Verlag, pp. 3–10, 1988b.

Nunez, P.L. Generation of human EEG by a combination of long and short range neocortical interactions. *Brain Topography.* 1:199–215, 1989a.

Nunez, P.L. Towards a physics of neocortex. In: *Advanced Methods of Physiological Systems Modeling, Vol. 2.* (V.Z. Marmarelis, Ed.) New York: Plenum Press, pp. 241–259, 1989b.

Nunez, P.L. Localization of brain activity with electroencephalography. In: *Magnetoencephalography: Advances in Neurology*. Vol. 54. (S. Sato, Ed.) New York: Raven Press, pp. 39–65, 1990a.

Nunez, P.L. Physical principles and neurophysical mechanisms underlying event related potentials. In: *Event Related Potentials of the Brain*. (J. Rohrbaugh, Johnson, R., Parasuraman, R., Eds.) New York: Oxford University Press, pp. 19–36, 1990b.

Nunez, P.L. and Pilgreen, K.L. The spline-Laplacian in clinical neurophysiology: a method to improve EEG spatial resolution. *J. Clin. Neurophysiol.* 8:397–413, 1991.

Nunez, P.L., Pilgreen, K.L., Westdrop, A.F., Law, S.K., and Nelson, A.V. A visual study of surface potentials and Laplacians due to distributed neocortical sources: Computer simulations and evoked potentials. *Brain Topography*. 4:151–168, 1991.

Nunez, P.L., Silberstein, R.B., Cadusch, P.J., Wijesinghe, R.S., Westdrop, A.F., and Srinivasan, R.A. A theoretical and experimental study of high resolution EEG based on surface Laplacians and cortical imaging. *Electroencephalogr. Clin. Neurophysiol.* 90:40–57, 1994.

Nunez, P.L. and Srinivasan, R.A. Implications of recording strategy for estimates of neocortical dynamics with EEG. *Chaos: An Interdisciplinary Journal of Nonlinear Science*. 3:257–266, 1993.

Penfield, W. and Jasper, H. *Epilepsy and the Functional Anatomy of the Human Brain*. Boston: Little, Brown, 1954.

Perrin, F., Bertrand, O., and Pernier, J. Scalp current density mapping: Value and estimation from potential data. *IEEE Trans. Biomed. Eng.* 34:283–288, 1987a.

Perrin, F., Pernier, J., Bertrand, O., and Echallier, J.F. Spherical splines for scalp potential and current density mapping. *Electroencephalogr. Clin. Neurophysiol.* 72:184–187, 1989.

Perrin, F., Pernier, J., Bertrand, O., Giard, M.H., and Enchallier, J.F. Mapping of scalp potentials by surface spline interpolation. *Electroencephalogr. Clin. Neurophysiol.* 66:75–81, 1987b.

Petsche, H. Personal communication, 1992.

Petsche, H., Pockberger, H., and Rappelsberger, P. Cortical structure and electrogenesis. In: *Dynamics of Sensory and Cognitive Processing by the Brain*. (E. Basar, Ed.) Berlin: Springer-Verlag, pp. 123–139, 1988.

Petsche, H., Pockberger, H., and Rappelsberger, P. On the search for the sources of electroencephalogram. *Neuroscience*. 11:1–27, 1984.

Plonsey, R. *Bioelectric Phenomena*. New York: McGraw-Hill, 1969.

Pockberger, H., Rappelsberger, P., and Petsche, H. Cognitive processing in the EEG. In: *Dynamics of Sensory and Cognitive Processing by the Brain*. (E. Basar, Ed.) Berlin: Springer-Verlag, pp. 266–274, 1988.

Poiseau, E., Dessimond, F., Scheuler, W., and Jobert, M. Coherence analysis of sleep EEG signals. Pan European Society of Neurology. Second Congress. Vienna, December, 1991.

Rappelsberger, P. and Petsche, H. Probability mapping: Power and coherence analysis of cognitive processes. *Brain Topography*. 1:46–54, 1988.

Regan, D. *Human Brain Electrophysiology. Evoked Potentials and Evoked Magnetic Fields in Science and Medicine*. New York: Elsevier Press, 1989.

Remond, A., Leséure, N., Joseph, J.P., Rieger, H., and Lairy, G.C. The alpha average. I. Methodology and description. *Electroencephal. Clin. Neurophysiol.* 28:245–265, 1969.

Roland, P.E. and Widen, L. Quantitative measurements of brain metabolism during physiological stimulation. In: *Functional Brain Imaging.* (G. Pfurtscheller, Lopes da Silva, F.H., Eds.) Toronto: Hans Huber, pp. 213–228, 1988.

Romani, G.L. and Rossini, P. Neuromagnetic functional localization: Principles, state of the art, and perspectives. *Brain Topography.* 1:15–21, 1988.

Rose, S. *The Conscious Brain.* New York: Vintage Books, 1976.

Rush, S. and Driscoll, D.A. Current distribution in the brain from surface electrodes. *Anesth. Analog.* 47:717–723, 1968.

Rush, S. and Driscoll, D.A. EEG electrode sensitivity: An application of reciprocity. *IEEE Trans. Biomed. Eng.* 16:15–22, 1969.

Scherg, M. Fundamentals of dipole source potential analysis. In: *Auditory Evoked Magnetic Fields and Potentials. Advances in Neurology.* Vol. 6. (M. Hoke, Grandori, F., Romani, G.L., Eds.) Basel: Karger, 1989.

Scherg, M. and Cramon, D. Two bilateral sources of the late AEP as identified by a spatio-temporal dipole model. *Electroencephogr. Clin. Neurophysiol.* 62:32–44, 1985.

Scherg, M. and von Cramon, D. Dipole source potentials of the auditory cortex in normal subjects and in patients with tempory lobe lesions. In: *Auditory Evoked Magnetic Fields and Potentials. Advances in Audiology.* Vol. 6. (M. Hoke, Grandori, F., Romani, G.L., Eds.) Basel: Karger, 1989.

Sem-Jacobsen, C.W., Bickford, R.G., Petersen, M.C., and Dodge, H.W. Depth distribution of normal electroencephalographic rhythms. *Proceedings of Staff Meetings of the Mayo Clinic.* 28:156–161, 1953.

Shaw, G.R. *Spherical Harmonic Analysis of the Electroencephalogram.* Ph.D. Dissertation. Alberta, Canada: The University of Alberta, 1991.

Sidman, R.D. A method for simulating intracerebral potential fields. The cortical imaging technique. *J. Clin. Neurophysiol.* 8:432–441, 1991.

Spehlmann, R. *EEG Primer.* New York: Elsevier, 1981.

Thatcher, R.W., Krouse, P.J., and Hrybyk, M. Cortico-cortical associations and EEG coherence: A two compartmental model. *Electroencephalogr. Clin. Neurophysiol.* 64:123–143, 1986.

Weinberg, H., Brickett, P., Robertson, A., Harrop, R., Cheyne, D.O., Crisp, D., Baff, M., and Dykstra, C. The location of source-systems in the brain: Early and late components of event-related potential. *J. Alcoholism.* 4:339–345, 1987.

Wikswo, J.P. and Roth, B.J. Magnetic determination of the spatial extent of a single cortical current source: A theoretical analysis. *Electroencephalogr. Clin. Neurophysiol.* 69:266–276, 1988.

Williamson, S.J. and Kaufman, L. Analysis of neuromagnetic signals. In: *Handbook of Electroencephalography and Clinical Neurophysiology* (revised series). Vol. 1. (A.S. Gevins, Remond, A., Eds.) Amsterdam: Elsevier, pp. 405–488, 1987.

Wood, C.C. Application of dipole localization methods to source identification of human evoked potentials. *Annals of the New York Academy of Sciences.* 388:139–155, 1982.

Yaglom, A.M. *Correlation Theory of Stationary and Related Random Functions. Vol. 1. Basic Results.* New York: Springer-Verlag, 1987.

Yan, Y., Nunez, P.L., and Hart, R.T. A finite element model of the human head: Scalp potentials due to dipole sources. *Med. Biol. Eng. Comput.* 29:475–481, 1991.

Yudofsky, S.C. and Hales, R.E. (Eds.). The American Psychiatric Press Textbook of Neuropsychiatry. Washington: American Psychiatric Press, 1992.

2

Toward a Physics of Neocortex

PAUL L. NUNEZ

Contributions of Physical Science in Electroencephalography

This chapter examines the brain in general and neocortex in particular as a distinct state of matter, somewhat as we would view solids, liquids, gases, plasma, or other more esoteric physical states often studied by physicists. This approach may elicit negative responses from those who associate it with materialism or extreme reductionism, in which everything we regard as uniquely human can be expressed in terms of physics. But we do not intend to presuppose anything about the relation between the mind and brain. Rather the philosophical position of this chapter is neutral. The general approach is to treat the available anatomic, physiologic, electroencephalographic (EEG), behavioral, and other data obtained at multiple hierarchical levels with sufficient respect to construct theories about the interrelations of these data and to see what additional experiments, especially in EEG, are suggested. In this manner, more about brain operation may be discovered from the new data, new or modified theories can be constructed, and the process then repeated. This, of course, is the general philosophy that has characterized scientific progress and has led, for example, to the discovery of physical properties of quasilinear (that is, subthreshold) membranes, followed by the extension of these ideas to account for highly nonlinear behavior, especially the propagation of action potentials. Although the former phenomena have close analogs in electric cable theory, the latter have no close relation to known physical systems. In a similar manner, we expect to find neocortical phenomena that are analogous to known physical systems as well as many other phenomena for which no analogs are adequate.

In the case of neocortex, many experimental data are available at large scales from scalp EEG recordings, data that are often correlated with the participant's clinical or psychologic state. These connections are discussed in Chapters 3, 4, 6, 7, 12, and 13. By analogy, a number of physical systems have been studied in which certain quantities are measured on a closed surface, quantities that vary with time and location in some complicated way. These stochastic field variables are not generally predictable, except perhaps in some statistical senses. Examples are air pressure, temperature, and velocity in the atmosphere, electron density, and electromagnetic field strength in the ionosphere, wave height in oceans, and seismic displacements at the earth's surface. Causes of the inherent randomness of these field variables include incomplete knowledge of rules governing the dynamics or of external input to the system. Another cause of the stochastic nature of systems is our inability to predict accurately the behavior of some nonlinear systems, even with the largest computers imaginable. Studies in the new field of chaos emphasize that precise long-range prediction in some systems is impossible (at least at small scales), even when the systems appear to be relatively simple. Chaotic behavior is explored in Chapter 10. Because several physical science disciplines are, in important ways, more advanced scientifically than the EEG field, the EEG researcher may wish to examine possible analogs and determine if specific physical methods can be useful in EEG studies.

Of course, physical science has critically affected EEG in several important ways. First, the hardware required to accurately record, filter, digitize, and store electric potentials in the microvolt range requires modern technology. With magnetoencephalography (MEG), which involves measurement of small magnetic fields (more than nine orders of magnitude below the earth's magnetic field), more advanced technologic achievements are required.

The second way in which physical science contributes unequivocally to EEG studies is in the interpretation of measured electric or magnetic fields in terms of underlying current sources. For example, standard EEG methods estimate tangential scalp currents that are related to neural source currents in nontrivial ways. The relation between these variables is governed by Poisson's equation (1.3); however, accurate solutions of the equation are difficult to obtain in practice because the boundaries and conductivities of different tissues are known imperfectly. This is true even for the forward problem; that is, estimating scalp surface potentials due to known neural sources. But at least accuracy can be improved continually as better volume-conductive models of the head are developed. In contrast, the unconstrained inverse problem, that is, estimating neural sources only from scalp surface potential distribution, has no unique solution. Thus constraints based on anatomic and physiologic considerations must be applied to estimate neural source activity (Nunez, 1981, 1990a, 1990b).

For many years, physical principles governing volume conduction in the head were largely ignored in EEG studies. Rather experimental techniques were based on EEG folklore, developed primarily through trial and error in thousands of EEG studies (Nunez, 1981). However every year more science and engineering expertise is added to EEG. For example, new methods to improve spatial resolution or to obtain constrained solutions to the inverse problem have been recently implemented in some locations, as discussed in Chapter 1. This new input from the physical sciences should substantially affect experimental design, including choices of reference electrode, density of electrode array, methods of data reduction, and interpretation of data in terms of the underlying neural sources. Apparently all but a few stubborn adherents to folklore-based EEG methods now accept the need for this kind of physical science input to EEG. Such developments can be expected to continue and perhaps accelerate.

A third way in which physical science can contribute to EEG is in the development of new pattern recognition methods to quantify brain states. This potential development is largely untapped in EEG. That is, current EEG quantification methods can be described as rather crude, ad hoc approaches that have minimal bases in the underlying behavior. The development of new pattern recognition methods, which are at least partly based on theoretical considerations of neocortical dynamic function, can profoundly affect research and clinical EEG. This issue is considered in more detail in the next section, and in Chapters 6, 7, 11, and 14.

A fourth reason why methods taken from the physical sciences may be valuable in EEG is evident. It is more difficult than the others to evaluate or define precisely but generally involves raising the intellectual level of the field. Talented people are likely to be attracted to intellectually stimulating endeavors. But clinical EEG typically involves reading page after page of EEG records in search of abnormal patterns that usually are defined only approximately. Although this aspect of clinical practice requires talent and training, electroencephalographers may regard it as a tedious exercise. Furthermore, clinicians and psychologists may perform EEG experiments with little or no theoretical framework. The arbitrary nature of these efforts does not encourage good science. By connecting EEG more closely to plausible models of neocortical function, interest levels in the EEG field can be raised considerably. Perhaps this can have a positive feedback effect by attracting more scientifically oriented clinicians, physiologists, psychologists, physicists, and engineers.

Effect of Theory on Experimental EEG

Our readers span the scientific spectrum from theoretical physics to clinical practice, with perhaps a few mathematicians and philosophers included as well. Whereas all presumably have a general interest in brain function, past experience has shown that the more experimentally oriented engineers, clinicians, or physiologists may have serious doubts about whether theoretical models of neurodynamics will be practical in the near future. But even descriptive models based only on questionable analogs to physical systems can have value. Furthermore, if theories of brain function can be developed that are based, at least in part, on realistic physiology and anatomy, a very positive influence can accrue to experimental science. Experience in the physical sciences especially suggests this outcome, even with theories later proved to be wrong.

To understand the important role of theory in science generally and EEG in particular, the impression held by some, that a "bad" theory is the same thing as a "wrong" theory, must be corrected. A theory that makes serious mathematical errors will almost certainly be judged as bad. However, most bad theories are bad simply because they do not really offer anything significant; that is, they fail to make predictions that can be tested. In contrast, good theories make predictions, ideally about the outcomes of several kinds of experiments; they contain the seeds of possible ultimate rejection.

All EEG scientists have ideas about how the brain works, and they choose experimental methods biased by these views. But, without reference to some model of brain function, the nature of their biases may not be communicated clearly to other scientists. This is especially likely when communication takes place across interdisciplinary fields. Thus, for example, some engineers and physiologists have viewed brain science as a "statics problem"; that is, given some recorded EEG activity, the scientist searches for the "source" of this activity. Indeed some important practical applications of localized activity exist that should be studied in this manner. But, as we suggest here using physiologically based theory, the study of brain dynamics, not brain statics, will probably yield the most insight into more general aspects of brain function. Thus we have defined one clear role for theoretical models in EEG—one of effective communication of scientific biases, which determine which experiments are performed. This will be a critical contribution to any field in which experimental methods move in and out of favor, depending perhaps on their promotion by a few influential scientists in the field. But many experimental designs are possible for any experimental study. Furthermore, the number of possible experimental studies is much larger (by many orders of magnitude) than the number that can actually be performed. Theories provide the conceptual framework required to make better experimental choices.

Another closely related purpose of theory in experimental science involves data reduction and methods of analysis. Suppose some experimental variable, perhaps scalp potential, is measured. We want to quantify this variable to relate it to psychologic or clinical state. Because the relation is complex, we are likely to look for some mathematical transformation of the data to simplify the analysis. That is, we hope the transformed data will bear a more obvious relation to brain state than does the raw data. Common examples are a representation of a time record by a Fourier series (that is a spectral analysis) or other expansion of temporal or spatial variables in series of basis functions (such as principal components analysis, Karhunen-Loeve expansion, and singular value decomposition). Estimation of Lyapunov exponent or correlation dimension of time series are more recent additions to time domain transformations.

In fact, data can be transformed in an infinite number of ways. Many such transformations are developed and applied, typically in a variety of mathematics, physics, and engineering subfields. Consider an arbitrary transformation, say the Q transformation (QT). A range of possibilities can be considered when evaluating QT:

1. When applied to EEG data, QT reveals information that would be difficult or impossible to obtain from the raw record. Spectral and coherency analysis of EEG time series or spline-generated surface Laplacians of spatial EEG data (which estimate local cortical potential) may be placed in this category.
2. Some suggest (usually by analogy to some physical system) that QT is useful in EEG. Thus QT is applied to data sets and papers are published, but whether

QT has actually revealed anything new and useful about EEG is unclear. Chapter 10 suggests that most estimates of correlation dimension of EEG data should probably be included in this category, although some of the new ways of looking at nonlinear systems may later move to the first category above.

3. The assumptions and limitations underlying QT are so obviously violated by EEG data that QT has no serious chance of being adopted in EEG. It may be just another mathematical method (among many) in search of an application, or it may be some method that has enjoyed success in applications to systems too dissimilar to the brain to be useful. Of course, its uselessness may not prevent its advocacy in EEG by those who have invested time in becoming experts in QT, writing papers, obtaining Ph.D degrees and so on. Methods that assume that evoked potentials consist of signal added to uncorrelated noise (that is, spontaneous EEG probably generated by much of the same neural tissue that generates evoked potentials) may belong in this category. (The brainstem auditory evoked response is an exception because different neural systems contribute to signal and noise.)

New QTs are proposed regularly in EEG by mathematicians and scientist-salesmen from inside and outside the EEG field. Sometimes the limitations of the QT procedure are discussed in detail and sometimes they are not. However someone (such as a journal referee) unfamiliar with QT often has difficulty judging its potential value to EEG. We can see, for example, how this process might have worked when spectral analysis became popular in EEG in the 1970s.

The application of spectral methods to EEG has no serious mathematical limitations, but this does not, of course, necessarily mean that it will be useful. Consider the example of very long ocean waves, the tides. Suppose an observer recorded the ocean level at some fixed location near the shore during a long period of time, perhaps 1 month. He would, of course, have a very complicated signal because of the stochastic nature of the many waves. However, if he were to coarse

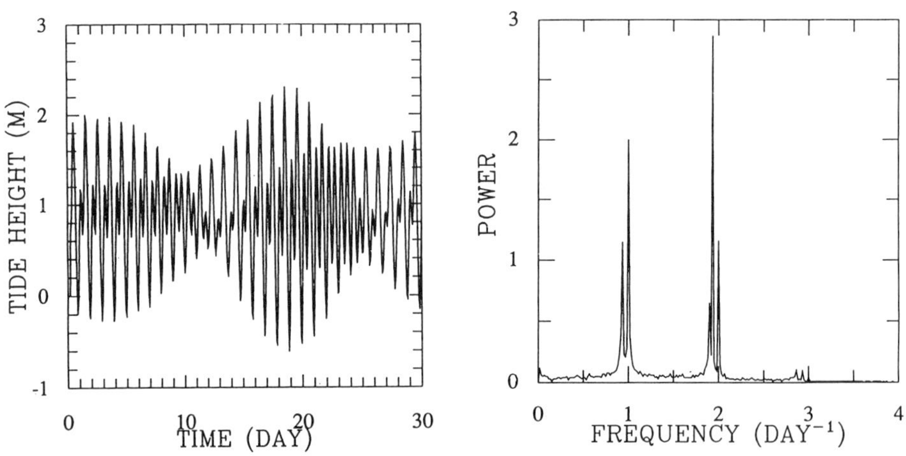

Figure 2-1. Left. "Smoothed" height of the tide off Los Angeles for January 1992. **Right.** Spectral analysis of smoothed data for the period January to June 1992.

grain his raw signal by computing a running time average during a period T of perhaps 1 hour, as in (1.1), he might obtain a smooth variation such as that shown in Figure 2-1a.

A plot of the ocean wave amplitude spectrum versus frequency is shown in Figure 2-1b. Suppose the observer had no idea of the cause of tides or even any idea of gravitational forces. Even in this state of scientific ignorance, he might guess correctly that tides are caused by actions of both the sun and moon because of the spectral peaks near periods of one half and one day. These underlying oscillations might be difficult or impossible to discover with noisy data. Given these arguments, the following suggestions can be made as a way of preliminary evaluation of the application of some new QT to EEG:

1. Try to determine whether the mathematical limitations of QT are consistent with certain kinds of EEG phenomena. Of course, this may be difficult because detailed statistical properties of EEG generally are not known. Thus step 2 is even more important.
2. Apply QT to several kinds of known systems that are postulated to have some similarities to neocortex. Consider the limitations of QT when applied to these known systems.

If QT can be shown to reveal more information about several kinds of known systems than can be obtained with existing methods, then perhaps it should be applied to EEG. If not, then there is no good reason to expect QT to be useful. This discussion suggests a second motivation for the use of theoretical models in EEG: The choice of known systems in step 2 requires determination of the systems that are likely to provide the best brain analogs.

The third motivation to use theoretical EEG models is the development of more effective pattern recognition algorithms. For example, if we can obtain a set of equations, which in some approximate sense describes a subset of EEG patterns, parameters in the equations can be fit to the EEG data. The parameters define brain state in a quantitative manner. The estimation of equivalent dipole location is a simple example of such fitting, in which five parameters indicating dipole location and orientation are determined, but this approach is probably applicable to only a few EEG phenomena. As the phenomena become more complex, quantification methods may require greater sophistication. Later chapters consider this issue in more detail.

A fourth motivation for EEG models is that they may help us understand how the brain processes information, regardless of whether EEG "waves" carry information or modulate the firing of neurons. We now know very little about neocortical dynamics. If theoretical models based on real physiology can be developed that yield even minimal agreement with observed properties of EEG, much progress will be achieved. However, until we can understand some of the more simple aspects of neocortical dynamics manifested in several EEG states, more complex processes such as the dynamics of cognition will probably remain largely beyond our reach.

Local and Global Phenomena and Linear Electrical Analogs

The issue of hierarchical level (that is, spatial scale) will probably be central to realistic theories of neocortical dynamic function. This subject is developed in detail in Chapter 14. As an introduction, we chose several physical analogs in this and the following sections to illustrate general ideas in a semiquantitative manner.

The first idea is distinction between local and global phenomena. We consider a local phenomenon to be one for which it is possible, in principle, to understand important aspects of the system dynamics only through knowledge of local properties. Predicting EEG frequency or, alternatively, some important measure of memory storage, given the properties of a cortical column, is an example. An electric circuit example, shown in Figure 2-2, consists of a large grid of circuit elements. First we imagine that we know little about the circuit elements except for the local $L_I C$ circuit (that is, the mesh) shown. What do we know about the time dependence of the current in this local circuit, given the limited information? The answer is that, in general, little or nothing can be said about the time dependence of this current. We gain little even if we are told that the same $L_I C$ mesh repeats itself throughout the grid but are not told the number of these meshes (that is we are not told the size of the overall system). However, an important special case occurs when the resistors R have sufficiently large resistance to prevent substantial current flow from outside into the local mesh. A local sensor (for example, ammeter) detects oscillations with dominant frequency equal to

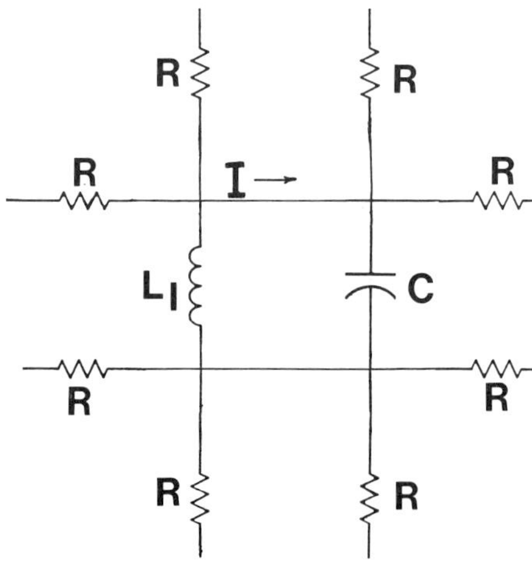

Figure 2-2. Large grid consisting of many circuit elements. One mesh consisting of a $L_I C$ circuit is shown. When the local mesh is isolated by allowing the surrounding resistances R to become large, local current oscillates with resonant frequency $\omega_0 = (L_I C)^{-1}$. However, when R is arbitrary, we cannot make predictions about local frequency based only on local circuit information. We remain ignorant, even if we know that the same mesh continually repeats itself, unless we also know the boundary conditions (such as the spatial extent of the system is both directions). These general considerations also may apply to neocortical circuits in which the degree of isolation is modified by external control parameters somewhat analogous to R. Such control can be achieved through chemical and electrical input from subcortical regions such as the brain stem activating system.

$(L_I C)^{-1}$, independent of the behavior of the large system. Based on anatomic observations, neocortical circuits are highly interconnected so that we may question the validity of EEG theories based on local circuit analogs. However, a known physiologic mechanism (lateral inhibition) may provide processes similar to the resistor R of the electric circuit, thereby localizing specific neural circuits corresponding to fixed physiologic states. This issue is considered in more detail in Chapters 5, 8, 12, and 13.

Local dynamic behavior of global phenomena are often determined by a larger system, possibly including global boundary conditions (for example, by the size and shape of the system). If, for example, the system of Figure 2-2 consists of known number of identical, repeating meshes as shown, the time dependence of the current in a local mesh can be predicted. However, if the resistors R have little resistance, so that local meshes are no longer isolated, oscillations will generally occur at many frequencies, none of which need be close to the local frequency $(L_I C)^{-1}$. Also the spectral content of the oscillations will tend to shift towards progressively lower frequencies as more identical meshes are added, that is as the size of the system increases.

A one-dimensional example of the local–global issue is the usual transmission line (for example, a coaxial television cable), but with ends connected to form a closed system as depicted in Figure 2-3. The coaxial cable consists of two conductors separated by a dielectric (partly insulating) material. With the coaxial line, outer and inner conductors are represented by a series resistance R and inductance L_I per unit length. The dielectric is represented by a capacitance C and conductance G per unit length (conductance is the inverse of resistance); the latter is included to account for current leakage across the dielectric. An applied voltage across any location of the transmission line propagates along the line with potential difference between inner and outer conductors governed by a simple wave equation. The propagation velocity v is determined by inductive and capacitive properties of the line, that is

$$v = (L_I C)^{-1/2} \tag{2.1}$$

The parameter associated with wave dispersion is the local frequency

$$\omega_0 = (RG/L_I C)^{1/2} \tag{2.2}$$

Because the transmission line forms a continuous closed loop, creating a disturbance (perhaps by passing a magnet over the line) causes standing waves of electric potential having normal mode frequencies ω_n given by the dispersion relation

$$\omega_n^2 = \omega_0^2 + v^2 k^2 \tag{2.3}$$

The dispersion relation for any wave phenomenon yields the relation between temporal (ω) and spatial (k) frequencies; the spatial frequencies are restricted in this example because the line forms a closed loop. Thus oscillations in the line are restricted to discrete temporal frequencies ω_n composed of a local frequency ω_0 (independent of the length of the line) and global frequencies $2\pi nv/L$, which

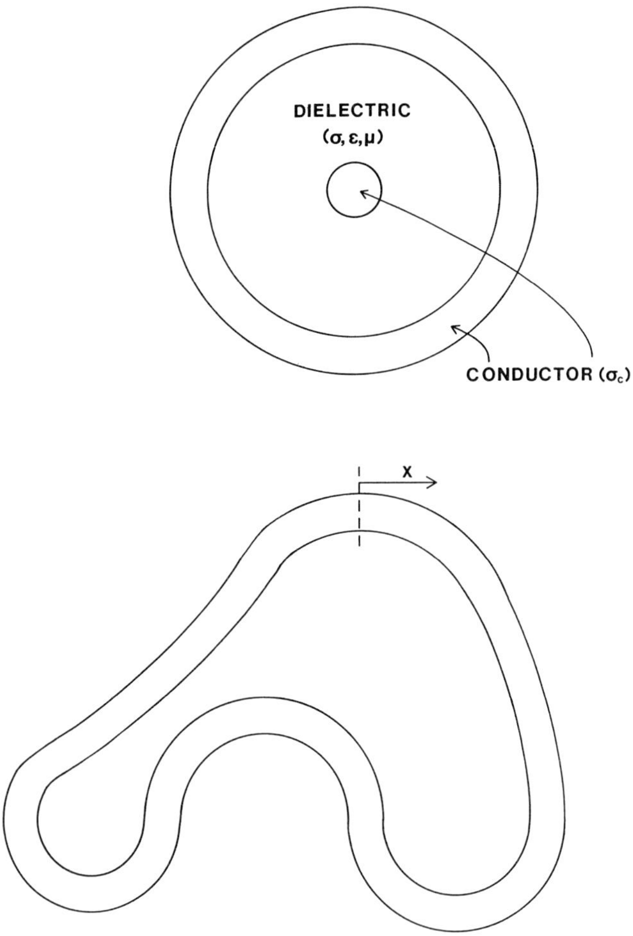

Figure 2-3. **Top**. Cross section of coaxial cable consisting of inner and outer conductors separated by dielectric (insulating) material. Conductive material is characterized by its conductivity (or resistance per unit length R). Dielectric is characterized by its conductivity or conductance per unit length G, permittivity (or capacitance per unit length C), and permeability (or inductance per unit length L_I). **Bottom**. Continuous length L of coaxial cable. Transmission lines are not usually designed like this, but an initial electromagnetic field disturbance with this geometry will produce standing waves of potential, with oscillation frequencies given by (2.3). Power distribution between the fundamental frequency ($n = 1$) and overtones ($n = 2, 3, 4, \ldots$) is determined by the spatial and temporal properties of the initial disturbance. This simple physical system illustrates a general principle that may apply to neocortex, that is, the distinction between local frequency ω_0, fully determined by a short length of the cable, and global frequency ($2\pi nv/L$), dependent on the propagation velocity v of electromagnetic waves and the length of the closed loop L. In neocortex, corticocortical action potential velocities are distributed over a relatively narrow range and the length L may be replaced by a surface area.

occur because of standing waves in a system closed on itself (periodic boundary conditions). In this analogy, neocortex of surface area L^2 is similar to a two-dimensional version of the transmission line of length L. Propagation velocity in corticocortical fibers is analogous to the transmission line velocity v, and local circuit oscillations in neocortex (perhaps at the macrocolumn or smaller scales) correspond to the local transmission line frequency ω_0.

Local theories of neocortical dynamics are considered in Chapter 5. In Chapter 11, local theories of neocortical dynamics, which predict EEG frequencies analogous to ω_0, are proposed to combine naturally with the global theory, which predicts EEG frequencies analogous to $2\pi nv/L$ in a manner somewhat similar to this combination in the transmission line and other physical systems. Of course, even these simplified EEG theories include many complexities not present in the transmission line example. Furthermore, the local–global theory is based on plausible anatomic and physiologic features. All model parameters are, in principle, measurable (no free parameters), and nothing is proved by analogy to physical systems.

External control of oscillations in the transmission line can be obtained by allowing the circuit parameters in (2.1) and (2.2) to be variable. External control of neocortical oscillations is provided by electrical and chemical input (neuromodulators) from subcortical structures, which changes control parameters of dynamic theories. These parameters are thought to change over time scales that are much longer than EEG oscillation times, so that parameters are treated as constants when the appropriate equations are solved. The control mechanisms of neocortex are discussed in Chapters 3, 4, 5, 13, and 14.

In addition, the manner in which transmission line power measured in voltage oscillations is distributed over the normal mode frequencies ω_n is determined by the initial conditions (by the path and how fast a magnet is passed over line, for example) with transient oscillations or by the input function with forced oscillations. Thus the power spectrum of voltage oscillations represents this input information; that is, it provides a crude mechanism for global memory storage.

Local and Global Phenomena and Nonlinear Analogs

The mechanical analog of the transmission line is the linear, stretched string with many attached linear springs, as shown in Figure 2-4 (Ingber and Nunez, 1990; Ingber, 1991; Nunez and Srinivasan, 1993). However, to make the analog more useful for neocortical studies, we allow local processes (the springs) to be nonlinear. In addition, we imagine a series of string displacement sensors, located outside a "blurring layer" analogous to the skull. The string displacement (analogous to modulation of cortical surface potential) is governed by

$$\frac{\partial^2 \Phi}{\partial t^2} - c^2 \frac{\partial^2 \Phi}{\partial x^2} + [\omega_0^2 + f(\Phi)]\Phi = 0 \qquad (2.4)$$

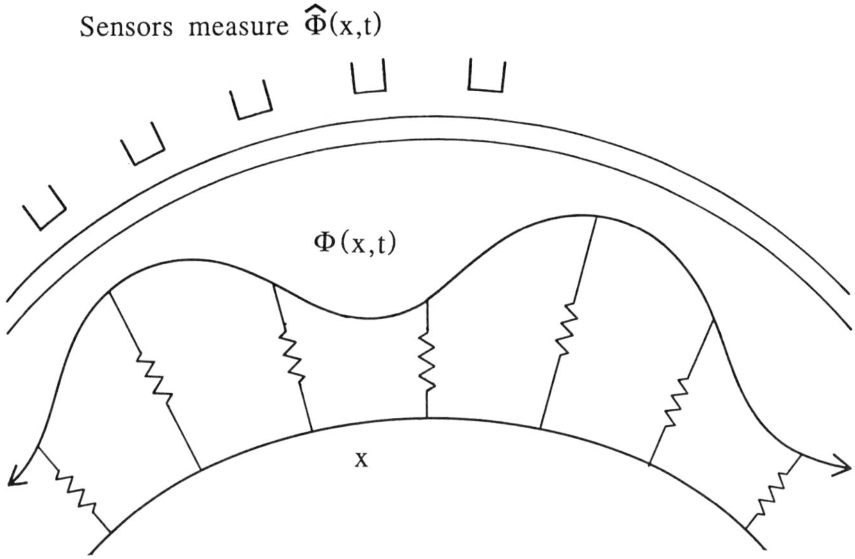

Figure 2-4. A linear stretched string is attached to nonlinear springs. The string forms a closed loop so periodic boundary conditions are appropriate. $\Phi(x, t)$ is string displacement (analogous to cortical surface potential). $\hat{\Phi}(x, t)$ is the estimate obtained by imperfect sensors (analogous to scalp potential). The sensors are located above a "blurring layer" (analogous to the skull). The linear or quasilinear string is imagined here as a metaphor for long-range neural interactions along corticocortical fibers. The nonlinear springs represent local circuit effects at macrocolumn or smaller scales. In the limiting case of linear springs, standing waves oscillate with frequencies also given by (2.3). Neocortical surface consists of 10^5 to 10^6 macrocolumns and 10^8 minicolumns.

Here the nonlinearity of the springs is described by the arbitrary function $f(\Phi)$. We seek a solution of the general form

$$\Phi(x, t) = \sum_{n=1}^{\infty} G_n(t)\sin(k_n x + \theta_n) \tag{2.5}$$

where the phases θ_n depend on initial conditions. With a closed loop of string or transmission line of length L, only an integer number of spatial wave lengths is allowed; that is,

$$k_n = \frac{2n\pi}{L} \qquad n = 1, 2, 3, \ldots \tag{2.6}$$

consistent with periodic boundary conditions. In the linear case, $f(\Phi) = 0$, and a solution to (2.4) is given by (2.5) with

$$G_n(t) = A_n \sin \omega_n t \tag{2.7}$$

and ω_n determined by the dispersion relation (2.3) for the transmission line. However, with the string and springs system, the velocity parameter v is (string tension/mass per unit length)$^{1/2}$, and ω_0 is the (spring constant/mass on the spring)$^{1/2}$. The dispersion relation is identical to that of the transmission line (2.3), except for the physical interpretation of parameters.

Consider now the relation between the actual string displacement Φ and the estimated displacement $\hat{\Phi}$, obtained with an imperfect set of sensors. The M sensors (analogous to scalp electrodes) are placed in a linear array with length that is typically a little less than one half the anterior-posterior circumference of the free (that is, not in fissures and sulci) cortical surface. The blurring layer acts to space average Φ; that is it acts as a low pass spatial filter. Chapter 1 showed that cortical EEG power is strongly attenuated with conventional methods (typically by 99%) between cortex and scalp when k_{max} is approximately 0.5 to 1.5 cm^{-1}. Because L is approximately 50 cm for the free cortical surface, (2.6) yields a crude estimate of the maximum eigenfunction that is observed experimentally with scalp recordings, that is, N is approximately 4 to 12. Thus with an abrupt cutoff of high spatial frequencies, the observed string displacement is given by

$$\hat{\Phi}(x, t) \sim \sum_{n=1}^{N} G_n(t)\sin(k_n x + \theta_n) \tag{2.8}$$

rather than by (2.5). With brain waves traveling in and out of fissures and sulci, the estimate of N is not changed because both L and the maximum observed wave number are changed by the same scale factor, which is of the order of two. We can be more precise about the macroscopic observable $\hat{\Phi}$ when this variable denotes scalp potential. That is, the spatial filtering properties of the volume conductor described by (1.20) suggest the expression

$$\hat{\Phi}(x, t) \cong \sum_{n=1}^{\infty} G_n(t)(k_n/k_1)^{-\sqrt{\delta}} \sin(k_n x + \theta_n) \tag{2.9}$$

This differs from (2.8) because a rolloff with high spatial frequencies is included in (2.9) rather than the abrupt cutoff of (2.8). The exponent $\sqrt{\delta}$ occurs because (2.9) expresses an amplitude variable, whereas (1.20) is a ratio of powers (that is, power is proportional to amplitude squared).

The nonlinear springs (or local equivalent circuit of the transmission line) are meant to be analogous to local circuit effects at the "mesoscopic" scale (between macro and microscopic) of the columnar structure of neocortex. The largest such column unit normally identified is the macrocolumn of diameter about 1 to 3 mm and containing 10^5 to 10^6 neurons and about 10^{10} synapses. Thus our minimum scalp wavelength equal to $2\pi/k_{max}$ is approximately 4 to 12 cm and spans about 10 to 100 macrocolumns. The terms "microscopic," "mesoscopic," and "macroscopic" are, by themselves, inadequate for use in the field of neocortical dynamics. For example, neuron–neuron intracortical interactions occur over about six orders of magnitude of spatial scale from the width of the synaptic cleft (10^{-6} cm) to the collateral dendrites of large pyramidal cells approximately 3 mm long, the scale that defines a macrocolumn, and surface parallel systems (about 6 to 8 mm) (Szentagothai, 1978). Furthermore, corticocortical interactions, whose fibers form most of the white matter, range from about 1 cm to 20 cm in humans (Braitenberg, 1978; Katznelson, 1981). Electrophysiologic measurements span about five orders of magnitude, ranging from microelectrode recordings at the single neuron level to scalp EEG (Petsche et al, 184; Nunez, 1981, 1990a). Thus spatial scales must be identified quantitatively in theoretical and experimental studies, as discussed in detail in Chapter 14.

Spatial scale can be described simply in general terms in connection with the string and springs model. In the proposed analogy to neocortex, the linear string is meant to represent interactions by means of long corticocortical fibers that carry action potentials with velocities in the typical range of approximately 6 to 9 m/second (Nunez, 1981; Katznelson, 1981). Under reasonable assumptions, these long-range interactions lead to linear or quasilinear integral equations (Nunez, 1974a, 1981, 1988, 1989a, 1989b; Nunez and Srinivasan, 1993; Katznelson, 1981; see also Chapter 11). Given these assumptions, what can we determine about the macroscopic observable $\hat{\Phi}(x, t)$, representing either estimated string displacement or scalp surface potential? We may guess that $\hat{\Phi}(x, t)$ can be described as a linear or quasilinear variable but influenced by local nonlinear behavior (because of springs or cortical columns) that crosses the hierarchical level from mesoscopic to macroscopic.

The string and spring model also illustrates the issue of "bottom up" compared with "top down" influences. For example, if we relax the string tension so that the velocity v becomes very small, the springs become decoupled, and each spring moves independently. The string is driven by the springs with negligible feedback from string to springs, which is a purely bottom-up influence and, in the linear case, oscillations occur at the local frequency ω_0. In neocortex, cutting the corticocortical fibers is somewhat analogous. Of course, this does not decouple macrocolumns because overlapping intracortical connections remain. However, it does remove important long-range influences, and the cutting of the callosal fibers (connecting the two brain hemispheres) causes a substantial decrease in EEG coherency between hemispheres (Nunez, 1981).

The opposite limiting case occurs when the spring constants relating force to displacement become very small. The feedback of spring forces on the string becomes small, and the springs are driven by the string, a purely top-down influence. A simple nonlinear spring driven by an external sinusoidal force can undergo chaotic motion (Ueda, 1980). Furthermore, several equations similar to (2.4) were studied numerically (Tabor, 1989), including equations motivated by studies in fluid mechanics (Lorenz, 1963), or the sine-Gordon equation describing Josephson-type transmission lines or relativistic field theory (Bishop et al, 1983; Tabor, 1989). Interesting behavior can be observed, including temporal chaos in the presence of stable, spatial structures (for example, solitons). However, the relation of microscopic chaos on macroscopic observables is generally not well understood. This issue is approached formally in Chapter 14 by integrating a critical mesoscopic variable over wave numbers k_n for $n > N$ to define a coarse-grained probability density function. Integration over fine-grained wave numbers smooths the influence of the k_n independent variables for $n > N$, effectively "renormalizing" dependent variables. This approach is similar to other modern studies of complex physical systems, in which the connection between variables defined at different scales is a central issue.

Standing Waves on Closed Surfaces

Issues related to neocortical interactions at microscopic and mesoscopic scales are very complex and will provide formidable challenges to theoreticians and experimentalists in the future. Ingber suggests that neocortex is the prototype medium for application of the new methods of nonlinear, nonequilibrium statistical mechanics, which were developed primarily since the 1970s (see Chapter 14). However, this section takes a more modest approach. We simply neglect all submacroscopic influence on the macroscopic scale; for example, we neglect the springs in our string and spring model, which is analogous to neglecting the local circuit delays in the neocortical model. In Chapters 5 and 11, local circuit effects are included in an approximate manner, but we focus here only on the effects of global boundary conditions. We do not suggest that local effects and nonlinearity are unimportant. Rather we want to consider only one set of issues at a time in this introductory chapter.

That standing waves occur in the brain may appear very speculative, especially to those neuroscientists who think in terms of locating centers of activity responsible for specific functions or EEG phenomena. Others, who take a more global or holistic view of brain operation, may be more receptive. Experimental support for the general standing wave concept, in which global boundary conditions and time lags due to corticocortical propagation play an important role, is emphasized in Chapters 3, 6, 11, 12, and 13. The reasons for early introduction are as follows:

1. Many neuroscientists are unfamiliar with the fundamental concepts of boundary conditions and wave interference except in the context of an (often) long-forgotten elementary physics course. This background is not sufficient for easy extrapolation to complex systems.
2. Experience with physical systems suggests that global boundary conditions usually make important, if not critical, contributions to system dynamics, whether the system is simple or complex. This fact may be obscured when theoreticians concentrate on a particular part of some problem, as with the famous Lorenz equations exhibiting chaotic behavior, which place minimal emphasis on boundary conditions in the actual physical system (see Chapter 10). By in large, however, theoretical studies of real systems (rather than mathematical abstractions) must include boundary conditions if agreement with experiment is to be achieved. This is apparently true of the actual physical system associated with the Lorenz equations, for example. Another example is provided by computer simulations of the dynamics of galaxies (Miller, 1992). The microstructure (trajectories of individual stars) predicted by these simulations varies dramatically with initial conditions; that is the system is chaotic. However, large-scale structures (star groups) are similar for different initial conditions and show radial standing wave phenomena ("breathing"). Nothing about brain anatomy or physiology obviously

distinguishes it from known physical systems in regard to the importance of boundary conditions. In fact, the extreme interconnectivity of the closed neocortical system appears to make global operation and boundary conditions especially important.

3. Physiologic parameters at large neural scales are known more accurately. Thus we can make quantitative predictions of EEG frequencies and other macroscopic observables based on parameters measured at macroscopic scales. Such comparisons of theory and experiment are more difficult to achieve at submacroscopic scales, in which we can become lost quickly in a myriad of unknown parameters.

4. The principal long-range goal of neocortical dynamic studies is to understand how brains process information. Our emphasis on EEG is due mainly to its ability to provide quantitative measures of cognitive processing, thereby providing a way to verify tentative theories. Specific cognitive events, indeed consciousness itself, evidently involves the global dynamics of brain in which the interactions between distributed systems (neural circuits, for example) is essential. Thus the global macroscopic theory of Chapter 11 and the multiple scale statistical theory of Chapter 14 contain many implications beyond narrow EEG issues. In contrast, local circuit theories may not have the same potential for extension to more general studies of higher brain function.

With these motivations in mind, consider still another physical analog, the spherical shell formed by the earth's surface and the bottom of the ionosphere, as indicated in Figure 2-5. The usual solution to Maxwell's equations for the resonant cavity in spherical geometry yields predicted normal mode frequencies of the electromagnetic field (Jackson, 1975) of

$$\omega_\ell = \sqrt{\ell(\ell + 1)}\,\frac{c}{R} \qquad \ell = 1, 2, 3, \ldots \tag{2.10}$$

where c is the velocity of light and R is the earth's radius. This is the two-dimensional analog of the dispersion relation (2.3). These "Schumann resonances" (named after the scientist who predicted them with theory) have theoretical mode frequencies of

$$f_\ell = \frac{\omega_\ell}{2\pi} \sim 10.6,\ 18.3,\ 25.8,\ \ldots\ \text{Hz} \tag{2.11}$$

→

Figure 2-5. **Top**. Spherical shell formed by the earth's surface and the bottom of the ionosphere. The resonant frequencies of f_ℓ depend on the velocity of light ($v = 3 \times 10^{10}$ cm/sec), the radius of the earth ($R = 6.4 \times 10^8$ cm), and the index ($\ell = 1, 2, 3, \ldots$) associated with the spherical harmonic standing wave patterns $Y_{\ell,m}(\theta, \phi)$. This resonant cavity exhibits normal mode frequencies of electromagnetic standing waves (Schumann resonances) expressed by (2.10); that is, $f_\ell = 10.6, 18.3, 25.8, 33.4, 40.9 \ldots$ Hz. Measured spectral peaks are close to these predicted values. **Bottom.** Brain-like structure imagined to result from mentally inflating the cerebral cortex to smooth the fissured surface. The spherical shell of white matter is filled with corticocortical axons with propagation velocity in the approximate range of 6 to 9 m/second (see Figure 2-6). The radius of the

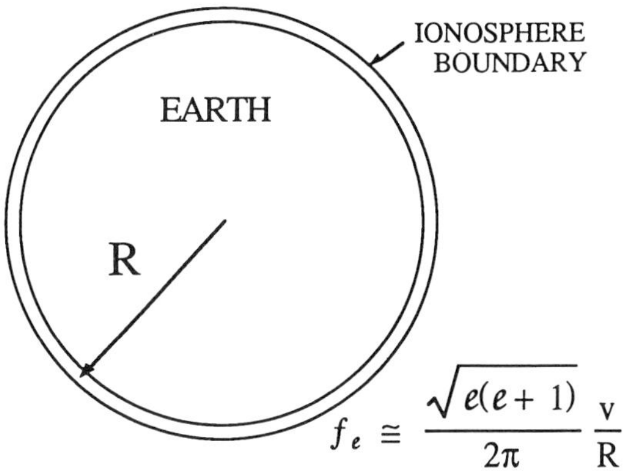

SCHUMANN RESONANCES

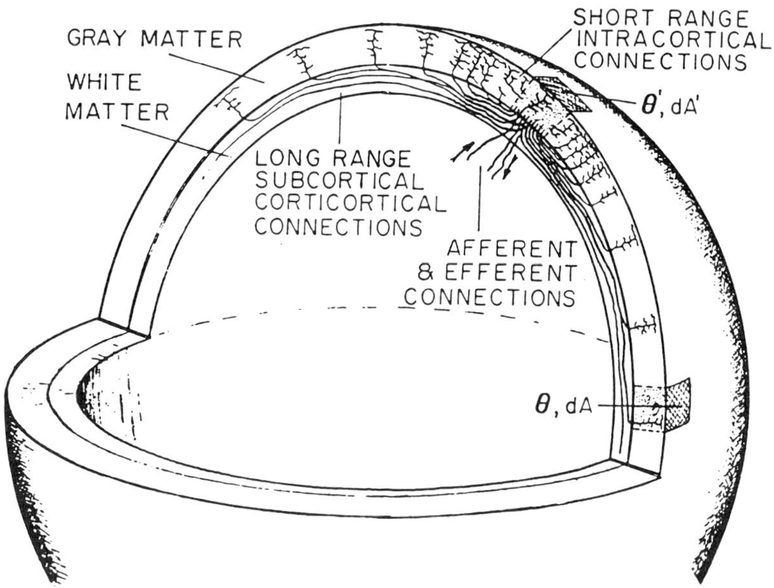

NEOCORTICAL RESONANCES

sphere is defined by the equivalent neocortical surface area; that is, R ~ 11 to 18 cm. The fundamental frequency (equation 2.10) estimated for putative nondispersive brain waves is then $f_1 \sim 7$ to 18 Hz. When estimated frequency is based on a single hemisphere, but with a more realistic shape (such as prolate spheriod), a similar frequency range is predicted for the fundamental mode. A physiologically based theory, developed in Chapter 11, makes similar predictions, except that the dispersion relation is more complicated and depends on at least one cortical control parameter that can change with physiologic state. (Reproduced with permission from Katznelson, 1981.)

that agree closely with the experimental values 1.28 f_ℓ, (Wagner and Balser, 1960). The correction factor is required because of the approximation of boundary conditions in the theory. Experimental spectra also indicate a dominance of the fundamental mode, with progressively smaller contributions from higher and higher overtones (modes). That the fundamental mode is close to the human alpha frequency is probably a coincidence, although it may be impossible to completely dismiss some subtle evolutionary coupling with the human brain. However, this apparent coincidence is unrelated to our reasons for predicting standing brain waves.

What have the Schumann resonances to do with the putative brain waves? Suppose we fill a spherical shell with fibers of different lengths that carry signals (action potentials) at much slower velocity and connect them to local relay circuits. Furthermore, we will scale down the system to the size of human neocortex, as indicated in Figure 2-5. In making this analogy, we must remember that specificity of connections between different regions is apparently important at small scales. However, at scales greater than 1 cm, every region may be connected to a large fraction of similar regions in the same hemisphere (Braitenberg, 1978; Nunez, 1981; Katznelson, 1981) implying some degree of homogeneity and isotrophy at macroscopic scales. The analogy to Schumann resonances may be less compelling when corticocortical connections are strongly anisotropic and inhomogeneous, (for example at small scales).

Estimates of the propagation velocity in myelinated corticocortical fibers are reviewed in Chapter 11 and in Katznelson (1981). Although the data have disparate sources, that is from direct measurements of velocity in the monkey and axon diameter histograms in humans, the agreement is good. The probability density function for (myelinated) corticocortical propagation peaks at about $v \sim 6$ to 9 m/second, with half-width of the distribution estimated to be about 3 m/second, as shown in Figure 2-6. Published estimates of neocortical surface area range from 1600 to 4000 cm^2 (Blinkov and Glezer, 1968; Mountcastle, 1979). This range corresponds to effective cortical radii (after mentally inflating the folded surface) of $R \sim 11$ to 18 cm. Equation (2.10) provides a crude estimate for the fundamental mode ($\ell = 1$) of possible "nondispersive brain waves" of

$$f_1 \sim 7 \text{ to } 18 \text{ Hz} \tag{2.12}$$

This frequency range is within a factor of about two of several human EEG states, such as resting with eyes closed (alpha), alpha coma, halothane anesthesia, and parts of sleep spectra, EEG phenomena that typically have high spatial coherency and sharp peaks in the spectra (as needed to unambiguously define "mode frequency" experimentally). Many other EEG states have complicated spectra, but in all states most surface EEG power measured with macroscopic electrodes in humans is less than 15 Hz on the scalp, with higher frequencies recorded from the cortex.

Although the estimate (2.12) may be another coincidence, it has enough physiologic and anatomic substance to have provided an incentive to look for EEG frequencies in this range if the estimate had been made before the first recording

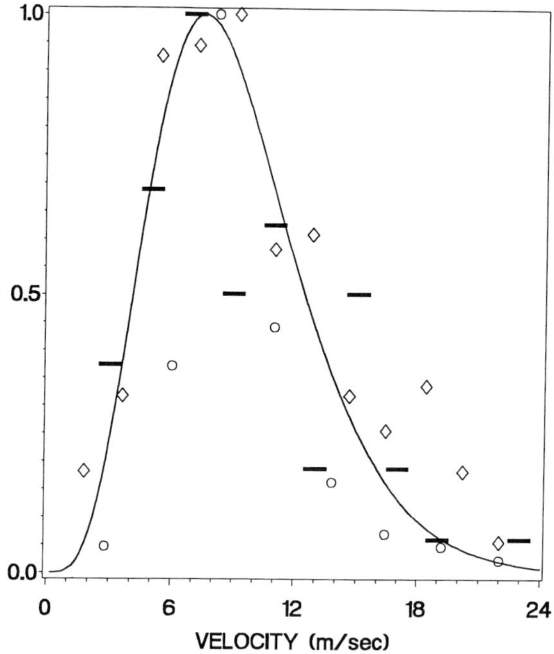

Figure 2-6. Estimated distribution of propagation velocity in myelinated corticocortical fibers. Three disparate sets of data were normalized for plotting on the same scale. Diameter histograms in humans (circles and diamonds) were used to estimate velocity based on the experimentally determined transformation v = 5.5 m/second per micrometer of axon diameter (Waxman and Bennett, 1972). Circle data were obtained from corpus callosum (Tomasch, 1954). Diamond data were obtained from frontal lobe (Bishop and Smith, 1964). Direct velocity estimates (bars) were obtained from callosal fibers of rhesus monkey (Swadlow et al, 1978). Additional data that are qualitatively consistent but could not be normalized accurately for this plot were omitted (for example, Blinkov and Glezer, 1968). Data were originally reviewed in Katznelson, 1981. The data were fit to the function $f(v) \sim v^n \exp(-av)$, with n equal to 4.5 (solid line).

of the human EEG in 1928. Of course, the specific mode frequencies (2.10), valid only for nondispersive waves in a spherical shell, have minimal physiologic basis; they would provide only crude frequency estimates, even if the general concept of standing waves in neocortex is correct. First, no reason is apparent for brain waves to be nondispersive (that is, travel with undistorted waveform). The dispersion relation equivalent to (2.10) must be based on interactions in the actual neocortical medium. Second, complicated boundary conditions are due to cortical geometry and inhomogeneity/anisotropy of corticocortical connections. Other major considerations are nonlinearity and local circuit effects. For example, multiple global modes allow for possible matching of global with local resonant frequencies, with different local resonances occurring in different parts of the brain. These issues are discussed in Chapters 3, 5, 6, 11, 12, 13, and 14.

Experimental Implications of Neocortical Standing Waves

No claim is made here that the relatively simple standing wave phenomena described previously approximate the complexity of neocortical dynamics. Rather we view these physical analogs as a means to estimate the possible effects of global boundary conditions on brain function. With this caveat in mind, we tentatively assume that some EEG phenomena are composed of linear or quasilinear standing waves and see what EEG behavior this assumption implies. It is perhaps surprising how many correct qualitative and, in several cases, semiquantitative predictions about disparate EEG experiments follow from this assumption. As further support for this general approach, plausible physiologic bases for this theory at large scales are described in detail in Chapter 11. As an introduction to this idea, a brief summary of several experimental connections follows:

1. An approximately correct prediction of the general frequency range of spontaneous EEG is obtained, as suggested in the section Standing Waves on Closed Surfaces. That is, the dispersive waves predicted by the physiologically based theory of Chapter 11 have lowest modes in the 10-Hz range, within a factor of about two.

2. As with all wave phenomena, a relation (or perhaps multiple relations) exists between spatial and temporal frequency. Normally we expect high temporal frequencies of "waves" to be associated more with high spatial frequencies. This is a possible reason for the attenuation of high temporal frequencies between cortex and scalp observed for spontaneous EEG. Direct evidence for the existence of dispersion relations for spontaneous EEG was obtained from frequency–wave number spectra (Nunez, 1974b, 1981). That is, the spectral density function $G(\omega, k)$ shows a tendency for high spatial frequencies to occur with high temporal frequencies, as suggested by Figure 2-7. In more recent work on spontaneous EEG, the spatially aliased power obtained with 5-cm electrode spacing was estimated using 2-cm electrode spacing (Shaw, 1991). The aliased power is plotted versus frequency in Figure 2-8, which shows a consistent power increase with frequency in four participants for frequencies greater than 10 Hz. This suggests the existence of a dispersion relation for this frequency range, which would be expected if the fundamental mode of the system is near to 10 Hz, with many closely spaced higher modes occurring, as in a typical resonant cavity with complicated geometry and inhomogeneous properties.

3. A relation exists between cortical surface area and EEG frequency. That is, the existence of standing wave phenomena suggests that, if all other influences are equal, larger systems produce lower normal mode frequencies. This prediction is supported by a study involving human alpha rhythm, as shown by Figure 2-9 (Nunez et al, 1977; Nunez, 1981).

Because mammalian cortices are similar, we could inquire whether the size–frequency relation can be applied to nonhuman mammals. This idea is complicated by the fact that the ratio of corticocortical to subcortical fibers is much higher in humans than in other mammals and by other important anatomic differences. Nevertheless, rough estimates of expected lower modes can be obtained from linear scale factors, which are the cube roots of the ratios of human to nonhuman brain weights. For example, the brain of the bottlenose dolphin

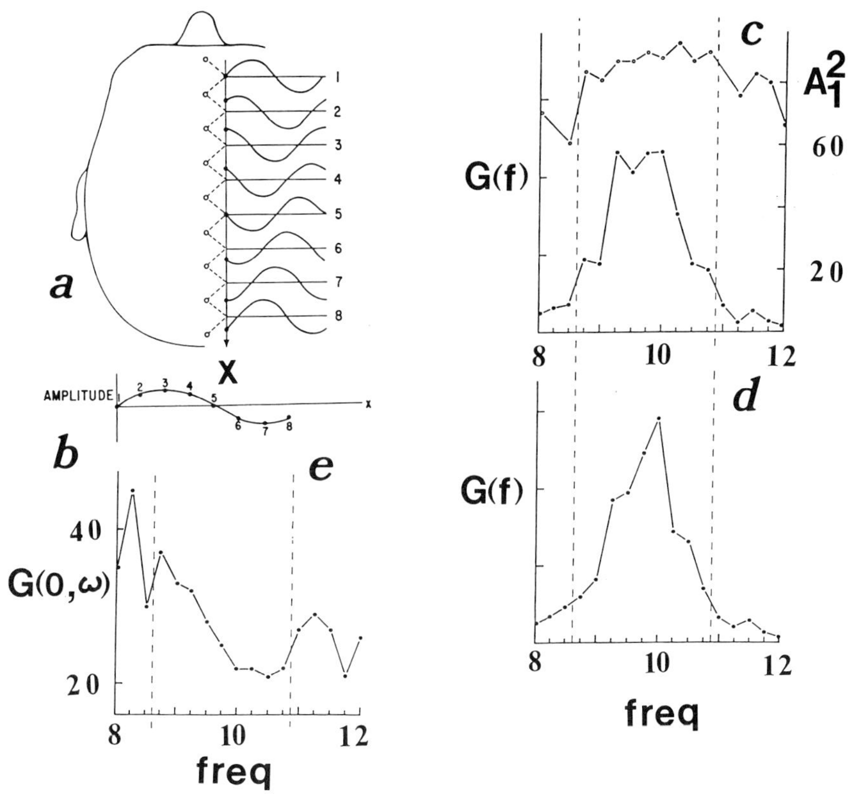

Figure 2-7. **a.** Electrode placement (open circles) used to record eight bipolar channels of alpha rhythm and calculate frequency–wave number spectra. Each channel shown produces a sine function with the same frequency but phase proportional to distance (x) along the midline. Center-to-center electrode spacing is 3 cm; effective electrode diameter is about 1 cm. A bipolar montage yields estimates of tangential electric field halfway between electrodes. Effective sampling length of array for the electric field is a = 24 cm. **b.** The amplitude at a fixed time (black dots) is shown to vary as a sine function in location to indicate a single wavelength approximately equal to the length of the electrode array. **c.** Power spectrum (lower curve) for channel 1 obtained from 4 minutes of highly peaked alpha rhythm (eyes closed, alpha index > 3.0; see Nunez, 1981 [subject MF]). A_1 is the coefficient of the first spatial principal component (orthogonal eigenfunction). **d.** Power spectrum for channel 8, same 4-minute record. **e.** Power in k = 0 band expressed as a percentage of total power. This general behavior of a shift in G(k, ω) toward higher wave numbers (k) as frequency increased through the alpha band was observed in all 13 participants studied in this manner. Because of the very limited spatial resolution at long spatial wavelengths, details of G(k, ω) were not obtained. (Reproduced with permission from Nunez, 1974b, 1981.)

typically weighs 1600 g (Ridgway, 1990); a typical human brain weighs 1350 g, so the linear scale factor is $(1350/1600)^{1/3} \sim 0.9$. Data on dolphin EEG are rare, but a typical, awake spontaneous EEG rhythm of 8 Hz has been reported (Ridgway, 1991). For the dog, this ratio is $(1350/70)^{1/3} \sim 2.7$. The dog exhibits a cortical EEG rhythm that peaks near 28 Hz in certain behavioral states (Lopes da Silva

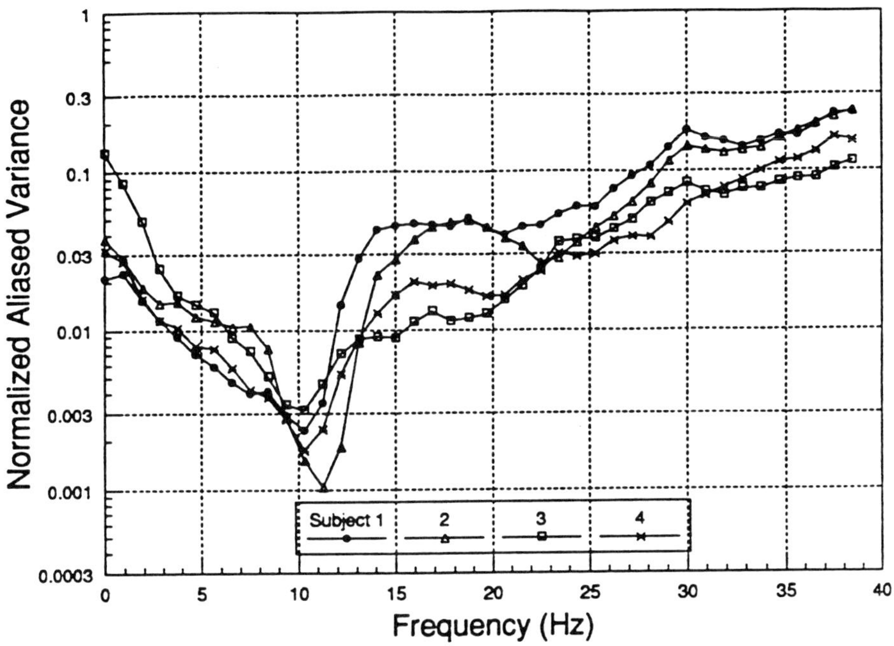
Normalized Aliased Variance
Frequency (Hz)
Subject 1
2
3
4

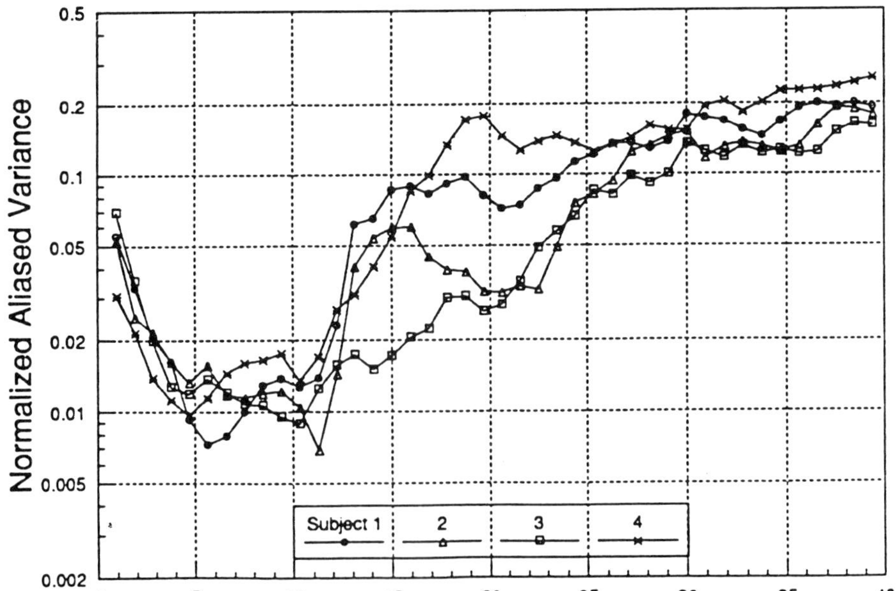
Normalized Aliased Variance
Frequency (Hz)
Subject 1
2
3
4

et al, 1970b), although we know of no evidence that this is a global mode. Also, driving the visual system of the dog with sine wave-modulated light produces a resonance-like peak in the same frequency range (Lopes da Silva et al, 1970a; Lopes da Silva and van Rotterdam, 1970b), which appears analogous to a similar effect in humans near 10 Hz (van der Tweel and Verduyn Lunel, 1965; Regan, 1988). Under halothane anesthesia, the dog may produce rhythms that are also about twice the frequency of the human halothane rhythm (Katznelson, 1981).

With the cat, the linear scale factor is $(1350/30)^{1/3} \sim 3.6$. A cortical rhythm of 35 to 45 Hz was recorded in the motor and parietal regions of alert cats (Bouyer et al, 1987), in rough agreement with predicted frequency ranges due only to size changes. The rhesus monkey has a linear scale factor of $(1350/90)^{1/3} \sim 2.5$. Electroencephalographic activity with a mean spectral peak of 30 ± 3.7 Hz was reported when the rhesus monkey accurately carried out a conditioned response (Freeman and Van Dijk, 1987). Again this EEG is generally consistent with the size–frequency relation.

The crude theoretical and experimental comparisons outlined above are, however, clouded by a 12-Hz rhythm in the dog, which is recorded in parts of the cortex and thalamus, is attenuated by opening eyes, and is apparently similar to the human alpha rhythm (Lopes da Silva and Storm van Leeuwen, 1978). Also alpha-like rhythms in the 10-Hz range have been recorded in the monkey. Possible explanations for dog and monkey rhythms in the 10-Hz range are that they are analogous to lower modes than the human alpha, are dominated more by local delays, involve nonlinear phenomena, or any combination of effects, some of which are discussed in Chapter 11. In any case, these estimates neglect many complications that are not accounted for by a transformation based only on size. In particular, different modes of rhythmic activity can be recorded from the same cortical sites, depending on the behavioral state of the animal (Lopes da Silva, 1991). Physiologists may tend to focus more attention on frequency ranges (such as alpha) of special importance in humans and thereby introduce some bias into the literature.

If all brains and neurons were exactly the same, except for size, a standing wave view of EEG based on corticocortical propagation would predict that all brains would produce the same normal mode frequencies. This follows because propagation velocity in myelinated corticocortical fibers is proportional to axon diameter. Thus, if axon diameter were to increase in proportion to brain size,

Figure 2-8. Spatially aliased EEG power as a function of temporal frequency, based on a spatial sampling (electrode spacing) of 5 cm. Aliased power is estimated based on comparison of data obtained with 2-cm spacing. Aliased power is minimal in the alpha frequency range (peak in the spectrum for eyes-closed data, upper record), indicating that the alpha range (also, 5 to 10 Hz for the eyes-open, lower record) is comprised of the longest spatial wavelengths (smallest modes k_n). The progressive increase of aliased power for higher frequencies is consistent with the existence of a dispersion relation; that is, higher spatial frequencies tend to occur with higher temporal frequencies. However, this effect only occurs for frequencies higher than alpha, as would be expected if the fundamental mode occurs in the alpha band. Data were obtained from electrodes placed on a 60-cm circumference of the head (average reference). The four plots show consistent behavior in four subjects. (Reproduced with permission from Shaw, 1991.)

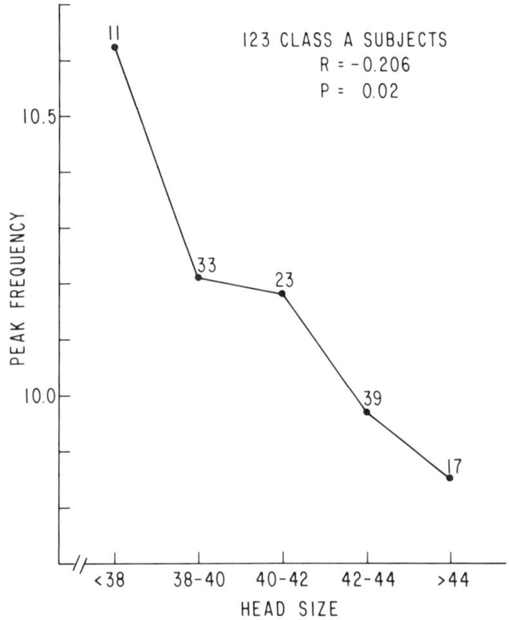

Figure 2-9. The relation of head size to peak alpha frequency is shown. Head size is defined as the cube root of the product of three linear measures. Peak frequency is determined by the peak power histogram. The black dots represent the average frequency of the local group of head sizes, as defined by the lower axis. The scatter diagram has a correlation coefficient $r = -0.206$ and significance $p = 0.02$. When head size is plotted versus "maximum frequency" (as determined by the peak power histogram), $r = -0.233$ and $p = 0.01$. See Chapter 12 for more details. (Reproduced with permission from Nunez et al, 1977.)

the propagation velocity and frequency would remain constant. Although axon diameter changes with mammalian species, the relation is not systematically related to brain size (Tower, 1954; Bok, 1959; Blinkov and Glezer, 1968). Based on the data cited above, we regard the nonhuman EEG data as inconclusive with regard to the general idea of standing waves in human neocortex.

More evidence comes from olfactory bulb data, which have been studied in a variety of species. Not all studies have obtained frequency spectra and some data show very broad spectra, thus limiting information on spectral peaks. Furthermore, we do not have exact information on olfactory bulb size. However, if we take the approximate frequency data (based mainly on zero crossings) at face value and assume that the olfactory bulb linear scale factor varies with the cube root of brain mass (which would be the case for similar brains), Figure 2-10 is obtained. Thus EEG frequencies in this neural system appear to be related to size of the system in the general manner expected with standing waves.

Freeman (1987, 1990) and co-workers proposed nonlinear theoretical models to explain olfactory bulb EEG. The arguments of this section neither support nor refute these models. Rather they suggest the important prediction that global (in this case an approximately spherical bulb with a diameter of several millimeters) boundary conditions may play an important role in EEG production. This idea should be considered in future theoretical models. In addition, this story illustrates the importance of theory to experiment. That is, if olfactory bulb investigators had considered the idea that a size–frequency relation might be important, estimates of these particular variables may have been considered more closely.

Another check of the idea of standing waves in olfactory bulb comes from the fact that its EEG rhythms are reported to originate at centers of activity and spread to other regions, somewhat like waves created by raindrops on a pond

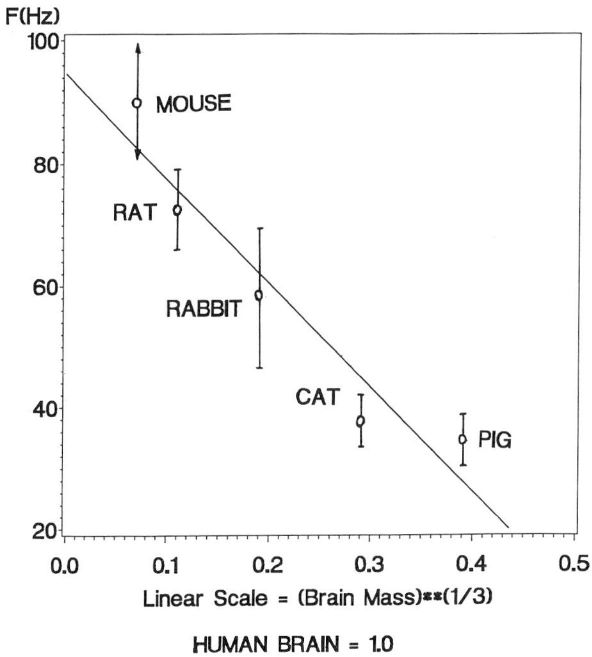

Figure 2-10. Olfactory bulb EEG frequency versus brain size. Cat and rabbit frequencies were obtained from Bressler and Freeman, 1980. Approximate data on mouse, rat, and pig (70 kg) were obtained by personal communication from Freeman in 1992 and 1994. (Earlier reports on rat data have been corrected based on recent experiments.) Frequency estimates were obtained from zero crossings. The linear scale is normalized so that the human brain size is 1.0 (see Table 2-1). The olfactory bulb does not change size in direct proportion to brain size. (For example, the human olfactory bulb is about the same size as the cat's.) However, the linear scale provides an approximate idea of relative bulb size in the species shown.

(Freeman, 1988, 1990). Although the underlying mechanisms that determine this spread are not understood, the "velocity of spreading" was estimated experimentally to be about 180 cm/second in the cat (Freeman, 1990). This figure can be compared with the expected surface velocity for nondispersive waves on a spherical surface using (2.10). That is, if waves of frequency f are approximately 40 to 50 Hz and correspond to the fundamental mode, surface propagation velocity in the olfactory bulb of radius R approximately 3 to 4 mm should be about

$$c = \sqrt{2}\pi R f_1 \sim 50 - 90 \text{ cm/sec} \qquad (2.13)$$

Because the experimental velocity is only a rough estimate and, in any case, the calculation (2.13) is based on the simplistic assumptions of linear, nondispersive waves, the agreement is fair.

4. Predictions of the resonant properties of neocortex agree, at least in some cases, semiquantitatively with experiment. Neocortical resonance is typically studied by driving the visual system with sine wave-modulated light. Of course,

many more complications are inherent in this type of study than in cases of resonance in simple mechanical or electrical systems. For example, we can control input to the retina, but this implies only partial control of input to the cortex because information is processed along the visual pathway. Furthermore, as in all systems having "significant" (defined more precisely in Chapter 9) spatial extent, resonance effects are expected to depend on the spatial and temporal properties of cortical input.

Despite these complications, we can consider the resonance response of relatively simple waves on a closed surface in relation to experimental evidence with EEG. However, rather than be limited by a spherical surface, we consider a slightly more complicated model—the prolate spheroid having a size and shape roughly similar to that of one brain hemisphere, but mentally "inflated" to account for fissures and sulci. The calculations required to determine normal mode frequencies for the prolate spheroid are outlined in Chapter 9. If a surface propagation velocity of 6 m/second is chosen (within the known range of 6 to 9 m/second for the bulk of action potential propagation in corticocortical fibers), predicted normal mode frequencies are those plotted in Figure 2-11b. The primary difference between spherical and prolate spheroidal models is a splitting of the $\ell = 1$ spherical mode into two separate modes, splitting of the $\ell = 2$ modes into three separate modes, and so on. The resonance response of the human brain to sinusoidally modulated light in one series of experiments (Regan, 1988) is shown in Figure 2-11a. Of course, the amount of resonance (the amplitude associated with each frequency component) should depend on the spatial distribution of cortical input (in relation to the nodes of the normal mode eigenfunctions), for example, in a manner analogous to power distribution in the closed transmission line. Figure 2-12 illustrates this idea, in which a prolate spheroidal shell is driven by transient input at two locations. The normal mode frequencies do not change when the input locations are changed because they are pure global phenomena. However, the power associated with each mode and the spatial properties of surface patterns change.

The agreement of Figure 2-11 is fair considering the crudeness of physiologic and anatomic data used in the theoretical calculations. Furthermore, nondispersive waves (those that do not distort as they propagate) have been assumed here for which no justification has been provided. (Dispersion relations are derived in Chapter 11.) In any case, this comparison involves no free parameters. We simply chose the surface propagation velocity in the correct range (6 to 9 meters/second) but also so that the two lowest modes ($\ell = 1$) line up approximately with the lower resonant frequency range. This procedure causes the higher resonant curve to line up roughly with the $\ell = 2$ modes. Again we have neglected many important details, including the possible importance of local resonant effects and nonlinearity. We should not imagine simple standing wave phenomena, but rather that this general idea is not implausible as a first guess. Neocortical resonance is an important but complicated issue considered in more detail in Chapter 6, with emphasis on apparent connections to standing wave phenomena and relations to cognitive processing. Of special interest are apparent nodal lines separating regions of neocortex. Chapters 3, 6, and 12 contain examples.

5. The global wave theory provides a possible partial explanation for the tuning of EEG by varying the depth of anesthesia. Using the simple example of wave

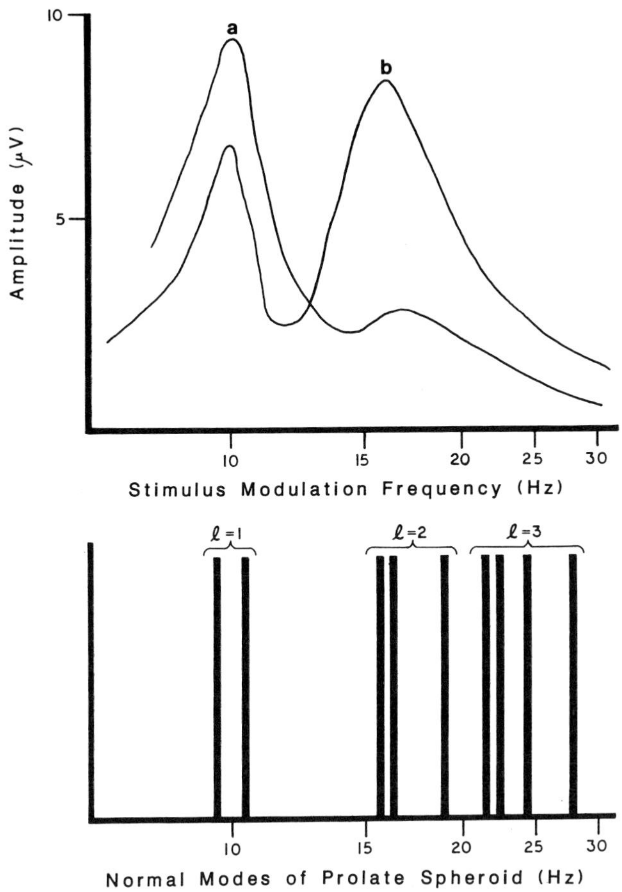

Figure 2-11. Top. Root-mean-square amplitude of steady-state scalp-evoked potential. Response of human brain to sine wave-modulated light, red on blue (a) and red (b). Centrally fixed stimulus field of 60 degrees subtense; mean retinal illumination, 3900 trolands; luminance modulation depth, 33%. Reproduced with permission from Regan, 1988. Other experiments on humans show that the response of the brain is sensitive to stimulus parameters. Also both linear and nonlinear responses apparently are possible depending on parameters and subject (Van der Tweel and Verduyn Lunel, 1965). **Bottom.** Lowest normal mode frequencies $\omega_{\ell m}$ (ℓ = 1, 2, 3) for nondispersive waves on the surface of a prolate spheroidal shell constructed with a medium with propagation velocity = 6 m/second, semimajor axis before stretching to account for fissures and sulci = 8.4 cm, stretching factor = 2.2, and eccentricity = 0.8. These data are based on estimates of propagation velocity in corticocortical fibers and actual shape of one brain hemisphere (Nunez, 1981). Uncertainty in the location of the lowest mode (assuming nondispersive waves) is perhaps a factor of two. Relative uncertainty of higher modes is probably less. When eccentricity is zero, normal mode frequencies are those of a spherical shell (equation 2.10), independent of m index. Departures from prolate spheriodal geometry or inhomogeneity–anisotropy of neocortical connections can be expected to cause further splitting of degenerate modes. Modes calculated from Helmholtz equation using classical methods (Morse and Feshbach, 1953). See Chapter 9 for more details. (Reproduced with permission from Nunez, 1989b.)

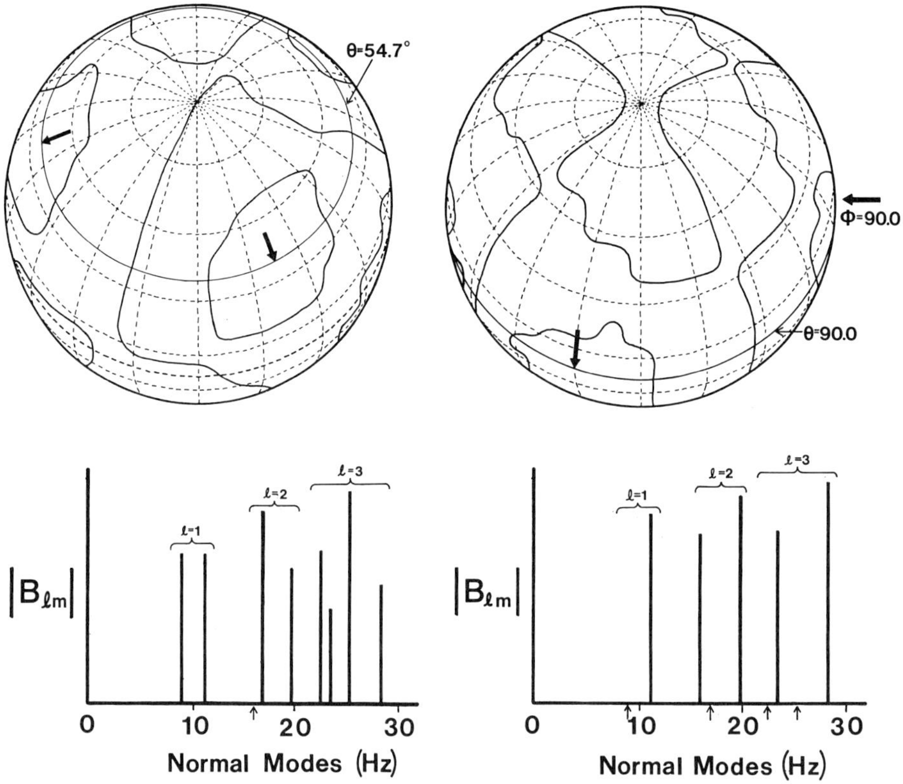

Figure 2-12. Spatial patterns and normal mode frequencies for standing waves in a prolate spheriodal shell, similar to Schumann resonances. Transient input (similar to lighting striking in the atmosphere) occurs at two locations, indicated by heavy arrows. Normal mode frequencies ($\omega_{\ell m}$, $\ell = 1, 2, 3, \ldots$ $m = 0, \ell$) are fixed; however, when input occurs on a nodal line of one of the eigenfunctions, the corresponding frequency does not occur in the resulting transient oscillation. For example in the left column, both inputs occur on the nodal line of the $\ell = 2$, $m = 0$ eigenfunction ($\theta = 54.7°$), so this mode (small arrow near 17 Hz) does not occur in the oscillation. In the right column, inputs occur at $\theta = 90°$ ($\phi = 0°$ and $90°$); these locations lie on the nodal lines of the four modes shown by small arrows. The higher modes ($\ell > 3$) are not shown. Power in all modes depends on the spatial extent of the input; that is, when each arrow refers to broad input, power is shifted toward lower modes. In contrast, delta function input excites all higher modes. The nodal lines shown represent linear combinations of eigenfunctions; however, they are partly idealized because of difficulties of plotting on prolate spheroidal surface. The coefficients $B_{\ell m}$ are the square roots of power in each mode. See Chapter 9 for more detail.

phenomena (nondispersive waves) described previously, resonant frequencies depend only on surface propagation velocity and system size. However, in the physiologically based theory developed in Chapter 11, an additional (control) parameter that measures the background excitability of the cortex also effects resonant frequency. Although the mechanisms by which anesthetic agents act on the central nervous system are not well understood, somehow they affect synaptic action, thereby changing average neocortical excitability.

Consider the scalp EEG spectrum recorded in a patient anesthetized with halathone, with inspired concentration changed with time as shown in Figure 2-13. The apparent EEG modes move up and down in a predictable manner

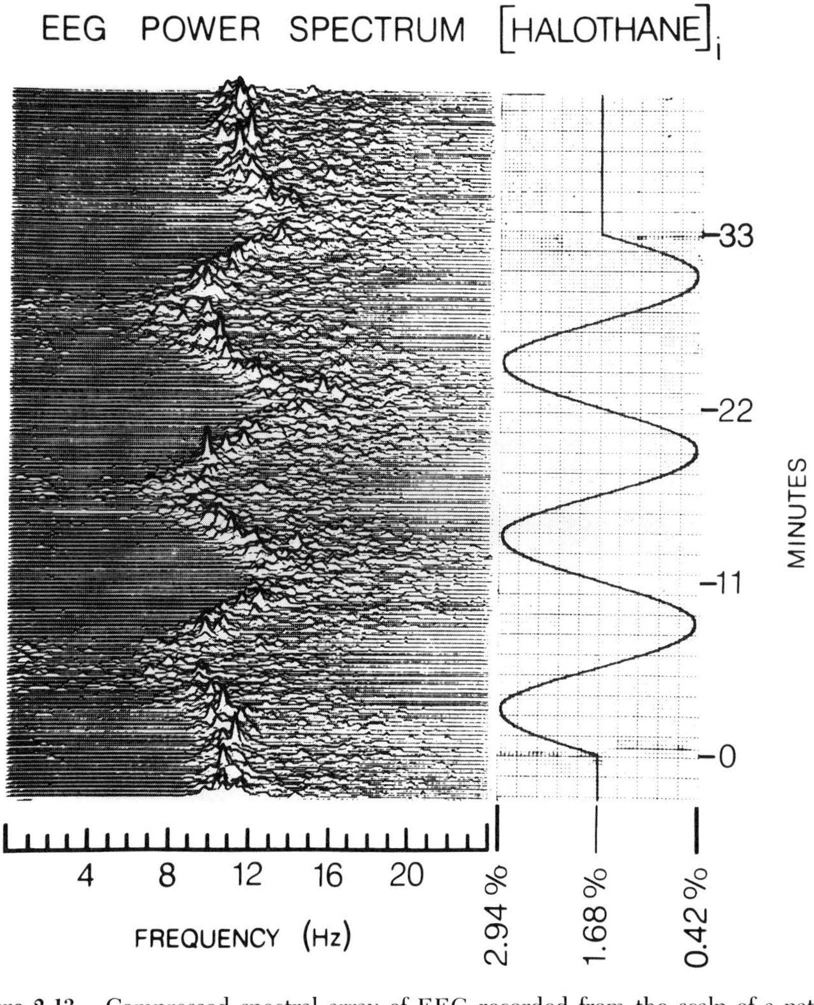

Figure 2-13. Compressed spectral array of EEG recorded from the scalp of a patient anesthetized with halothane. Inspired concentration of halothane varies over a period of 33 minutes, as indicated by the plot at right. One channel of eight channel recording is shown. Other channels reveal similar spectra; EEG is of large amplitude and spatially coherent over the entire scalp. Data from one experimental subject in a study of about 10 subjects is shown. All subjects showed the same qualitative behavior of EEG, but with quantitative differences in number and intensity of apparent modes, which increase and decrease in frequency as halothane concentration is changed. (Reproduced with permission from Stockard, 1976 and Nunez et al, 1977.)

with concentration. Furthermore, this EEG is spatially coherent over the entire scalp, as would be expected of simple standing waves. In Chapter 12, it is argued that these data exhibit a mode scanning property, in the sense that certain cortical states are more efficient for certain modes (Katznelson, 1981), a result consistent with the standing wave theory of Chapter 11. In addition, the halathone rhythm in the dog exhibits a somewhat similar behavior, but at about twice the dominant human frequencies. This observation is reasonably consistent with the linear scale factor of about 2.8 required to convert human to canine frequencies, in the idealized case in which frequency differences are due only to brain size differences.

6. Crude estimates of phase and group velocities obtained from scalp-recorded EEG are in about the same range as corticocortical propagation velocities (6 to 9 m/second). For example, in one study of phase and coherence of scalp-recorded EEG in 189 children, the average (calculated over time and participants) phase shift between anterior and posterior scalp regions in the alpha frequency band translated to a phase velocity of $\omega/k \sim 6$ m/second (Thatcher et al, 1986). In a different type of study of multichannel EEG involving one-dimensional frequency–wave number spectra, a very crude approximation of apparent group velocity of alpha rhythm was obtained; that is, $d\omega/dk \sim 4$ to 24 m/second (Nunez, 1981). The difference between phase and group velocities is discussed in Chapters 1 and 12.

The accuracy of these estimates is severely limited by the poor spatial resolution usually obtained in conventional scalp recordings and by confounding effects of multiple waves traveling in different directions. However, in another study these difficulties were overcome in part by recording both EEG and MEG evoked by diffuse sine wave-modulated light. This experiment resulted in progressive phase shifts of both EEG and MEG with distance from the visual cortex, which is discussed in Chapter 6. The phase shift was corrected to account for waves traveling along the folded cortical surface and translated to a phase velocity of $\omega/k \sim 5$ to 13 m/second. These cortical delays, which involve only large-scale source activity, are apparently due to action potential propagation in corticocortical fibers. These data are discussed in more detail in Chapters 6 and 12.

7. The general view of EEG taken by electroencephalographers, who record primarily from the human scalp, is often different from that of physiologists, who record EEG almost exclusively from inside the cranium of animals (such as rats, dogs, and cats). Aside from species differences, a substantial difference of spatial scale is involved, as discussed in Chapter 1. As a result, human scalp recordings have a more global character; physiologists tend to think more locally about EEG than do clinicians. Although widespread, spatially coherent activity obviously occurs in several anesthetic, coma, and sleep states in humans, it is less obvious in the normal waking state. The human alpha rhythm appears to be somewhat of an intermediate case, with perhaps a mixture of local and global underpinnings. However, global contributions to its character are evident in certain experiments, as discussed in Chapters 3 and 12.

Consider, for example, the estimate of front to back coherency, obtained with the electrode array of Figure 2-7 and shown in Figure 2-14. Unlike the subject of Figure 2-7, the EEG in these participants showed weak spectra peaks in frontal regions. However, the front to back coherency was large in the alpha band, over a scalp separation of 21 cm. A critical issue in coherency estimates

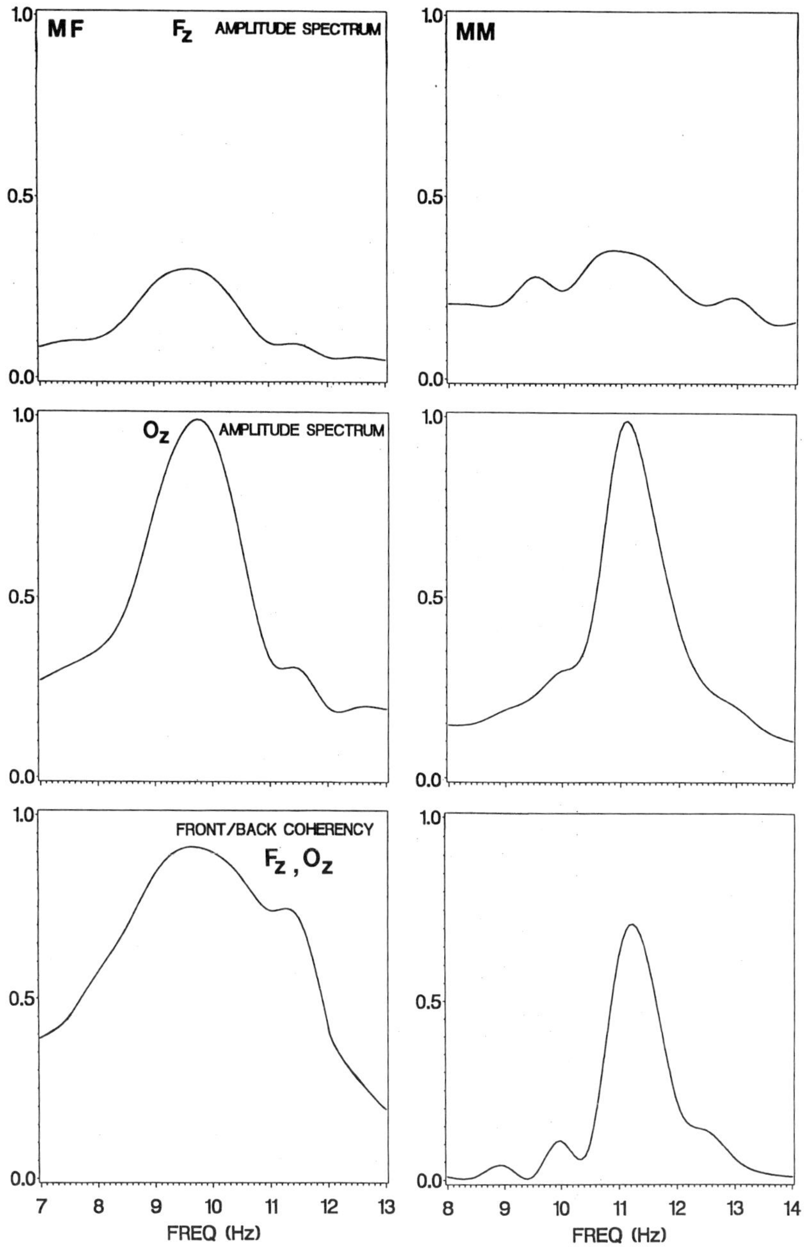

Figure 2-14. Amplitude spectra obtained from resting, eyes-closed EEG records (approximately 2 minutes), recorded with bipolar montage shown in Figure 2-7a. Subjects MF and MM with alpha index set to 1.8 to remove suspected artifact (see Nunez, 1981). Upper plots are obtained from frontal region (channel 1); middle plots from posterior region (channel 8). Lower plots are front–back coherency obtained from the same data. The coherency between two locations separated by 21 cm is high over the alpha band. Spectra for subject MF are similar to those obtained in Figure 2-7, except the alpha index is lower here, that is, more epochs are used in the analysis.

obtained from the scalp is the removal of erroneous high coherence due only to volume conduction, as shown in Figure 1-7 using Laplacian electrode arrays. In the experiment illustrated in Figure 2-14, volume conduction contributions to coherency were largely eliminated using close (3-cm) bipolar recordings, a strategy that works well for coherency estimates between distant locations, as discussed in Chapter 3.

8. The proposed emphasis on global dynamics and top-down influences on local and regional circuits provides a new conceptual framework for brain studies. In this view brainstem neuromodulators alter control parameters which mediate the amount of cortico-cortical coupling so that brain states switch between more local and more global dynamics. Selective changes in local and global control may be due to different transmitters which act in different cortical layers. These ideas were recently developed by Silberstein and are presented in Chapter 13. It is suggested that several disease states may be manifestations of pathological hypocoupling or hypercoupling of neocortical tissue.

By themselves, any one of the apparent agreements between the crude global theory and experiment cited above could easily be coincidence. However, as a whole, they provide strong support for the important influence of global boundary conditions on several common EEG phenomena. Questions of how closely actual EEG resembles linear or quasilinear standing waves (as opposed to spatial structure dominated by strongly nonlinear effects) or the relative importance of local circuit effects remain mainly unanswered. However, a strong motivation for the theoretical efforts of this book is guiding new experimental design. Some of the theoretical–experimental connections cited here are so crude because investigators were unaware of possible influence of global boundary conditions and possible standing wave phenomena, thereby missing opportunities to test these ideas.

Recently, studies using a physiologically based theory (Nunez, 1989a; see also Chapter 11) suggested that both local and global effects can result in EEG phenomena with peaked frequency spectra approximating that observed in humans. This combined local-global theory indicates that both long and short wavelength phenomena can occur in the same frequency range (due to multiple branches of the dispersion relation) as a natural consequence of known anatomic and physiologic features. Thus any of the multiple global modes can be matched with local modes in any particular region of neocortex (and perhaps olfactory bulb), perhaps facilitating a global (top-down) influence on local EEG frequencies that vary from place to place in the brain as a result of changing local control parameters. This matching of local resonances with particular global modes may have several advantages, as considered in Chapters, 3, 11, 13, and 14.

This speculation about matching of local and global modes (or effective time constants) does not explain why oscillatory behavior is even necessary. But data obtained from recent experiments in cat visual cortex show that individual neurons have oscillatory responses to nonoscillatory visual stimuli in the frequency range of 40 to 60 Hz (Gray et al, 1989). Neurons in spatially distributed columns can synchronize their oscillatory responses. Common input from subcortical structures was dismissed as the cause of this synchronization. Rather tangential intracortical and corticocortical connections are the apparent anatomic substrates for this phenomenon. These physiologists suggest that synchronization may provide a

> mechanism for the extraction and representation of global and coherent features of a pattern . . . Synchronization of oscillatory responses may however also have a more general function in cortical processing because it is a powerful mechanism for establishing cell assemblies that are characterized by the phase and frequency of their coherent oscillations.

This idea correlates well with the general concept of multiple global modes providing a top-down influence on local or regional circuits in cortical and subcortical structures. It is discussed further in the context of the physics of music in Chapter 3, and the physiologically based theories of Chapters 11 and 14. The means by which neuromodulators may selectively change local and global control parameters and the implications of these ideas in neuropsychiatry are discussed in Chapter 13.

Neocortical Structure

Many volumes have been published on the neural structure (morphology) of neocortex. Our description in the next few sections is, of necessity, an abbreviated summary, with emphasis on general quantitative properties that appear most important to neocortical dynamics at macroscopic scales most closely related to scalp EEG.

A salient feature of neocortex is the relative lack of specificity of intracortical connections as compared with other neural structures, such as cerebellum. Therefore it may be best to avoid the term "neural circuit" (at least at small scales), which appears inadequate to describe the high degree of interconnectivity illustrated in Figure 2-15. For example, a recent study by Braitenberg and Schuz (1991) estimated an average 4-cm axon length for each of the 10^7 mouse cortical neurons, a length longer than the diameter of the mouse brain. Another illustration of the extreme interconnectivity of neocortical tissue is the estimate of about 4-km axon length per cubic millimeter by these anatomists. Furthermore, any cortical neuron lies within no more than two or three synapses of any other cortical neuron because of the many corticocortical fibers forming most of the subcortical white matter. These and other quantitative anatomic arguments prompted these anatomists to note the apparent lack of specificity of connections (at least at small scales) and to conclude that "A picture of the cortex emerges as a device for the most widespread diffusion and most intimate mixing of signals which is compatible with the natural limitations of nerve cells" (Braitenberg and Schuz, 1991).

This skeptical view of the neural circuit in neurophysiology at small scales is also supported by the existence of multiple methods for information transfer that can occur in nervous tissue, especially over short distances (Bullock, 1980). These include reciprocal synapses directly between adjacent dendrites (Rall and Shep-

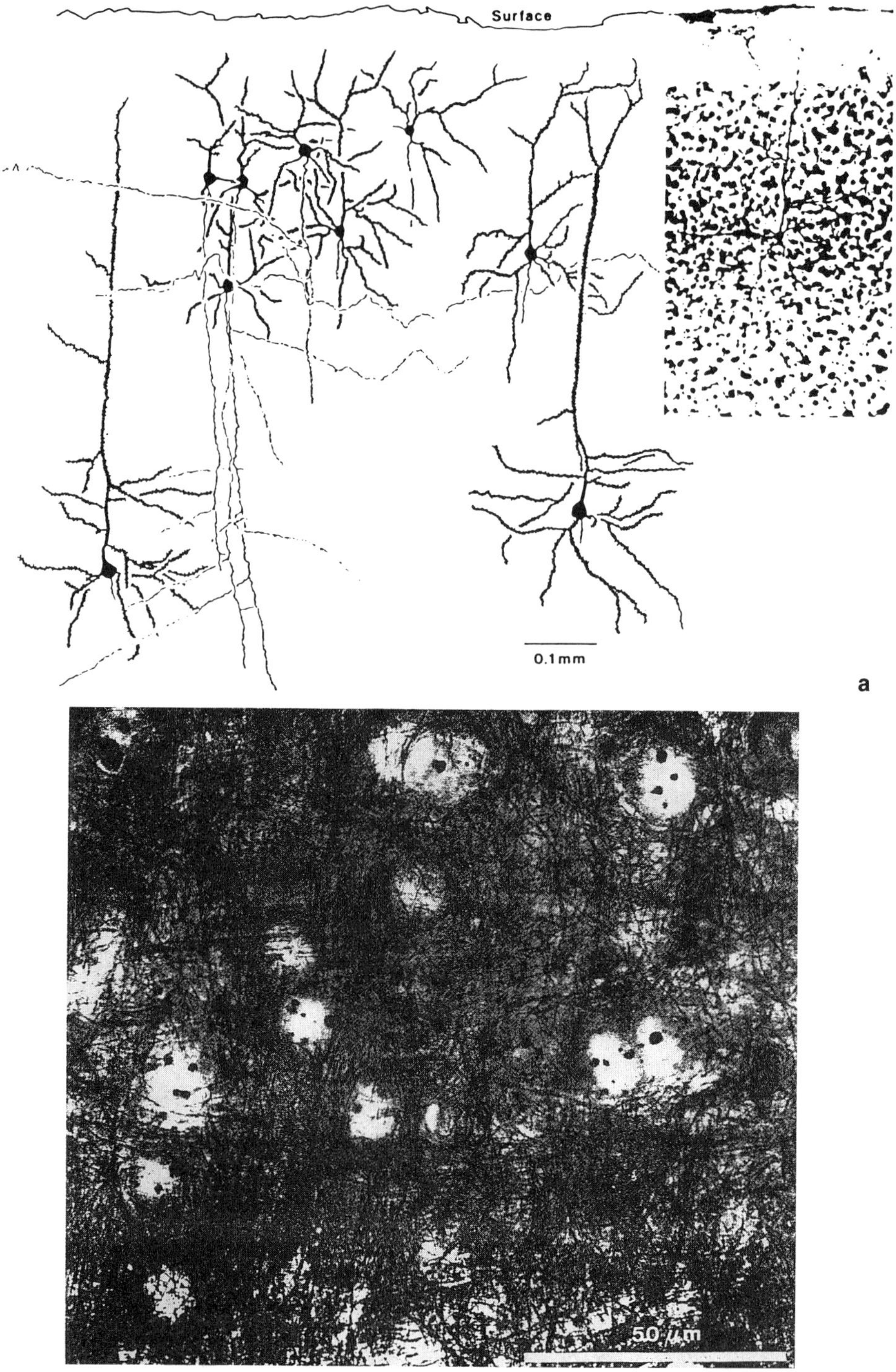

Figure 2-15. *Legend on facing page*

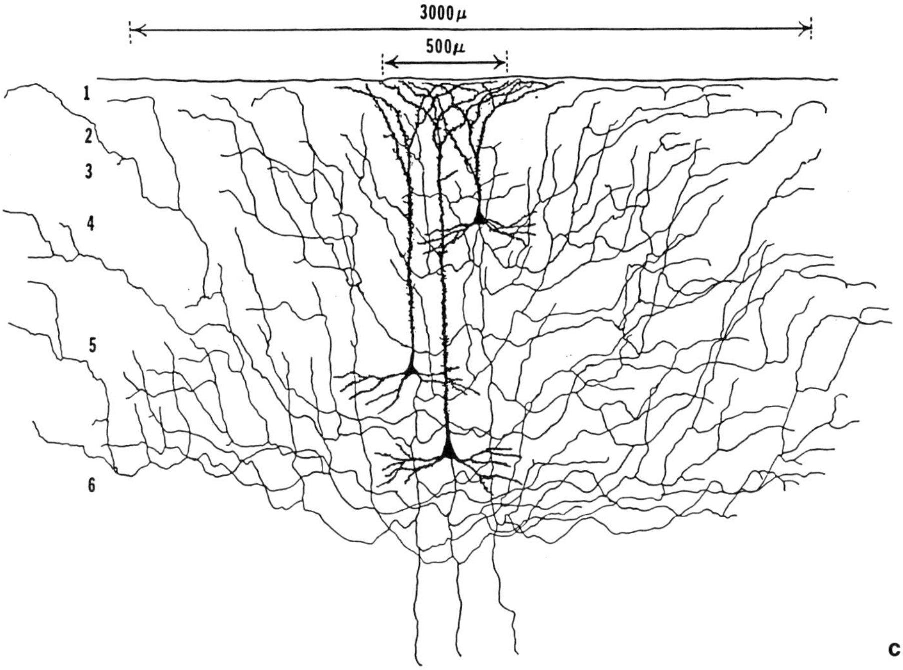

c

Figure 2-15. **a.** Pyramidal cells from one Golgi preparation in their correct relative position. The Golgi method consists of silver (black) impregnation of whole neurons, which can be viewed against a transparent background of unstained tissue because only a few of the local neurons are stained (Rakic, 1979). Their location in depth varies between layer II and layer VI. In some, the descending axons and the axon collaterals are also stained. The photomicrograph on the right shows one Golgi-stained pyramidal cell at the same magnification among a multitude of cell bodies counterstained with a Nissal stain. This is a reminder of the actual density of neurons in the cortex, of which the Golgi picture on the left gives a misleading impression. (Reproduced with permission from Braitenberg and Schuz, 1991). **b.** Reduced silver stain of the mouse cortex. The staining of axons is fairly complete, whereas the staining of dendrites and neural cell bodies is suppressed, except for some lumps inside the nuclei. The density of axons on such preparations is greater than 1 km/mm^3. (Reproduced with permission from Braitenberg and Schuz, 1991.) **c.** Recurrent collaterals are shown surrounding three pyramidal cells in neocortex. Each cell may send 3 to 10 of these axon branches to distances as great as 3 mm. This spatial scale provides one definition of the macrocolumn. (Reproduced with permission from Scheibel and Scheibel, 1970.)

herd, 1968), fast chemical transport, and the passive spread of extracellular fields that can excite adjacent neurons (Taylor and Dudek, 1984a, 1984b). These data prompted Bullock to suggest the idea of a neural throng, which is not a circuit in the usual sense but rather a mass of tissue that supports many complex interactions within its volume. His analogy is to a "very densely packed social gathering with more structure and goals than a mob." A somewhat similar concept from the physical sciences is collective interactions, as in hot plasma systems in which many kinds of waves interact simultaneously with each other and with individual particles. The extreme complexity of neural interactions at small scales, in which dynamic function is determined largely by physiologic parameters of unknown magnitudes, provides substantial motivation for the development of macroscopic theories of neocortical dynamics. This view is taken in the same spirit as that used to derive more macroscopic and phenomenologic approaches to other complex systems, such as plasma dynamics, electromagnetic field interactions and quantum effects in DNA molecules, macroeconomic systems and so forth.

The high degree of integration in neural tissue motivated some neuroscientists, notably Freeman (1975), to view brain operation at hierarchical levels above the single neuron—the neural mass. Properties of a neural mass differ as much from those of a neuron as neuron properties differ from those of a patch of membrane. When synaptic interactions within a neural mass are sufficiently dense, we expect the mass to show macroscopic properties that are relatively independent of its exact inner circuitry. Neither the macroscopic properties nor interactions between neural masses can be understood at the level of the individual neuron, any more than the physical concepts of temperature or viscosity can be explained in terms of a single water molecule. In addition, the rules of interaction of neural masses at one spatial scale may differ considerably from interactions at other scales. This general idea was exploited to derive theories of mass action (that is, the dynamics of units of neural tissue, defined at many spatial scales), as described in later chapters. As a complement to this work, the studies described in Chapter 14 address the derivation of rules of interaction at progressively larger scales from rules at smaller scales.

Much of the information on neocortex has been obtained from nonhuman mammals, and we must be careful when generalizing these data to humans. Fortu-

Table 2-1 Linear Scale Factors for Mammalian Brains

Species	Linear Scale
Mouse	0.07
Rat	0.11
Rabbit	0.19
Cat	0.27
Dog	0.37
Rhesus monkey	0.41
Chimpanzee	0.65
Man	1.00
Bottle nose dolphin*	1.06
Elephant	1.64
Fin whale	1.71
Sperm whale*	1.80

Adapted with permission from Tower, 1954 and from Ridgway*, 1990. (Two estimates were obtained from Ridgway, the rest from Tower.)

nately, however, considerable similarity exists between the cerebral cortices of different mammals. In fact, it is difficult for an anatomist to distinguish slides of cortical neurons taken from mice, cats, dogs, cows, monkeys, and humans (Braitenberg, 1972). Of course, substantial differences of scale exist. Cortical thickness varies from an average of about 0.8 mm in mice to 2 or 3 mm in humans. Brain size, and more importantly for our purposes, neocortical surface, varies more than this. Table 2-1 lists the relative linear scale factors for several mammalian brains. Scale factor is defined such that it is proportional to (brain weight)$^{1/3}$, with the human brain arbitrarily assigned a value of 1. Thus, if all brains were identical except for size, we could calculate the relative size of any brain structure by taking a simple ratio of factors located in column two. Although many differences exist besides size, this procedure allows for a reasonable first guess, which will be adequate for some purposes. However, a dramatic enlargement of neocortex relative to the rest of the brain distinguishes primates from other mammals and humans from other primates (Mountcastle, 1979) so that scale factors can be applied only with care.

Another parameter available from these studies is the approximate number density of cortical neurons. To a reasonable approximation (Tower, 1954; Nunez, 1981)

$$\text{number density} \sim (\text{linear scale factor})^{-1} \tag{2.14}$$

The decrease in number density with brain size occurs in parallel with increased cortical thickness in a manner that keeps the total number of neurons within a neocortical column remarkably constant among mammalian species. We have not found equivalent data on dolphins and whales; they may be exceptions to this rule.

Cortical neurons are oriented perpendicular to the cortical surface and arranged in columns that show large-scale homogeneity and isotropy in directions tangent to the surface. Neocortex has a stratified appearance because of differences in the relative densities of different types of neurons at different cortical depths, that is layers I through VI, as depth increases. To first approximation, cortical neurons can be divided into two major types, pyramidal cells and interneurons. Pyramidal cells, which occupy cylindrical volumes, account for more than three quarters of neocortical neurons. Most interneurons (for example, stallate cells) occupy more spherical volumes (Sholl, 1956; Bok, 1959; Braitenberg, 1978). Because of their large size (and by implication large dipole moments) and parallel orientation, pyramidal cell current sources are thought to make the dominant contribution to surface EEG (Lopes da Silva and Storm van Leeuwen, 1978; Nunez, 1981).

Nearly every pyramidal cell sends an excitatory axon into the white matter, and most of these re-enter the cortex at some distant location in the same hemisphere (corticocortical fibers) or opposite hemisphere (commissural fibers, primarily callosal fibers). Other efferent axons may provide feedback to midbrain regions or send signals to muscle fibers (Braitenberg, 1978). In addition, multiple branches of the axon (typically 3 to 10 branches, called "recurrent collaterals") stay within the cortex and provide excitatory input to local regions within a 3-mm radius, as shown in Figure 2-15c (Scheibel and Scheibel, 1970). Multiple synapses between the same two neurons are rare; thus each pyramidal cell makes synaptic contact with about as many other pyramidal cells as it has synapses.

The average number of synapses per cortical neuron is about 10^4, with large pyramidal cells of humans receiving as many as 8×10^4. Pyramidal neurons are the primary intracortical cells with excitatory axons (Braitenberg and Schuz, 1991); that is, interneurons are mainly inhibitory. In mice, cortical synapses are 90% excitatory, and pyramidal cell-to-pyramidal cell connections represent 75% of all synapses (Braitenberg and Schuz, 1991). Pyramidal cells and their synapses are the most numerous neurons, provide a mechanism for nonlocal neocortical interaction (through corticocortical axons), and apparently generate the large dipole moments required to produce cortical surface potentials of sufficient magnitude be measured on the scalp (Nunez, 1981). More quantitative estimates are considered in Chapter 11 as related to the global wave theory.

Neuronal input occurs over dendrites and cell body (about 10% of input surface). In cats, the number of basal dendrite branches from a single neuron that intersects concentric spherical surfaces surrounding the cell body decreases with distance (according to Sholl, 1955):

$$\text{number of branches} \sim \exp(-\lambda \times \text{radial distance}) \tag{2.15}$$

where $\lambda \sim 350 \text{ cm}^{-1}$ is the characteristic length constant. The number of branches of the apical dendrites also decreases monotonically with distance but is better fit to a power law.

The arguments of this section and cited references indicate a neocortical medium exhibiting strong interconnectivity between individual neurons, with specific "circuitry" perhaps due mainly to chance. Also implied is a large redundancy of circuitry, which perhaps should be anticipated because adult humans are reported to lose approximately 10^5 neurons each day without dramatic functional loss. Thus the action of any single neuron can, at best, have a minimal effect on higher brain functions. Apparently we must look to larger spatial scales for the basic operational units of neocortical dynamic function.

Neocortical Modules

Neocortical neurons are arranged in overlapping modular units or columns of different sizes, with column axes oriented perpendicular to the cortical surface. These modular units are excellent candidates for theoretical treatment of neocortex in terms of neural mass action. An important modular unit is the corticocortical column shown in Figure 2-16. The corticocortical column may span the 2- to 3-mm cortical thickness in humans and has a diameter of about 0.3 mm (Szentagothai, 1979). This modular unit is defined by the spatial extent of its extracortical input. Cortical axons that are not specific sensory afferents (for example, ipsilateral association fiber or callosal axon from contralateral cortex) provide multiple excitatory synaptic input to the corticocortical column relatively uniformly over the depth of cortex, but with more synaptic contacts in layer I.

Perhaps 4000 neurons are found in the corticocortical aborization column (module), of which perhaps 3400 are pyramidal cells. Each of the pyramidal cells sends an axon into the subcortical layer of white matter; most of these axons re-enter the cortex at some distant location. The white matter in humans consists mainly of about 10^{10} corticocortical fibers (Braitenberg, 1978). The remaining white matter is composed of commussural fibers crossing between hemispheres (perhaps 2%, mostly callosal) and afferent and efferent axons between cortex and several midbrain regions, mainly the thalamus (perhaps 1%). This extreme dominance of corticocortical over thalamocortical connections in humans is notably less characteristic of other mammals and may be an important feature in making the human brain "human" (Braitenberg, 1978). This issue is addressed in more detail in a later section.

There are about 10^{10} neocortical neurons, or about 2×10^6 corticocortical columns. Recent estimates suggest that approximately 85% of cortical neurons are pyramidal cells (Braak and Braak, 1986; Braitenberg and Schuz, 1991); nearly all send connections to other parts of neocortex. Based on these data, each corticocortical column receives on average about 2500 to 6500 excitatory axons and several times this number of synaptic inputs from nonlocal cortical regions. Each module may project many fibers to the same secondary module. Thus, it has been conjectured that each module projects to perhaps 10 to 100 other modules and receives input from the same number (Szentagothai, 1978; Eccles, 1984). This is still a much higher degree of interconnectivity than normally implied by "circuit." However, the number of units connected to any one unit is 100 to 1000 times lower than the corresponding number at the single neuron level.

A burst of action potential discharge from corticocortical columns produces excitatory input to other corticocortical columns by association and callosal projections (Eccles, 1984). It is useful to add that distant cortical regions are excited only after time delays that depend mainly on the rise times of postsynaptic potentials in target neurons (apparently of about 1 to 10 ms) and on delays due to finite velocity of action potential propagation. Because the latter global delays depend on separation distances between cortical regions, they are distributed over a relatively broad range. For example, with typical action potential propagation velocities in myelinated axons of 6 to 9 m/second, time delays along the short U fibers (~1 cm) connecting adjacent gyri are about 1 ms, delays that may be negligible with respect to postsynaptic potential rise times. Alternately, delays along the long axons (~20 cm) connecting frontal and occipital regions are about 20 to 30 milliseconds. Evidence discussed in Chapter 11 suggests that a considerable fraction of callosal (and by implication corticocortical) fibers may be nonmyelinated with propagation velocities of only 10% to 20% of that of myelinated fibers of the same diameter. In this case, time delays between remote cortex may extend to the range of several hundred milliseconds.

Some of the secondary modules in homologous or association cortex are sufficiently excited, in turn, to send excitatory input to tertiary modules, and so on

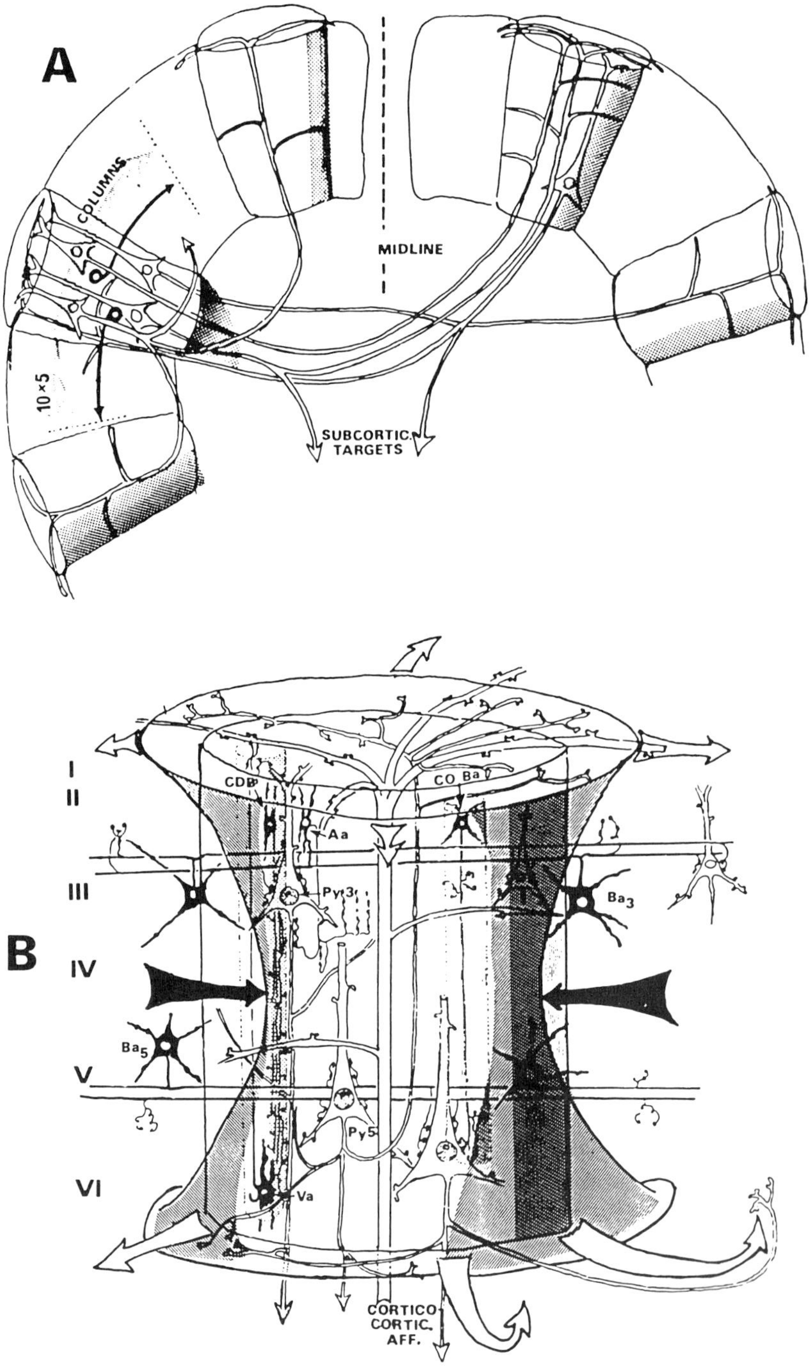
A
COLUMNS
10×5
MIDLINE
SUBCORTIC.
TARGETS
B
I
II
III
IV
V
VI
CDB
CO Ba
Aa
Py 3
Ba$_3$
Ba$_5$
Py 5
Va
CORTICO
CORTIC.
AFF.

(Eccles, 1984). The system of massive positive feedback is not a general feature of gray matter. Rather it is a distinctive characteristic of neocortex. In cerebellar cortex, for example, all known feedback loops involve inhibitory synapses (Braitenberg and Schuz, 1991). The positive feedback of neocortex causes a spreading excitation pattern. The spreading is apparently neither random nor like a traveling wave at the sub-millimeter scale. Rather it is determined by the specific interconnections that allow for the sequential excitation of columns that may jump from place to place. However, corticocortical fibers consistently tend to project more densely to close regions than to remote cortical regions. This suggests the possibility of traveling waves at large scales (~1 cm) based on corticocortical interactions, an issue alluded to previously and considered in more detail in Chapter 11. Given this situation, one plausible way to view neocortex is as a

←

Figure 2-16. Diagram illustrating the modular architectonics principle of the neocortex. **A**. The two halves of the cerebral cortex, connected over the midline by the fiber system of the corpus callosum. Three columnar modules are shown on the left and two on the right side. Corticocortical connectivity occurs at larger distances by the axons of pyramidal cells that arborize in the whole space of one column. Ipsilateral corticocortical columns originate from pyramidal cells of the superficial layers (II–III), while callosal fibers may originate from any layer II–VI. The main axon of the layer V pyramidal cell is directed toward subcortical targets. Local intracortical connectivity is indicated in the middle left column by hatched arrow. Excitatory spread is little known, highly specific, and varies greatly according to cortical area; inhibition (indicated in full black) is probably more stereotypic within cortical areas and may stretch over 10^5 neighboring corticocortical columns. **B**. A stereoscopic view of a single corticocortical column, with a diameter of 200–300 μm and stretching through the entire depth of the cortex. (For reasons of space, the transverse diameter is greatly exaggerated.) Lamination of the cortex is indicated at left margin in roman numerals. A corticocortical afferent arborization is placed into the axis of the large cylinder. Its terminal arborization in layer I exceeds the limits of the cylindrical space shown. One or two representative pyramidal cells are drawn in some detail (Py_3 for a layer III and Py_5 for a layer V pyramidal cell). The cell labeled Py_5 illustrates a cell type that sends several ascending collaterals specifically to layer I, but this is not typical for pyramidal cells, whose collaterals are distributed more generally in the deeper cortical layers. Horizontal spread of inhibition occurs mainly by two rows of large basket cells (full black and Ba_3 for the upper row situated at the border of laminate III–IV, and the lower row Ba_5 at the border of laminae IV–V). More strictly localized vertical inhibition is indicated by the two smaller cylinders (minicolumns, inset). The cylinder at right corresponds to a specific type of basket cell with columnar distribution (CoBa). The cylinder at left illustrates mutual vertical inhibition (or disinhibition) between the upper and lower layers affected by specific cells and a vertically ascending inhibitory cell (Va) in the bottom layers. (Throughout the diagram outlining indicates excitatory elements or affects; full black, inhibitory elements or effects.) The "hourglass" shape of the module indicates the dynamic distortion of the original cylindrical module by the tendency of excitation to spread toward neighboring columns in lamina I and VI (large outline arrows) and horizontal inhibitory effects (large black arrows) acting mainly upon the middle layers (III, IV, and V). The main end control of pyramid cell activity is secured by a specific inhibitory cell type, the axoaxonic (Aa) neurons. (Reproduced with permission from Szentagothai, 1987).

system involving the dynamic interaction of 10^6 overlapping corticocortical columns on a two-dimensional surface, rather than 10^{10} neurons in three dimensions. Although this assumption that corticocortical columns are functional units in which inner circuitry can be ignored in some applications is an enormous simplification of potential dynamic behavior, we are left with an immense number of possibilities for the development of spatio-temporal patterns.

A summary of primary inputs (all excitatory) to the corticocortical column (module) is given by Eccles (1984).

1. The axon collaterals of pyramidal cells of adjacent modules, as shown in Figure 2-15c. These extend outward from each pyramidal cell to a radius of approximately 3 mm and define a relatively large spatial scale of neural mass action, the macrocolumn.

2. The surface parallel intracortical axons of layer I. These tangential fibers are formed by the bifurcation of axons that ascend in a module and extend over a radius of perhaps 6 to 8 mm. Because some of these axons are extensions of corticocortical and thalamic fibers, the idea that input from a single afferent axon is confined to a radius of 300 μm must be regarded as only a first approximation. Martinotti cells were identified as the origin of many of the surface parallel fibers, and they are thought to be excitatory. Very small nonmyelinated axons as long as 1 cm can apparently add time delays in the range of several tens of milliseconds due only to slow axon propagation.

3. Thalamocortical inputs. All areas of neocortex receive this input, but it is particularly dense in primary sensory cortex. Specific thalamic inputs tend to concentrate on cells of layer IV and the deeper parts of layer III. Earlier anatomic studies emphasized mapping and reciprocity, in which connections from specific thalamic regions target specific cortical regions, and thalamus-to-cortical connections are matched by cortical-to-thalamus connections. However, more recent studies indicate a paucity of direct relations between a given thalamic nucleus and a given cortical region (Goldman-Rakic, 1988). Rather individual thalamic nuclei project to widespread cortical areas and a given cytoarchitectonic region receives afferents from multiple thalamic nuclei.

Several scientists proposed EEG theories based on thalamocortical feedback circuits while ignoring corticocortical connections. In humans, however, thalamocortical fibers contribute no more than about 1% of the total number of afferents that enter any large region of cortex. Most of the remaining afferents are corticocortical fibers, thereby providing strong support for the idea that "(human) cortex is largely a reflexive machine, working on its own output" (Braitenberg 1977, 1978). The bias in most neuroanatomic literature favoring thalamocortical interactions over corticocortical interactions is apparently due to the larger relative importance of thalamocortical fibers in the lower mammals most often studied by anatomists and to our paucity of understanding of the structure and function of the corticocortical system.

Included in the thalamocortic input category are diffuse cortical inputs originating in the brainstem, inputs that are necessary to keep the cortex awake. This input provides one mechanism for external control of the background state of neocortex, (for example, the ease with which an average neuron with fixed input fires an action potential). Cortical control by subcortical structures is discussed in the context of conscious state in Chapters 3, 4, 5, and 13.

4. The corticocortical and callosal (and other crossing fibers) inputs. Inputs are distributed over all layers of cortex. A reciprocity of callosal connections facilitates large coherency of scalp EEG between homologous regions of the two hemispheres, although asymmetry of the two neocortical hemispheres with respect to standard scalp locations complicates EEG observations (Myslobodski et al, 1991). The section called "Global Integration of Neocortical Function" below and Chapter 11 consider this long-range system in more detail.

The description of neocortex described in this section, consisting of interacting corticocortical columns, is interesting and appears to be valuable as a reasonable first approximation. However, several important features are omitted. First, no role for inhibitory neurons is elucidated. Second, the specific spatial scale of these modular units is emphasized. We expect interactions to occur simultaneously at other spatial scales but with generally different rules for interaction.

Multiple Scales of Cortical Mass Action

The minicolumn with a diameter of about 20–50 μm (Figure 2-16B) also has been proposed as a basic functional unit of neocortex (Mountcastle, 1979; Szentagothai, 1979). Minicolumns can be defined by the characteristic lateral spread of axons of inhibitory interneurons. The axons of these cells run along minicolumn axes with very short lateral spread so that interneurons are more densely connected along the axes than in tangential directions. This anatomic description is supported by physiologic experiments using small, extracellular electrodes. Extracellular potentials at different locations along the axes are highly correlated, whereas lateral shifts of the electrodes beyond the minicolumn diameter cause lower correlations. The minicolumn diameter is also less than the typical spatial extent of the extracellular field generated at the soma when an action potential is fired (Abeles, 1982). Thus we can postulate nonsynaptic interaction between neurons within the same minicolumn. The usual concept of neural circuitry may be especially inaccurate at this or smaller scales.

A minicolumn spanning the entire cortical thickness contains about 110 neurons, lined up along its axis. This figure is remarkably constant, both for different cortical areas and different species of mammals, except for striate (that is, primary visual) cortex that contains about 260 neurons (Mountcastle, 1979). The interneurons receive excitatory input from pyramidal cells, are themselves excited, and provide inhibitory (that is negative feedback) to the pyramidal cells. They also provide inhibitory input to other inhibitory cells within the same minicolumn, with a resulting indirect excitatory affect on pyramidal cells (Szentagothai, 1979). Thus the open question of how many interneurons have excitatory synapses may not be of direct value to macroscopic dynamic theories because inhibition of inhibitory interneurons may have an effect on pyramidal cells similar to direct excitation. Anatomic and physiologic data support the hypothesis that the corticocortical column (module) is functionally subdivided into approximately 100 minicolumns. The minicolumns sharpen the boundaries of modules by inhibiting pyramidal cells of adjacent modules, thereby limiting dynamic action to more local regions (Mountcastle, 1979; Eccles, 1984). Thus we can conjecture that they play a role somewhat analogous to the resistors of the circuit shown in Figure 2-2, which limit the effects of distant parts of the circuit on local currents.

Still another processing unit, the macrocolumn with a diameter of approximately 0.5 to 3 mm has been identified in neocortex. This range of spatial scale of operation is defined by several authors in terms of structure or function (Mountcastle, 1979). For example, specific locations in the visual field (or on the retina) are mapped to specific locations on visual cortex. A block of visual cortex with a diameter of 1 to 2 mm (of many possible cross-sectional shapes) apparently contains just enough neural circuitry to process information about its region of the visual field, for all line orientations in the visual field and for both eyes (Hubel and Wiesel, 1962). These hypercolumns (as named by the authors) are subdivided into subunits of ocular dominance columns with diameters of approximately 0.4 mm, which apparently allow for separation of function and partial mixing of separate information obtained by each eye. This information spreads to more distant cortical regions along corticocortical fibers for higher-order processing. For example, 16 distinct visual areas (including frontal regions) were discovered in the cortex of owl monkey (Allman and Kaas, 1971).

Somewhat similar schemes have been proposed for other sensory cortex. For example, stimulation of specific peripheral nerves produces neural activity in specific parts of somatosensory cortex at the macrocolumn scale. Other parameters of the stimulus, such as strength, modality, and so on, determine neural action in specific macrocolumn subunits, which may or may not be mapped topographically within the macrocolumn. We can speculate that these subunits have a range of sizes from the minicolumn to larger scales. In this view, the minicolumn is an irreducibly small processing unit of the neocortex (Mountcastle, 1979).

Another experiment that affects the macrocolumn scale involves the amplitude of EEG measured from the surface of cortex using electrodes of different sizes. If all neurons in a mass of cortex were synchronously active, EEG amplitude would be approximately independent of electrode size. However, such high synchrony occurs only in epilepsy. For normal brain operation, higher amplitudes are obtained with smaller electrodes over certain ranges of electrode diameter due to less cancellation of positive and negative contributions (Abeles, 1982; Nunez, 1981, 1990a). The manner and range over which this amplitude variation occurs can be used to determine estimates of "synchrony" (or effective correlation length) at different scales of columnar interaction. A study of EEG recorded from mouse cortex (Abeles, 1982) concluded that the region of statistically homogeneous generator properties extends to 3 to 4 mm (the macrocolumn scale). Furthermore, based on this study, macrocolumns were thought to be divided into 10^4 subpopulations, each of which exhibits highly correlated activity within itself. The scale of these subpopulations is about that of the minicolumn.

For historical reasons we adopted the macrocolumn label, but we consider it to be a general spatial scale of neural interaction rather than columns of exact cross-sectional size or shape. This scale is defined anatomically by the spatial extent of the axon collaterals of the large pyramidal cells of Figure 2-15. Because the density of these branches decreases with distance, it might be more natural to define a macrocolumn more precisely, for example, by the average distance at which the number of axon branches decreases to one half its maximum value. This "characteristic interaction distance" is probably about 1 or 2 mm. However, such precise quantitative information is not available, so we defined the macrocolumn scale as covering a mass of neocortical tissue of arbitrary cross-sectional shape with a diameter of 0.5 to 3 mm. These neural masses contain about 10^5 to 10^6 neurons, 10^3 to 10^4 minicolumns, and 10 to 10^3 corticocortical columns. A summary of spatial scales of neural interaction is shown in Table 2-2.

The next step up in the neural hierarchy may be defined loosely in terms of cytoarchitectural criteria, that is numbers and types of cells at various cortical depths that are observed in different regions of neocortex. Broadman (1909) subdivided each human brain hemisphere into approximately 50 regions, as shown in Figure 2-17; the numbering system is still used today. Some Broadman regions correspond closely to primary sensory areas; most have unknown functional importance. If we take 3000 cm^2 as a typical surface area of both hemispheres (more than one half in fissures and sulci), the linear scale associated with a Broadman area of average size is about 5 cm and contains approximately 10^8 neurons. This scale is also close to the spatial resolution obtained with high-resolution EEG scalp recordings. That is, along the free surface with new high-resolution EEG

Table 2-2 Spatial Scales of Human Neocortex

Structure	Typical Diameter (mm)	Number of Neurons	Description
Minicolumn	3×10^{-2}	10^2	Spatial extent of inhibitory connections
Corticocortical column (module)	3×10^{-1}	10^3 to 10^4	Width of aborization column of corticocortical afferents, i.e., input scale for specific long-range connections
Macrocolumn	0.5 to 3.0	10^5 to 10^6	Extent of axon collateral system of single pyramidal cell, i.e., spatial scale for intracortical excitatory output; hypercolumn scale in visual cortex
Regional scale	50	10^8	Average length of corticocortical fibers, i.e., one spatial scale for long-range excitatory output; typical scale of cytoarchitectonic (Broadman) area; EEG must be correlated over area of this size to be measurable on scalp without averaging
Lobeal scale	170	10^9	Ten lobes defined in relation to prominate sulci and gyri; scale of conventional EEG recording methods
Hemisphere	400	10^{10}	Longest corticocortical fibers

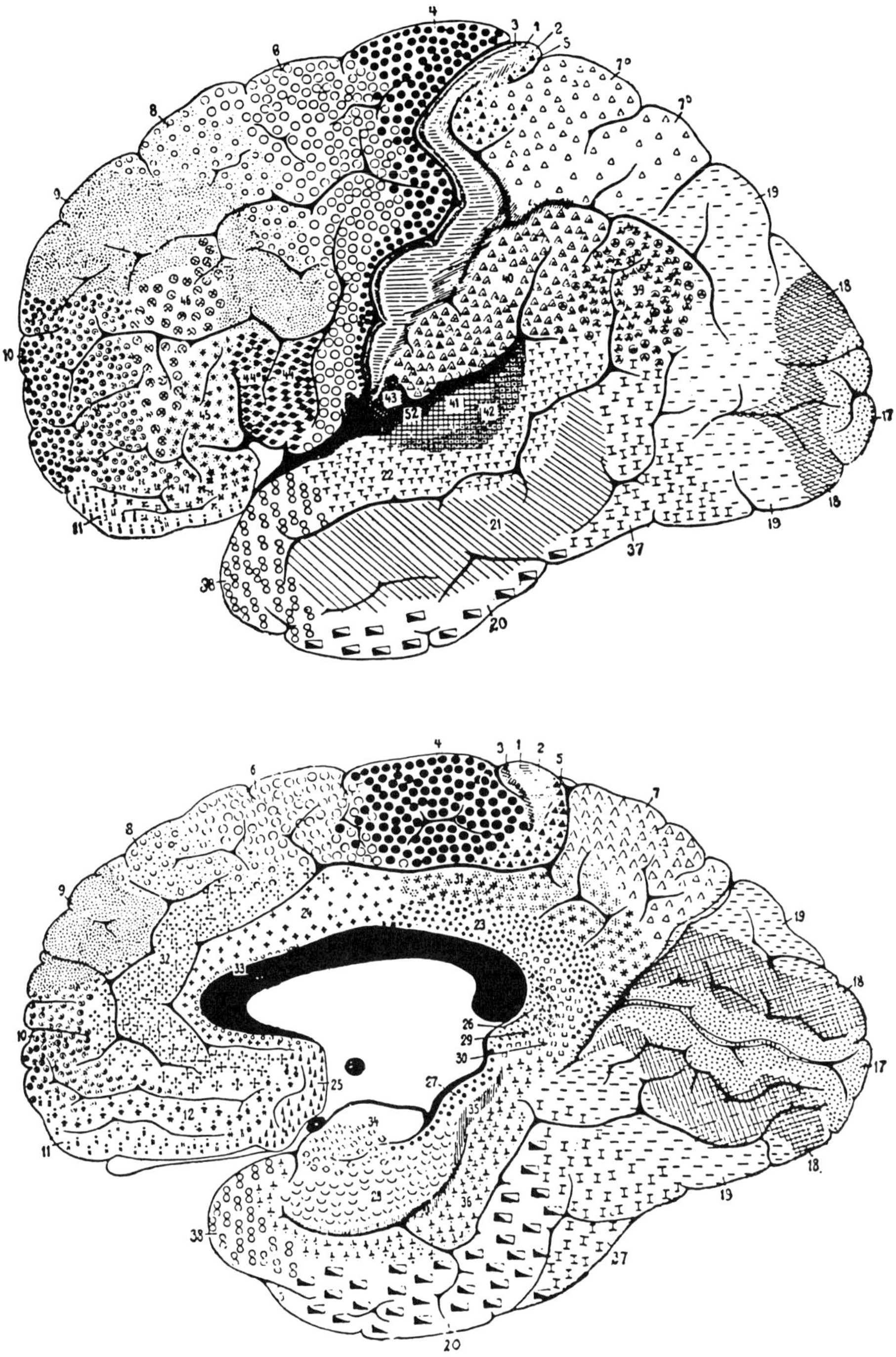

Figure 2-17. Broadman's map of regions of human cerebral cortex. Top. Lateral view. Bottom. Medial view. (Reproduced with permission from Jones, 1987).

methods discussed in Chapter 1, 1- to 3-cm resolution apparently can be obtained. Magnetoencephalography may better resolve sources tangential to the scalp, but extracranial resolution is, in either case, limited by the separation between sensor and sources ($\sim$1 cm). We refer to 5 cm as the regional scale of neocortical dynamics. This scale is also close to the average length of corticocortical fibers in humans.

Ten major subdivisions of neocortex are defined partly in relation to the most prominent sulci and gyri, that is, the frontal, precentral, parietal, occipital, and temporal lobes of each hemisphere. Boundaries generally coincide with those of the Broadman areas so that the latter are subunits of lobes. The linear scale associated with the average lobe is about 17 cm. This length is about the length of the longest corticocortical fibers in humans. Finally, the linear scale associated with a single brain hemisphere is $\sqrt{3000/2} \sim 40$ cm.

In Chapter 1, polarization vectors **P**(x, y, t) defined at several columnar scales were proposed as plausible measures of neocortical state. If we are to study neocortical state with scalp electrodes, which have rather poor spatial resolution, we should ask whether this coarse-grained spatial data can have much relation to behavioral or cognitive state. Experimental evidence that coarse-grained spatial EEG is correlated to state is presented in Chapters 3 to 7. However, we can approach this question from a theoretical direction to determine if such coarse-grained correlations could have been anticipated before such experiments were attempted.

We can guess that choices between fine- and coarse-grained spatial patterns involve compromises. The former apparently allow for more brain states whereas the latter are favored by more redundancy, fewer physical constraints on connections, and so on. Suppose for illustrative purposes that global neocortical state can be defined (in some nontrivial sense) by a distribution of binary states of each unit (column). That is, in each unit the polarization vector (approximately the space-average current source density) is either up or down. Thus, if neocortex is divided into M subunits, there are 2^M possible states. If global state is defined only by the states of the 10 major lobes, there are already 1024 possible global states at each instant in time. If state is determined at the regional scale (Broadman areas), there are $2^{100} \sim 10^{32}$ states. To put this number into perspective, note that it is in the general range of the number of large grains of sand that could be packed into the volume of the earth. If state is defined at the macrocolumn scale, the number of global states is $2^{10,000} \sim 10^{3162}$. For comparison, the number of electrons that could be packed into the volume of the known universe is about 10^{120}. This is a microscopic number compared with the number of possible global states defined at macrocolumn or smaller scales.

The purpose of this numeric exercise is not, of course, to suggest how the brain actually works. Rather we suggest that there is no obvious requirement for neocortex to hide all, or even most, of its secrets in small spatial scales not accessible to experimental study from the scalp. We are more likely to have a different problem, one of recording massive amounts of data from many regions and integrating this information to form meaningful quantitative measures of global neocortical function. If we extend the data cited at small scales to larger scales, we can conjecture small patterns within larger patterns, which occur within still larger patterns, and so on, with different information about behavioral or cognitive states coded at different scales. The general idea of state determined by relatively large-scale spatial patterns (as compared with the size of the system) is also supported by recent reports that specific odors are coded in global patterns on the surface of olfactory bulb (Freeman, 1987).

Physics or Neuroscience at Multiple Length Scales

Many physical, chemical, and social systems consist of interacting units at the microscopic level. These interactions can involve nearly any form of information transfer at small scales, such as forces between gas molecules, communication among persons in a social system, or synaptic action between neurons or cortical columns. An open system has, in addition to the internal interactions, external input from the environment. A few macroscopic variables can be defined that characterize much of what is of interest about the system, that is, variables that can be measured directly. When the external input takes on specific character (that is, control parameters attain critical values), macroscopic states may undergo radical changes, called "phase transitions." Possible examples are the transition from laminar to turbulent flow of a fluid at high Reynolds number (due perhaps to high flow velocity), loss of magnetization of a ferromagnetic at high temperature, political revolution due to reduced external food supply (Weidlick and Haag, 1983), or transition from the awake to sleeping state due to removal of brainstem input. These complex systems are the province of nonlinear, nonequilibrium statistical mechanics. Close analogies often exist at the macroscopic level between disparate systems, even when they are composed of different functional units with different interactions at the microscopic scale. The science of these dynamic phenomena in multicomponent systems was labeled "synergetics" by Haken (1983).

With neocortical interactions, the existence of several distinct scales makes the simple distinction between "microscopic" and "macroscopic" insufficient. That is, different spatial scales in neocortex are distinguished by important anatomic and physiologic characteristics, as summarized in Table 2-2. Thus different rules govern interactions at different hierarchical levels. For example, short-range inhibitory synaptic action is clearly important for interactions between minicolumns, whereas long-range excitatory synaptic action may dominate interactions between corticocortical columns. Interaction at the macrocolumn scale may involve short-range inhibition, short- and intermediate-range intracortical excitation, and long-range excitatory (corticocortical) interactions.

An important goal of the emerging field of neocortical physics is to relate rules of interaction across hierarchical levels. For example, we may want to predict statistical properties of macroscopic human potentials (perhaps recorded from the scalp) from a combination of theory and electrophysiologic recordings obtained at smaller scales in animal cortex. Rather than trying to understand the cortex in terms of the interaction of 10^{10} neurons or 10^8 minicolumns, an ideal theory would allow us to move progressively up the spatial scale, with rules at each hierarchical level derived from those at the next lower level (Ingber and Nunez, 1990). In this manner, we would try to create a manageable theory appropriate for the scale of a particular experiment. This is the general approach of Ingber (1982, 1983, 1984, 1985, 1991), who developed a comprehensive and ambitious theory of the "statistical mechanics of neocortical interactions," described in detail in Chapter 14. This work complements other approaches; that is, phenomenologic theories in which plausible input-output relations at higher levels of neural tissue are suggested, and subsequent predictions are made of the outcomes of specific EEG experiments. This latter approach was noted previously and is considered in more detail in Chapters 5 and 11. These two general theoretical approaches are analogous to the simultaneous and independent developments of kinetic and fluid dynamic theories of gas, for example.

The issue of hierarchical level in neocortex is partly analogous to problems encountered in physical media having multiple-length scales for interaction between functional units of the media (Ma, 1976; Wilson, 1979). The latter reference, an excellent popular account by a physicist who received a Nobel prize for his contribution, provides several general ideas that appear to apply to neocortex. Consider, for example, the two-dimensional lattice shown in Figure 2-18 that may, in this account, represent either a region of ferromagnetic material or neocortical surface. In the magnetic case, each location in the lattice shows the magnetic dipole moment associated with a single atom. A filled space represents a positive dipole moment and a blank space indicates a negative dipole moment. At high temperatures (Figure 2-18b), the dipole moments are random so that a macroscopic region produces no net magnetization. When the temperature decreases to the Curie point, the dipole moments of individual microunits become highly correlated to produce a net magnetization in the material (Figure 2-18a). However, fluctuations at smaller scales persist below the Curie temperature, and all scales of length must be included in any comprehensive theory of the ferromagnet. Wilson's graphic description reminds us immediately of the multiple scales of neocortex, that is,

> Small fluctuations are not suppressed; they merely become fine structure superimposed on the larger one. An ocean of positive dipole moments may contain an island of negatives, which, in turn, surrounds a lake of positives with an islet of negatives.

The dramatic increase in apparent correlation length when the Curie temperature is obtained is due only to nearest-neighbor interactions. That is, a molecule with a positive dipole moment influences adjacent molecules so that they have a greater than even probability, depending on temperature, of also having positive dipole moments. When this probability becomes sufficiently high, as occurs at the Curie temperature when the influence of random molecular vibration is reduced, long-range order emerges from short-range interactions. Wilson's contribution, the renormalization group, is a method to construct theories to cross

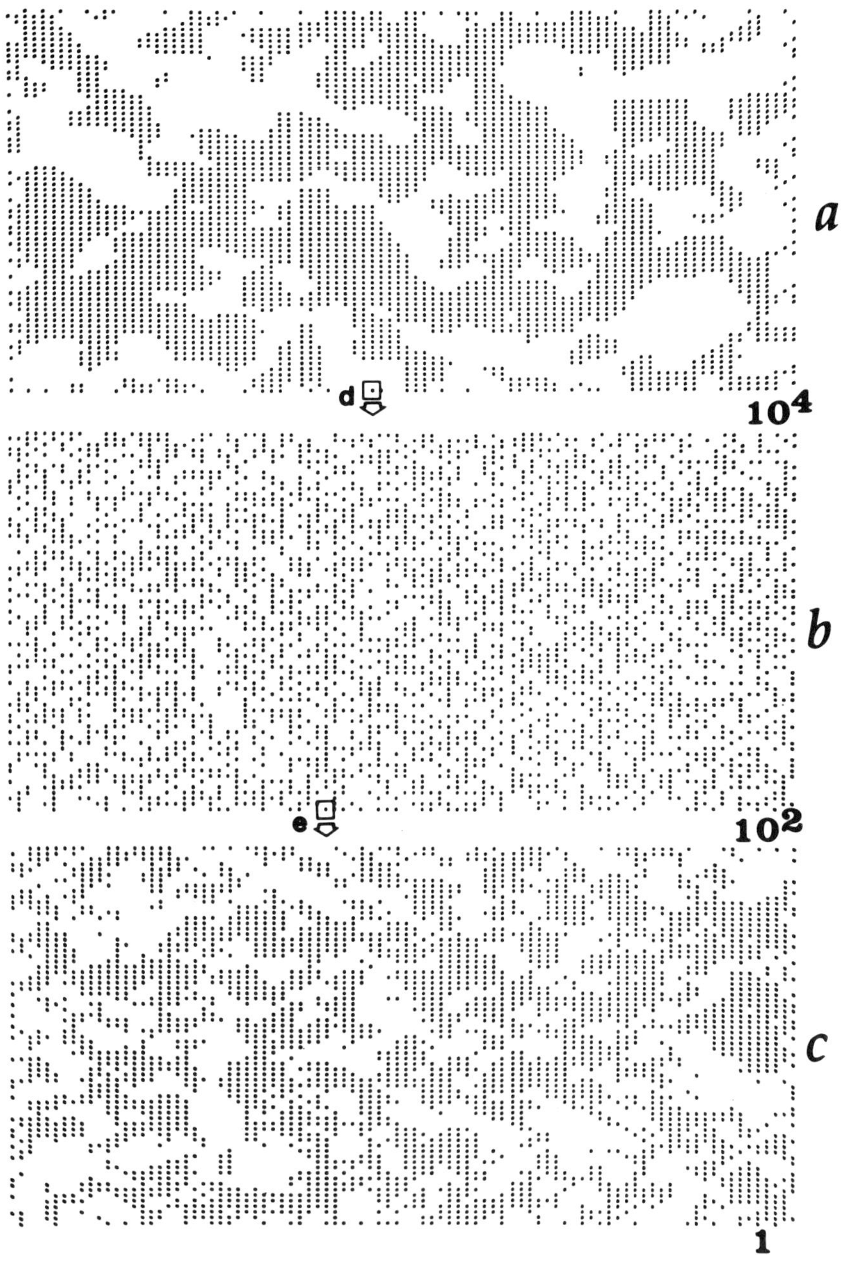

Figure 2-18. Lattice of units representing magnetic dipole moment vector in ferromagnetic materials or instantaneous polarization vector in neocortical columns at different scales. The appropriate vector can, in general, change continuously, but for illustration a filled space indicates a positive vector and a blank space indicates a negative vector. In the magnetic example, (a) represents a material with temperature below the Curie

hierarchical levels. That is, a theory of ferromagnetism is obtained by dividing a large problem with multiple-length scales into a sequence of smaller problems, each of which is confined to a single scale. For example, the lattice of microunits might be divided into M miniunits, each consisting of N contiguous microunits. The magnetic dipole moment of the m th miniunit may be expressed as the average of the dipole moments of the N microunits, P_n, that is

$$\hat{P}_m = \frac{1}{N}\sum_{n=1} P_n \qquad m = 1, M \tag{2.16}$$

This procedure is illustrated in Figure 2-18 at locations d and e with N = 6300 microunits. The original lattice of microunits (c) is replaced by a lattice of miniunits (b), and the problem advances one level in the hierarchy. This procedure may be repeated so that the lattice of miniunits is replaced by a lattice of mesounits (a), which is replaced in turn by a lattice of macrounits, and so on. The success of the renormalization group is in allowing calculation of the rules governing interactions at one level from the rules that apply at lower levels. Some mathematical features of the renormalization group have been applied to neocortex (Ingber and Nunez, 1990). In the statistical mechanical treatment of neocortex (Ingber, 1983, 1984), analogs of temperature (in magnetic materials) might be neuromodulators of synaptic activity, which may be incorporated in control parameters. Of course, the analogy between magnetic materials and neocortex cannot be considered precise. One caveat is that the renormalization group treatment requires continuity across scales on each side of the Curie temperature. In neocortex, different scales may have quite different interaction rules, so EEG theory, for example, is expected to require more specific connections to the appropriate columnar scale, as illustrated in Chapter 14. Also corticocortical fibers or long intracortical fibers should enhance long-range correlations that might be barely supported by the shorter range columnar interactions, as discussed in Chapters 1, 11, and 14.

Figure 2-18 also may be used to illustrate neocortical dipole fields at three successive spatial scales. The units (a) exhibit a long effective correlation length, the units (b) a short correlation length, and the units (c) a moderate correlation length; that is, the dipole field cannot be described by a single correlation length. Correlation functions estimated from the experimental data depend on the size and location of the sensor. This point appears to be poorly understood in elec-

←

point (magnetized) and (**b**) represents an unmagnetized material at high temperatures. In the neocortical example, three spatial scales are depicted, spanning roughly four orders of magnitude. A highly correlated dipole layer at perhaps the regional column scale (**a**) is examined more closely by expanding small region (d) to reveal quasi-random dipole layer at intermediate scale (**b**), which is, in turn, examined more closely by expanding region (e) to obtain moderately correlated dipole layer at perhaps the sub-minicolumn scale. This figure is for illustration only; it is not based on any neurophysiologic calculations. (Reproduced with permission from Nunez, 1989b, based partly on description in Wilson, 1979.)

trophysiology, in which recordings span five orders of magnitude of spatial scale. For example, intracortical connections might produce patches of moderately correlated minicolumns (c). Perhaps the corticocortical modules simultaneously produce patterns of uncorrelated activity (b), whereas macrocolumns produce activity (polarization for example) of high correlation (a). This situation could change with physiologic state. These ideas are only descriptive; they are not based on any neocortical theory. However, the complexity of neocortical dynamics, including the fact that synaptic interaction lengths span seven orders of magnitude, make such general speculation plausible.

We have good reasons to believe that spatial scale considerations partly account for the differing views of brain dynamics held by physiologists and electroencephalographers. The former record potentials at sub-macrocolumn scales, often at sub-minicolumn scales. But the character of spatial patterns (for example, coherency) is scale dependent. To take an example from a different field, we can note that the pattern of human population density (and its dynamics) in a neighborhood is different from the highly clumped patterns of humans in cities, as observed at global scales.

Global Integration of Neocortical Function

Neuroscience in this century has been influenced strongly by the idea that the brain develops in phylogeny (that is, through evolution) by the successive addition of more parts. In this view, each new addition has been accompanied by more complex behavior and, at the same time, imposed regulation on more primitive parts of the brain (Mountcastle, 1979). Thus the brainstem (the "reptilian brain"), limbic system, and neocortex form three distinct levels, both in spatial organization and in terms of evolutionary development, with the lower structures perhaps retaining many of their former functions (McLean, 1977). Or, expressed in the more colorful language of Koestler (1967), "when a psychiatrist treats a patient, he is dealing with three creatures, an alligator, a horse, and a man." Although much of this view remains intact, other developments support a more global concept. As expressed by Mountcastle, "the brain is a complex of widely and reciprocally interconnected systems and the dynamic interplay of neural activity within and between these systems is the very essence of brain function." In this section, we focus mainly on connections between different parts of neocortex and conclude with some rough quantitative ideas about the possible importance of these interactions compared with interactions of neocortex with subcortical structures.

→

Figure 2-19. **a.** A few of the corticocortical fibers in human brain obtained by dissection. The total number of corticocortical axons is about 10^{10}; that is, for every axon shown, there are another 100 million not shown. **b.** Horizontal section of human brain showing callosal axons connecting homologous regions of the hemispheres. (Reproduced with permission from Krieg, 1963.)

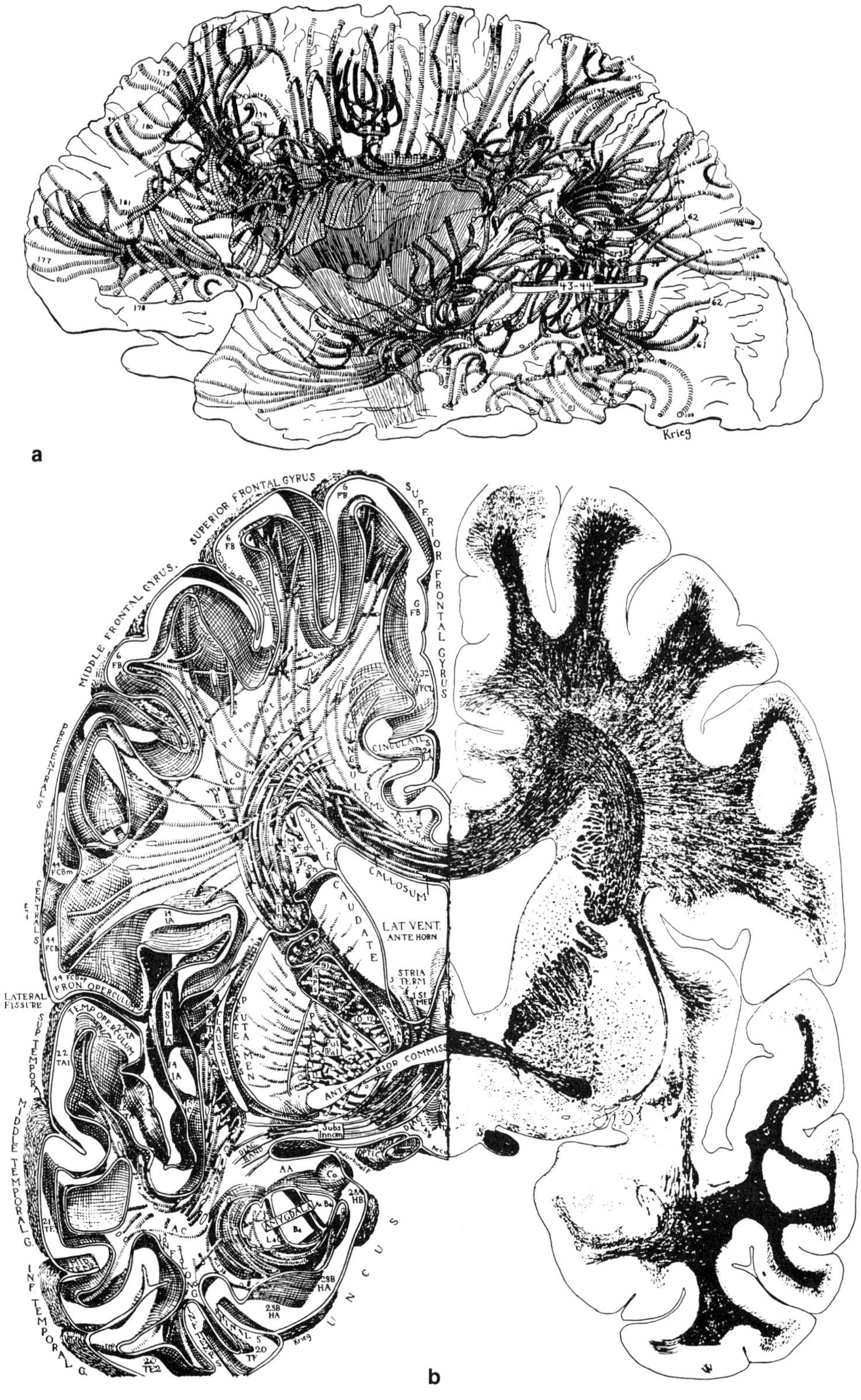
a
Krieg
43-44
b
SUPERIOR FRONTAL GYRUS
MIDDLE FRONTAL GYRUS
PRECENTRAL S
CENTRAL S
LATERAL FISSURE
FRON. OPERCULUM
TEMP. OPERCULUM
INSULA
CLAUSTRUM
PUTAMEN
CAUDATE
CALLOSUM
CINGULATE S
LAT VENT. ANTE HORN
STRIA TERM
ANTERIOR COMMISS
AMYGDALA
UNCUS
MIDDLE TEMPORAL G.
INF TEMPORAL G.

Nonlocal interactions between cortical regions are mainly accomplished by connections of the corticocortical (that is, association) fibers. These axons range in length from less than 1 cm (the U fibers connecting adjacent gyri) to the total length (through the white matter) between frontal and occipital lobes, or about 20 cm. Some of these fibers obtained by dissection of fresh human brain are shown in Figure 2-19a (Krieg, 1963, 1973). Remember, however, that the total number of corticocortical fibers is roughly equal to the number of pyramidal cells, that is, about 10^{10}. Thus, for every axon shown in Figure 2-19a, another hundred million are not shown. In addition, about 2×10^8 commissural (mostly callosal) fibers connect the two brain hemispheres (Tomasch, 1954), and a few are shown in Figure 2-19b.

The remaining fibers of the white matter layer of the human brain are composed of connections between cortex and midbrain, but these fibers contribute no more than a few percent to the total (Braitenberg, 1977, 1978; review by Katznelson, 1981). No compelling anatomic data requires the corticocortical fibers to be substantially less efficient than the diffuse thalamocortical projections in exciting modules (Katznelson, 1981; see also Chapters 9 and 11). Thus human neocortex may be regarded as a structure that is far more strongly coupled to itself than to subcortical structures. Qualitative descriptions in the anatomic literature that emphasize the large number (about 10^8) of diffuse thalamocortical afferent fibers are somewhat misleading in this regard, at least when applied to human neocortex. Note also that the total number of specific sensory axons that provide cortical input is about 2×10^6 (Blinkov and Glezer, 1968), that is, 1 or 2 for every 10,000 corticocortical fibers. These specific afferents are concentrated in a few small areas, that is, primary sensory cortex, and terminate mainly in layer IV. The specific afferents are apparently more strongly coupled to neocortex than are the corticocortical or diffuse thalamocortical input systems.

The specific connectivity of the corticocortical fibers also has been studied by injection of radioactive tracers into cortex that are transported along axons to their terminal branches (Goldman and Nauta, 1977; Kunzle, 1978). These connections are widely distributed, mainly over ipsilateral cortex. There are also dense connections to mirror-image areas of contralateral cortex and fewer diffuse contralateral connections. These connections form repetitively appearing lateral patches approximately 300 to 500 μm wide, that is at the scale of the modules (corticocortical columns) discussed previously. Connection density tends to decrease with distance from the injection site, although quantitative information on the distribution of connections is minimal. Quantitative data on this fiber distribution is considered in Chapter 11 in connection with the global theory.

Despite a paucity of detailed quantitative information concerning the distribution of corticocortical fibers, several interesting estimates have been made by the cortical anatomist Braitenberg (1978, 1979). For example, he imagines division of neocortex into M separate compartments of equal area. We noted the apparent specificity of corticocortical connections between modules with diameters of about 0.3 mm. However, we can imagine an increase in the size of the M compartments such that every compartment can be connected to every other compartment, given a fixed number of connections N. As illustrated by Figure 2-20, the number of compartments defined in this manner is obtained from

$$M = N^{1/2} \tag{2.17}$$

Estimates of neuron number density in human neocortex vary from 1 to $2 \times 10^4/\text{mm}^3$ (Tower, 1954). The average thickness of human cortex is about 2.5 mm; the average of reported surface areas is about 3000 cm^2 (Mountcastle, 1979). These data provide an estimate of neuron surface density of 2 to $5 \times 10^4/\text{mm}^2$ or 6 to 15×10^9 total neurons in the cortex. About 85% of cortical neurons are pyramidal cells (Braitenberg, 1978; Braitenberg and Schuz, 1991), and approximately 95% of these pyramidal cells send an axon into the white matter (Sholl, 1956). Thus the number of corticocortical axons in humans is $N \sim 10^{10}$, and the number of "square root compartments" is $M \sim 10^5$. Each square root compartment sends about 10^5 axons into the white matter, more than 95% of which re-enter the same cortical hemisphere at a distant location (Braitenberg, 1978).

Each square root compartment in humans has a diameter of about 2 mm, the typical size of a macrocolumn. In mouse cortex, the diameter of the square root compartments is about 0.17 mm (Braitenberg and Schuz, 1991). These authors note that in both humans and mice the square root compartments have about the same diameter as the largest dendritic trees, the structures that provide most of the cell surface for synaptic input. Based on the total volume of white matter, the average length of the corticocortical axons in humans is estimated to be a few centimeters (Braitenberg, 1978), although accurate data on the distribution of fiber lengths has not been obtained. However, in one experiment involving mice, the distribution of corticocortical axons was continuous over the range 1 to 7 mm, with broad peaks near 2 and 4 mm and an average length of about 3 mm (Brai-

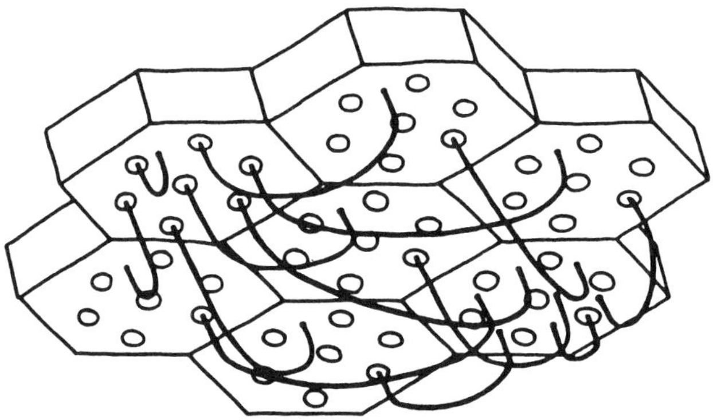

Figure 2-20. Square root compartments, defined so that each compartment can send at least one axon to every other compartment. Neocortical surface is imagined to be divided into M compartments. Given a fixed number of axon connections N, the number of square root compartments is $M = N^{1/2}$. In this simple example, 49 fibers are required for each of the seven compartments to be connected by one fiber to each of the other compartments. (Reproduced with permission from Braitenberg, 1978.)

tenberg and Schuz, 1991). If we apply a linear scale factor based only on brain size (Table 2-1), the corresponding human length range would be about 1 to 10 cm, with an average length of 4 cm. However, some human corticocortical fibers are as long as 20 cm (Kreig, 1963, 1973). The mouse has an unfolded cortical surface, whereas the folding of human neocortex introduces an additional linear scale factor of about two (Nunez, 1981). If this additional factor of two is included, the amplified estimate based on mouse data yields the correct maximum length of human fibers. These data are considered in more quantitative detail in Chapter 11.

The average diameter of human corticocortical axons is approximately 2 μm (Tomasch, 1954; Bishop and Smith, 1964; Blinkov and Glezer, 1968; review by Katznelson, 1981). Thus the maximum possible number of axons crossing the gray-white matter interface of a 4 mm^2 human square root compartment is about 10^6. If we allow a specificity of connections at the macrocolumn scale that requires some compartments to accept more than the average number of inputs and some spacing between axons to minimize "short circuits," these estimates suggest that axon diameters are not very different from the maximum possible, given a fixed geometry and number of connections. Signal propagation velocity is proportional to myelinated axon diameter and axons of the peripheral nervous system are typically much larger (20 μm or more) and produce faster signals (100 m/seconds or more). Thus there is a compromise between signal speed and connectivity. Apparently evolution has opted for increased connections and massively parallel processing rather than speed of serial processing in mammalian neocortex.

Although the number of corticocortical connections to different compartments of human cortex is sufficiently large so that every compartment at the macrocolumn scale could be connected to every other compartment, no evidence suggests this. However, given these numerical estimates and the radioactive tracer studies reviewed in Chapter 11, a reasonable guess is that each macrocolumn compartment is connected directly to perhaps 10% or more of other similar compartments within the same hemisphere. This percentage should increase rapidly as the spatial scale of compartments increases, so the point at which every compartment is connected to nearly every other compartment in the same hemisphere appears to be between the macrocolumn (a few millimeters) and regional scales (a few centimeters). Direct evidence from retrograde axonal transport studies suggests nearly complete intrahemispheric interconnectivity at the regional scale. For example, regions of prefrontal cortex and posterior parietal cortex both project to the same targets in more than 12 distinct cytoarchitectonic regions (Goldman-Rakic, 1988).

Suppose, for purposes of illustration, that each macrocolumn receives input from and sends output to 10% of the other macrocolumns in the same hemisphere (connections to 10^3 to 10^4 other macrocolumns), in addition to a lesser number of connections to widespread locations in the ipsilateral hemisphere. The amount of interconnectivity is 10 to 1000 times greater than that estimated between corticocortical columns (perhaps 10 to 100 interconnections between modules). Thus a neural network view of neocortex suggests degrees of interconnectivity that depend critically on spatial scale: high connectivity between pyramidal cells (10,000), moderate at the modular scale (10 to 100), high at the macrocolumn scale (1,000 to 10,000), and low at very large (lobeal) scales (10). We can, of course, only speculate about the importance of different degrees of interconnectivity at different scales for higher brain function. However, it appears prudent to consider them if we seriously want to understand EEG and shed light on the relation between mind and brain.

What Makes the Human Brain Human?

Consider one of the oldest and most central questions of neuroscience. What distinguishes the human brain from that of other mammals? This question leads us immediately to an apparent paradox. Expressed succinctly, cognitive processing, indeed most, if not all of our conscious experience, apparently depends on the operation of neocortex. But there is very little difference in the cortical morphology (structure) of different mammals. This striking similarity even includes a constant number of neurons within the minicolumn. Larger brains will, of course, have more of these units to interact with one another. However, this does not explain why we are the neuroscientists rather than the elephants, dolphins, and whales, all of which have larger brains covered by folded cortices that look (at least superficially) much like human cortex. We can, of course, form arguments based on the ratio of brain to body weight (Jerison, 1973); however, this kind of study contributes little to the functional question of how human brains produce more complex behavior.

The view expressed by Mountcastle (1979) and many others, that is, that the dynamic interaction between brain subsystems "lies at the very essence of brain function," suggests that we look as closely at the long-range connections as we do at the subsystems themselves. Thus Braitenberg (1977, 1978) noted an important quantitative difference between mammalian species in the fraction of axons entering (and leaving) the cortex that originate (or terminate) in other cortical regions, that is, the ratio expressed in the following equation:

$$R = \frac{\text{number of corticocortical input fibers}}{\text{number of midbrain input fibers}} \tag{2.18}$$

Although we have no data based on actual fiber counts, estimates of lower bounds on the fraction of corticocortical fibers have been made based on the surface areas of cortex and major subcortical regions that border white matter (Braitenberg, 1977, 1978). These and other data have been compiled and summarized by Katznelson (1981), as shown in Figure 2-21.

The area ratio plotted in the lower part of Figure 2-21 represents a rough estimate of the ratio (2.18). Thus the number of midbrain fibers in the rat is roughly equal to the number of corticocortical fibers. In contrast, the portion of corticocortical fibers in humans is at least 95% according to these estimates. In fact, the data suggest that the number of corticocortical connections becomes a progressively larger fraction of the total fiber population leaving and entering

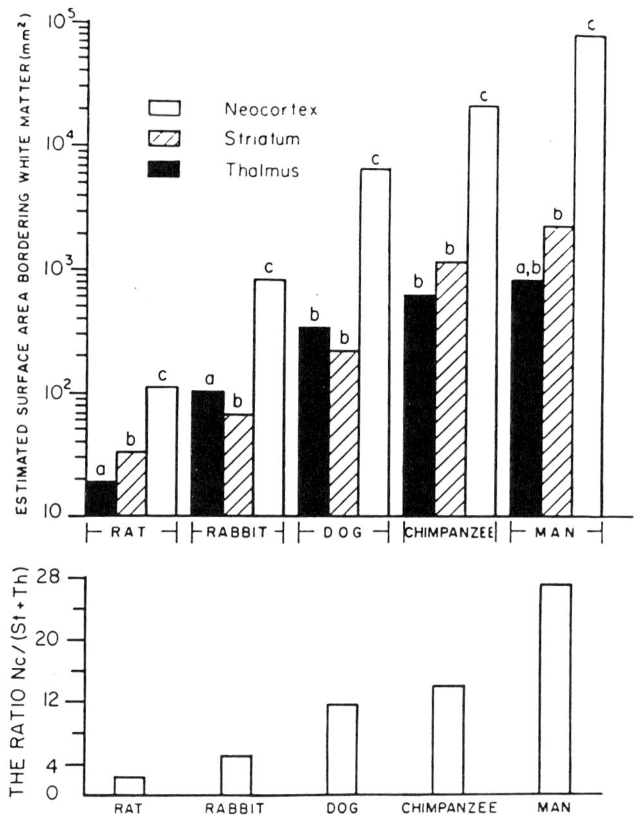

Figure 2-21. Upper. Comparative estimate of surface area bordering white matter in brain structures in a series of mammals. Lower case letters correspond to the estimation method: (**a**) Estimates based on stereotaxic atlases of the thalamus for man, rabbit, and rat. (**b**) Surface estimates based on volumetric data and shape of the corresponding structures. (**c**) Cortical surface area bordering white matter is the cortical surface. **Lower**. The ratio of neocortical surface area to surface area of the thalamus and striatum, that is, an estimate of the ratio of corticocortical to midbrain inputs (equation 2.18). (Reproduced with permission from Katznelson, 1981, based partly on discussion in Braitenberg, 1977, 1978 and Braitenberg, personal communication to Nunez in 1992.)

neocortex as the mammal moves up the phylogenetic scale (Katznelson, 1981). Of course these results are due primarily to disproportionate increases in cortical surface area in higher mammals. However, they appear to have a more direct connection to information processing and potential complexity of function when viewed in this manner.

We have not found sufficient quantitative data to make estimates equivalent to those of Figure 2-21 for mammals with brains larger than human brains, that is elephants, dolphins, and whales (see Table 2-1). However, mean cortical surface area in several studies of bottlenose dolphins was about 60% higher than that of a similarly sized population of human brains. This compares with an increased volume of about 20%. Thus the dolphin brain was determined to be more convoluted than the human brain (Ridgway and Brownson, 1984; Ridgway, 1990), which counters the popular myth that humans have the most convoluted of all brains. Studies of several midbrain regions of the dolphin also have shown large increases over equivalent human midbrain structures. Therefore the corresponding behavior of the ratio plotted in Figure 2-21 is unclear.

Two other anatomic differences between human and dolphin brain are important. Cortical thickness in bottle nose dolphins is only 1.3 to 1.8 mm, about one half that of human neocortex (Ridgway, 1990). Thus the corticocortical columns, proposed as basic units of neocortical function, have less volume for corticocortical synaptic input. Specific thalamocortical input fibers in humans tend to concentrate in layer IV and in the deeper parts of layer III, whereas corticocortical inputs are widely distributed in cortical depth (Szentagothai, 1978). Perhaps a reduced cortical thickness implies less relative density of corticocortical connections than thalamocortical connections. In any case, the corpus callosum of bottlenose dolphins has a cross-section that is apparently no more than 35% of that of a human brain of the same size, which implies much greater hemispheric independence in dolphins than in humans (Ridgway, 1990, 1991). These anatomic data are consistent with the remarkable EEG finding that each dolphin hemisphere can apparently sleep while the other is awake (Mukhametov et al, 1977). We will return to this and human data related to issues of conscious experience in Chapter 3.

The apparent relation between phylogenetic scale and relative long-range interconnectivity of neocortex may or may not hold when scrutinized in a detailed study of larger brains using new methods of quantitative anatomy (such as magnetic resonance imaging). However, the smaller relative importance of cortical-midbrain connections in humans unites the global and evolutionary brain views noted previously. That is, the degree of relative isolation of neocortex from midbrain is a species-dependent quantitative issue. These estimates also make intuitive sense in other ways. For example, we probably believe that we are more intelligent than our pet dogs. But in what sense are we smarter? Our olfactory cortex is certainly not "smarter," any more than our primary visual cortex is likely to be smarter than that of a hawk. However, it may be that more "complete" (in some sense that we barely understand) integration of many cortical modules, most having unknown functions, is an important part of what makes the human brain "human." In addition, feedback between neocortex and midbrain may have relatively less importance in humans than in lower mammals. We are more human than horse-like or alligator-like. This general view also is supported by some EEG studies involving measured coherence between widespread cortical regions in humans and other mammals (Livanov, 1977). These studies highlight the importance of corticocortical interactions in establishing synchronous potentials, whereas subcortical influences were reported to have more importance in animal studies.

Summary

Neocortex can be viewed as a distinct state of matter and studied using methods derived from many branches of science, including physics and engineering. These particular fields are emphasized because they have often been ignored or misused by neuroscientists generally and electroencephalographers in particular. The usual approach of neural networks does not seem to apply very closely to neocortex, at least at small scales. Specific linear and nonlinear physical systems are described in the context of important concepts such as global boundary conditions, nonlinear effects, chaos, standing waves, phase transitions, self-organization and spatial scale interactions. Relations to experimental data are emphasized rather than abstract variables. In particular, the EEG experimental implications of neocortical boundary conditions are emphasized.

The neural structure of neocortex is described with special emphasis on columns of various size and corticocortical interactions. Neocortical dynamics at multiple spatial scales is discussed and comparisons made to complex physical systems that apparently have somewhat similar properties. The brain view proposed is that the "dynamic interplay of neural activity within and between its subsystems is the very essence of brain function" (Mountcastle, 1979), as indicated symbolically in Figure 2-22. Thus, rather than a neural network, the brain can be described more aptly as a neural social system. This idea is extended further in Chapter 3 in connection with the mind–brain issue. An important way to obtain new quantitative measures of neocortical state is by measuring different spatial–temporal statistical properties of EEG and evoked potentials.

Several metaphors from other fields have been adopted. However, real theories of neocortical dynamics, rather than metaphors, begin with known anatomy and physiology. Then they try to make reasonable guesses about which physiologic parameters are most important to the dynamics. Inherent in this process is the

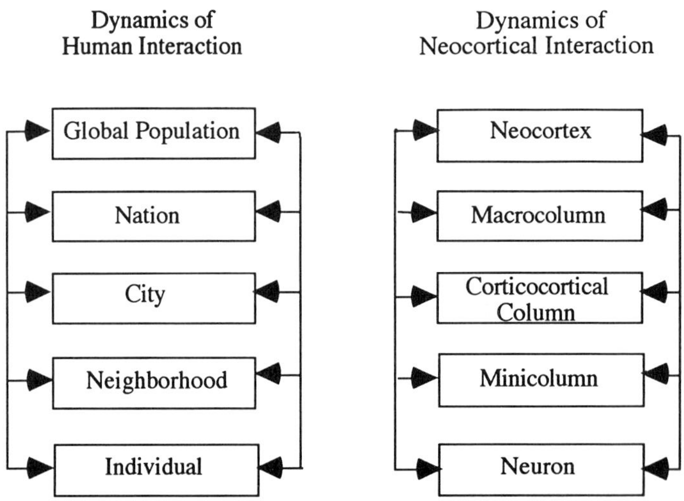

Figure 2-22. Dynamic behavior in complex systems is characterized typically by interactions at the same scale and across scales. Entities in the right column may be viewed as smaller scales of entities in the left column. See Chapter 3 for discussion of sociologic metaphoric links to neocortical dynamics.

question of spatial scale, such as at which level of the hierarchy should connections to experimental data be attempted. Based on these decisions, a set of equations can be derived from some oversimplification of real anatomy and physiology. Solutions to the equations may provide some insight into the dynamics and suggest new kinds of experiments. The new experiments may lead to modifications or complete rejection of the original theory.

However, the process described above sometimes leads to confusion in the neurosciences because of two distinct approaches to "modeling" of the nervous system:

1. Theories based on plausible concepts of physiology and anatomy may be developed, as described in the previous paragraph, in which no free parameters occur. That is, all parameters are in principle, measurable. In certain limiting cases (such as when some parameter is small), the equations may reduce to a set that describes some known physical system, such as spin glasses, hot plasma, and so on. It is then of interest to note the analogy, because many of the consequences of the known set of equations may have been discovered. Thus we may develop a new understanding of neocortical dynamics that, however, can be expected to apply only to certain limiting cases (such as brain states). This is the approach taken in Chapters 5, 11, 13, and 14.
2. Metaphoric links may be developed between neural and physical systems. That is, we may guess at possible similarities, as we do in Chapters 1 to 3. Artificial neural networks perform a similar function. These metaphors may have considerable value in facilitating communication between disparate fields. However, they should not be called "theory," if only because of the enormous difference in potential value to neuroscience (not to mention intellectual effort) required to construct realistic theory as opposed to metaphoric descriptions. Metaphoric descriptions can be expected to go in and out of favor rather quickly. Theory provides a relatively stable foundation on which to build.

Unfortunately, many neuroscientists do not seem to distinguish easily between theory and metaphoric description. The tendency to place everything containing mathematics into a single category is disturbing. It is safe to say that this attitude is a great source of frustration for anyone trying to develop serious theory. Perhaps the first test of any new mathematical description relating to neocortical dynamics includes identifying the following: the physiological parameters (if any) of the "theory"; and predictions made by the "theory" and their dependence on these parameters. In this manner, genuine theories perhaps can be distinguished from metaphoric descriptions, even when the mathematics is obscure or beyond the reader's grasp.

Computer simulations of artificial neural networks cannot contribute substantially to a conceptual framework for neocortical dynamic function unless such networks are convincingly allied with real physiology. Real neurons in human neocortex are so numerous and strongly interconnected that division into manageable subsystems is not easily justified. Furthermore, dynamic behaviors of artificial networks depend on a myriad of connection parameters that must be determined in order to yield genuine theoretical predictions. Despite these limitations, artificial neural networks provide compelling metaphors for emergent behavior based on global dynamic patterns which may have important aspects in common with neocortex (Amit 1989). Modified networks, in which functional units consist of neural masses rather than single neurons, may eventually cross the line between metaphor and theory (Liley and Wright, 1994; Wright and Liley, 1994). It is suggested throughout this book that cognitive events may involve continual reforming of functional neural networks within a background of global dynamic behavior (standing waves, for example). Perhaps realistic models of such networks will eventually be developed at intermediate scales (such as corticocortical columns).

References

Abeles, M. *Local Cortical Circuits.* New York: Springer-Verlag, 1982.

Allman, J. and Kaas, J. Representation of the visual field in striate and adjoining cortex of the owl monkey (aotus trivirgatus). *Brain Res.* 35:89–106, 1971.

Bishop, A.R., Fesser, K., Lomdahl, P.S., and Trullinger, S.E. Influence of solutions in the initial state of chaos in the driven, damped sine-Gordon system. *Physica.* 7D:259–279, 1983.

Bishop, G.H. and Smith, J.M. The size of nerve fibers supplying cerebral cortex. *Exp. Neurol.* 9:483–501, 1964.

Blinkov, S.M. and Glezer, I.I. *The Human Brain in Figures and Tables.* New York: Plenum Press, 1968.

Bok, S.T. *Histonomy of the Cerebral Cortex.* New York: Elsevier, 1959.

Bouyer, J.J., Montaron, M.F., Vahnee, J.M., Albert, M.P., and Rougeul, A.Anatomical location of cortical beta rhythms in cat. *Neuroscience.* 22:863–869, 1987.

Braak, H. and Braak, E. Ratio of pyramidal cells versus non-pyramidal cells in the human frontal isocortex and changes in ratio with aging and Alzheimer's disease. In: *Progress in Brain Research.* (E. Fliers, Mirmiran, M., Van Gool, W.A., and Van Haaren, F., Eds.) Amsterdam: Elsevier, pp. 185–212, 1986.

Braitenberg, V. Comparison of different cortices as a basis for speculation on their function. In: *Synchronization of EEG Activity in Epilepsies.* (H. Petsche and Brazier, M.A.B., Eds.) New York: Springer-Verlag, pp. 47–63, 1972.

Braitenberg, V. *On Texture of Brains.* New York: Springer-Verlag, 1977.

Braitenberg, V. Cortical architectonics: General and areal. In: *Architectonics of the Cerebral Cortex.* (M.A.B. Brazier and Petsche, H., Eds.) New York: Raven Press, pp. 443–465, 1978.

Braitenberg, V. and Schuz, A. *Anatomy of the Cortex. Statistics and Geometry.* New York: Springer-Verlag, 1991.

Broadman, K. *Vergleichende Lokalisationslehre dere Grosshirnrinde in Ihrer Prinzipien dargestellt auf Grund des Zellenbaues.* Leipzig: Barth, 1909.

Bullock, T.H. Reassessment of neural connectivity and its specification. In: *Information Processing in the Nervous System.* (H.M. Pinsker and Willis, W.D., Eds.) New York: Raven Press, pp. 119–220, 1980.

Eccles, J.C. The cerebral cortex: A theory of its operation. In: *Cerebral Cortex, Vol. 2, Functional Properties of Cortical Cells.* (E.G. Jones and Peters, A., Eds.) New York: Plenum, 1984.

Freeman, W.J. *Mass Action in the Nervous System.* New York: Academic Press, 1975.

Freeman, W.J. Analytic techniques used in the search for the physiological basis of the EEG. In: *Handbook of Electroencephalography and Clinical Neurophysiology.* (Revised series) Vol. 1. (A.S. Gevins and Remond, A., Eds.) New York: Elsevier, 1987.

Freeman, W.J. Nonlinear neural dynamics in olfaction as a model for cognition. In: *Dynamics of Sensory and Cognitive Processing by the Brain.* (E. Basar Ed.) Berlin: Springer-Verlag, 1988.

Freeman, W.J. On the problem of anomalous dispersion in chaotic-chaotic phase transitions of neural masses, and its significance for the management of perceptual information in brains. In: *Synergetics of Cognition.* (H. Haken and Stadler, M., Eds.) New York: Springer-Verlag, 1990.

Freeman, W.J. and Skarda, C.S. Spatial analysis, nonlinear dynamics and perception: The neo-Sherrington view. *Brain Res. Rev.* 10:147–175, 1985.

Freeman, W.J. and van Dijk, B.W. Spatial patterns of visual cortical fast EEG during conditioned reflex in a rhesus monkey. *Brain Res.* 422:267–276, 1987.

Goldman, P.S. and Nauta, W.J.H. Columnar distribution of cortico-cortical fibers in the frontal association, limbic, and motor cortex of the developing rhesus monkey. *Brain Res.* 122:393–413, 1977.

Goldman-Rakic, P.S. Changing concepts of cortical connectivity: Parallel distributed cortical networks. In: *Neurobiology of Neocortex.* (P. Rakic and Singer, W., Eds.) New York: Wiley, pp. 177–202, 1988.

Gray, G.M., Konig, P., Engel, A.K., and Singer, W. Oscillatory responses in cat visual cortex exhibit inter-columnar synchronization which reflects global stimulus properties. *Nature.* 338:334–337, 1989.

Haken, H., *Synergetics*, New York: Springer, 1983.

Hubel, D.H. and Wiesel, T.N. Receptive fields, binocular interaction, and functional architecture in the cat's visual cortex. *J. Physiol.* 160:106–154, 1962.

Ingber, L. Statistical mechanics of neocortical interactions. I. Basic formulation. *Physica.* D(5):83–107, 1982.

Ingber, L. Statistical mechanics of neocortical interactions. Dynamics of synaptic modification. *Physical Rev.* A(28):395–416, 1983.

Ingber, L. Statistical mechanics of neocortical interactions. Derivation of short-term memory capacity. *Physical Rev.* A(29):3346–3358, 1984.

Ingber, L. Statistical mechanics of neocortical interactions: Stability and duration of the 7 ± 2 rule of short-term memory capacity. *Physical Rev.* A(31):1183–1186, 1985.

Ingber, L. Statistical mechanics of neocortical interactions: A scaling paradigm applied to electroencephalography. *Physical Rev.* A(44):4017–4060, 1991.

Ingber, L. and Nunez, P.L. Multiple scales of statistical physics of the neocortex: Application to electroencephalography. *Mathematical and Computer Modelling.* 13:83–95, 1990.

Jackson, J.D. *Classical Electrodynamics. 2nd Ed.* New York: Wiley, pp. 360–364, 1975.

Jerison, H.J. *Evolution of the Brain and Intelligence.* New York: Academic Press, 1973.

Jones, E.G. Broadman's Areas. *Encyclopedia of Neuroscience*, Vol. 1 (G. Adelman, Ed.) Boston: Birkhaüser, pp. 180–181, 1987.

Katznelson, R.D. Normal modes of the brain: Neuroanatomical basis and a physiological theoretical model. In: *Electric Fields of the Brain: The Neurophysics of EEG.* (P.L. Nunez, Author) New York: Oxford University Press, 1981.

Koestler, A. *The Ghost in the Machine.* New York: Macmillan, 1967.

Krieg, W.J.S. *Architectronics of the Human Cerebral Fiber Systems.* Evanston, IL: Brain Books, 1973.

Krieg, W.J.S. *Connections of the Cerebral Cortex.* Evanston, IL: Brain Books, 1963.

Kunzle, H. An audioradiographic analysis of the efferent connections from the premotor and adjacent prefrontal regions (areas 6 and 9) in Macaca fascicularis. *Brain Behav. Evol.* 15:185–234, 1978.

Liley, D.T.J. and Wright, J.J. Intracortical connectivity of pyramidal and stellate cells: Estimates of synaptic densities and coupling symmetry. *Network: Computation in Neural Systems,* 5(2): 175–189, 1994.

Livanov, M.N. *Spatial Organization of Cerebral Processes.* New York: Wiley, 1977.

Lopes da Silva, F. Neural mechanisms underlying brain waves: From neural membranes to networks. *Electroencephalogr. Clin. Neurophysiol.* 79:81–93, 1991.

Lopes da Silva, F.H., van Rotterdam, A., Storm van Leeuwen, W., and Tielew, A.M. Dynamic characteristics of visual evoked potentials in dog. I. Cortical and subcortical potentials evoked by sine wave modulated light. *Electroencephalogr. Clin. Neurophysiol.* 29:246–259, 1970a.

Lopes da Silva, F.H., van Rotterdam, A., Storm van Leeuwen, W., and Tielew, A.M. Dynamic characteristics of visual evoked potentials in the dog. II. Beta frequency selectivity in evoked potentials and background activity. *Electroencephalogr. Clin. Neurophysiol.* 29:260–268, 1970b.

Lopes da Silva, F.H. and Storm van Leeuwen, W. The cortical alpha rhythm in dog: the depth and surface profile of phase. In: *Architectonics of Cerebral Cortex.* (M.A.B. Brazier and Petsche, H., Eds.) New York: Raven Press, pp. 319–333, 1978.

Lorenz, E.N. Deterministic non-periodic flow. *Journal of Atmospheric Science.* 20:130–141, 1963.

Ma, S.K. *Modern Theory of Critical Phenomena.* Reading, MA: Benjamin/Cummings, 1976.

McLean, P. On the evolution of three mentalities. In: *New Dimensions in Psychiatry: A World View.* Vol. 2. (S. Arieti and Chrzanokowski, G., Eds.) New York: Wiley, 1977.

Miller, R.H. Experimenting with galaxies. *American Scientist.* 80:152–163, 1992.

Morse, P.M. and Feshbach, H. *Methods of Theoretical Physics.* Vol. 2. New York: McGraw-Hill, p. 1502, 1953.

Mountcastle, V.B. An organizing principle for cerebral function: the unit module and the distributed system. In: *The Neurosciences 4th Study Program.* (F.O. Schmitt and Worden, F.G., Eds.) Cambridge, MA: MIT Press, 1979.

Mukhametov, L.M., Supin, A.Y., and Polyakova, I.G. Interhemispheric asymmetry of the electroencephalographic sleep in dolphins. *Brain Research.* 134:581–584, 1977.

Myslobodsky, M.S., Coppola, R., Bar-Ziv, J., and Weinberger, D.R. Adequacy of the international 10-20 electrode system for computed neurophysiologic topography. *J. Clin. Neurophysiol.* 7:507–518, 1990.

Nunez, P.L. The brain wave equation: A model for the EEG. *Mathematical Biosciences.* 21:279–297, 1974a.

Nunez, P.L. Wave-like properties of the alpha rhythm. *IEEE Trans. Biomed. Eng.* 21:473–482, 1974b.

Nunez, P.L. *Electric Fields of the Brain: The Neurophysics of EEG.* New York: Oxford University Press, 1981.

Nunez, P.L. Global contributions to cortical dynamics: Theoretical and experimental evidence for standing wave phenomena. In: *Dynamics of Sensory and Cognitive Processing by the Brain.* (E. Basar, Ed.) New York: Springer-Verlag, 1988.

Nunez, P.L. Generation of human EEG by a combination of long and short range neocortical interactions. *Brain Topography*. 1:199–215, 1989a.

Nunez, P.L. Towards a physics of neocortex. In: *Advanced Methods of Physiological Systems Modeling*. Vol. 2. (V.Z. Marmarelis, Ed.) New York: Plenum Press, pp. 241–259, 1989b.

Nunez, P.L. Localization of brain activity with electroencephalography. In: *Magnetoencephalography: Vol. 54. Advances in Neurology*. (S. Sato, Ed.) New York: Raven Press, pp. 39–65, 1990a.

Nunez, P.L. Physical principles and neurophysiological mechanisms underlying event related potentials. In: *Event Related Potentials of the Brain*. (J. Rohrbaugh, Johnson, R., Parasuraman, R., Eds.) New York: Oxford University Press, pp. 19–36, 1990b.

Nunez, P.L., Reid, L., and Bickford, R.G. The relationship of head size to alpha frequency with implications to a brain wave model. *Electroencephalogr. Clin. Neurophysiol.* 44:344–352, 1977.

Nunez, P.L. and Srinivasan, R.A. Implications of recording strategy for estimates of neocortical dynamics with EEG. *Chaos: An Interdisciplinary Journal of Nonlinear Science*. 3:257–266, 1993.

Petsche, H., Pockberger, H. and Rappelsberger, P. On the search of the electroencephalogram. *Neuroscience*. 11:10–27, 1984.

Rakic, P. Genetic and epigenetic determinants of local neuronal circuits in the mammalian central nervous system. In: *The Neurosciences 4th Study Program*. (F.O. Schmitt, Worden, F.G., Eds.) Cambridge, MA: MIT Press, pp. 109–127, 1979.

Rall, W. and Shepherd, G.M. Theoretical reconstruction of field potentials and dendrodendritic synaptic interactions in olfactory bulb. *J. Neurophysiol.* 31:884–915, 1968.

Regan, D. Human visual evoked potentials. In: *Handbook of Electroencephalography and Clinical Neurophysiology. Vol. 3 (Revised edition)*. (T.W. Picton, Ed.) New York: Elsevier, 1988.

Ridgway, S.H. The central nervous system of the bottlenose dolphin. In: *The Bottlenose Dolphin*. (S. Leatherwood, Reeves, R.R., Eds.) New York: Academic Press, 1990.

Ridgway, S.H. Personal communication, 1991.

Ridgway, S.H. and Brownson, R.H. Relative brain sizes and cortical surface areas of odortocetes. *Acta Zoologica Fennica* (Helsinki). 172:149–152, 1984.

Scheibel, M.E. and Scheibel, A.B. Elementary processes in selected thalamic and cortical subsystems—the structural substrates. In: *The Neurosciences: 2nd Study Program*. (F.O. Schmitt, Ed.) New York: Rockefeller University Press, pp. 443–457, 1970.

Shaw, G.R. Spherical Harmonic Analysis of the Electroencephalogram. Ph.D. Dissertation. Alberta, Canada: The University of Alberta, 1991.

Sholl, D.A. The Organization of the Cerebral Cortex. New York: Wiley, 1956.

Stockard, J.J. Epileptogenicity of General Anesthetics. Basic Mechanisms and Clinical Significance. Ph.D. Dissertation. San Diego: University of California at San Diego, 1976.

Swadlow, H.A., Rosene, D.L., and Waxman, S.G. Characteristics of interhemispheric impulse conduction between prelunate gyri of the rhesus monkey. *Exp. Brain Res.* 33:455–467, 1978.

Szentagothai, J. The neuron network of the cerebral cortex: A functional interpretation. *Proc. Roy. Soc. Lond.* B201:219–248, 1978.

Szentagothai, J. Local neuron circuits of the neocortex. In: *The Neurosciences 4th Study Program*. (F.O. Schmitt and Worden, F.G., Eds.) Cambridge, MA: MIT Press, pp. 399–415, 1979.

Szentágothai, J. Architectonics, modular, of neural centers. *Encyclopedia of Neuroscience, Vol. 1.* (G. Adelman, Ed.) Boston: Birkhaüser, pp. 74–77, 1987.

Tabor, M. *Chaos and Integrability in Nonlinear Dynamics.* New York: Wiley, 1989.

Taylor, C.P. and Dudek, F.E. Excitation of hippocampal pyramidal cells by an electrical field effect. *J. Neurophysiol.* 52:126–142, 1984a.

Taylor, C.P. and Dudek, F.E. Synchronization without active chemical synapses during hippocampal afterdischarges. *J. Neurophysiol.* 52:143–155, 1984b.

Thatcher, R.W., Krause, P. J., and Hrybyk, M. Corticocortical associations and EEG coherence: a two compartmental model. *Electroencephalogr. Clin. Neurophysiol.* 64:123–143, 1986.

Tomasch, J. Size distribution and number of fibers in the human corpus callosum. *Anat. Rec.* 119:119–135, 1954.

Tower, D.B. Structure and functional organization of mammalian cerebral cortex: the correlation of neuron density with brain size. *J. Comp. Neurol.* 101:19–52, 1954.

Ueda, Y. Steady motions exhibited by Duffing's equation: A picture book of regular and chaotic motions. In: *New Approaches to Nonlinear Problems in Dynamics.* (P.J. Homes, Ed.) Philadelphia: SIAM, pp. 311–322, 1980.

Van der Tweel, L.H. and Verduyn Lunel, H.F.E. Human visual responses to sinusoidally modulated light. *Electroencephalogr. Clin. Neurophysiol.* 18:587–598, 1965.

Wagner, C.A. and Basler, M. Observations of earth—ionosphere cavity resonances. *Nature.* 188:638–641, 1960.

Waxman, S.G. and Bennett, M.V.L. Relative conduction velocities of small myelinated and non-myelinated fibers in the central nervous system. *Nature New. Biology.* 238:217–219, 1972.

Weidlick, W. and Haag, G. *Concepts and Models of a Quantitative Sociology.* New York: Springer-Verlag, 1983.

Wilson, K.G. Problems in physics with many scales of length. *Sci. Am.* 241:158–179, 1979.

Wright, J.J. and Liley, D.T.J. A millimetric scale simulation of electrocortical wave dynamics based on anatomical estimates of cortical synaptic density. *Network: Computation in Neural Systems*, 5(2), 191–202, 1994.

3

Mind, Brain, and Electroencephalography

PAUL L. NUNEZ

This chapter provides a variety of introductory information to readers who lack backgrounds in either biology or the physical sciences. In particular, the mind–brain issue and its connection to electroencephalography (EEG) is considered as an introduction to studies of cognition presented mainly in Chapter 4 (spontaneous EEG), Chapter 6 (steady-state evoked potentials), and Chapter 7 (transient evoked potentials). A brief section on subcortical control of neocortex by neuromodulating systems introduces this topic as it is discussed in Chapters 4, 5 and 13. Additional analogs to physical systems are provided as background for theories of neocortical dynamic function considered primarily in Chapters 5, 11, 12, and 14, with the additional goal of making tentative connections between neocortical dynamics and cognitive studies.

Chapters 8 to 10 provide physical and mathematical background for the theoretical efforts of Chapters 11 and 14. They also make important connections to quantitative neurophysiology. For example, negative feedback in both linear electric circuits and neural tissue is discussed in Chapter 8, thus supplementing discussions of local neural circuits in Chapter 5. Chapter 9 considers the general idea of spatial interactions in physical and neural systems that are approximated as continuous media. Nonlinear systems analysis is introduced in Chapter 10, with special emphasis on biological examples.

Some new data on spontaneous EEG is presented in this chapter that also appear to be consistent with the proposed theoretical framework. Specifically the general idea that certain EEG phenomena (such as alpha rhythm) result from a combination of local or regional circuit effects and global standing waves is suggested by high-resolution images of neocortical magnitude and phase patterns of potential estimated from 64-channel scalp recordings. Furthermore, cognitive processing appears to involve a general shift from more global to more local operation, as indicated by decreased overall coherence obtained when a cognitive task is performed. This qualitative view does not, of course, suggest that cognitive tasks are localized to specific regions of neocortex. Rather a plausible interpretation of the spontaneous EEG data is that cognition involves specific neocortical "circuitry" (at least at very large scales) that may, nevertheless, be distributed over widespread cortical regions. These pilot data appear to be generally consistent with the well-known studies of cognition using transient evoked (or event-related) potentials performed during the last 15 years by Gevins and colleagues, as summarized in Chapter 7. Chapter 6, on steady-state evoked potentials by Silberstein, also supports these general ideas on cognition and the proposed framework of dynamic properties.

This chapter also includes some highly speculative material. No sweeping claims about brain operation are implied. Rather certain ideas about brain operation that appear consistent with data presented in later chapters are suggested. These postulates provide a useful, if tentative framework for further study.

Input-Output in Cerebral Cortex

A succinct overview of brain function is shown in the diagram of Figure 3-1. As a very first approximation, we can regard the brain as a system with certain inputs

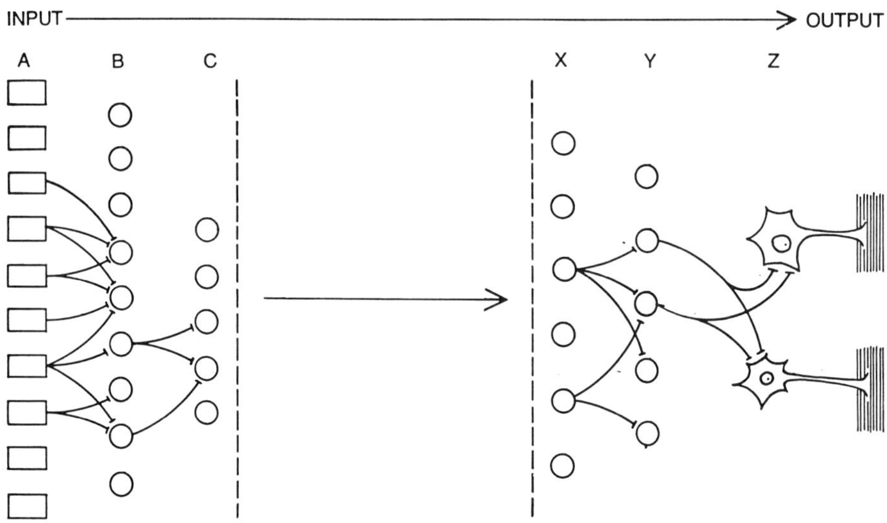

Figure 3-1. Overall organization of the brain is indicated in a rough caricature that suggests the flow of information from the input of sensory signals by receptor cells (A) to the eventual output by motor neurons (Z) terminating on muscle cells. The outputs of receptors and neurons usually branch to send diverging signals to the next stage. Most neurons receive converging inputs, both excitatory and inhibitory, from earlier stages. We know something about the importance of the connections near the input end of the brain (B, C) and near the output end (X, Y). We know much less about the workings of regions in between, which comprise most of the brain. (Reproduced with permission from Hubel, 1984.)

(sensory information) and outputs (motor activity). This view is, of course, greatly oversimplified. As described by Hubel (1984), signals move mainly from left to right in the diagram; however, lateral connections also occur between cells at many stages, as does feedback, or connections from right to left. The same sensory information between input and output can take many possible paths. Thus the number of synaptic relay stations between receptors and muscles may be large or as few as two or three. Physiologists know something about operations close to the input and output ends but very little about operations in between. This lack of knowledge is especially pervasive with neocortical dynamic function.

Time delays between input and output (that is, the response that can be clearly related to known input) can range from a few milliseconds to hundreds of milliseconds or longer. Very short delays are associated with reflex and may not involve the cerebral cortex at all, as with spinal cord reflexes. In contrast, long delays typically involve cognitive processing. It takes some time for an input signal to reach a person's conscious awareness, perhaps as much as 500 milliseconds (Deecke et al, 1976; Libet, 1987).

Another oversimplified aspect of the situation shown in Figure 3-1 is the implied view of the brain as a black box with certain inputs that cause outputs, such as a stimulus-response system in the vernacular of psychology or simply a system using engineering terminology. But this view may have merit only in certain limited cases. First, outputs often occur without any discernible input, and many stimuli elicit no apparent motor response (Harth, 1982). Some argue, however, that such distinctions between engineering systems and the brain are quantitative rather than qualitative; that is, they are the result of vast differences in complexity of the brain and known physical systems. The human stimulus-response view implies that freedom of action and many other aspects normally regarded as "human" are only illusions. The branch of psychology that places more emphasis on the stimulus-response approach to humans is called behaviorism. Skinner (1971) refined early behaviorist ideas by stressing the idea that reinforcement strengthens a response, making it more probable. A newer view of learning called cognitivism emphasizes the role of memory in altering behavior, although the two ideas are not incompatible (Petri and Mishkin, 1994).

One general, qualitative view of what occurs between the input and output ends of the diagram in Figure 3-1, based on anatomic and physiologic studies of cortex and association (that is, corticocortical) connections, was expressed by Pandya and Yeterian (1985);

> As sensory input arrives at the cerebral cortex, it first passes through successive stages of intramodality elaboration, allowing progressively more complex discrimination of stimulus features. Subsequently, by a series of further interconnections, this already elaborated complex information is conveyed to multimodal areas for intersensory integration. In turn, the information is relayed to paralimbic and limbic structures for investment with emotional tone and for memory consolidation. Finally, it is the frontal lobe regions where both sensory and limbic

> influences are integrated in preparation for the organism to execute behavior appropriate to environmental and internal factors.

An expanded view of frontal cortical function is suggested in Chapter 7:

> Although the frontal cortex plays a pivotal role in these high-level (cognitive) processes, it would be simplistic to consider the frontal lobes as only executive in nature. Rather many areas probably are involved in a constellation of rapidly changing functional networks that provide the delicate balance between stimulus-locked behavior and purely imaginary ideation.

Dynamic Analogs of Brain Function

Although the descriptions above are fair representations of the beliefs of many neuroscientists, the vague characterization shows the lack of depth of our understanding of the actual dynamics of neocortical function. Furthermore, the temporal sequence of events implied by the first view is based partly on extrapolation from sequential processes that occur in subcortical regions, especially in peripheral nervous system. But, the anatomic and physiologic data cited in Chapter 2 suggest that the effect of cortical input spreads through neocortex in perhaps 50 to 100 milliseconds. Consciousness awareness of sensory input may occur only after times longer by perhaps a factor of five to ten when multiple feedback mechanisms between remote cortical and subcortical regions have been activated. Thus our subjective conscious experience is strongly correlated with the global dynamics of brain, with neocortex playing a dominant role. Furthermore, the notion of sequential activation of association cortex may deteriorate quickly. Recall, for example, that any two cortical neurons are separated by no more than two or three synapses so that, as a general rule, every neuron "knows" the state of all other cortical neurons (Braitenberg and Schuz, 1991). As a result of these considerations, several neuroscientists noted the apparent analogy between neocortex and complex physical systems with regard, for example, to the important properties of self-organization (Freeman and Skarda, 1985; Freeman, 1987), multiscale interactions (Ingber, 1981, 1991; Nunez, 1981; Ingber and Nunez, 1990), and global boundary conditions (Nunez, 1974a, 1981, 1989a; Katznelson, 1981).

A simple example of multiscale interactions is provided by the string-springs system shown in Figure 2-4, except that for the arguments of this section, the string does not have to be linear. The string-springs system also illustrates the issue of causal interactions across hierarchical levels of dynamic function. This analogy is appropriate if each spring corresponds to one of the columnar structures of neocortex. Thus the number of springs imagined is about 100 to 10,000 (in one dimension), depending on column size. Two limiting cases occur for which causal descriptions are accurate.

1. When string tension is sufficiently small, the feedback of string motion (analogous to large-scale behavior in the brain) on the springs (analogous to small-

scale behavior) is negligible. Thus an accurate view is that spring motion causes the motion of the string. This is strictly a "bottom up" influence across spatial scales. Furthermore, motions of different springs are uncorrelated (that is, incoherent or asynchronous) because the mechanism for information transfer between springs was removed by making the string limp.

2. When spring constants (which measure stiffness of springs) are sufficiently small, the feedback of spring motion on the string is negligible. Thus an accurate view is one in which the string causes (or drives) the springs. This is a "top down" influence across spatial scales. This case also differs from that above because spring motion will, in general, be correlated due to the unifying influence of string motion, which is partly restricted by global boundary conditions.

When the physical parameters of the system assume arbitrary values, motion of the string and spring system involves an ongoing transfer of information in both directions across spatial scales. We can no longer identify either the springs or the string as causal agents; rather we can speak only of the dynamic interaction between the string and springs. This example illustrates some typical behavior of complex systems and, as suggested in several discussions of this book, may help alert us to possible kinds of brain behavior.

The string-springs analog has the important property of relative simplicity. For example, numerical solutions of the equations of motion have been obtained and a variety of behavior described quantitatively, such as temporal chaos coexisting with stable spatial structure (Nunez and Srinivasan, 1993; see also Chapter 10). However, this system is too simple to mimic other complex behavior that may be important in brain science. Thus we turn to another analog, the human global social system, which consists of the dynamic interaction of 5×10^9 human brains. Obviously, with this colossal advance in system complexity, we are describing a system that mostly prohibits quantitative analysis. However, it has been argued convincingly that social systems show many of the same general attributes as complex physical systems, including self-organization and multiscale interactions (Weidlick and Haag, 1983).

For most of human history (a few hundred thousand to a million years), human brain interaction has occurred almost exclusively through local sensory exchange. Nonlocal mechanisms, such as smoke signals, carrier pigeons, and especially journeys of explorers often have had critical effects on history. However, the bulk of information transfer has been mainly local; that is, influence between distant populations have occurred largely by transfer through people and places in between. A dramatic change occurred with the invention of the printing press and later with the widespread use of radio and television. A more recent example is the growing use of electronic mail connections among scientific groups. Thus the human dynamic system has undergone a fundamental change of character during a period equal to only 0.01% of its history. We live in this narrow time window. We note the analogy of nonlocal interactions in neocortex through the corticocortical system, which has been cited as an important contributor to human behavior and consciousness, as discussed in Chapter 2. We can also speculate about the implications of massive new nonlocal interactions for humanity as a whole.

A second apparent similarity of the human global system to brain dynamics is that of multiscale interactions, such as interactions between individuals, families, neighborhoods, cities, and countries. In the string-springs system and many other simple physical systems, the dynamics can be separated into microscopic and macroscopic categories without finer distinction. However, many complex physical systems and the human global system are characterized by many hierarchical levels of interaction, as indicated in Figure 2-22. Interactions occur between different entities at the same scale and across scales. For example, persons (such as political leaders, writers, scientists, business leaders, criminals) often cause critical changes at higher levels (even directly at the global level), thereby providing "bottom up" influences across spatial scales. However, the suggested causality is only a crude approximation because these critical persons are also formed and continually influenced by their environment. Furthermore, individuals are simultaneously and directly influenced by multiple higher and lower scales, ranging from the human global system (and perhaps higher) to systems composed of single cells and smaller units. A continual flow of information occurs across scales.

The limiting case approximation that emphasizes the causal role of individuals is sometimes called the "great man theory of history," a concept having some common ground with the putative "grandmother cell" of neurophysiology. But more realistic brain analogs occur at scales above the single neuron level. These are relatively small structures that effect critical influences on global brain function, such as the general activating system of brainstem and thalamus (controlling sleep-waking), Wernicke's and Broca's areas of cortex (required for different language functions), and hippocampus (important for long-term memory storage). Dramatic changes in the character of physical systems (such as transitions from water to ice, magnetized to nonmagnetized) are called "phase transitions" (Haken, 1982). In the human global system, we use labels such as "industrial revolution," "world war," and so on to indicate phase transitions. The critical macroscopic parameters that have dominant influence on phase transitions in physical systems are called "control parameters." A change in control parameters (such as by changing the temperature of a fluid system) may cause phase transitions. After this new order has emerged, the system has changed in essential respects and new variables, called "order parameters," are needed to describe it. New order parameters typically emerge after each phase transition. Order parameters governing war and peace may involve food or oil supply, religious fervor, monetary inflation, personal ambition, and so on. Obviously we have no quantitative theory of social systems that allows precise prediction of phase transitions. However, advantages may exist in fields such as economics, politics, and so on to adopting some of the terminology and conceptual framework from physical systems for which more precise prediction is possible.

A third important aspect of complex systems having sociologic counterparts is self-organization (Prigogine and Stengers, 1984; Nicolis and Prigogine, 1989). In closed physical systems (that is, having no outside influences), the second law of thermodynamics ensures that entropy can only increase; that is, order (in a technical sense defined in Chapter 10) must decrease continually toward equilibrium.

However, systems with external input (such as energy, information) can be far from equilibrium. Such physical systems are typically studied with new methods (developed during the last 20 years) of nonequilibrium statistical mechanics, as described in Chapter 14. Examples of self-organization in physical systems are Jupiter's great red spot, earth hurricanes, and spatial pattern formation due to chemical reactions in a laboratory dish. In fact, the development of living molecules in the primordial sea is believed to be a highly developed example of self-organization.

Roughly speaking, self-organization is due to some positive feedback mechanism that may draw a disproportionate share of energy, mass, and so on, into a local region. The typical example in social systems is urbanization. For some reason (such as local water supply or perhaps a random fluctuation), a particular location has a higher population density than its surroundings. Others living outside this new "town" see advantages of moving in, such as safety, commerce, labor specialization, and social interaction. As more persons move in, the advantages continue to grow, thereby attracting still more persons until (presumably) the disadvantages of crime, crowding, pollution, and so on overcome the advantages. Freeman (1987) obtained evidence for self-organization in olfactory bulb, in which specific odors have signatures expressed as specific spatial patterns on the surface. Neocortical function may involve self-organization in a somewhat similar manner (Freeman, 1990). A partial switch from global standing waves to distributed or local circuit operation (associated with a cognitive task, for example) may be a form of self-organization.

A fourth apparent similarity between brain and social systems is that of nonlocal temporal interactions, called "non-Markovian" interactions in the physical sciences. Much information, in the form of written texts, can be retrieved from libraries, which provides one-way communication of earlier ideas from the living and the dead. Again this type of information access is a very recent development in human history. The analogy to storage of large amounts of information in human long-term memory is compelling. In contrast, the information capacity of short-term memory is severely limited and appears to have a more Markovian character. A theoretical basis for short-term memory is suggested in Chapter 14.

Music, Violins, and Physics

Metaphoric links between mind, brain, and scientific method and music, violin, and physics are suggested as a starting point for discussion. We first consider the violin as a brain analog. In this manner, we can forge a few connections between the issues of scale interactions, standing waves, neural plasticity, multiple structures, pacemakers, and EEG resonance. As with the sociologic metaphor, we want to carry analogy as far as possible without deciding in advance how seriously to regard it. We are not attempting to describe how brains work in any general sense but rather introduce some ideas about how brains may sometimes work, an exercise that, in turn, may suggest new kinds of experiments to test new ideas.

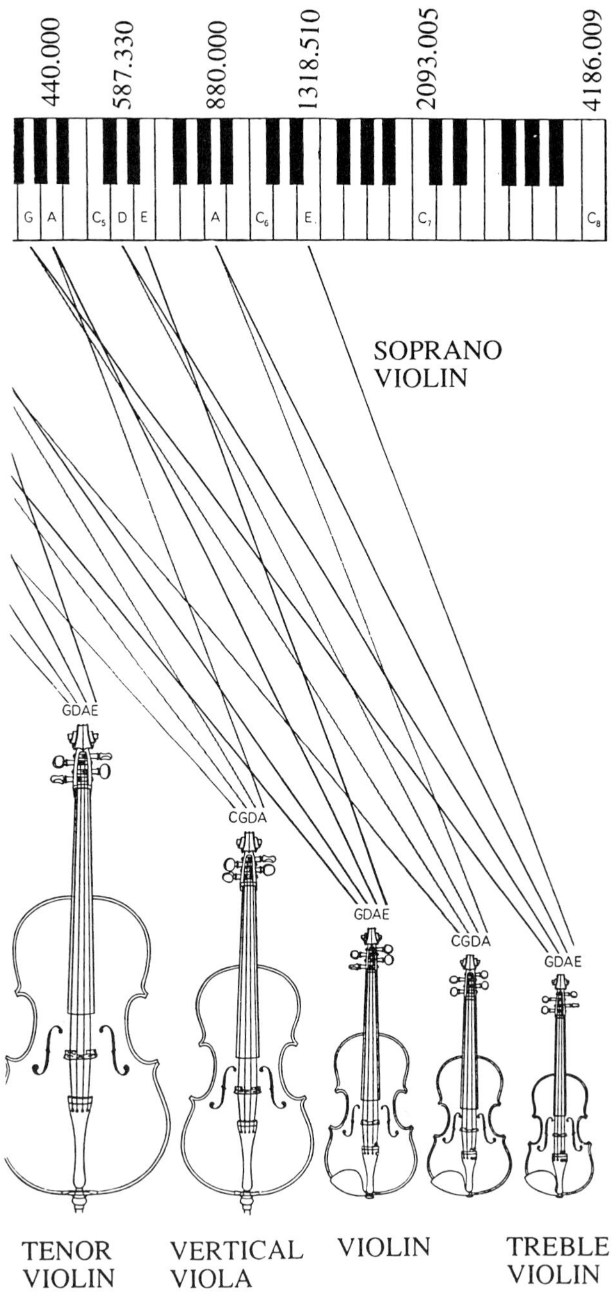

Figure 3-2. Smaller members of the violin family. The bass and cello are not shown. Large instruments generally produce a lower range of frequencies due to increased string length and larger bodies. However, several other features contribute to frequency range. Each member has four strings with different fundamental frequencies, as indicated by the piano keyboard. Numbers along the keyboard indicate notes to which the four strings of each instrument are tuned; frequencies are given in Hz. (Reproduced with permission from Hutchins, 1962.)

The violin family of musical instruments evolved during many centuries, by "natural selection" rather than by scientific analysis. The violin itself reached its present form in the sixteenth century and stabilized by the end of the eighteenth century (Taylor, 1965). The violin consists mainly of four strings, a wooden body, and a bridge, as shown in Figure 3-2. Each string (labeled GDAE) has its own fundamental mode frequency determined by its length, tension, and mass per unit length. (In the guitar, effective string length can be altered by moving the frets.) Each string generally vibrates at a mixture of frequencies consisting of the fundamental mode and overtones (called "partials" by musicians). In the special case of a string vibration, the overtones are, to close approximation, integral multiples of the fundamental frequency; that is, the overtones are harmonics. The first overtone is the second harmonic, the second overtone is the third harmonic, and so forth. The manner in which the amplitude of a string is distributed over the harmonics is determined by how and where it is plucked in the example of the guitar, in which case transient oscillations are created in the string. The violin example is similar except that the bow remains in constant contact with the strings and forced oscillations are produced at some combination of mode frequencies, which depends on the skill of the musician, that is, how and where he or she moves the bow.

The strings themselves produce very little sound. The body of the musical instrument is required to amplify string vibrations so they can be heard. This occurs through energy transfer from strings to body through the bridge. However, different overtones of the strings are amplified selectively. This selectivity is due primarily to the properties of the resonant cavity formed by the wood body. (The term "resonant cavity" can be applied to many wave media and geometry in which boundary conditions dictate allowed spatial eigenfunctions. These need not be physical hollow cavities, as in the example of musical instruments.) Both the wood and air vibration contribute to the sound. The complex shape of the body creates a multiplicity of modes (that is, resonant frequencies), which are overtones of the fundamental mode of the violin body. These overtones are generally not harmonics of the body's fundamental frequency. Thus those string modes that match body modes are amplified most efficiently by the body and make the largest contributions to the resulting musical sound. The frequencies and corresponding amplitudes of the overtones determine the quality or timbre of the sound.

Because the modes of vibration produced by string and body have independent origins, there is no guarantee that any of the modes will match exactly. To produce a better match, the body must be constructed to act as a resonant amplifier that responds over a relatively broad band of frequencies. Two methods can accomplish this (Taylor, 1965): (1) Design a body with heavy damping to broaden the resonance peak, as illustrated by Figure 8-2, or (2) make the body more complex to produce more closely spaced modes. An example of this general phenomenon in resonant cavities is changing the spherical shell to a prolate spheroid shell, as shown in Figure 2-12. Another example is coupled oscillators with either equal or different resonant spectra, as shown in Figure 8-5.

Because each violin string has its own fundamental mode and set of overtones, independent of the other strings, these resonant modes are more local than the body modes. To enhance our analogy to local and global processes in neocortex, we can imagine a musical instrument with millions of small strings (a "super piano") representing neocortical columnar dynamics. The degree of coupling between local string modes can be varied by changing control parameters (such as when the musician pushes different piano pedals). In this manner, many string modes could be created at many different spatial scales of operation. However, only those string modes that matched the global body modes would contribute substantially to the musical sound.

In addition to the basic operation of musical instruments, additional subtle effects, called "formants" occur due to nonuniform resonance or amplification; these may distinguish two apparently identical instruments. Variations in body wall thickness is a possible cause. Others include slight alterations in overtone frequencies after repeated use, that is, plasticity. ("Violins seem to get better after being played for a century or so." [Taylor, 1965]). We can wonder if a somewhat analogous effect occurs in brain. Repeated excitation of global modes, which are proposed to be determined by corticocortical propagation velocity and boundary conditions, may influence local time scales at the synaptic level, an idea apparently consistent with general notions of neural plasticity.

Fundamental and overtone frequencies occur as a result of interference between waves traveling in different directions that combine to form standing wave patterns. These spatial patterns are called the "eigenfunctions" of the system. In the examples of the violin, one-dimensional patterns are created in the strings, and two-dimensional patterns occur in the body surface. The two-dimensional patterns may be observed directly by placing sand on the surface of a vibrating body, as shown in Figure 3-3 (Saunders, 1948). The sand accumulates along nodal lines (lines of zero motion) of the eigenfunctions (or linear combination of eigenfunctions). If the body is excited in just the right way (as determined by the spatial properties of the exciting force), single modes can be excited. Thus, for each temporal frequency, a corresponding spatial pattern occurs, or spatial frequency with one-dimensional standing waves.

The concept of spatial frequency is not precise in systems with complicated two- or three-dimensional shapes because the eigenfunctions are no longer sinusoidal. However, the general idea that high spatial frequencies correspond to high temporal frequencies is preserved. For example, in the violin body, low tones occur with a spatial pattern consisting of a few large areas having equal signs of deflection at any fixed time; high tones correspond to patterns with many such small areas. This effect is also illustrated by patterns in the spherical shell (Figure 2-12) or more simply for the rectangular drum membrane, as illustrated in Figures 9-4 and 9-5. Evidence that brain waves may exhibit this general kind of behavior is presented in Chapters 2, 6, 11, and 12, although in contrast to simple physical waves, higher eigenfunctions are predicted to contribute to fundamental brain wave frequencies. Possible standing waves of EEG (generally composed of a combination of eigenfunctions) are illustrated in this chapter.

Because resonances in the body and strings of instruments in the violin family

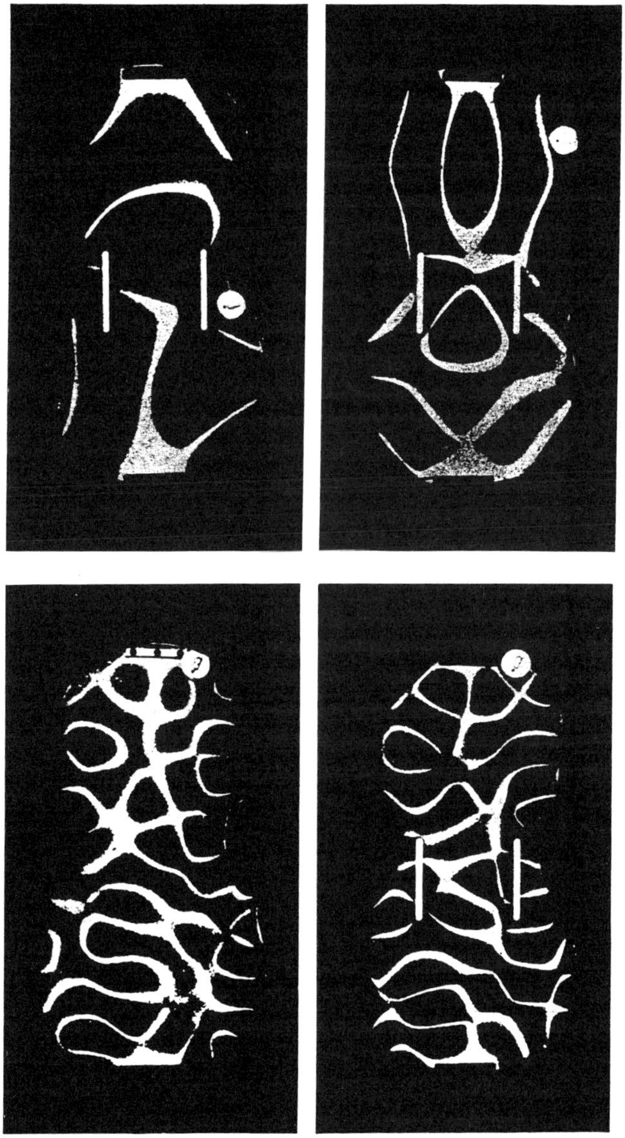

Figure 3-3. Patterns produced by covering a violin-shaped brass plate with sand and drawing a violin bow across its edge. When the plate vibrates, sand concentrates along the nodal lines, which here result from a linear combination of eigenfunctions. Motion on either side of a nodal line is out of phase. Bowing the plate at various points, indicated by the circular marker, produces different combinations of vibration frequencies with corresponding spatial patterns. Low frequencies occur with a pattern of a few large areas, whereas high frequencies occur with many small areas. (Reproduced with permission from Saunders, 1948.) Similar EEG patterns on the cortical surface are shown in this and other chapters.

are due to standing waves, we expect that if two instruments are similar except in size, the larger will produce the lower range of frequencies. And this is generally true (Hutchins, 1962). The violin has a length of 60 cm and an orchestral range of 196 to 2,000 Hz, whereas the cello has a length of 115 cm with range of 65 to 700 Hz. The large bass has an even lower range. Exact frequency ranges depend on the details, however. For example, the four violin strings are tuned to the fundamental frequencies (Hz) 195.998 (G), 293.665 (D), 440.000 (A), and 659.225 (E). The main resonance (the one most easily excited by string motion) of the wood body is close to that of the A string. In addition, resonances at lower frequencies are associated with the air motion inside the body. Furthermore, a subharmonic resonance at one half the main wood resonance normally improves the quality of lower tones. Thus the relatively simple example of harmonic overtones in each of the four strings does not accurately describe the violin's sound, which depends on other factors, including the complex pattern of modes produced by the body and the details of coupling between strings and body. Other possible effects that may be important in similar resonant systems are nonlinear interactions between frequency components (such as combination tones, described in Chapter 10) and feedback from body to strings. When the latter effect is sufficiently large, we can no longer think of the strings as driving the cavity resonances. Rather there is a single integrated system involving complex interactions between different parts of the system.

A physiologic basis for wave interference and global standing waves is described in detail in Chapter 11. Briefly, this phenomenon mainly requires that each neural mass have a relatively large number of synapses so that the modulation of synaptic action within the tissue mass exhibits an approximately linear relation to modulation of action potential input. Thus the analysis applies most clearly to relatively large spatial scales. Wave propagation requires only that signals are transferred between two locations in a time roughly proportional to the distance between locations. One basis for such signal propagation at large scales is provided by the corticocortical axons. Direct experimental evidence for macroscopic waves traveling in the correct velocity range (5 to 13 m/second) is presented in Chapters 6 and 12. Standing waves are generally expected in closed systems, in which waves traveling in one direction on the surface can interfere with waves traveling in other directions, as in the examples of the spherical or prolate spheroidal surfaces discussed in Chapter 2. Whether waves are actually observed in any such system depends on the magnitude of wave damping. In neocortex, wave damping is proposed to be determined by the relative contribution of inhibitory and excitatory synaptic action, as measured by the magnitudes of external control parameters.

An old idea in EEG is that dominant frequencies are due to subcortical "pacemakers" that drive the cortex (Andersen and Andersen, 1968), as depicted in Figure 3-4. Partial support for this idea is provided by experiments involving either surgery or drugs that block interactions between cortex and a midbrain structure, such as the thalamus. Ideally this procedure would be somewhat analogous to removing the bridge in the violin so energy from string vibrations can no longer excite cavity resonances. One of the problems in evaluating the concept

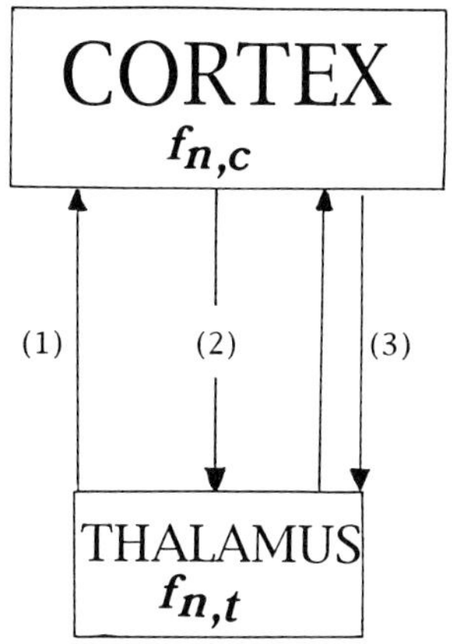

Figure 3-4. Symbolic representation of three kinds of cortex–thalamus interaction. (1) Thalamus is assumed to produce its own set of characteristic frequencies $f_{n,t}$ (n = 1, 2, 3 . . .) that are imposed on neocortex; that is, the usual "pacemaker" idea. (2) Cortex produces characteristic frequencies $f_{n,c}$ that are imposed on thalamus. (3) Dynamic interaction between cortex and thalamus. If coupling is sufficiently strong, the characteristic frequencies can no longer be identified with a single structure.

of pacemaker origins of EEG is that this term is often used simply to explain away phenomena that are poorly understood. To avoid such tautologies, the word "pacemaker" may be defined more precisely as a mass of neural tissue that produces signals with characteristic spectral peaks due only to neural interactions within the mass. These resonant frequencies may then provide input into a second neural system (the neocortex) in which the same spectral peaks are recorded, that is, case 1 of Figure 3-4. Given this definition, the following objections can be made to most pacemaker explanations of EEG data.

1. The pacemaker idea typically attributes some resonant frequency to a small mass of interacting neurons with little justification for why that particular frequency is produced. No mechanism is elucidated for changing frequency with physiologic state or cortical location.
2. Although neurons in the thalamus may produce resonances, cortical neurons are, by implication, not allowed this privilege. In the violin analog, the spectra of actual sounds produced depend as much on cavity as string resonances. Many of the same cavity resonances could be excited if white noise input were to replace driving by the strings (although the quality of the sound would suffer greatly). Thus the violin strings are not labeled very accurately as "pacemakers" of musical sounds, although they do produce similar frequencies.
3. The thalamic pacemaker concept disallows the possibility that resonances are due to important interactions between thalamus and cortex, which in this case, must be considered a single system. Obviously blocking these feedback circuits will eliminate or alter resonances. However, such outcomes are not necessarily evidence for pacemakers.
4. Many of the experiments that block thalamocortical interactions also block corticocortical interactions because both fiber systems form the white matter. Action potential propagation in corticocortical axons provides a plausible mechanism for neocortical resonances. Thus interference with the normal operation of these axons should affect EEG frequencies. Again such outcomes do not necessarily provide evidence for pacemakers.
5. The overall background state of neocortex is controlled by chemical and

electrical input from the brainstem. Interference with this input affects cortical EEG. This does not, however, necessarily imply a brainstem pacemaker. For example, there is evidence that brainstem lesions alter the damping but not dominant frequencies of EEG observed in cats (Wright and Kydd, 1984).

A legitimate question concerning any EEG data that exhibit spectral peaks is whether these peaks occur because of neocortical resonance or subcortical pacemakers, or whether they depend critically on interactions between cortical and subcortical regions, as illustrated by Figure 3-4. One way to resolve this issue involves driving a sensory system of an animal with sine wave-modulated input and recording the steady-state response at midbrain and cortical locations. If resonance is observed only at the cortical level, this structure would be implicated as the origin of resonance. However, if resonance was observed at both subcortical and cortical locations, we might not be able to determine whether the resonance was due only to the subcortical structure or its dynamic interaction with cortex and other structures. Unfortunately there is a paucity of this type of data. The issue of localized pacemaker compared with distributed circuit origins of resonance is considered further in Chapters 5 and 13.

It may be difficult to separate local from global resonances experimentally. Locally measured properties may be partly or largely due to global, that is "top down" influences, as illustrated in Figure 2-4. A second possible reason involves neural plasticity. It has long been suspected that learning changes brain structure at the synaptic level. For example, there is the "Hebb rule," a postulate that suggests that more active synapses are strengthened by their enhanced activity. Given this view, global resonances, which are partly determined by boundary conditions, might alter local circuit time constants over some developmental period. Because the brain apparently operates locally and globally simultaneously, there may be distinct advantages for a system with matching local and global resonances (or time constraints), in a manner somewhat analogous to the matching of string and body resonances in the violin. This issue is considered more quantitatively in Chapters 13 and 14.

To extend analogs between violin and the neocortical theories of Chapters 11 through 14 further, a more complex version of the violin must be imagined. For example, interactions across spatial scales in a musical instrument might involve placement of many very small (that is, mesoscopic) strings inside the body or attaching them to the strings in the manner of the string-spring system shown in Figure 2-4. These might respond to very high frequencies, created by high overtones of the body or string or by nonlinear interactions between lower modes. The system dynamics then involves a continual exchange of energy across scales, but coupling between scales is more efficient over certain frequency ranges. However, this analogy is imperfect, partly because neocortical dynamics at different scales evidently involve much of the same neural tissue.

Although most essential functions of the violin apparently involve only linear behavior, nonlinear interactions are an essential feature of the statistical methods of Chapter 14. In contrast, the analysis of Chapter 11 is primarily linear. However, an interesting quasilinear case is described in Chapter 11 in which each spatial mode (that is, eigenfunction) follows a separate limit cycle in time, but the total oscillation is still expressed by a linear superposition of spatial modes.

The Brain as a Low Pass Filter

We have used several metaphors to suggest ways in which the brain (or neocortex independently) acts as a multiple band pass filter. The preferred frequency ranges of EEG observed in different physiologic or clinical states of the brain appear to have some similarity to the usual resonant frequencies found in complex physical systems. An additional salient characteristic of human and other vertebrate EEG is its low pass behavior (Bullock, 1977). Most power in a typical vertebrate EEG lies below 100 Hz. With humans and other large mammals, nearly all EEG power is below 50 Hz. In contrast, invertebrate EEG typically contains substantial relative power above 100 Hz. Also invertebrates rarely produce the "slow oscillations" (below 20 Hz) with peaked spectra that are characteristic primarily of humans and several other mammals in specific behavioral states. Much of the vertebrate "slow oscillations" reported in the literature have spectra that can be described as $1/f^n$ noise, such as random noise that has been passed through a low pass filter. These EEG are not good candidates for linear, global resonances.

A reasonable conjecture is that the high-frequency EEG observed in invertebrates is dominated by the firing of individual neurons (Bullock, 1977). In contrast, we can guess that slow oscillations, sharply peaked frequency spectra, or both result mainly from the collective interaction of many neurons made possible by the high degree of interconnectivity of more complex systems. This does not imply that single neurons cannot undergo slow oscillatory changes of transmembrane potential. However, the primary contribution to EEG recorded with electrodes of moderate to large size (perhaps 1 mm to 1 cm) results from many coherent sources, as discussed in Chapter 1. High coherence usually implies high interconnectivity, and high interconnectivity suggests the importance of system dynamics at scales much larger than that of single neurons.

The possible origins of low pass EEG behavior are discussed in several contexts in this book. For convenience, refer to the following summary.

1. Temporal filtering as a byproduct of spatial filtering. If high temporal frequencies occur with high spatial frequencies (as with most wave phenomena), any mechanism that space averages EEG signals will also remove high temporal frequencies. Space averaging over larger regions occurs as intracranial electrode size increases. Also space averaging increases as the electrode is moved further away from the sources or placed on the other side of a high-resistance medium such as skull. This effect is discussed in Chapters 1 and 2.

2. Temporal filtering by the capacitive properties of dendrites. The core conductor model of a single neuron with branched dendrites may be used to predict the response (the soma transmembrane potential) to synaptic input in the dendritic tree as a function of frequency. Chapter 9 shows that the response decreases

to about one half its zero-frequency maximum at frequencies in the 50-Hz range. This result agrees semiquantitatively with EEG observations.

3. More efficient coupling of input functions to the lower modes of a global oscillating system. The usual resonant cavity has an infinite number of modes (that is, resonant frequencies). However, physically realistic inputs may excite mainly the lower modes because of their spatial and temporal properties. For example, diffuse spatial input primarily excites lower modes. This is true of the Schumann resonances (electromagnetic standing waves near the earth's surface) discussed in Chapters 2 and 10. This issue of diffuse compared with localized input is considered in the context of steady-state visual-evoked potentials in Chapter 6.

4. Low pass dynamics of standing waves due to a spread of the distribution of corticocortical axon velocities. The standing waves in simple physical systems discussed in Chapters 1 to 3 depend on specific, discrete velocity parameters that characterize the wave medium. However, when the underlying velocity is distributed, as in Figure 2-6, new phenomena occur. In particular, wave damping may become more dependent on wave number so that higher modes are more heavily damped. This is illustrated for hot plasma waves in Chapter 9 and for the putative brain waves in Chapter 11.

5. Important contributions of higher spatial modes to lower frequency ranges. Normally this only occurs in nonlinear systems, as with subharmonics discussed in Chapter 10. However, the linearized brain wave equations, derived from neocortical physiology in Chapter 11, have an unusual property for linear waves when solved on the surface of a sphere: Many spatial modes can contribute power to the frequency range of the fundamental and first overtone. (This effect is not predicted for brain waves in an infinite one-dimensional closed loop.)

Human Consciousness and Artificial Intelligence

Many books and articles have been written on the relation between the mind and brain. This copious output apparently results from a combination of widespread interest and paucity of knowledge of the subject in any scientific context. The latter condition allows great diversity of opinions that cannot be easily debunked. We do not try to summarize this material, but a few recent references are noted: A review of many of the philosophical and scientific issues is presented in Churchland (1986). Other approaches having a greater physical science flavor are given by Harth (1982) and Penrose (1989). An issue of *Behavioral and Brain Sciences* (December 1990) contains interesting feedback on the Penrose book from several cognitive and computer scientists. A critical review of exaggerated claims of artificial intelligence that contains arguments concerning possible mind–brain connections is provided by Dreyfus (1979). The role of attractor neural networks as brain metaphors is described by Amit (1989).

Perhaps the first point to be emphasized concerning the mind–brain issue is that each of us has no direct experience of any consciousness other than our own. We infer that others share similar kinds of internal experiences mainly because they look, behave, and talk as we do. We believe that other persons are aware of their own existence, thoughts, and environment just as we are. However, when human differences are increased, as for example by not sharing a common language, our understanding of the internal states of others will decrease sharply. In extreme, but not uncommon cases, persons may dehumanize others based on differences of language, religion, appearance, and so on. We typically assume some level of consciousness in most living humans and higher mammals, but we have no real idea of the subjective experiences of animals, except by anthropomorphic extension. We certainly have no satisfactory working definition of "nonhuman consciousness."

Because of the modern interest in computers and artificial intelligence (AI), the traditional mind–brain issue now has a relatively new focus. Thus, we turn now to the Turing test, named for the famous English mathematician. Turing (1950) proposed an operational test to determine if a computer possessed "intelligence comparable to that of a human." Two sealed rooms are imagined, one containing a person while the other holds the computer. The observer communicates with the two rooms using a computer keyboard. If after a long period of typing questions and receiving replics, we cannot determine which room holds the computer, Turing proposed that the computer should be regarded as having human-level intelligence.

Although Turing apparently suggested this test as an operational definition of human level intelligence, some others have treated it as a test for consciousness. But, in the absence of any experimental test for nonhuman consciousness, we have no way to determine whether "human intelligence" implies "consciousness." The philosopher Searl (1980a, 1980b) argued that passage of the Turing test need not involve consciousness at all. In particular, Searl criticized the position known as "strong AI," the view that mental states of some sort can be attributed to the logical functioning of any computational device, that is, one that carries out well-defined sequences of operations called algorithms. According to this view, human consciousness appears as something new because of the extreme complexity (in some ill-defined sense) of brain computation. Searl's position is illustrated by different versions of what he calls the "Chinese Room Argument."

In one version of the Chinese room, a sequence of Chinese symbols is fed into a room containing English-speaking occupants who do not understand Chinese. The sequence of symbols may represent a question asked in a Turing test, for example. The occupants of the room have an extensive set of instructions written in English for manipulating Chinese symbols. Thus the room occupants can supply excellent answers to the questions using only the English instructions (that is, the algorithm), thereby passing the Turing test even though individual occupants have no knowledge of Chinese or the questions asked. Thus, in Searl's view, it is absurd to attribute any understanding of the questions to the "creature" (the interacting inhabitants) inside the room.

The following is an objection to Searl's argument: To mimic operations of complexity in any sense similar to that of the human brain, the number of room occupants required to perform symbolic manipulation in reasonable time should be large. Suppose we choose a sufficiently large "room" with the number of inhabitants perhaps close to the earth's total population. In addition, give these people exceptional abilities to communicate as individuals and as groups, that is, with interactions across spatial scales. This would, of course, require a very complex algorithm. Then the inhabitants apparently become analogous to the individual neurons of a single human brain. We do not expect our neurons to be individually conscious; rather consciousness appears to be an emergent property dependent on the dynamic interaction of many neurons. Thus the fact that the individual inhabitants of the Chinese room do not understand Turing test questions may not preclude some sort of emergent group consciousness that does "understand" the questions because of the dynamic interaction of the inhabitants. Although this may seen implausible, the only requirement for consciousness of which we are relatively confident is that of system complexity. Thus we cannot easily exclude the possibility that sentient beings might emerge in systems with complexity exceeding that of a single human brain, such as human social systems. We have no reason to assume that humans would be aware of the existence of such beings. We will return to this point in the next section.

A view associated with much less controversy is "weak AI," the belief that computers can be developed to mimic human mental processes, as evidenced by their behavior. The principal controversies concerning weak AI concern how much of human activity can be simulated and how fast this will occur. One apparent paradox is that past predictions (from perhaps 20 to 30 years ago) of future computational speed, storage, and cost of computers have been generally too pessimistic whereas, simultaneously, predictions of future abilities to perform human-like functions have been overly optimistic. One possible explanation is that advances are inherently more difficult for software than for hardware. Another is that new hardware (such as parallel processing or neural network computers) is required for more realistic simulations of human behavior.

An interesting perspective on how intelligent life evolved has been developed in a monograph concerning mechanical vehicles that move on a surface (Braitenberg, 1984). The vehicles are relevant because of the complex behavior they exhibit although they have very simple, easily analyzed internal structures. To an outside observer who knows nothing of their inner workings, the vehicles appear to exhibit fear, aggression, love, goal-directed behavior, and many other human characteristics; that is, they exhibit a "synthetic psychology." Similar ideas were expressed in a popular science fiction novel by Hogan (1983) in which a race of robots marooned on Titan for several million years exhibited genetic variability, competition, natural selection, and adaptation, apparently a form of life. These works of fiction were probably inspired by the famous writings on cybernetics by Wiener (1961). They are of special relevance to arguments of strong AI versus weak AI because they emphasize how difficult, if not impossible, it may be to resolve arguments about intelligence and consciousness based only on external observation of computer behavior.

Some argue that we are far from computer intelligence that is sufficiently developed to pass the Turing test. However, this belief appears to be based primarily on imagined tests involving comparisons of the computer with very intelligent, healthy adults. But, what about comparisons with mentally retarded, autistic, schizophrenic, or lobotomized persons or even healthy young children? Do we not allow such persons some measure not only of human-level intelligence but also consciousness? If so, then passage of a "weak Turing test," perhaps one in which the computer cannot be distinguished from a 3- or 4-year-old child, may be close at hand. The issue then becomes very much a quantitative one—that of determining what level of human intelligence a computer can simulate.

The Turing test may provide important information about similarities between machine and human intelligence but probably little information about consciousness. Although system complexity appears to be a necessary condition for consciousness, we have no evidence to support the idea that it is a sufficient condition. To return to the music and violin metaphor for mind and brain, violins are substantially more complex than a simple vibrating string; however, much more than complexity of the musical instrument is required to produce music. This suggests that consciousness may occur only in small subsets of systems having seemingly equivalent complexity. We have general ideas of how to determine complexity but no knowledge of the rules that may distinguish "conscious music" from "nonconscious noise" in complex systems. For example, perhaps some general physical condition, such as the matching of local and global time constants, is required. In any case, as phrased by Wilensky (1990), we should be skeptical that "pretheoretical notions like consciousness will emerge unscathed from our future scientific endeavors. Even the most cherished commonsense notions about time, space, and energy have undergone drastic revision in the course of science. It would be astonishing if concepts like consciousness did not."

Multiple Scales of Human Consciousness

The pessimism surrounding studies of "nonhuman consciousness" expressed in the previous section does not imply that all arguments about consciousness are concerned only with metaphysical questions, that is, those outside the province of science. Perhaps there is no more impressive example of the successful scientific approach to human consciousness than the famous studies of split-brain patients by Sperry (1974, 1982) and coworkers (Bogen et al, 1965; Gazzaniga and LeDoux, 1978). Human brains are separated into two hemispheres connected by commissures. The largest of these is the corpus callosum, containing about 2×10^8 axons crossing in both directions. Other smaller connecting structures include the anterior, posterior, and hippocampal commissures. The brain is undivided at the brainstem, which apparently allows for transfer of some information at this level before and after surgery.

The subjects of the split-brain studies consist of a group of patients with epilepsy so severe that it can not be controlled by medication or unilateral surgery (removal of several centimeters from the tip of the temporal lobe, for example). The split-brain operation, called "midline cerebral commissurotomy," eliminates cross-communication between cerebral hemispheres but leaves both hemispheres otherwise intact and functioning independently. Other versions of the operation leave some crossing fibers (such as the anterior commissure) intact. The operation often has been successful in reducing seizures, apparently by preventing the spread of epileptic electrical activity between hemispheres. However, with the many fibers sectioned, we would expect severe postoperative brain deficits to occur. However, a surprising paucity of symptoms has been observed, that is, speech, verbal intelligence, motor coordination, personality, and other standard measures were largely unchanged.

One test that should reveal dramatic differences is the interhemispheric coherency of EEG, which is expected to decrease dramatically after commissural fibers are cut. Although very little EEG data on split-brain patients has been published, one pilot study of three patients showed intrahemispheric coherencies substantially lower than those of healthy persons (Nunez, 1981). However, preoperative EEG coherency data were not available so no direct comparison of preoperative and postoperative states could be obtained. (Coherency measures are not yet part of standard, clinical EEG studies.)

Lateralization of function in a typical right-handed person is illustrated in Figure 3-5. This is a greatly oversimplified view of neocortical asymmetry, a general principle that has been documented by a long history of behavioral and cognitive deficits in patients with unilateral brain damage (Witelson, 1987). More recently, studies of healthy persons with a single anesthetized hemisphere have increased these data. These studies did not show that specific functions, such as language, are confined to one hemisphere. Rather they show that specific neural tissue in one hemisphere may be critical for anything approaching normal function. For example, an isolated left hemisphere can carry out normal mental calculations, but the isolated right hemisphere is typically limited to calculations involving simple additions of sums less than 20 (Sperry, 1974). Functional asymmetry apparently results from specialized methods of information processing in each hemisphere, or perhaps from differences of specialization between only certain parts of each hemisphere. These data are also consistent with the idea presented in Chapters 7 and 13 that specific, but widely distributed, regional circuits are associated with certain kinds of cognitive processing. Any such circuit may have elements in both hemispheres, but critical "nodes" may be confined to a single hemisphere.

Figure 3-5 shows that visual information from both eyes, but only in the right visual field, enters only the left hemisphere. Conversely, the left visual field projects only to the right hemisphere. In healthy persons, this information is available to both hemispheres because of signal transfer through the commissural fibers. In split-brain patients, however, each hemisphere functions independently in most conscious mental activities; that is, each disconnected half appears to have a "mind of its own" (Sperry, 1974).

A typical experimental design is depicted in Figure 3-6. The words "key" and "ring" are flashed to the right and left hemispheres, respectively. One "subject" (i.e., the left, speaking hemisphere) reports having seen the word "ring" but denies having seen the word "key" or of feeling any object presented to the left hand (which projects to the right, mute hemisphere). However, when asked to

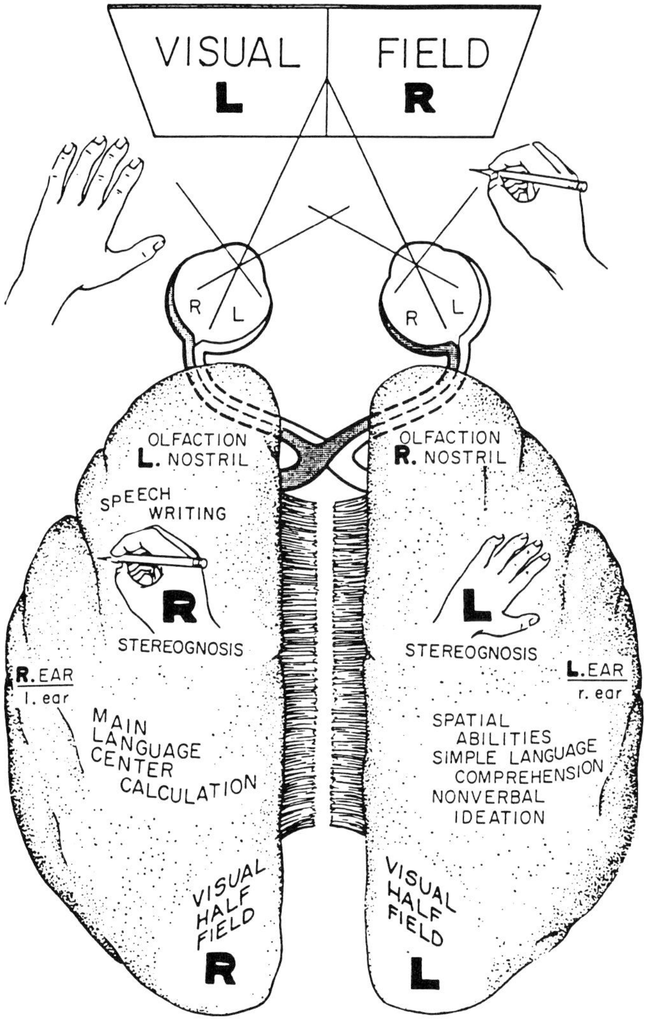

Figure 3-5. Simplified view of brain functions separated by split-brain surgery. A summary using data for neuroanatomy, cortical lesions, and postoperative testing. (Reproduced with permission from Sperry, 1974.)

retrieve an object flashed to the left visual field (key), the other "subject" (right hemisphere) correctly picks the key with the left hand, even though the left hemisphere denies having seen it. Some have objected to the idea of two separate minds in one brain, by denying consciousness to the right brain, for example. However, many nonverbal tests and a few studies of brains having bilateral speech, in which each hemisphere is anesthetized separately, provided strong evidence that each hemisphere is a distinct conscious entity. We also note several patients with complete removal of the (dominant) left hemisphere (Smith, 1966; Gott,

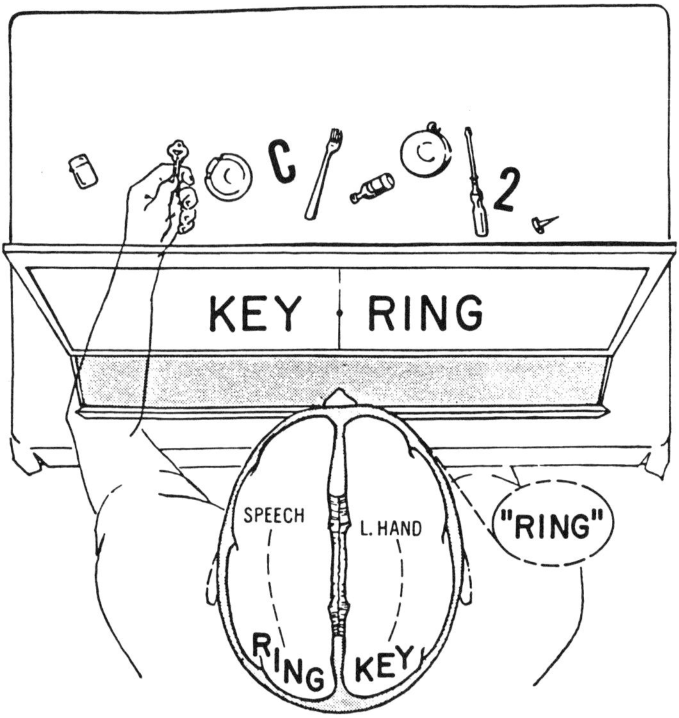

Figure 3-6. Sample split-brain responses: Subject reports (through speaking left hemisphere) having seen only the visual stimulus flashed to the right half of screen and denies having seen left-field stimulus or recognizing objects presented to the left hand. At the same time, the left hand correctly retrieves objects named in the left field for which the subject verbally denies having any knowledge. When asked to name the object selected by the left hand, the speaking hemisphere refers to the stimulus shown in the right field. (Reproduced with permission from Sperry, 1974.)

1973; Burcklund and Smith, 1977) who clearly retained communication abilities and certainly gave the strong impression of being conscious.

Strong emotions produced in one hemisphere of split-brain patients tend to spread easily into the opposite hemisphere, presumably through intact brainstem connections or feedback from peripherical reactions such as blushing, giggling, facial expressions, and so on (Sperry, 1974). Thus emotional events appear to exert a general unifying influence on the separated hemispheres. For example, in one case, a picture of a nude woman was flashed to the right hemisphere of a young woman patient (Gazzaniga and LeDoux, 1978). Her reaction was to blush, giggle, and hide her face. When asked to explain why she was laughing, she replied, "I don't know . . . nothing . . . oh, that funny machine." Another example illustrates a case in which two hemispheres seemed to disagree on behavior (Sperry, 1966): "The patient and his wife used to refer to the "sinister left hand" that sometimes tried to push the wife away aggressively at the same time that the hemisphere of the right hand was trying to get her to come and help him with something."

Although this anecdotal evidence would be difficult to evaluate in isolation, it is apparently consistent with hard data. These and many more studies not described here suggest the following generalization of split-brain patients that presumably applies also to healthy persons, but to a lesser extent (Gazzaniga and LeDoux, 1978; Gazzaniga, 1985):

> The conscious verbal self is not always privy to the origin of our actions, and when it observes the person behaving for unknown reasons, it attributes cause to the action as if it knows but in fact it does not . . . There are multiple mental systems in the brain, each with the capacity to produce behavior, and each with its own impulses for action, and these systems are not necessarily conversant internally.

This short review of a few of the many split-brain and related experiments is meant primarily as a superficial introduction for readers unfamiliar with the field. The studies add some credence to reports of multiple personality in psychiatric patients with intact commissures, cases that might otherwise be dismissed as elaborate acting. These afflictions, called "dissociation of the personality" in contemporary psychiatry, have varying and controversial interpretations (Dennett, 1987). The split-brain data show an interesting consistency with the dolphin EEG sleep studies cited in Chapter 2, suggesting that one hemisphere can sleep while the other is awake, an elegant solution to the problem of how dolphins can both breathe and sleep. These data emphasize that widely accepted concepts concerning the identity of "self" may not hold up under the microscopy of experimental evidence. The data strongly suggest that levels of significant conscious experience can be attained by neural subsets that comprise only about one half of total brain tissue, although interpretations of these data are not unanimous. It is not unreasonable to believe that smaller subsets of neural tissue may manifest rudimentary consciousness. We are faced with the (perhaps uncomfortable) idea that consciousness may be a continuous variable, partly dependent on the size and complexity of the neural interactions that support it.

Apparently consciousness that is not so dissimilar from that of healthy persons can occur at spatial scales below that of the intact human brain, such as in lower mammals, patients with severe loss of neocortical tissue, or single hemispheres of split-brain patients. By implication, it is not unreasonable to ask whether consciousness might then occur at scales larger than the human brain. I know of no scientific evidence of large-scale intelligence. However, as indicated by the example of the human global system, it is not obvious that we could ever know of the existence of such creatures. Furthermore, there are serious problems with extrapolating the idea of human consciousness to larger scales. We simply do not know how to define consciousness at large scales in a scientific context any more than we can unambiguously define "consciousness" for computers.

A favorite science fiction story by the astronomer Hoyle (1957) illustrates some of the issues concerning identity of self, neural complexity, and integration in single brains. A large, black cloud approaches our solar system. It displays inexplicable behavior in reaction to repeated attempts to study its physical properties by probing with electromagnetic fields. Reluctantly the scientists are forced to accept the only possible explanation—the cloud is intelligent! The next question addressed by the scientists is whether there are many or only a single intelligence within the cloud. They argue that the cloud has developed highly effective methods of communication by means of electromagnetic fields among its parts. That is, nonlocal communication may take place between transmitters emitting signals in specific, multiple frequency ranges and receivers tuned to specific multiple frequencies, which only partly overlap those of any given transmitter. The process imagined is similar to a society with many television channels and many television sets tuned to different channels. Thus specificity of communication between distant locations is achieved. This process is equivalent to specificity of corticocortical connections between distant locations of human neocortex. Because the rate of information transfer between individual parts of the black cloud is so high, subclouds cannot be thought of as individual intelligences. This conclusion follows because all thoughts and emotions "experienced" by any part are quickly communicated to the whole.

By analogy, neocortical columns apparently do not operate as isolated units. However, in important cases, synaptically excited columns cause surrounding tissue to have enhanced inhibitory synaptic action, thereby limiting local (that is, intracortical communication). In this manner, a neocortical column can be isolated from contiguous columns and simultaneously communicate with distant columns through the excitatory corticocortical axons. Humans presumably maintain individual identities only by limiting communication with others in the global system. In special cases, the usual barriers to communication are abnormally weak, at least over short time periods. Possible examples are revival meetings, rock concerts, athletic teams in intense competition, encounter groups, soldiers in combat, some marriages, mobs, and entire nations caught up in nationalistic or religious fury. Although it is speculative to interpret "group consciousness" in any scientific context, the general idea does not appear to be inconsistent with the little we know about human consciousness. Certainly many have had subjective experiences as part of a group that were very abnormal. Because most of what we know of consciousness is through personal subjective experience, it does not make sense to ignore it, despite the enormous difficulties in interpretation and extrapolation.

The speculative idea of group consciousness was introduced as a metaphor for integrative action of neocortex and to illustrate how far we are from a scientific framework that encompasses nonhuman consciousness, such as with putative computer consciousness. However, a reasonable argument can be made in favor of group intelligence. Consider, for example, the interaction of a collection of scientists in some field. Communication may occur through written and spoken language and through figures, graphs, electronic mail, and so on. In physics and engineering, a critical part of this communication involves mathematics. Knowledge is also advanced through multiscale interactions. Individual scientists pass on information, as do groups of different sizes who collectively developed it. Important synergistic aspects of this process provide part of the motivation for cooperative activity. The critical role of mathematics in creating this synergy in several scientific fields perhaps partly explains what physicist Eugene Wigner (1974) called "the unreasonable effectiveness of mathematics" in describing the physical world. That is, mathematics involves the communication of detailed, quantitative concepts that would otherwise be impossible. A similar argument can be made for the communication of emotional experience through various artistic media; music is the most widely appreciated example.

Rumblings from Modern Physics

Speculations by nonphysicists concerning possible relations between mind and brain typically neglect any consideration of modern physics (such as that by Churchland, 1989). In contrast, when physicists engage in such speculations, modern physics may appear to be the central issue (such as in Penrose, 1989). The view adopted in this book is based primarily on physical ideas of a classical nature. To some degree, this choice of emphasis on classical concepts is based on pedagogic considerations; that is, analogs are useful mainly to compare known and unknown systems. Because many readers are unfamiliar with the intricacies of, for example, quantum mechanics, metaphoric links between brain and quantum systems may have very limited use. There are, however, several reasons to include a few remarks on modern physics:

1. Quantum mechanics makes effective use of classical wave concepts, but the physical interpretation of these waves is entirely new. The idea of determinism, that certain forces cause a particle to move in a predictable manner described by Newton's law, is replaced by probabilistic laws. In particular, Schrodinger's equation (9.45) governs the spatial–temporal behavior of the quantum wave function. The wave function is deterministic; that is, Schrodinger's equation has exact solutions. However, the wave function does not yield the location of a quantum particle but rather the probability of finding it near some location. If the probability function (equal to the wave function times its complex conjugate) is highly localized, we can be relatively sure of its location. However, when the probability function is spread out in space, much less information about location is available. The fact that a familiar mathematical framework can be applied so successfully to entirely foreign phenomena is a dramatic demonstration of Wigner's "unreasonable effectiveness of mathematics" in science. This general view may be an important epistemologic contribution to neuroscience.
2. An astounding view of the universe has emerged through developments in relativity and quantum mechanics in this century. For example, the notion that an entity (such as an electron) moves along a continuous trajectory is replaced by the idea of motion consisting of discrete jumps from place to place. That is, the electron can move between two locations without ever occupying the space in between. Such quantum jumps are common in elements of modern electronic

circuits, for example. It seems as if reality consists of successive frames of a motion picture (Bohm, 1951). An electron is observed at different locations in different frames, but its location between frames has no meaning. Motion at macroscopic scales gives the illusion of continuity in a manner analogous to our impression when viewing a motion picture.

The new ideas run so counter to intuition based on daily experience that, when first encountered, they seem more aligned with witchcraft than science. Speculative ideas such as conscious computers or black clouds may appear almost mundane compared with some of the concepts forced on us by quantum mechanics. The difference is that quantum mechanics is based on a large body of experimental evidence and forms the foundation for much of late twentieth century technology. An appreciation of the grand conceptual leap required in the transition from classical to quantum systems may give us some vague feeling for how far from current views neuroscience eventually may lead. Such humbling recognition will perhaps make us especially skeptical of attempts to "explain away" (that is with tautology) data that do not merge with common notions about consciousness, such as multiple conscious entities in a single brain, hypnosis, and so on.

3. The atomic world, as described by quantum mechanics, has a holistic nature that is foreign to classical thinking in physics. In any experiment, the observer and system being studied are joined in a new and intimate way associated with the quantum mechanical wave function. This strange connection formed a basis for speculation about possible links between observer consciousness and the physical world. Although I am unaware of any hard evidence for the existence of such links, there are some intriguing hints about possible ties (see, for example, Barrow and Tipler, 1988). Given our modest understanding of mind–brain relations, it seems reasonable to cast a large net, which includes aspects of modern physics, in the hope of adding something important to the knowledge base.

4. Modern theories of the universe appear in the form of fundamental information barriers. Relativity, quantum mechanics, and the second law of thermodynamics limit the speed or amount of information transfer observed in different physical situations. The human brain is a machine for processing massive amounts of information. Evidently limits on information transfer must occur for humans to remain individuals. We can only speculate about possible connections between these information barriers.

States of Human Consciousness

Different states of human consciousness have been defined by a variety of measures, such as behavioral manifestations, electrophysiologic recordings (including EEG and evoked potentials), biochemical levels, physical aspects of body (posture, muscle tension), mental alertness (as measured by tests of cognitive performance, for example), or by reports of introspection. However, the concept of a distinct conscious state seems to be most useful when applied to conditions in which objective and quantitative measures are consistent with qualitative behavior and internal experience. Several states do exhibit reasonably direct connections between behavioral or cognitive measures, internal experience, and EEG measures.

Table 3-1. Behavioral States and Cognitive Levels Correlated with Electroencephalographic Measures

Cognitive processing
Selective or general attention
Relaxed wakefulness
Drowsiness
Rapid eye movement (REM)
Sleep stages I to IV
Partial or generalized seizures
Light to deep anesthesia
Coma
Death

Modified from D.B. Lindsley. Activation, Arousal, Alertness, and Attention. In: *Encyclopedia of Neuroscience*, Vol. 1. (G. Adelman, Ed.) Boston: Birkhäuser, pp. 3–6, 1987.

Table 3-1 provides a useful but oversimplified view of these human states represented as a one-dimensional continuum.

Several caveats regarding Table 3-1 are needed. First, EEG measures that distinguish between the first three states are more difficult to obtain and often are controversial. For example, serious experimental obstacles are often associated with large intersubject variability (due partly to different cognitive styles) and separation of brain from nonbrain electrical activity (artifact). Nevertheless, several

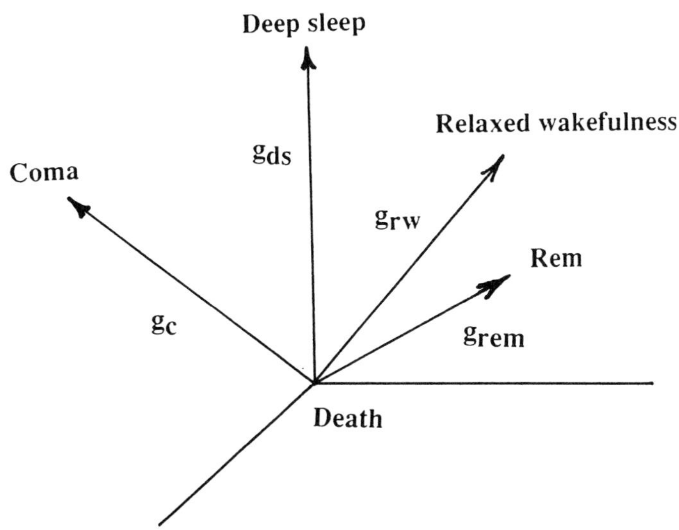

Figure 3-7. Multidimensional representation of consciousness, symbolic only. The plot indicates that many measures can be used to define brain state. The vectors g are represented in a space of dimension equal to the number of defining measures. (Modified with permission from Hobson, 1989.)

robust EEG differences between the first three states have been verified, as discussed later in this chapter and in Chapters 4, 6, and 7. Many new and robust EEG measures of awake, mental states probably will be discovered soon, due in no small part to improved spatial resolution, as discussed in Chapter 1. Another caution regarding Table 3-1 is the inference, which is only partly correct, that states listed in close proximity have overlapping characteristics, thereby providing justification for the one-dimensional continuum. Actually, states that appear close together with one measure may be far apart based on other measures; that is, states of human consciousness are more accurately represented in a multidimensional space (Hobson, 1989), as shown symbolically in Figure 3-7.

Differences in EEG patterns in states beginning with "relaxed wakefulness" are typically robust, especially when viewed in a single person, but also between persons. States of deep sleep (stages III and IV), moderate to deep anesthesia, and some comas are typically characterized by large-amplitude, low-frequency (often below 3 Hz), near-sinusoidal oscillations, which are easily recorded over the entire scalp. There are, however, exceptions such as alpha coma and moderate depth of halothane anesthesia, in which large amplitude, spatially coherent oscillations in the 4- to 16-Hz range occur, also over the entire scalp. Furthermore, additional frequency peaks are often evident in the spectra (perhaps other overtones in the standing wave interpretation). Each anesthetic has its particular spectral signature, which also varies somewhat among patients. Drowsiness is characterized by alpha drop-out, in which the sinusoidal alpha rhythm of moderate amplitude is typically replaced by a low-amplitude, broad-spectrum signal. The EEG associated with drowsiness is more like that of brain death (a flat EEG trace) than are some EEG coma patterns, an observation that reminds us of the difficulties in interpretation due to the multidimensional character of brain states.

Sleep and waking states are thought to be regulated by the general activating system, located in the brainstem and in other subcortical structures, as indicated by Figure 3-8. Seminal observations in this area of neuroscience consisted of electrical stimulation of the brainstem of the cat using implanted electrodes. Small currents awakened a sleeping cat in a manner similar to normal arousal from sleep (Magoun and Moruzzi, 1949). In humans, loss of consciousness or coma caused by head trauma or lesions is now closely associated with damage in the brainstem. The classic reticular formation is composed of a dense collection of neurons along the axis of the brainstem with short dendrites and axons. An auditory, visual, somatosensory, or olfactory stimulus causes action potentials to travel along the axons of the appropriate sensory pathway. As these signals pass the brainstem, synaptic input is provided to the reticular formation and other subcortical structures along axon branches, whereas other synaptic input enters primary sensory cortex. The function of the reticular formation was long believed to be that of general arousal of the cortex. However, most of the reticular projections to cortex were later found to follow classic anatomic patterns, with synapses in the thalamus en route to cortex. The classic role of the reticular activating system was replaced by those of specific neurotransmitter systems, with cell bodies in brainstem, pons, and diencephalon (review by Bloom, 1988). These systems project monosynap-

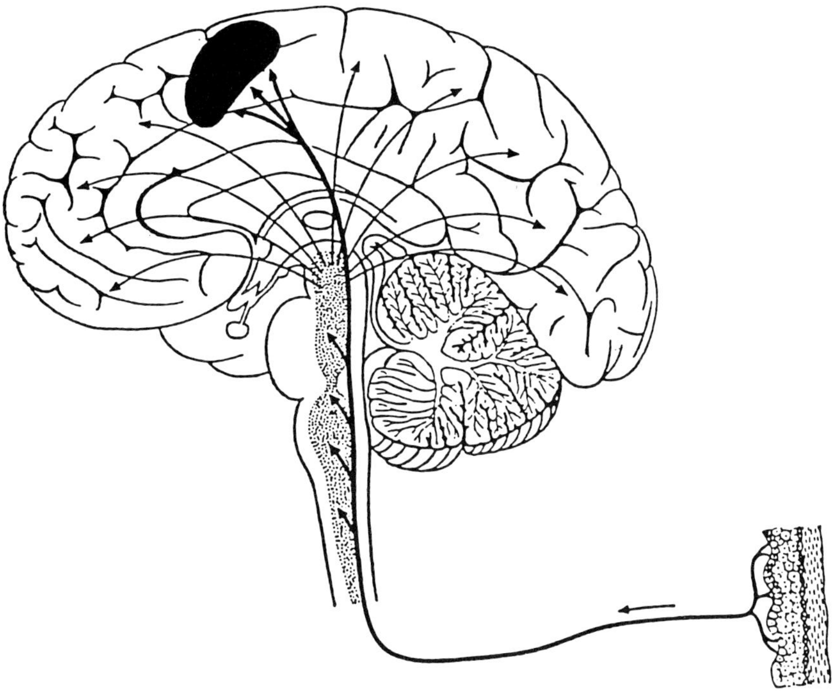

Figure 3-8. The general activating system of the brainstem and other subcortical structures. The modern view replaces that of the classical reticular activating system. The background state of neocortex is controlled from below with different neuromodulators. See Bloom, 1988 for review. (Reproduced with permission from French, 1948.)

tically to neocortex carrying transmitters directly to widespread regions of neocortex. The neurotransmitters, which apparently can have general excitatory, inhibitory, or more specific effects on target neurons of neocortex, are called neuromodulators when applied in this manner.

The complex role of neuromodulators in controlling the state of neocortex is discussed in more detail in Chapters 4, 5, and 13. However, a common example of arousal is provided from EEG studies in which an awake person shows loss of alpha rhythm during a drowsy period. An unexpected laboratory noise (such as a ringing telephone) will cause activation of the cortex. Robust alpha rhythm production closely follows the noise. A telephone ring sometimes causes alpha blocking in an alert subject; that is, it is possible for similar stimuli to cause successive changes from drowsy to relaxed wakefulness to attentive. The attentive and drowsy EEG patterns are often more similar to each other than to the alpha rhythm of relaxed wakefulness. The attentive state typically has more high-frequency activity than does the drowsy state.

The rapid eye movement (REM) stage of sleep is more closely associated with dreaming than are other stages (Hobson, 1989). REM is sometimes called paradoxical sleep because the cortex is activated; that is, EEG patterns are much closer to those of waking state than to other sleep stages, whereas muscle activity is inhibited. The general activating system "turns on" neocortex while "turning off" the spinal cord. If normal deactivation of the motor neurons that execute movement does not occur during rapid eye movement sleep, sleep walking, sleep talking or tooth grinding may occur. The EEG in sleep and other states of consciousness are described in more detail in Chapter 4.

Methods to Analyze Spontaneous EEG

To prepare the reader for experimental studies described in the next section, we describe several methods for data analysis applied to simulated data. The first example is provided by Figure 3-9, which shows two simulated waveforms, $X_1(t)$ and $X_2(t)$, during a 2-second interval. Both are composed of the sum of two sinusoidal oscillations at frequencies of 5 Hz and 12 Hz , with relative amplitudes of 1 and 2, respectively. The waveforms also contain random noise terms, each with a relative amplitude of 5. Amplitude spectra are obtained by sampling the waveforms at 160 Hz, obtaining fast Fourier transforms for each 1-second epoch, and averaging over 176 seconds, using identical procedures applied to actual EEG data (see the next section). The estimates of amplitude spectra for the two waveforms are nearly identical; one is shown at the lower left in Figure 3-9. Thus, by averaging over many 1-second epochs, the two frequency peaks emerge from the background noise, with the 12-Hz peak showing twice the amplitude over background noise as the 5-Hz peak.

Amplitude spectra provide information about the frequency content of signals but no information about relative phase relations. The coherency between signals $X_1(t)$ and $X_2(t)$ is a correlation coefficient (squared) expressed as a function of frequency, which measures the phase consistency of two signals. In this example, the phases of sinusoidal oscillations at 5 Hz (based on 1-second epochs) were varied randomly between $\pm 18^0$, whereas the phases of oscillations at 12 Hz were varied randomly between $\pm 180^0$. As a result, the estimated coherency between $X_1(t)$ and $X_2(t)$ was 0.5 at 5 Hz, but 0 (that is, incoherent) at 12 Hz and 0 at all other frequencies (because of added white noise). Coherency estimates are independent of amplitude, so that it is possible to obtain high coherencies over parts of the spectrum with small amplitudes or low coherencies at frequencies with large amplitudes. If two noise-free signals have a constant-phase relation (regardless of the phase difference) at some frequency, the coherency between the two signals at this frequency is always 1.

The accuracies of spectral and coherency estimates depend on the number of epochs used in the average. An approximate relation for the 95% confidence interval for the power spectrum G(f) or coherency $\gamma^2(f)$ is expressed in Bendat and Piersol's (1986) equation,

$$\frac{1}{1 + 2\varepsilon} \leq \frac{\hat{S}(f)}{S(f)} \leq \frac{1}{1 - 2\varepsilon} \tag{3.1}$$

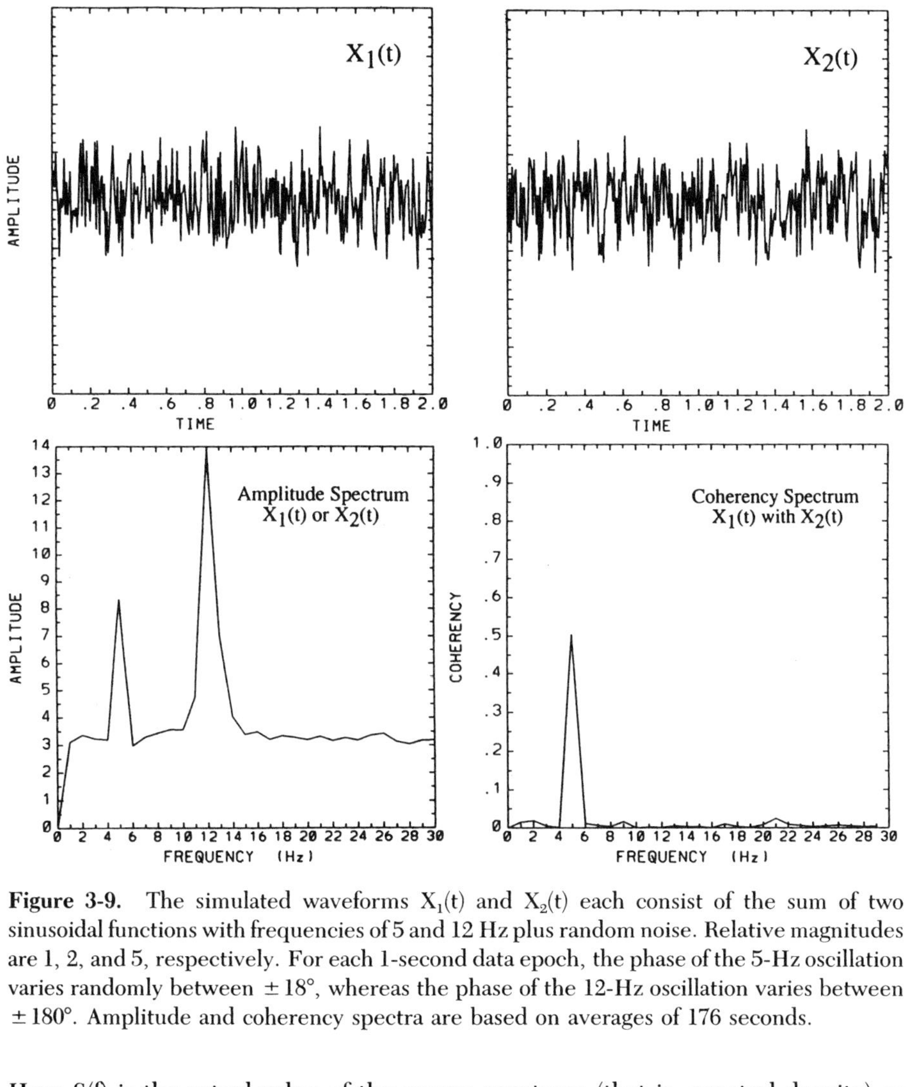

Figure 3-9. The simulated waveforms $X_1(t)$ and $X_2(t)$ each consist of the sum of two sinusoidal functions with frequencies of 5 and 12 Hz plus random noise. Relative magnitudes are 1, 2, and 5, respectively. For each 1-second data epoch, the phase of the 5-Hz oscillation varies randomly between ± 18°, whereas the phase of the 12-Hz oscillation varies between ± 180°. Amplitude and coherency spectra are based on averages of 176 seconds.

Here S(f) is the actual value of the power spectrum (that is, spectral density) or coherency at some frequency, a quantity that is never known exactly. $\hat{S}(f)$ is the estimate of S(f), and ε is the normalized root-mean-square error. With power spectra, normalized root-mean-square error may be estimated from

$$\varepsilon_G \sim \sqrt{\frac{1}{N}} \tag{3.2}$$

N is the number of epochs averaged to obtain $\hat{S}(f)$, and the estimate is reasonably accurate for $N > 25$. For example, if we obtain the estimate $\hat{G}(f_0) = 100$ (arbitrary units) at frequency $f = f_0$ based on $N = 176$ epochs, the 95% confidence interval for power at frequency f_0 estimated from (3.1) and (3.2) is

$$87 \leq G(f_0) \leq 118 \tag{3.3}$$

With a given set of data, we can always increase the number of epochs N by submitting shorter epochs to the Fourier transform. However, frequency resolution equals (epoch length)$^{-1}$ so that, for example, a 1-second epoch length yields 1-Hz resolution, a 2-second epoch length yields 0.5-Hz resolution, and so on. Thus spectral estimates (such as power, coherency, phase spectra) always involve tradeoffs between confidence interval and frequency resolution. If epoch lengths are 1 second, the estimate (3.3) applies approximately to the frequency band $f_0 \pm 0.5$ Hz. With the same set of data, we can narrow the 95% confidence interval using epochs of 0.5-second length and N = 352 epochs; however, with this change, our spectral estimates apply to the broader band $f_0 \pm 1.0$ Hz.

An estimate of the 95% confidence interval for coherency also may be obtained from (3.1), but the estimate of normalized root-mean-square error depends on coherency (Bendat and Piersol, 1986)

$$\varepsilon_{\gamma^2} \sim \sqrt{\frac{2}{N}}\,\frac{[1 - \gamma^2(f)]}{|\gamma(f)|} \tag{3.4}$$

In using (3.4), actual coherency is here approximated by estimated coherency, and the approximation is reasonably accurate for $\varepsilon_{\gamma^2} \leq 0.2$. Relations (3.1) and (3.4) may be combined to obtain the following 95% confidence intervals based on N = 176 epochs, examples that are useful when actual EEG data are discussed in the next section:

$$\begin{aligned} \hat{\gamma}_{12}^2 &= 0.8 \qquad 0.76 \leq \gamma_{12}^2 \leq 0.84 \\ \hat{\gamma}_{12}^2 &= 0.5 \qquad 0.43 \leq \gamma_{12}^2 \leq 0.59 \\ \hat{\gamma}_{12}^2 &= 0.2 \qquad 0.14 \leq \gamma_{12}^2 \leq 0.32 \end{aligned} \tag{3.5}$$

Thus, when coherency estimates of approximately 0.1 or 0.2 or more are obtained using averages of 176 epochs, we can be relatively certain that such estimates are not due to statistical fluctuations; this is, the signals in question are correlated at the frequency in question. These results are consistent with the simulation of Figure 3-9, in which all 29 coherency estimates (at integer frequencies) outside the coherent 5-Hz band are less than 0.05.

We list the following potential sources of erroneous high-coherence estimates in EEG studies:

1. Statistical fluctuation, discussed above.
2. Volume conduction. We are interested in coherency between neural current sources, but EEG measures scalp currents that have been distorted by the head volume conductor. Thus incoherent sources can produce coherent scalp potentials (Nunez, 1981; Nunez and Pilgreen, 1991).
3. Reference electrode effects. Common activity at the reference electrode causes correlated signals.

4. Algorithm effects. Some Laplacian and cortical imaging algorithms that are adopted to reduce volume conduction effects may introduce false coherency estimates because of their global character; that is, estimates of some variable at any one location may depend on potentials measured at every point within the electrode array (Biggins et al, 1991).

Fortunately, remedies are available for each of these sources of error. We showed that statistical errors are small if many data epochs are averaged. Most

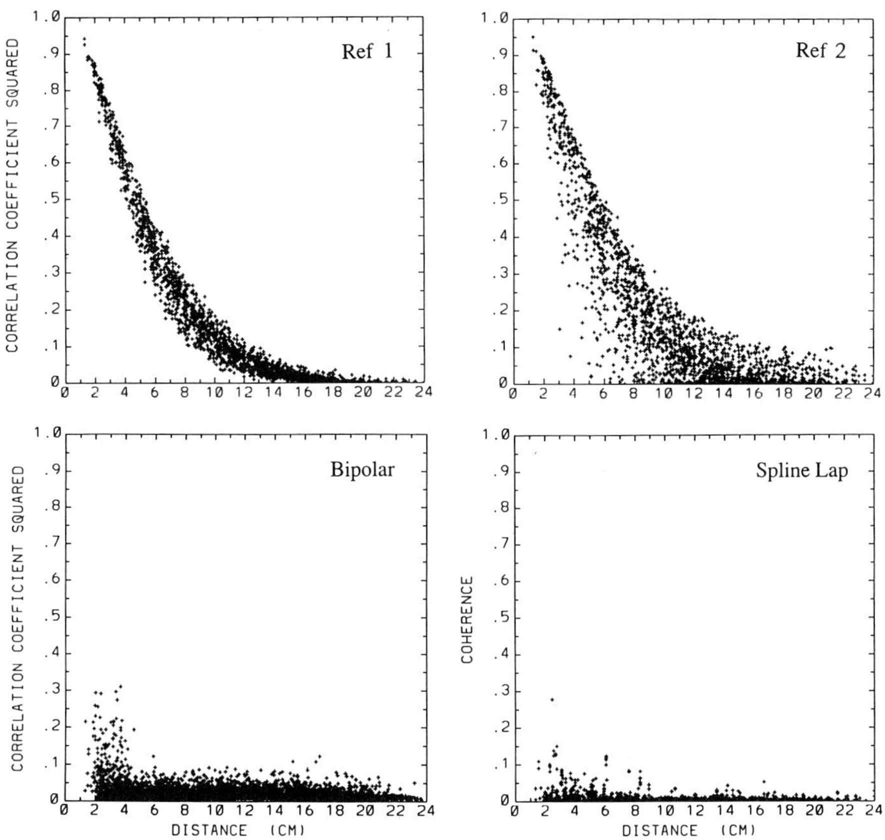

Figure 3-10. Simulations of scalp correlation coefficients (squared) due to 4200 random (uncorrelated) radial dipole sources in the cortex. Correlation coefficients between 2016 pairs of scalp locations are estimated based on 500 random source distributions. In the upper row, raw potential correlation coefficients (squared) are plotted as a function of electrode separation distance (measured in centimeters). Reference 1 is on the bottom of the sphere; reference 2 is at the location of an ear. The erroneous high correlations shown at distances less than about 10 cm are due only to volume conduction effects. Approximately 12,000 bipolar pairs (not containing a common electrode) were used to obtain the plot in the lower left corner. Spline-Laplacian estimates were used to obtain the plot in the lower right corner. Methods illustrated in the lower row remove most of the erroneous high coherency due to volume conduction at distances greater than about 4-cm.

volume conduction and all reference electrode effects are apparently eliminated using either close bipolar recordings or Laplacians, as illustrated in Figure 3-10. In these simulations, 4200 random dipole sources are located in the cortex of a three-spheres theoretical model of the head. Scalp potential distributions due to 500 source distributions can be calculated using this model. Correlation coefficients can be obtained between all pairs of electrode positions (64 × 63/2 = 2016); these positions are nearly identical to those used in the experiments discussed in the next section. Correlation coefficients squared are plotted versus distance in a manner analogous to the EEG coherency versus distance plots of the next section.

The plot in the upper left corner of Figure 3-10 shows the result of a simulation with the reference (reference 1) on the bottom of the sphere. Reference 2 is at the approximate location of an ear. The underlying sources are uncorrelated; that is, the erroneous high correlations of scalp potential shown for electrode separation distances up to 10 or 12 cm are due to volume conduction and (for reference 2) reference electrode effects. In the lower left corner, bipolar correlations are shown. This plot was constructed by forming bipolar potentials involving all electrode pairs closer than 5 cm and calculating all correlation coefficients between bipolar potentials not containing a common electrode. Approximately 12,000 correlation coefficients were obtained in this manner. Bipolar recordings should therefore remove most erroneous high coherence due to volume conduction at distances greater than about 4 cm. (Distances are measured between the midpoints of electrode pairs with bipolar simulations.) Use of nearest-neighbor or spline-Laplacian algorithms also tends to remove errors due to volume conduction although we must use global algorithms with care.

Dynamic Structure of EEG

This section describes recent observations of EEG dynamics using high-resolution methods. The data were recorded at the Swinburne Centre for Applied Neurosciences in Melbourne, Australia and studied at Tulane University, New Orleans, Louisiana. Some of the results presented here duplicate EEG observations made by many EEG scientists during the past 60 years. Other results are new. Scalp potentials were recorded using a unique 64-channel system developed by the Melbourne group (see Chapter 6). Spring-loaded electrodes were fit through a hard, shielded, spherical-shaped helmet. Electrode placement and impedance checks require about 20 minutes. A balanced neck reference electrode was chosen to minimize EEG contributions and electrocardiographic artifact to the reference channel. Automatic rejection of artifact is based on amplitude criteria and calculation of nearest-neighbor correlations. However, these data apparently were very "clean," because less than 1% of the data were rejected because of suspected artifact. Furthermore, most of the spatial patterns described refer only to the 1-Hz band width at 10 Hz, for which the signal-to-noise ratio is high. Thus we can be relatively confident that the dynamic properties described reflect neocortical dynamic function rather than artifact.

We describe a pilot study of two distinct brain states occurring in a single subject. However, most if not all of the general results obtained in this subject probably also apply to many others. In the control state, the subject is relaxed, with eyes closed and silently counts his breaths (the "resting state"). This procedure was followed to minimize random thoughts and thereby provide a more constant control state for comparison with other states. In the "cognitive state," the participant silently summed the series (1+2+3+4+ . . .) during three separate periods of 1 minute each. The cognitive states were interspersed with resting states, also of 1-minute duration. This particular mental calculation was chosen because it is more difficult than several other calculations reported in other similar studies (such as counting backward by sevens) but not so difficult that frequent errors and loss of concentration occurred. In this manner, we tried to maximize differences between control and cognitive states. Of course, investigators

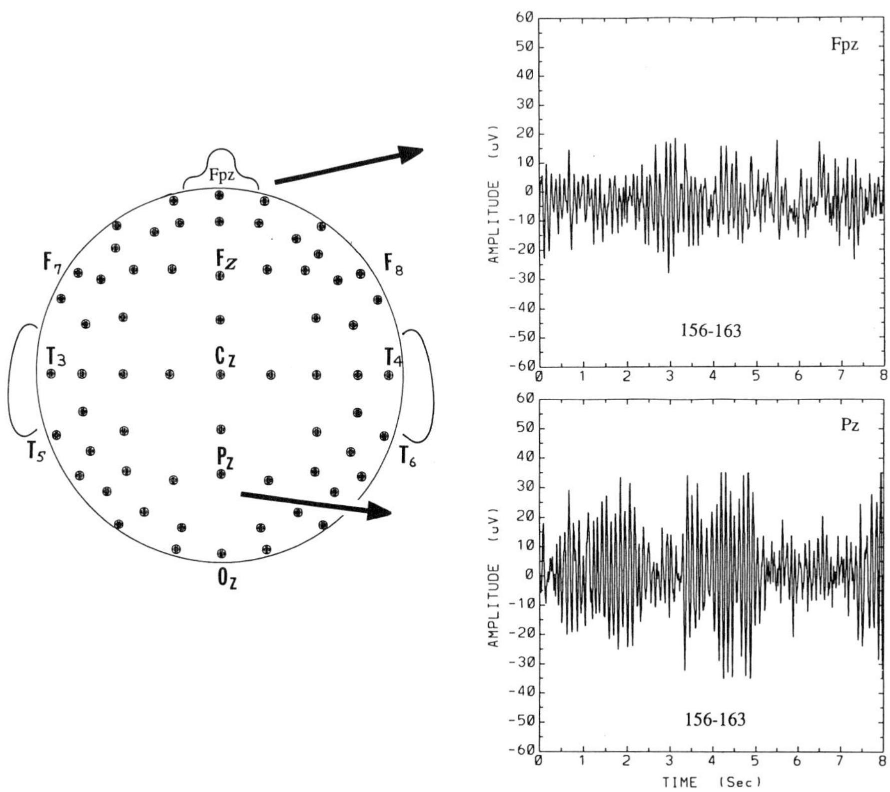

Figure 3-11. Electrode array (*left*) used to record alpha rhythm (*right*). These data were recorded by the Melbourne group using a balanced neck reference. See also Chapter 6; Silberstein et al, 1990; and Nunez et al, 1994.

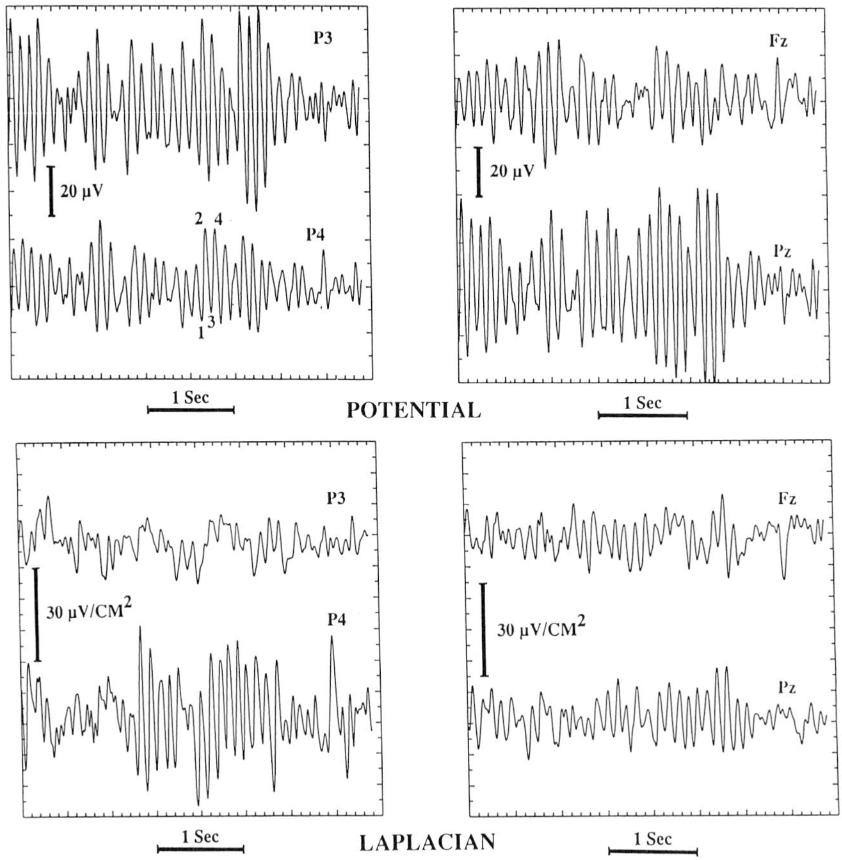

Figure 3-12. Four (of 64) channels of alpha rhythm potential recorded with a neck reference are shown in the upper row. Waveforms were digitized at 160 samples/second. Potentials at the 64 electrodes were used to calculate the spline-Laplacian at each time and three-point smoothing used to obtain corresponding Laplacian waveforms in the lower row. The unprocessed scalp potentials represent low pass spatially filtered estimates of cortical potential, as indicated in Figure 1-28. The four extrema of the P4 potential (upper left) labeled 1 through 4 indicate times at which potential (Figure 3-13) and Laplacian (Figure 3-14) maps were obtained.

must check that the subject consistently follows prescribed mental procedures. In this study, this control was accomplished using the author as subject.

The electrode array and 8 seconds of raw data recorded during the control state from anterior and posterior scalp are shown in Figure 3-11. This is the classical alpha rhythm that may occur in bursts of larger and smaller amplitudes, as illustrated by the parietal-midline (Pz) electrode record. In other participants, amplitude may be more constant. This near-sinusoidal oscillation is apparent in posterior regions in about 95% of persons when resting with eyes closed. The

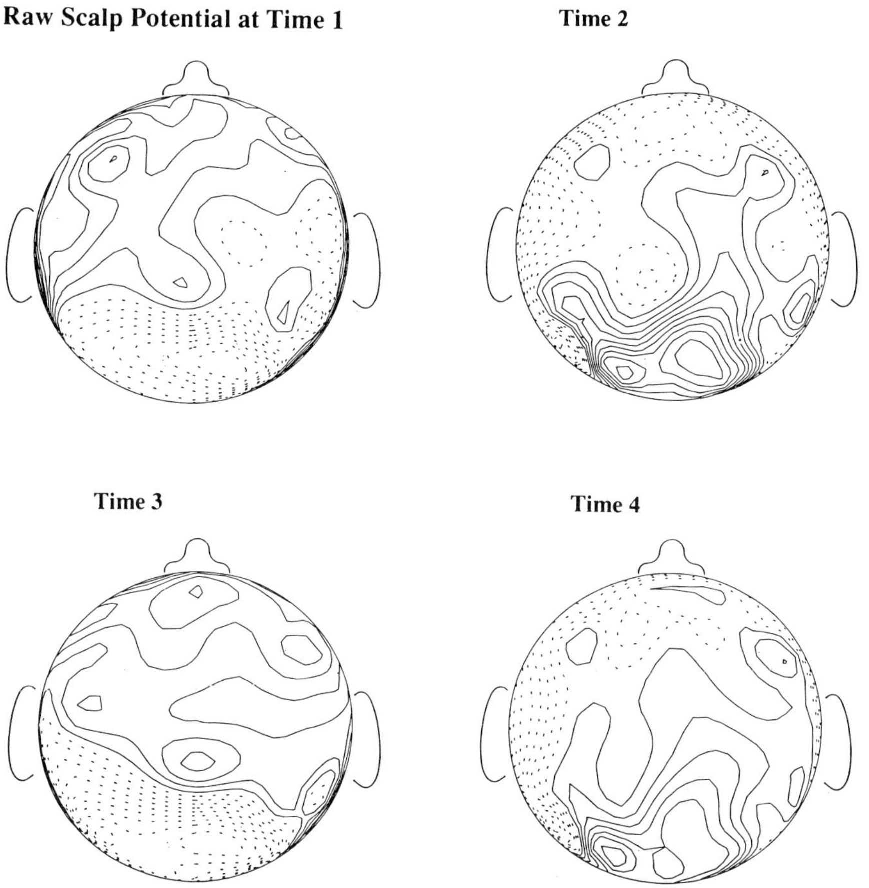

Figure 3-13. Plots of scalp potential at maxima and minima of P4 potential shown in Figure 3-12. Potentials at the 64 electrode locations were submitted to a spline interpolation which produced potential estimates at 613 surface locations. Contour lines were plotted using potential at the 613 locations without further interpolation. The dynamic behavior can be interpreted as standing waves composed mainly of low spatial frequency components (small indices ℓ of the spherical harmonic functions).

frontal alpha shown apparently depends on minimizing "intensity" of mental activity; for example, it is enhanced by the relaxation exercise of silent breath counting.

Spatial properties of alpha rhythm were studied with several methods. Figure 3-12 (upper row) shows 4 seconds of unprocessed potential data in 4 channels. These 4 seconds were free of obvious artifact in all 64 channels. The data were digitized at 160 samples/second. Each time slice was submitted to the spline-Laplacian and the resulting waveform smoothed over 3 consecutive time points to produce the Laplacian waveforms shown in lower row. These waveforms are most likely produced by local cortical sources space-averaged over several square

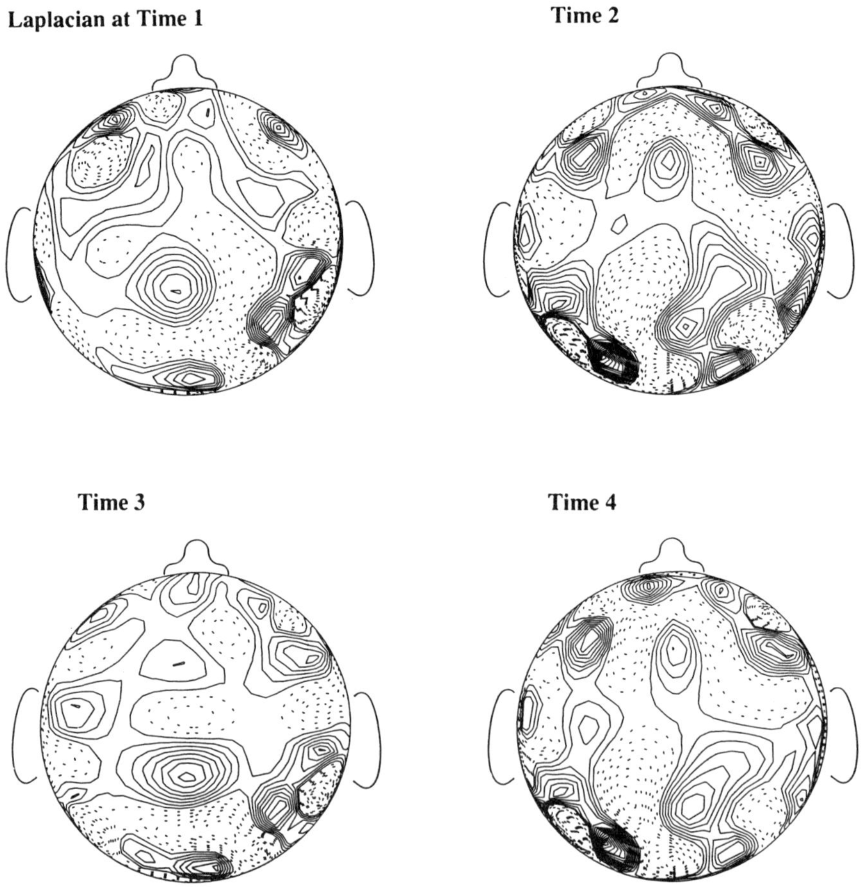

Figure 3-14. Spline-Laplacian maps of the same time slices shown in Figure 3-13. The dynamics can also be interpreted as standing waves, but with more relative contribution from higher spatial frequencies (large ℓ indices of the spherical harmonic functions). Cortical image estimates based on a four concentric spheres model of the head yield approximately the same spatial patterns (Nunez et al, 1994).

centimeters of cortical surface near each electrode. In contrast, the raw potential waveforms represent cortical sources space averaged over much larger regions, perhaps tens or hundreds of square centimeters, with possible contributions from subcortical sources.

Four extrema of the P4 potential waveform (labeled 1 through 4 in Figure 3-12) were chosen to produce the instantaneous potential maps shown in Figure 3-13. The corresponding Laplacian maps are shown in Figure 3-14. Cortical image maps based on a four concentric sphere model (not shown) are quite similar to the Laplacian maps as discussed in Chapter 1 (Nunez et al, 1994). Maps at negative potential peaks (1 and 3) are quite similar to each other, as are maps at positive potential peaks (2 and 4). This occurs in both the potential and Laplacian maps in a manner consistent with neocortical standing waves. In this view, the potential maps display mainly low spatial frequencies (ℓ indices equal to 0 through 2 of the special harmonics), whereas the Laplacian maps show higher spherical harmonics, as suggested by the volume conductor calculations of Figure 1-28.

Spatial properties of the resting (that is, control) alpha rhythm were studied in more detail as follows. Raw EEG recorded from each of the 64 channels were edited for artifact based on two separate criteria: amplitude and nearest-neighbor correlation. Data points with magnitude greater than the three–root-mean-square magnitude for the channel tested were identified as possible artifact. Furthermore, if the correlations between any channel and its four nearest-neighbors were less than a certain value (based on experience with similar data), artifact was suspected. These criteria were established using preliminary studies, including visual inspection, purposeful introduction of known artifact, and theoretical volume conduction considerations (Silberstein et al, 1990; Nunez et al, 1994). Suspected artifactual data were replaced by nearest-neighbor interpolated data, except when coherency estimates were involved. In this case, suspect channels were excluded from the analyses. Fewer than 1% of raw data points were replaced in this manner.

Fourier transforms of waveforms obtained at each of the 64 electrode sites yielded 64 real and 64 imaginary coefficients at 10 Hz, corresponding approximately to the middle of the band (9.5 to 10.5 Hz) containing most of the signal. Based on separate studies, this procedure is thought to remove nearly all artifact remaining after editing the raw data because most known artifact contributes primarily in the delta frequency range (0 to 4 Hz). Of course, artifact contribution at 10 Hz is always possible. For example, muscle activity is broad band (Nunez, 1981); however, signal-to-muscle noise ratio in the 9.5- to 10.5-Hz band is very high in these data. We emphasized the discussion of artifact here despite our general intention in this book to avoid detailed discussions of experimental methods. This exception is needed because of the frequent publication of EEG cognitive studies to which artifact is suspected to have made a large contribution.

The sets of real and imaginary 10-Hz Fourier coefficients were submitted to spline-Laplacian and cortical imaging algorithms, thereby estimating real and imaginary spatial maps of cortical surface potential. We report only on spatial properties of spline-scalp potential and spline-Laplacian maps because the corresponding cortical image maps are similar to the Laplacian maps; that is, they have typical correlation coefficients in the 0.8 to 0.9 range (Nunez et al, 1994).

Magnitude and phase at 10 Hz were obtained in the usual manner from the Fourier coefficients:

$$\mathrm{Mag}_{ij} = (\mathrm{Real}_{ij}^2 + \mathrm{Imag}_{ij}^2)^{1/2} \tag{3.6}$$

$$\mathrm{Phase}_{ij} = \tan^{-1}\left(\frac{\mathrm{Imag}_{ij}}{\mathrm{Real}_{ij}}\right) \tag{3.7}$$

The subscripts $i = 1{,}178$ and $j = 1{,}64$ refer to each 1-second epoch and electrode position, respectively. Absolute phase for each 1-second epoch is arbitrary and depends only on the temporal position of each sinusoidal waveform sampled. Thus the phase for each epoch and electrode position is rotated so that phase is forced to zero at electrode position Pz. In this manner, we can realistically compare phases between both epochs and electrode positions.

Magnitude and phase plots of spline-Laplacians based on three successive 1-minute epochs of resting data (10 Hz) are shown in Figure 3-15. One question addressed concerns the temporal stability of these patterns at different temporal scales; that is, how much do they vary from minute to minute or from second to second? Potential and Laplacian maps are stable at the 1-minute scale, as shown in Figure 3-15. This stability of 1-minute patterns was quantified using the first minute as a template and calculating magnitude and phase correlation coefficients for five successive 1-minute epochs of resting alpha rhythm (only two are shown here). All of these correlation coefficients are greater than 0.9.

A few Laplacian maps based on 1-second epochs are shown in Figures 3-16 and 3-17. The stability of these maps is shown in Figure 3-18, which indicates the evolution of correlation coefficients obtained by comparing templates formed by the 3 minutes of data depicted in Figure 3-15 with a succession of 1-second maps covering the same 3 minutes of data. Note the apparent periodicity in correlation coefficient variations, mostly between 0 and 0.8; that is, at about every 6 seconds, the spatial patterns of magnitude and phase change to new patterns for roughly 1 second but then return to patterns more similar to that obtained with the 3-minute average. We can speculate that this underlying rhythm is related to the breathing cycle; however, data discussed in the section EEG Dynamics During a Cognitive Task, below, do not appear to support this. A more extensive study of these data yields the following summary of alpha magnitude and phase at 10 Hz.

Magnitude

Scalp potential magnitudes based on data averaged over many seconds suggest dominant regions of coherent sources in posterior cortex, a result consistent with classical views of alpha rhythm as generated by posterior "generators." However, many 1-second epochs suggest the presence of important central and frontal coherent source regions. The Laplacian magnitude plots for 1-second epochs reveal these source regions more clearly. Based on experience with simulated data using concentric spheres models (Nunez, 1981; see also Chapter 1), we interpret these regions as relatively large areas of more highly correlated source activity. That is, alpha rhythm sources may occur over the entire cortex (and in some subcortical regions), but our EEG methods are most sensitive to large, coherent neocortical dipole layers. We can postulate that dipole layers which are less correlated with contiguous tissue are more involved in specific "circuit" operation, and that the portion of neocortical surface involved in such circuits is increased with cognitive processing. Interruption of coherent activity (such as by eye opening or cognitive tasks) is predicted by simulations to cause substantial reduction in magnitudes (Nunez, 1981; Nunez et al, 1991; see also Chapter 1). This prediction is, of course, consistent with a voluminous alpha rhythm literature and supports long-held no-

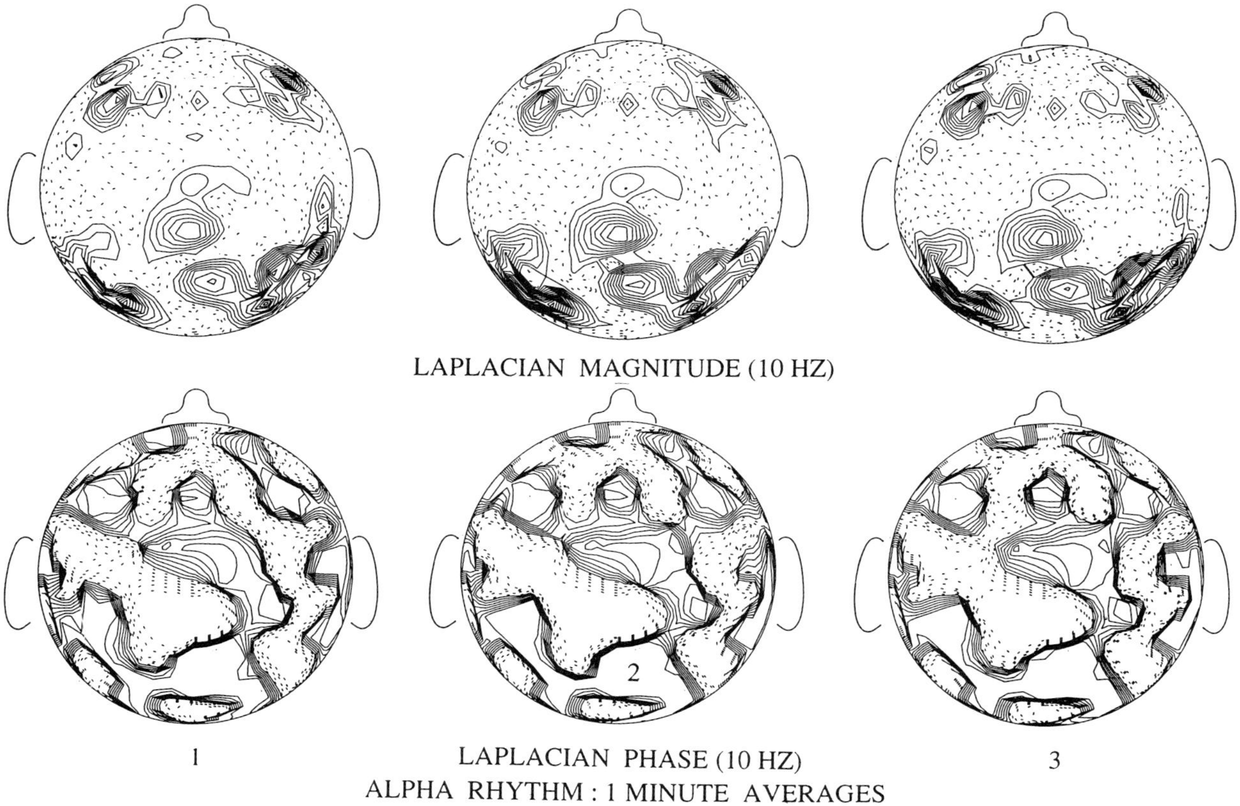

Figure 3-15. Average spline-Laplacian magnitude and phase plots at 10 Hz for 3 consecutive 1-minute periods of resting alpha rhythm. Solid lines in magnitude plots are above-average magnitude; dotted lines are below-average magnitude. Maximum potential magnitude in the 1-Hz band is 6 microvolts (not shown). Maximum spline-Laplacian magnitude is about 2 microvolts per square centimeter. Cosine (phase) is also plotted. Solid lines are positive and dotted lines are negative. Phase is rotated for each epoch so that cosine (phase) at Pz is always equal to 1. Contour intervals are 0.15 (dimensionless).

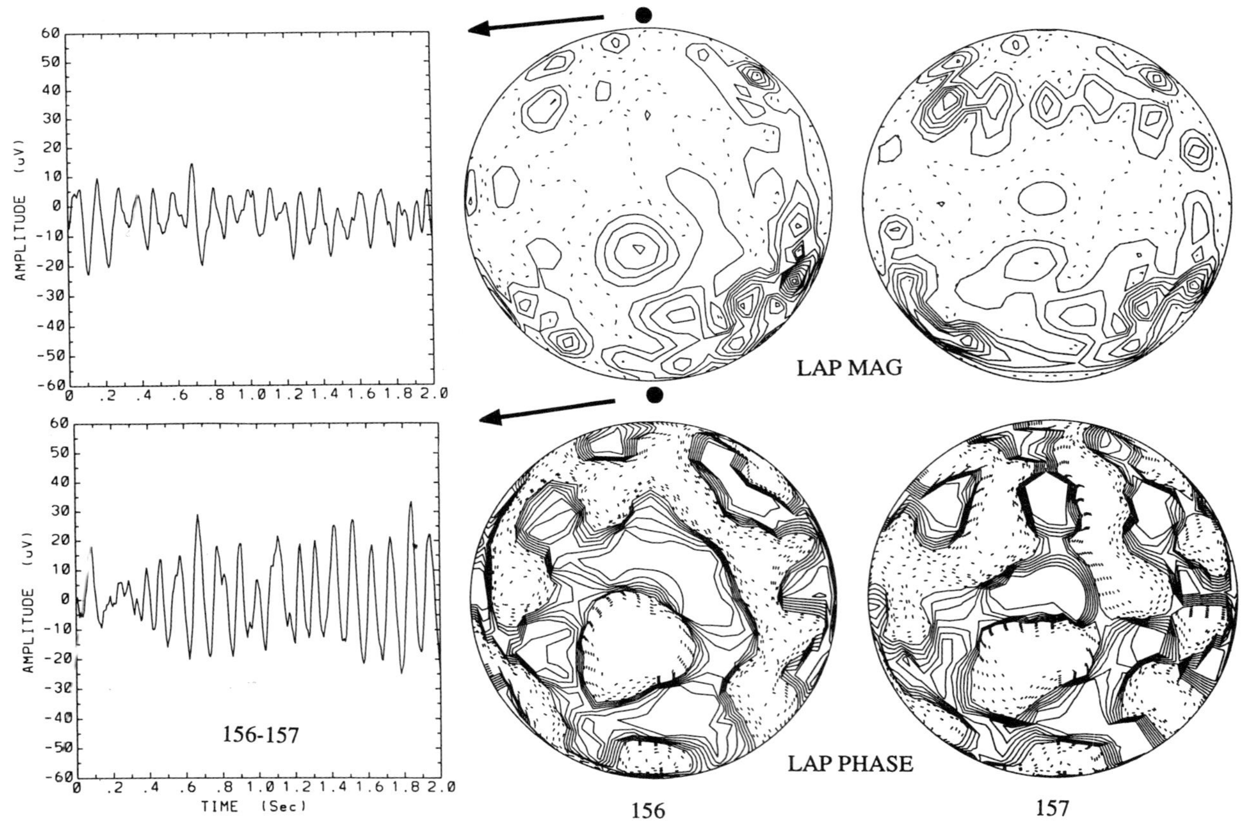

Figure 3-16. Alpha rhythm recorded on anterior (*top*) and posterior (*bottom*) scalp is shown at left. Spline-Laplacian magnitude and phase plots for two successive 1-second epochs are shown at right.

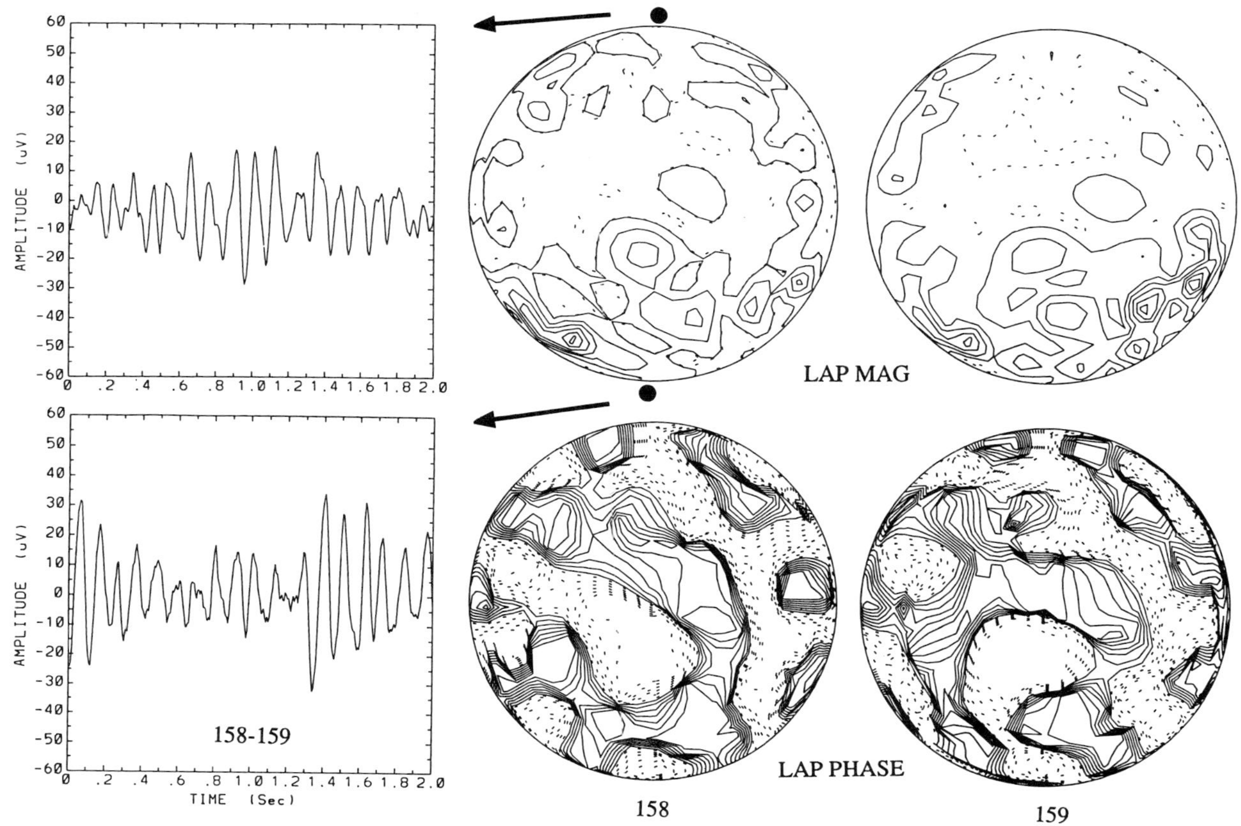

Figure 3-17. Alpha rhythm for 2 seconds following data shown in Figure 3-16.

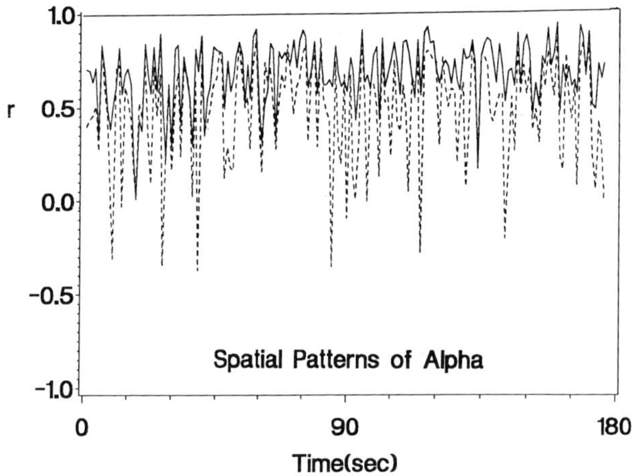

Figure 3-18. Variations in correlation coefficients between Laplacian magnitude and phase based on successive 1-second epochs of alpha rhythm compared with template magnitude and phase maps based on the entire 3-minute record average (template shown in Figure 3-15). Magnitude (solid line) and cosine phase (dashed line) correlations are shown. Data were recorded while the subject was in resting state.

tions that large amplitude rhythms involve "synchronous" sources. Thus the term "desynchronized rhythm" is often used in the EEG literature to denote amplitude reduction (see Chapter 4).

Phase

Scalp potential phase plots based on 1-second epochs show relatively gradual phase changes, nearly always less than 90° over the entire scalp and often much less than this. Phase changes are most gradual over regions of large scalp magnitude but generally show larger gradients over regions of lower scalp magnitude. This result is expected if large scalp magnitudes occur over large dipole layer correlated source regions. In contrast to the gradual phase changes of scalp potential, Laplacian (or cortical image) phase nearly always exhibits multiple, abrupt phase changes of 180° over a few centimeters. Significant correspondence occurs between boundaries separating regions of large phase difference (apparent nodal lines) and boundaries separating regions of relatively large and small magnitude. These apparent nodal lines may be evidence for standing waves in neocortex, as discussed in detail in Chapters 6, 11, and 12. Finally, the structure of alpha rhythm (both magnitude and phase) on 1-second time scales is quasi-stable and is very stable on 1-minute time scales when brain state is held relatively constant, that is the "resting state" in which the subject slowly counts breaths.

Coherence estimates between multiple pairs of scalp locations were obtained using 176 seconds of EEG recorded during the control (resting) state. The 10-Hz

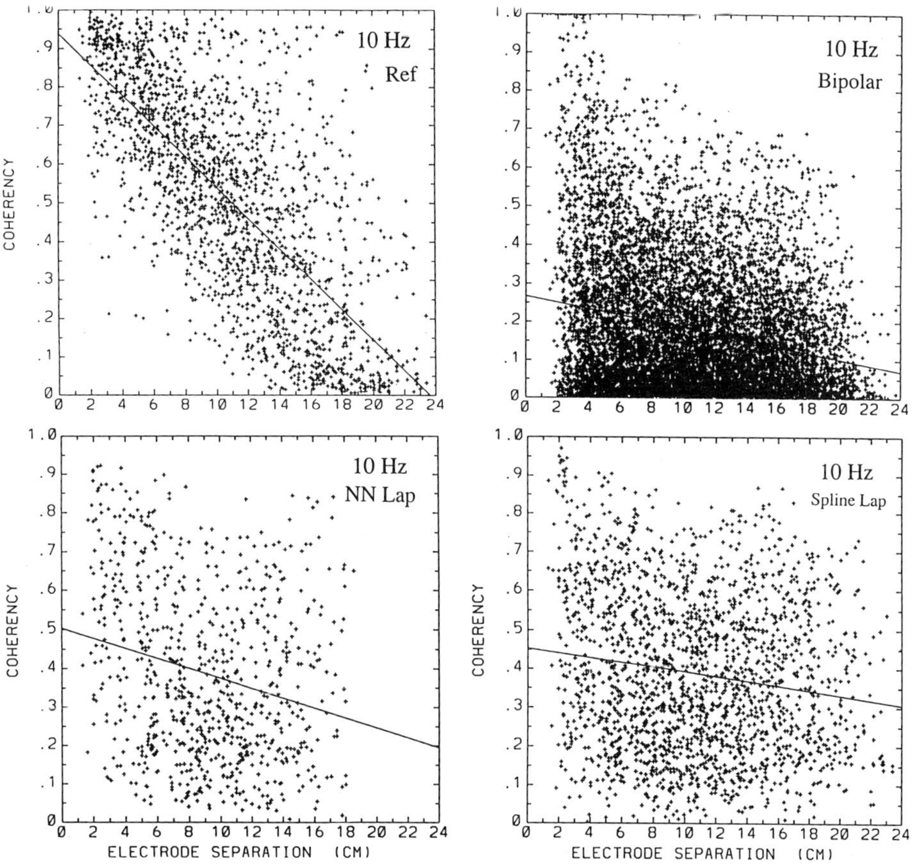

Figure 3-19. Coherency at 10 Hz is plotted versus electrode separation distance based on 3 minutes of resting alpha rhythm data (64 channels). Raw scalp potential coherency (neck reference) is shown at upper left. Coherency obtained with all bipolar pairs having electrodes closer than 5 cm and no electrodes common to pairs of data channels is shown at upper right. Nearest-neighbor Laplacian (5 electrode) coherencies are shown at lower left. The relatively small number of points occurs since edge electrodes and electrodes common to different Laplacians are excluded. Spline-Laplacian coherencies (global) are shown at lower right. Coherency is essentially correlation coefficient squared. These data may be compared directly with the simulations shown in Figure 3-10 which are based on uncorrelated cortical sources.

coherence is plotted versus electrode separation in Figure 3-19. The unprocessed data (neck reference) shows many high-coherency estimates at interelectrode distances greater than 10 cm. This is in contrast with the simulation studies illustrated in Figure 3-10, in which scalp correlation coefficients (squared) due to uncorrelated sources were predicted to be less than 0.2 at distances greater than 10 cm. However, we must consider possible contributions from the reference electrode that might cause erroneous high-coherence estimates even though these data were recorded with a "distant" (neck) reference.

Approximately 12,000 bipolar coherencies, which are independent of reference electrode, were obtained in a manner similar to that used in the simulations of Figure 3-10. Again, many high-coherence estimates are obtained at distances greater than 10 cm. Finally, nearest-neighbor Laplacian (excluding common electrodes) and spline-Laplacian coherency for the same data are shown in Figure 3-19. Spatially coherent source activity over scalp distances of 10 or 20 cm is not unusual in these data. A few example plots of bipolar coherency versus frequency are shown in Figures 3-20 and 3-21. These estimates are all based on 176 one-second epochs so that statistical errors are small, as shown by the example confidence intervals (3.5). Furthermore, these bipolar coherencies all apply to locations greater than 10 cm; that is, reference electrode contamination is zero and volume conduction effects are very small in the data of Figures 3-20 and 3-21.

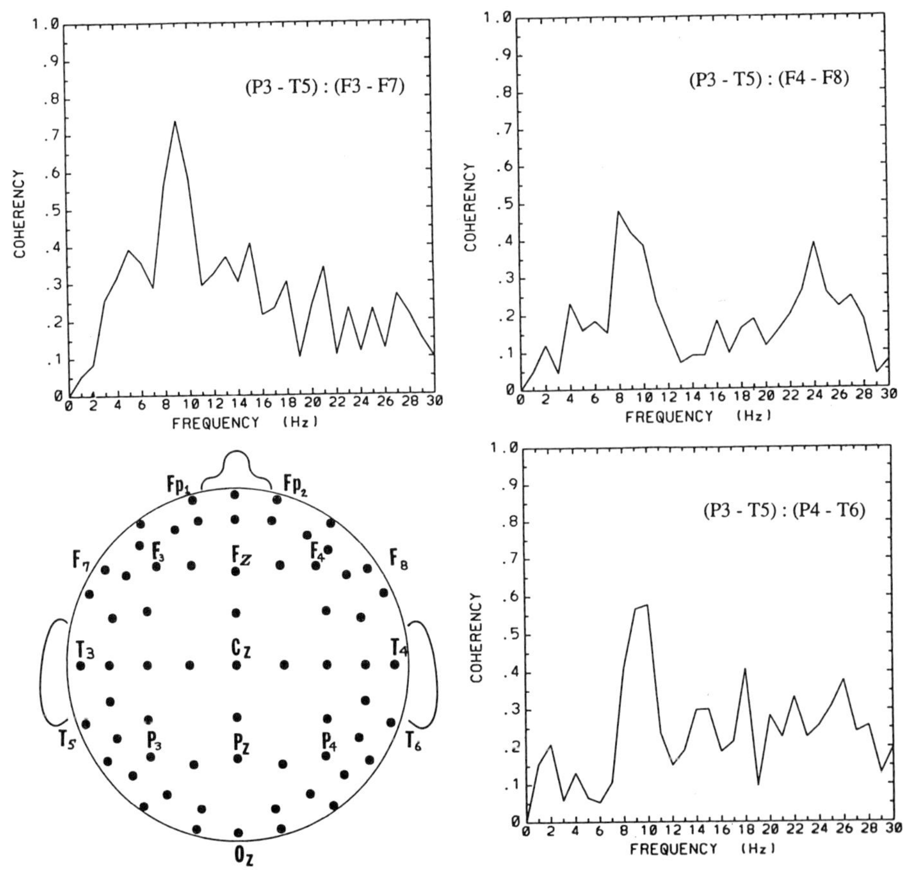

Figure 3-20. Coherency spectra for bipolar recordings from several scalp regions separated by more than 10 cm. Coherency estimates are based on 3 minutes of resting alpha rhythm. Volume conduction and statistical fluctuation errors are very small; reference electrode errors are zero. Thus high-coherency estimates are thought to be due only to high neocortical source coherency.

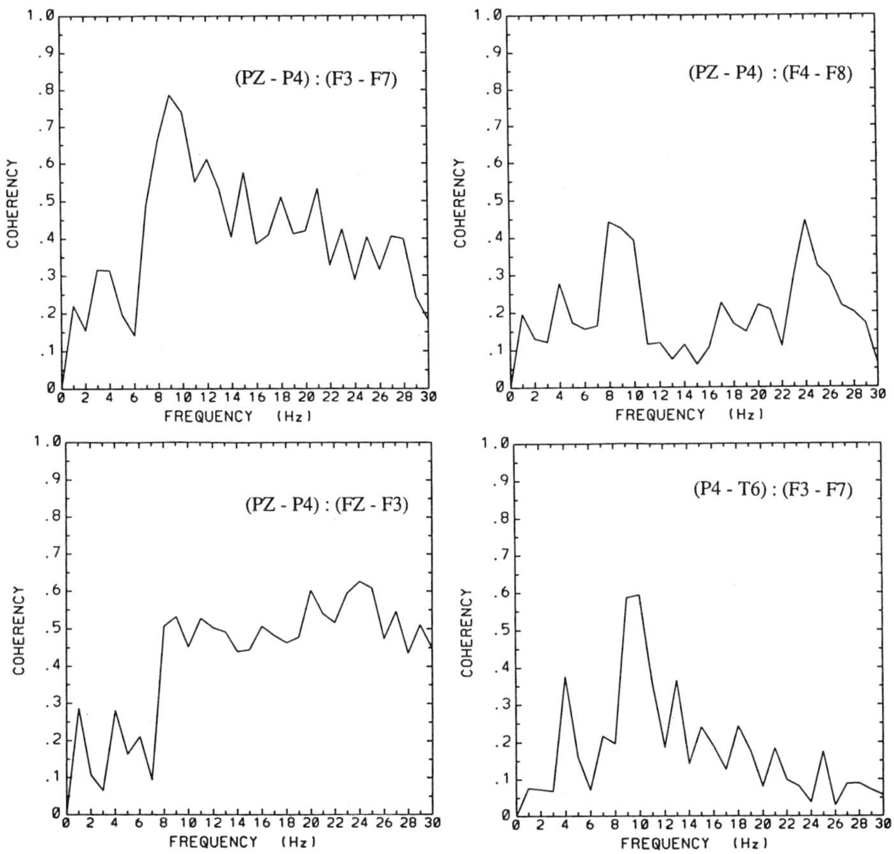

Figure 3-21. Additional bipolar coherency spectra. See Figure 3-20.

Coherencies are generally higher near 10 Hz, but there are many examples of high coherence at other frequencies. Coherency peaks ranging from 0.4 to 0.8 are common.

The coherency spectra also show that volume conduction effects have indeed been minimized. That is, volume conduction is independent of frequency, so erroneous high coherency can be expected to contribute uniformly over the spectrum. The existence of wide spectral bands with low coherency provides an upper limit on coherency errors caused by volume conduction.

Coherency also may be studied using Laplacian estimates to remove volume conduction and reference electrode effects. However, we must be careful with global spline estimates that may provide erroneous high coherence due to the algorithm itself (Biggins et al, 1991). Here we show Laplacian coherency using the following procedure: Twelve electrodes in the vicinity of locations P3, P4, F3, and F4 are used to form four separate local spline-Laplacian estimates for the posterior and anterior regions of each hemisphere. The six regional coherencies resulting from these Laplacian estimates are shown in Figure 3-22. Because the

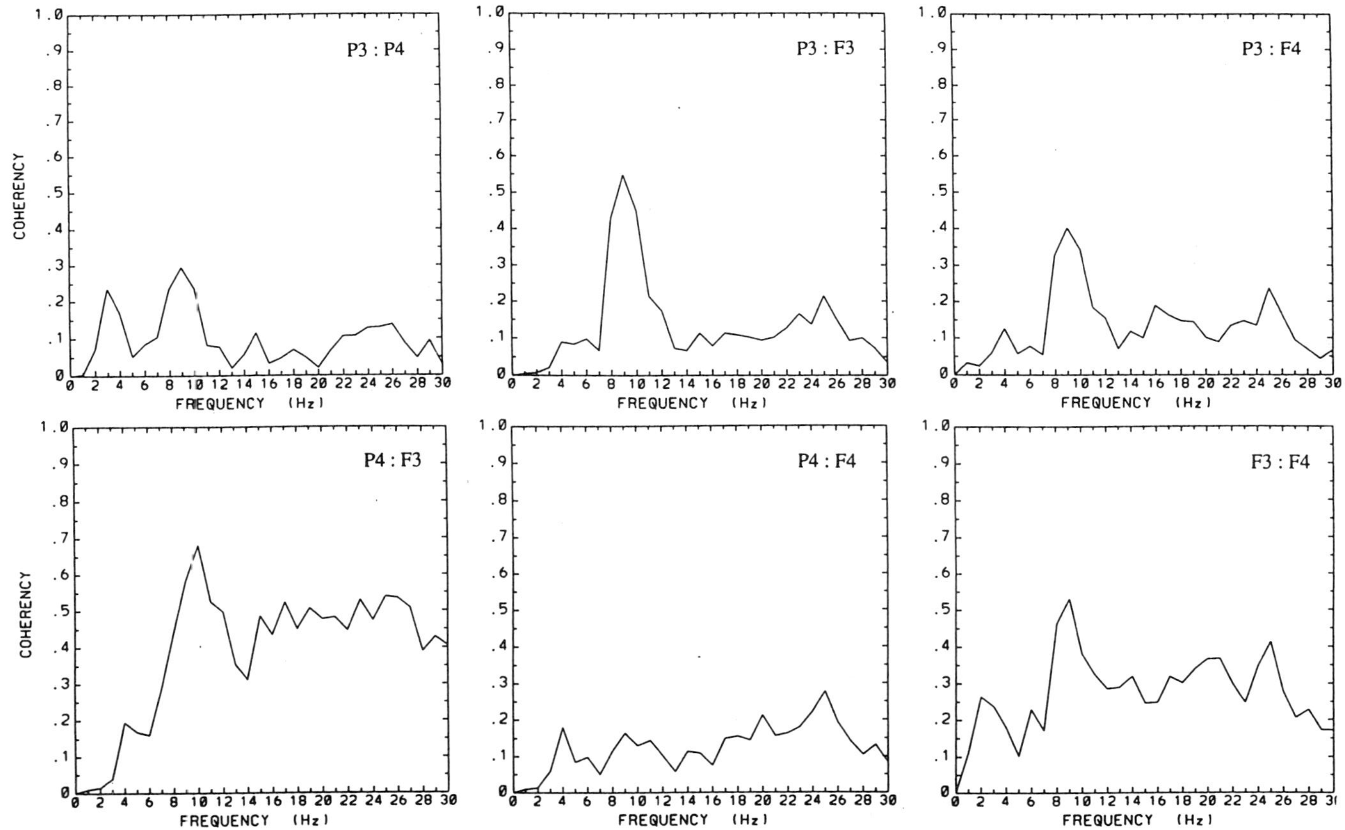

Figure 3-22. Local spline coherency spectra. Local Laplacian estimates were obtained by fitting potentials recorded for 12 local electrodes. In this manner, Laplacians were obtained for the four major scalp regions centered approximately at P3, P4, F3, and F4. The six coherency spectra were based on 3 minutes of resting alpha rhythm. Local splines were used to eliminate possible erroneous high-coherency estimates due to global spline functions (see Biggins et al, 1991). Since the Laplacian is a low-pass filter, it may remove low spatial frequency source coherency in addition to that caused by volume conduction; that is it may produce erroneous low coherency estimates.

four Laplacian estimates involve no common electrodes, erroneous high coherency due only to the spline algorithm cannot occur.

The bipolar and Laplacian coherency estimates are applicable to different parts of the spatial spectrum, as discussed in Chapter 1. Because coherencies at one spatial scale need not match coherencies at other scales in complex systems (see Figure 2-18), we cannot claim that reference, bipolar, or Laplacian coherencies are the most accurate representations of dynamic source activity. That is, methods that remove erroneous high coherency caused by volume conduction by spatially filtering the data also remove actual source coherency that occurs at the same spatial scale.

The following is a plausible (but not unique) interpretation of the EEG coherency results obtained here. If we imagine multiple, distributed neocortical circuits, we may expect pairs of electrode positions that mainly record source activity from the same circuit to produce higher coherencies than pairs recorded from different circuits. Thus a specificity of coherence patterns with respect to frequency band and location is implied. It is not uncommon to find electrode pairs separated by large distances to have higher coherencies than other coherencies obtained from closer positions. This is often observed in the EEG data, regardless of the method of spatial filtering. In addition, the presence of a single, global neocortical network, with activity either in separate regions or superimposed on specific circuits, tends to produce relatively high coherence over large regions of neocortex. These are the putative standing wave oscillations. If cognitive processing involves the recruitment of more specific circuits than operate in the resting state, an overall decrease in neocortical coherency would be expected, but certain specific coherencies associated with the new circuits may increase. This generally observed result is discussed in the next section.

We have been purposely vague about the exact nature of these circuits. However, we have in mind "circuit elements" at something between macrocolumn and regional scales, with interelement communication between distant elements occurring mainly through corticocortical axons, and the isolation of local tissue required to create different multiple circuits occurring at different times provided by lateral inhibition. Each element in these imagined macroscopic circuits is then a neural mass containing between perhaps 10^6 and 10^8 neurons. Of course, we expect simultaneous activation of circuits at smaller scales, which produce potential patterns not directly accessible from scalp recordings. Physiologic bases for such circuits are considered in Chapters 5, 8, and 13. The means by which small-scale neural activity may cross hierarchical levels to produce observable effects at large scales are discussed in Chapter 14.

EEG Dynamics During a Cognitive Task

The spatial–temporal properties of EEG obtained while counting breaths (six 1-minute periods of "resting state") are compared here with EEG recorded while summing a series (three 1-minute periods of "cognitive state"). Laplacian mag-

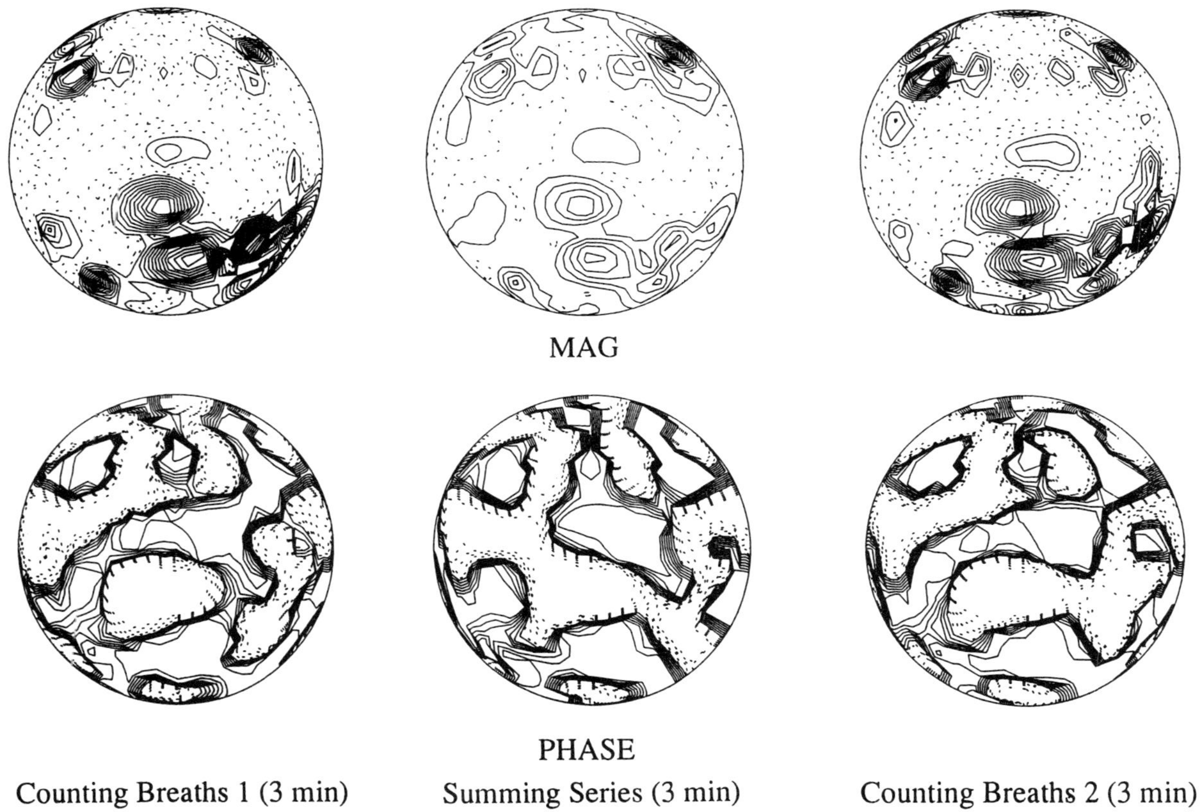

Figure 3-23. Spline-Laplacian magnitude and phase maps. Maps for two 3-minute periods of resting alpha rhythm are shown in the right and left columns. Maps for 3 minutes of alpha recorded during a cognitive task are shown in the middle column.

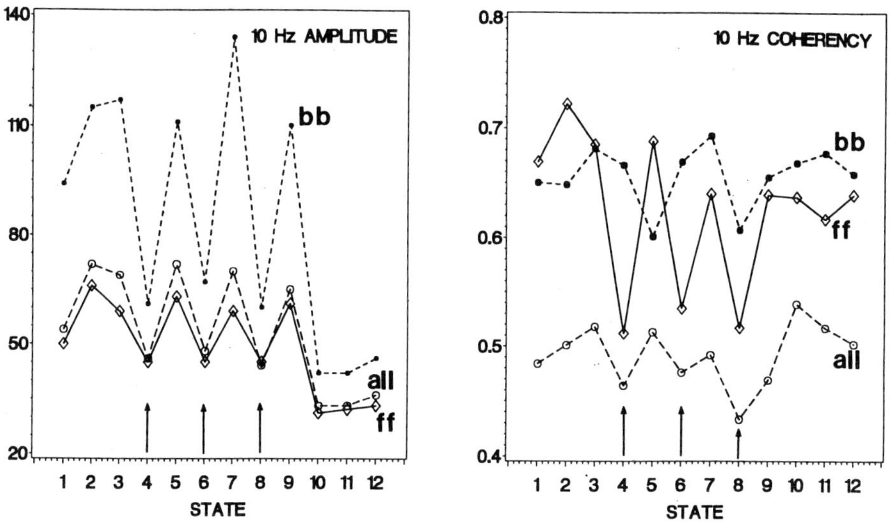

Figure 3-24. Root-mean-square amplitude and coherency as a function of brain state. States 1, 2, 3, 5, 7, and 9 are resting (counting breaths) states, each 1 minute long. States 4, 6, and 8 (arrows) are "cognitive states" (summing a series), each 1 minute long. States 10, 11, and 12 involve driving the visual system with 10-Hz sinusoidal modulated light (eyes open, resting). In these studies, four channels were flagged for possible artifact during parts of the recording and were excluded. Channels bb refer to 16 electrode positions over extreme posterior scalp; ff refers to 28 electrode positions over approximately the anterior half of the scalp. "All" refers to all 60 (64 − 4) electrode positions. Amplitudes and coherencies are averaged over positions within each subgroup. The strongest changes during cognitive states were large decreases in magnitude in posterior electrodes (bb) and large decreases in coherency in frontal-to-frontal coherencies (ff).

nitude and phase plots for two 3-minute resting periods and one 3-minute period of cognitive task are shown in Figure 3-23. Comparison of the cognitive task period with the resting periods indicates that magnitude and phase maps are similar except for an overall reduction in magnitude during the cognitive state (center column).

In addition to global map changes with cognitive state, changes over smaller regions of the scalp are evident. Figure 3-24 illustrates root-mean-square amplitude and coherency changes in three separate groups of channels: bb (the 16 most posterior channels excluding four that were flagged by the artifact rejection algorithm as having possible artifact), ff (the 28 most anterior electrodes), and "all" (all 64 − 4 = 60 electrodes). Root-mean-square amplitudes of unprocessed scalp potential are shown for each of these electrode groups in Figure 3-24 (left) as a function of state number. Resting states are 1, 2, 3, 5, 7, and 9. Cognitive states (arrows) are states 4, 6, and 8. "Evoked states" 10, 11, and 12 involve driving the visual system with diffuse sine wave-modulated light at 10 Hz (see Chapter 6 for discussion of experimental methods). There is an unambiguous decrease in EEG amplitude during both cognitive and evoked states, but the largest changes occur at posterior positions. The amplitude decreases during cognitive states are typically called "alpha blocking," although the alpha rhythm remains relatively robust during cognitive tasks in this subject.

The 10-Hz coherencies for the same electrode groups are also shown in Figure 3-24 (right). In this case, bb refers to the average of all back to back coherencies ($16 \times 15/2 = 120$), ff refers to all frontal to frontal coherencies ($28 \times 27/2 = 378$), and "all" refers to all ($60 \times 59/2 = 1770$) coherencies. The frontal to frontal coherencies show robust decreases during the three cognitive states (4, 8, 6), that is, from average coherencies of approximately 0.7 to average coherencies of 0.5.

Amplitude spectra obtained from frontal and parietal locations were also obtained. In this case, 3 minutes of resting were compared with the 3 minutes of cognitive task. Electrode positions over the back of the head generally show well-defined peaks near 10 Hz in either state, but with amplitude diminished by about 40% during the cognitive task. Well-defined alpha peaks also occur in most frontal locations during the resting state, but these spectral peaks may be obscured by relative increases in low-frequency contributions. These spectra are typical of those observed in chaotic systems, as discussed in Chapter 10. Unfortunately, we cannot be entirely sure that data outside the alpha band are uncontaminated by artifact, although obvious artifact was rejected with the experimental protocol. However, this general spectral signature is probably an accurate representation of neocortical dynamics of cognition in this subject.

To quantify changes in spatial patterns, Laplacian magnitude and phase patterns based on an average of 3 minutes of resting data (Figure 3-15) were used as standards of comparison. Correlation coefficients between these "standard" maps and maps based on 1-second epochs were calculated for 6 consecutive minutes, with resting and cognitive states alternating every minute. These correlation coefficients are plotted in Figure 3-25, with the upper solid line referring to magnitude correlations and the dashed line referring to phase correlations. Magnitude correlation coefficients vary primarily between 0.3 and 0.7 in the data shown in Figure 3-25. In the same data, phase correlations are mainly between 0.2 and 0.5 during resting periods (counting breaths) and slightly lower during cognitive periods. The root-mean-square magnitudes at 10 Hz, averaged over 64 electrodes, are plotted (solid line) in the lower part of each figure and show that magnitudes are generally lower during the cognitive task but that substantial second-to-second variation in magnitude occurs for all 1-minute periods.

These data indicate that spatial patterns are quasi-stable at 1-second scales during resting and cognitive states. By this we mean that both magnitude and phase conditions are moderate for second-to-second pattern comparisons. That is, patterns vary considerably from second to second; however, pattern changes are not random, so moderate positive phase and magnitude correlations are obtained. The reductions in correlation between standard maps and maps based on 1-second epochs usually occur at about every 6 seconds during both resting and cognitive states. This effect is not obviously related to breathing cycles, which were somewhat longer during resting periods than during cognitive periods.

Although much of this data is consistent with known properties of alpha rhythm,

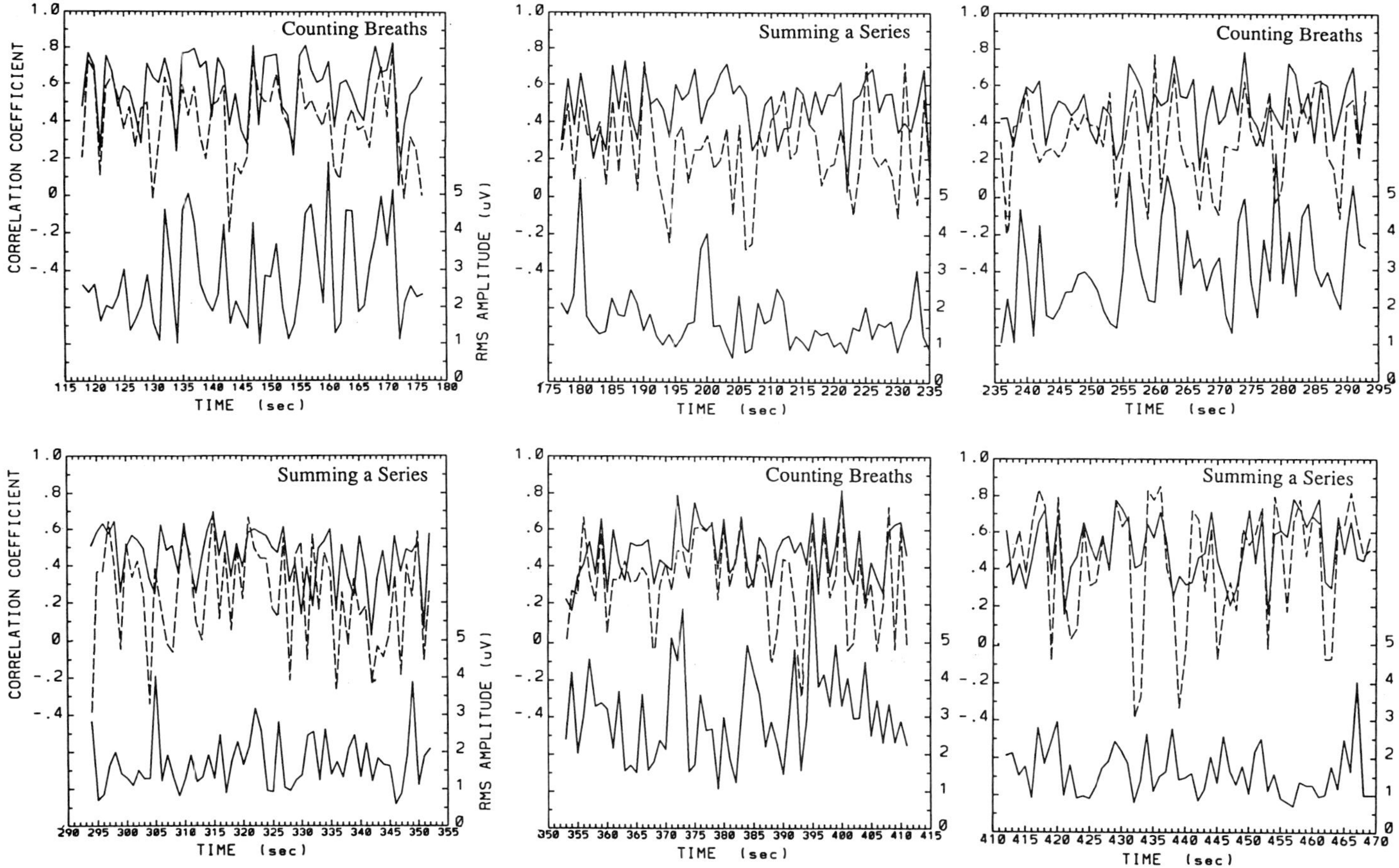

Figure 3-25. Correlation coefficients based on comparisons of successive 1-second epochs with template Laplacian maps shown in Figure 3-15. States 3 to 8 of Figure 3-24 are shown. Upper plots show magnitude (*solid line*) and phase (*dashed line*) correlation coefficients. Lower solid line shows second-to-second changes in root-mean-square magnitude of the 64-channel data.

our results have several advantages over many traditional studies: better artifact rejection, better spatial resolution, more quantitative analysis of data, and direct comparison with simulation studies to aid in interpretation. In addition, several new properties of alpha rhythm are suggested, although these new results must be regarded as tentative because of the limited number of subjects studied at this time.

We have applied modern engineering methods to record and analyze EEG during a cognitive task so as to demonstrate robust EEG differences between brain states. However, our methods may not be appropriate for many cognitive studies. For example, cognitive scientists might want to follow state changes over much shorter times than the 1-minute epochs used here. Or, they might want to study EEG effects of tasks more closely related to specific cognitive theories. However, such choices typically involve critical compromises between engineering and cognitive science. For example, the reduction in data associated with shorter epochs may reduce the statistical significance of EEG differences between different states, many cognitive tasks introduce EEG artifact, and so on. These issues are discussed in more detail in Chapters 6 and 7.

EEG and Neocortical State: A Tentative Qualitative Model

During the past 60 years, proposed physiologic bases for EEG have frequently been labeled either "pacemaker" or "reverberating circuit theories." Generally these explanations have been so lacking in realistic physiology and anatomy and quantitative substance that they should be considered tautologies. For example, we can read of different putative pacemakers for different rhythms. One obvious trouble with this idea is that different pacemakers must apparently be imagined for each of the hundreds of distinctly different EEG states easily observed from the human scalp, with little indication of how they turn on and off, of the physiologic time constants that support characteristic EEG frequencies, or of how they interact. Thus, in many writings, substitution of some other word, such as "gremlin," for "pacemaker," does not detract from the already minimal information conveyed. Although the pacemaker idea may be useful for some EEG phenomena, the arguments in the section Dynamic Analogs of Brain Function discussed previously suggests that applicability of this idea may be quite limited. In addition, the term "reverberating circuit," as used in the EEG literature, is not well defined; it will be avoided in subsequent discussions, although several of the mechanisms we propose may be similar to those of proponents of this idea.

If an EEG theory is to be considered substantive rather than tautologic, it must address the following core issues. (1) The neural tissue required to generate characteristic EEG frequencies: Although characteristic frequencies have often been recorded in small masses of neural tissue, the critical issue of dependence of these frequencies on external interactions is rarely addressed. (2) The physiologic time constants that support these particular frequencies. (3) The means by which spatial–temporal patterns change with physiologic state. We would, of

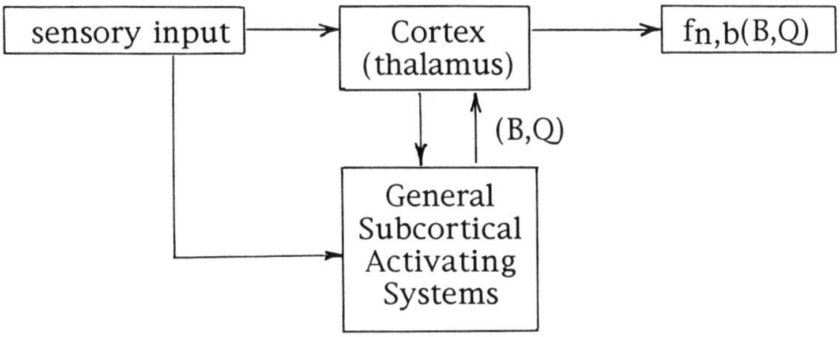

$f_{n,b}(B,Q)$	Characteristic frequencies (overtones)
$n = 1,2,...$	Linear normal mode or quasilinear limit cycle mode
$b = 1,2,3$	Global or local branches of dispersion relation
B	Global control parameter (phase transitions)
Q	Local control parameter (phase transitions)
$\gamma_{n,b}(B,Q)$	Wave damping, mode selectivity

Figure 3-26. A qualitative model for EEG production that encompasses several theoretical efforts by different scientists.

course, prefer that our models accomplish more, especially in making predictions of EEG properties not yet measured. However, these core issues can be regarded as minimum requirements for any preliminary theoretical description of EEG.

A composite qualitative model for EEG generation is illustrated in Figure 3-26. The qualitative description of this section is based on the combined theoretical work of several scientists who have directly addressed the question of EEG origins. Supporting quantitative developments are presented in Chapters 5, 6, 8, 11, 12, 13, and 14. Because physiologic parameters with poorly known magnitudes are involved, we cannot make precise comparisons with experiment. However, several qualitative and semiquantitative connections to experiment are presented in following chapters. Important features that distinguish these different EEG theories are (1) Local versus global generation; that is, "bottom-up" versus "top-down" mechanisms; and (2) Linear, quasilinear, or fully nonlinear approaches.

The diagram of Figure 3-26 is designed to encompass local and global EEG generation and linear and quasilinear interactions in neural tissue. Thus it includes the possibility of pacemakers in the thalamus driving neocortex or, perhaps more realistically, dynamic interaction between cortex and thalamus. It also includes the effects of global boundary conditions and propagation along corticocortical fibers. Although the full nonlinear approach in Chapter 14 includes ideas not shown in Figure 3-26, it encompasses several important limiting cases of general nonlinear, nonequilibrium complex systems. Many distinctions between individual theories are viewed here as quantitative rather than qualitative issues, depending on the relative values of physiologic (control) parameters. General qualitative features of the composite EEG model outlined in Figure 3-26 are listed as follows, beginning with interpretation in the context of linear systems (1 to 4) but including extension to nonlinearity (5 to 7).

1. Characteristic EEG frequencies $f_{n,b}(B,Q)$ occur because of local delays (such as rise and decay times of postsynaptic potentials) and global delays due to finite propagation velocity in corticocortical axons. The subscript (n) indicates specific spatial patterns (eigenfunctions) and corresponding normal mode frequencies, that is, the fundamental and overtones. To simplify the notation, a single subscript (n) is used to identify different eigenfunctions of the complicated two-dimensional geometry of cortical surface—(n) represents the subscripts (ℓ) and (m) for the spherical or prolate spheroid surfaces.

2. EEG frequencies also depend on the value of the second subscript (b) which denotes a particular branch of the dispersion relation. Physiologically, the physical terminology "branch of the dispersion relation," means that different kinds of brain waves can exist simultaneously in the same tissue and interact with each other. Analogous phenomena do not occur in simple physical systems such as the stretched string of Chapter 2 or the violin discussed previously; however, multiple branches of dispersion relations are well known in complex systems such as hot plasma, in which several kinds of waves can exist simultaneously in the same underlying medium. In the specific, local–global theory of Chapter 11, multiple branches occur due only to global effects, and an additional branch occurs because of local circuit delays. The modulation of synaptic action, which is expected to parallel modulation of spontaneous EEG, may be approximated by

$$H \sim \sum_{b} \sum_{n} A_{n,b} e^{-\gamma_{n,b}(B,Q)t} \sin[2\pi f_{n,b}(B,\ Q)t + \phi_{n,b}] \tag{3.8}$$

3. In the limiting case of a brain with zero local delays, the characteristic frequencies $f_{n,b}(B,Q)$ are due only to corticocortical propagation delays, that is, the usual linear, normal mode frequencies. Many closely spaced frequencies can occur, but they are the same at all locations of neocortex. In the opposite limit of zero global delays, a single characteristic frequency occurs ($n = 1$, $b = 1$) at each local tissue mass (or specific, distributed circuit), but this frequency can vary between locations because of changes of the local control parameter Q or fixed differences in tissue properties.

4. The background state of neocortex (and perhaps thalamus) is controlled by diffuse chemical and electrical input from the general activating system by causing changes in the global (B) and local (Q) control parameters. These measure general levels of cortical excitability; that is they are approximately proportional to the number of additional action potentials fired by a tissue mass for each additional excitatory synaptic input from other cortical tissue. The local and global control parameters Q and B are related but can change independently given the variety of possible electrical and chemical control mechanisms acting at different cortical layers which are available to the general activating system (see Chapter 13). Dramatic changes of state in physical systems (such as steam/water/ice/, laminar/turbulent fluid flow) are called "phase transitions" caused by changes in external

control parameters (such as temperature, fluid velocity). A term similar to "phase transition" is "bifurcation," which normally refers to a change in the dynamics of a system of equations as the result of parameter changes. Such equations may or may not describe real physical systems. In neocortical systems, the control parameters (B, Q), or others in more comprehensive theory, may cause changes in physiologic state (such as awake/sleeping, REM/non-REM, resting/epileptic seizure) in an analogous manner.

5. These ideas based mostly on linear theory can be extended to include quasilinear phenomena. In one limiting case described in Chapter 11, each spatial mode undergoes its own limit cycle oscillation; however, the modulation of synaptic activity is still expressed by a linear sum of spatial modes, as in equation (3.8), with periodic but generally nonsinusoidal time dependence. Limit cycles are well-established nonlinear phenomena that occur in a variety of physical systems (such as nonlinear circuits). Generally limit cycles occur when damping parameters are amplitude dependent and can change sign. Small amplitude oscillations then increase with time, whereas large amplitudes decrease; in either case they become part of a limit cycle. Some systems have multiple limit cycles, in which case change of background state (bifurcation due to changes in control parameters B or Q) may cause transitions between limit cycles. In contrast to linear systems, these transitions involve an amplitude-dependent change of frequency. In the parlance of modern nonlinear systems theory, limit cycles are special cases of attractors. That is, a system in the "basin of a particular attractor" (due to the magnitudes of control parameters) tends to "fall into" that attractor. Although the quasilinear version allows for new and interesting phenomena, it is often possible to make plausible estimates of characteristic frequency ranges based only on linear theory. An example of this is the famous Van der Pol circuit discussed in Chapter 10.

6. Given the extreme complexity of neocortical interactions, linear or quasilinear descriptions are probably inadequate for any general theory of neocortical function. Rather we can view cases 1 to 5 as crude approximations, which may nevertheless be useful. For example, we can often predict the main spectral peaks in weakly chaotic systems using only linear theory, as discussed in Chapter 10. Several good reasons exist to look first at relatively simple models, one of the most important being that they typically involve fewer physiologic parameters. For example, numerical solutions of complicated nonlinear equations may not be very illuminating unless conclusions are robust with respect to parameter changes over the range of physiologic uncertainty. Fully nonlinear approaches to neocortical dynamics are considered in Chapter 14.

7. Figure 3-26 may partly illuminate the relation between spontaneous EEG and evoked potentials. Some neuroscientists have postulated that transient, cortical evoked potentials can be viewed as the "ringing" (damped oscillation) of a resonant system. There is, in fact, experimental support for this idea, although evoked potential phenomena are more complex than the simple transient responses of linear electric circuits (Basar, 1980; Basar et al, 1987; Wright et al, 1990). For example, in a linear system with spatial extent, the combination of

modes (n) excited by the external stimulus depends on the spatial properties of the inputs, as discussed in Chapter 9.

Summary

Various dynamic analogs of brain function are proposed. The idea behind this metaphoric approach is not to provide an accurate view of brain operation in any general sense. Rather these analogs are suggested as limiting cases of brain function corresponding to certain EEG states. In particular, the physics of the violin family is outlined in connection with characteristic EEG frequencies, standing waves, and putative "pacemakers." Possible causes of the low-pass behavior of EEG recorded in vertebrates are listed. A sociologic metaphor continues our emphasis of Chapters 1 and 2 on spatial scale interactions in neocortex and introduces concepts generally used in the study of complex systems, such as phase transitions and self-organization.

Mind–brain relations are considered in the contexts of computer intelligence and split-brain patients. The idea of large-scale intelligence is introduced partly as a metaphor of neocortical dynamic function at multiple scales and partly to illustrate how little we know about the possibilities for "nonhuman consciousness." A few speculative remarks on possible connections between quantum mechanics and consciousness are added.

States of human consciousness that are revealed with various measures are considered as points in a multidimensional space. This emphasizes that states that are similar using some measures may be much different when quantified with other measures. A model system of EEG generation is outlined in a qualitative manner. The model is sufficiently general to encompass most theories proposed for EEG, with local and global and linear and quasilinear effects included. State changes are believed to be controlled by input from the general activating system of the brainstem and other subcortical structures, which alters global and local control parameters. Such state changes may be similar to the phase transitions observed in complex physical systems.

The general dynamic structure of large-scale spontaneous EEG is studied using 64-channel data, for which suspected artifact is removed with modern engineering methods. High-resolution algorithms are used to estimate cortical surface potential. Magnitude and phase plots of scalp and cortical potentials are obtained. Coherency patterns are presented. Differences in dynamic patterns at time scales in the 100 millisecond to 1-minute range and differences between resting and cognitive states are outlined. The experimental data are considered in the context of a qualitative neocortical model consisting of specific, distributed circuits and global standing waves, which may operate simultaneously. A partial switch between more global operation during resting states and more dominance of specific circuits during cognitive states is implied. The general idea has experimental support from the cognitive studies outlined in Chapters 6 and 7. Regional circuits, which are intermediate between local and global networks, are considered in Chapter 13.

Relations between cognitive processing and changes of EEG pattern on shorter time scales (such as, a few tens of milliseconds) are described in a series of studies by Lehmann et al (1987) and Wackermann et al (1993). Because of the tradeoff between frequency and time resolution, these studies of "brain microstates" concern spatial changes within broad frequency bands. However, the resulting improvement in temporal resolution provides a means to view potential patterns which change over short times and may correspond to distinct functional "microstates" of the brain. Such ideas are consistent with our earlier discussion of local and distributed circuits operating within the global dynamic system with state changes mediated by local and global control parameters. Data which support the idea that local and global control parameters may be altered by different neuromodulators are presented in Chapter 13.

References

Amit, D.J. *Modeling Brain Function. Attractor Neural Networks.* New York: Cambridge University Press, 1988.

Andersen, P. and Andersen, S.A. *Physiologic Basis of the Alpha Rhythm.* New York: Appelton, 1968.

Barrow, J.D. and Tipler, F.J. *The Anthropic Cosmological Principal.* New York: Oxford University Press, 1988.

Basar, E. *EEG Brain Dynamics: Relations Between EEG and Evoked Potentials.* New York: Elsevier, 1980.

Basar, E., Basar-Eroglu, C., Roschke, J., and Schutt, A. The EEG is a quasi-deterministic signal anticipating sensory-cognitive tasks. In: *Brain Dynamics.* (E. Basar and Bullock, T.H., Eds.) Berlin: Springer-Verlag, pp. 43–71, 1987.

Bendat, J.S. and Piersol, A.G. *Random Data. Analysis and Measurement Procedures, 2nd Ed.* New York: Wiley, 1986.

Biggins, C.A., Fein, G., Raz, J., and Amir, A. Artifactually high coherences from using spherical spline computation of scalp current density. *Electroencephalogr. Clin. Neurophysiol.* 79:413–419, 1991.

Bloom, F.E. What is the role of the general activating systems in cortical function? *Neurobiology of Neocortex.* (P. Rakic and Singer, W., Eds.) New York: Wiley, pp. 407–421, 1988.

Bogen, J.E., Fisher, E.D., and Vogel, P.J. Cerebral commissurotomy, a second case report. *JAMA.* 194:1328–1329, 1965.

Bohm, D. *Quantum Theory.* New York: Prentice-Hall, 1951.

Braitenberg, V. and Schuz, A. *Anatomy of the Cortex, Statistics and Geometry.* New York: Springer-Verlag, 1991.

Braitenberg, V. *Vehicles. Experiments in Synthetic Psychology.* Cambridge, MA: MIT Press, 1984.

Bullock, T.H. *Introduction to Nervous Systems.* San Francisco: W.H. Freeman, 1977.

Burcklund, C. W. and Smith, A. Language and the cerebral hemispheres. *Neurology* 27:627–633, 1977.

Churchland, P.M. *Neurophilosophy*. Cambridge, MA: MIT Press, 1986.

Deecke, L., Grotzinger, B., and Kornhuber, H.H. Voluntary finger movement in man, cerebral potentials and theory. *Biol. Cybern.* 23:99–112, 1976.

Dennett, D.C. Dissociation of the personality. In: *The Oxford Companion to the Mind*. New York: Oxford University Press, pp. 160–164, 1987.

Dreyfus, H.L. *What Computers Can't Do, (2nd Ed.)* New York: Harper and Row, 1979.

Freeman, W.J. Analytic techniques used in the search for the physiological bases of the EEG. In: *Handbook of Electroencephalography and Clinical Neurophysiology. (Revised Series). Vol. 1.* (A. Gevins and Remond, A., Eds.) New York: Elsevier, 1987.

Freeman, W.J. Consciousness as physiological self-organizing process. *Behavioral and Brain Sciences.* 13:604–605, 1990.

Freeman, W.J. and Skarda, C.S. Spatial analysis, nonlinear dynamics and perception: The neo-Sherrington view. *Brain Res. Rev.* 10:147–175, 1985.

French, J.D. The reticular formation. *Sci. Am.* 54–60, May 1957.

Gazzaniga, M.S. and LeDoux, J.E. *The Integrated Mind.* New York: Plenum, 1978.

Gazzaniga, M.S. *The Social Brain: Discovering the Networks of the Mind.* New York: Basic Books, 1985.

Gott, P.S. Cognitive abilities following right and left hemispherectomy. *Cortex.* 9:266–273, 1973.

Haken, H. *Evolution of Order and Chaos.* New York: Springer-Verlag, 1982.

Harth, E. *Windows on the Mind: Reflections on the Physical Basis of Consciousness.* New York: William Morrow, 1982.

Hobson, J.A. *Sleep.* New York: W.H. Freeman, 1989.

Hogan, J. *Code of the Lifemaker.* New York: Ballantine Books, 1983.

Hoyle, F. *The Black Cloud.* New York: The New American Library, 1957.

Hubel, D.H. The brain. *Sci. Am.* 241:39–47, 1979.

Hutchins, C.M. The physics of violins. *Sci. Am.* 207:79–93, 1962.

Ingber, L. Statistical mechanics of neocortical interactions: A scaling paradigm applied to electroencephalography. *Phys. Rev.* 44(A):4017–4060, 1991.

Ingber, L. Towards a unified brain theory. *Journal of Social and Biological Structure.* 4:211–224, 1981.

Ingber, L. and Nunez, P.L. Multiple scales of statistical physics of neocortex: Application to electroencephalography. *Mathematical and Computational Modelling.* 13:83–95, 1990.

Katznelson, R.D. Normal modes of the brain: Neuroanatomical basis and a physiological theoretical model. In: *Electric Fields of the Brain: The Neurophysics of EEG.* (P.L. Nunez) New York: Oxford University Press, 1981.

Lehmann, D., Ozaki, H., and Pal, I. EEG alpha map series: Brain microstates by space oriented adaptive segmentation. *Electroencephalogr. Clin. Neurophysiol.* 67:271–288, 1987.

Libet, B. Consciousness: conscious, subjective experience. *Encyclopedia of Neuroscience.* 1:271–275, 1987.

Magoun, G. and Moruzzi, H. Brain stem reticular formation and activation of the EEG. *Electroencephalogr. Clin. Neurophysiol.* 1:455–473, 1949.

Nicolis, G. and Prigogine, I. *Exploring Complexity.* New York: W.H. Freeman, 1989.

Nunez, P.L. The brain wave equation: A model for EEG. *Math Biosciences.* 21:279–297, 1974a.

Nunez, P.L. Wavelike properties of the alpha rhythm. *IEEE Trans. Biomed. Eng.* 21:473–482, 1974b.

Nunez, P.L. *Electric Fields of the Brain: The Neurophysics of EEG*. New York: Oxford University Press, 1981.

Nunez, P.L. Generation of human EEG by a combination of long and short range neocortical interactions. *Brain Topography*. 1:199–215, 1989.

Nunez, P.L. and Pilgreen, K.L. The spline Laplacian in clinical neurophysiology: A method to improve EEG spatial resolution. *J. Clin. Neurophysiol.* 8:397–413, 1991.

Nunez, P.L., Pilgreen, K.L., Westdrop, A.F., Law, S.K., and Nelson, A.V. A visual study of surface potentials and Laplacians due to distributed neocortical sources: Computer simulations and evoked potentials. *Brain Topography*. 4:151–168, 1991.

Nunez, P.L. and Srinivasan, R.A. Implications of recording strategy for estimates of neocortical dynamics with electroencephalography. *Chaos: An Interdiciplinary Journal of Nonlinear Science*. 3:257–266, 1993.

Nunez, P.L., Silberstein, R.B., Cadusch, P.J., Wijesinghe, R.S., Westdrop, A.F., and Srinivasan, R.A. A theoretical and experimental study of high resolution EEG based on surface Laplacians and cortical imaging. *Electroencephalogr. Clin. Neurophysiol.* 90:40–57, 1994.

Pandya, D.N. and Yeterian, E.H. Architecture and connections of cortical association areas. In: *Cerebral Cortex. Vol. 4. Association and Auditory Cortices.* (A. Peters and Jones, E.G., Eds.) New York: Plenum, 1985.

Penrose, R. *The Emperor's New Mind.* New York: Oxford University Press, 1989.

Petri, H.L. and Mishkin, M. Behaviorism, cognitivism and the neuropsychology of memory. *Amer. Scientist.* 82:30–37, 1994.

Prigogine, I. and Stengers, I. *Order Out of Chaos: Man's New Dialogue with Nature.* New York: Bantum Books, 1984.

Saunders, F.A. Physics and music. *Sci. Am.* 179:32–41, July 1948.

Searl, J.R. Minds, brains, and programs. *Behavioral and Brain Sciences.* 3:417–457, 1980a.

Searl, J.R. Intrinsic intentionality. *Behavioral and Brain Sciences.* 3:450–456, 1980b.

Silberstein, R.B., Schier, M.A., Pipingas, A., Ciorciari, J., Wood, S.R., and Simpson, D.G. Steady-state visually evoked potential topography associated with a visual vigilance task. *Brain Topography*. 3:337–347, 1990.

Skinner, B.F. *Beyond Freedom and Dignity.* New York: Knopf, 1971.

Smith, A. Speech and other functions after left (dominant) hemispherectomy, *J. Neurol. Neurosurg. Psychiatry.* 29:467–471, 1966.

Sperry, R.W. Brain bisection and mechanisms of consciousness. In: *Brain and Conscious Experience.* (J. C. Eccles, Ed.) New York: Springer-Verlag, 1966.

Sperry, R.W. Lateral specialization in the surgically separated hemispheres. In: *The Neuroscience 3rd Study Program.* (F.O. Schmitt and Worden, F.G., Eds.) Cambridge, MA: MIT Press, pp. 5–19, 1974.

Sperry, R.W. Some effects of disconnecting the cerebral hemispheres. *Science.* 217;1223–1226, 1982.

Taylor, C.A. *The Physics of Musical Sounds.* New York: Elsevier, 1965.

Turing, A.M. Computing machinery and intelligence. In: *The Mind's Eye.* (D.R. Hofstadter and Dennett, D.C., Eds.) New York: Basic Books, pp. 53–69, 1981. Originally published in 1950.

Wackermann, J., Lehmann, D., Michel, C.M., and Strick, W. Adaptive segmentation of spontaneous EEG map series into spatially defined microstates. *Internat. J. Psycholphys.* 14:269–283, 1993.

Weidlich, W. and Haag, G. *Concepts and Models of a Quantitative Sociology.* New York: Springer-Verlag, 1983.

Wiener, N. *Cybernetics or Control and Communication in the Animal and the Machine. 2nd Ed.* Cambridge, MA: MIT Press, 1961.

Wigner, E.P. The place of consciousness in modern physics. In: *Consciousness and Reality.* (C. Muses and Young, A.M., Eds.) New York: Avon Books, 1974.

Wilensky, R. Computability, consciousness, and algorithms. *Behavioral and Brain Sciences.* 13:690–691, 1990.

Witelson, S.F. Brain asymmetry, functional aspects. In: *Encyclopedia of Neuroscience. Vol. 1.* (G. Adelman, Ed.) Boston: Birkhäuser, pp. 152–156, 1987.

Wright, J.J., Sergejew, A.A., and Stampfer, H.G. Inverse filter computation of the neural impulse giving rise to the auditory evoked potential. *Brain Topography.* 2:293–302, 1990.

4

Physiologic, Medical, and Cognitive Correlates of Electroencephalography

KENNETH L. PILGREEN

Since the first electroencephalographic (EEG) recordings, electroencephalographers have been interested in the relation between EEG and the behavioral state of the person studied (Berger, 1929). Such relations are observed at many spatial and temporal scales. Anatomically, they span molecular, cellular, locally specialized neuronal network, and whole-brain levels. Each of these levels of analysis has specific electrical and behavioral correlates. As noted in Chapters 1 and 3, the temporal resolution of EEG spans all anatomic and functional scales and makes it a particularly useful tool in behavior analysis. Behavioral states consist of varied states of arousal, including the different stages of sleep.

The term "EEG" as we commonly use it refers to electrical activity measured at the scalp that arises from neurons in the cerebral cortex. This includes activity that arises spontaneously or in response to sensory stimuli, although the latter are more commonly known as "evoked potentials" (EP). Spontaneous EEG activity is generally believed to result from the summation of inhibitory (IPSP) and excitatory (EPSP) postsynaptic potentials of underlying regions of cerebral cortex (Nunez, 1989). This activity fluctuates with time at locations on the surface of the scalp. The amplitude at any given time for any particular location depends on the orientation of many coherent sources that fluctuate with time, as discussed in Chapter 1. The term "source" generally refers to the electrical activity of groups of neurons that produce the measured EEG. As depicted in Figure 1-4, neuronal activity in the depths of sulci typically contributes minimally to scalp-recorded electrical activity.

Evoked potentials consist of electrical responses to a sensory stimulus and usually are described as purely dependent on attributes of the stimulus. Event-related potentials (ERP) depend more on internal factors related to the cognitive set of the person studied. The latter type of activity could include such variables as level of motivation, such as for reward, which exists as a dimension within the waking state. Spontaneous ("background") EEG also may vary within this cognitive dimension. The actual electrical signal in EPs is thought to be generated by neural sources similar to those described for spontaneous EEG, with possible contributions from action potentials in the case of brainstem evoked potentials (Nunez, 1990).

Molecular and Cellular Basis of EEG

Electroencephalography as commonly measured is the result of a complex pattern of pyramidal cell activity with some contributions from granule and glial cells in the cerebral neocortex (Speckmann and Elger, 1987). A generalized neuron is depicted in Figure 4-1, with its anatomic processes and different types of synapses. The organization of the neocortex is complicated (see Chapters 1, 2, and 5), consisting of six distinct layers as seen with the light microscope (Figure 4-2). Cellular variation within each of these layers constitutes the basis for the Broadman map in Figure 2-17. Figure 4-2 shows four examples of neocortex from distinct anatomic locations. Note the differences in cell number, size, and type among the regions according to layer. These different areas have functional specificity, but even within these areas, variation of function occurs with no clear anatomic differences (Douglas and Martin, 1990). Variance in quantitative aspects of afferent (entering) and efferent (leaving) fiber tracts may account for this apparent paradox (Creutzfeld, 1977). These tracts carry the axons that link disparate brain regions (that is, cortical–cortical associations) and the "outside world." This latter example is an observation at the largest spatial and functional scales.

The pyramidal cells are the largest cells in the cerebral cortex, and the largest of them are found in the primary motor strip. These Betz cells control muscles in the leg. Specific inputs tend to terminate at stereotyped locations on the pyramidal cell, as shown in Figure 4-3. Specific thalamic inputs terminate on the apical dendrite near the soma in layer 4 and long-range cortical inputs terminate on the distal portion of the apical dendrite in layers 2 and 3. The thalamus provides the primary routing to cerebral cortex from other regions of the brain, including the basal ganglia, cerebellum, limbic system, and multiple specific brainstem nuclei. These nuclei consist of small groups of neurons with varying orientation; their "random" orientation is one reason why brainstem evoked potentials of any modality are of much lower amplitude than background electrical activity. Auditory, vestibular, and gustatory (taste) inputs to neocortex arise in the brainstem, whereas olfactory inputs enter through limbic connections. Visual inputs are represented by an almost direct route through two separate areas of thalamus—specifically the pulvinar and lateral geniculate body with termination in the occipital cortex. The thalamus is depicted in Figure 4-4 with its inputs, local relays, and outputs to neocortex (see also Table 4-1). Although there are reciprocal connections between neocortex and thalamus, most neocortical outputs leave through multiple routes and influence every other region of the brain and spinal cord.

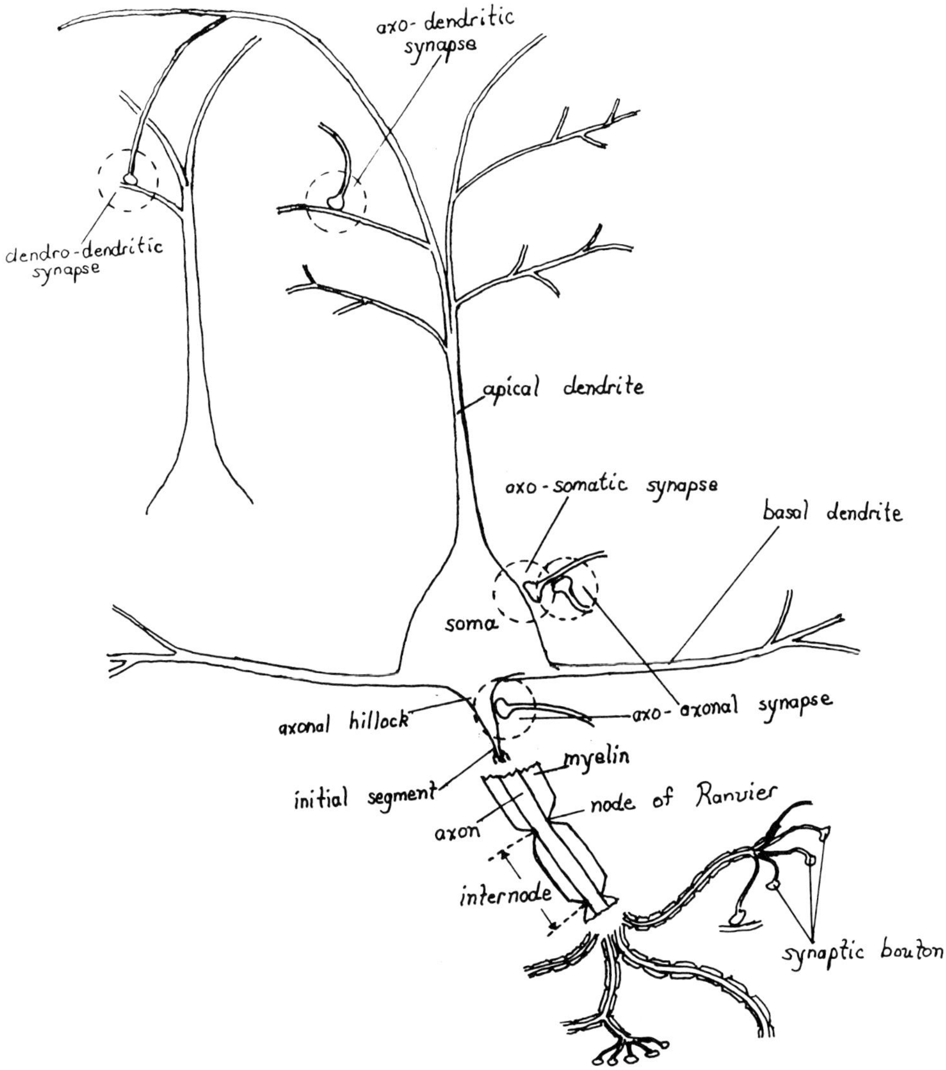

Figure 4-1. Generalized pyramidal cell showing cellular and macromolecular aspects of anatomy. Axodendritic synapses are usually excitatory (glutamatergic, for example), whereas axosomatic and axoaxonal synapses tend to be inhibitory ($GABA_A$). Apical dendrites extend toward the brain surface and then branch to interact with many other neurons through dendrodendritic synapses. Recurrent axonal collaterals also have excitatory synapses on the basilar dendrites of neighboring pyramidal cells. The nodes indicate an area on the axon that is not sheathed by myelin and is the location of most axonal ionophores.

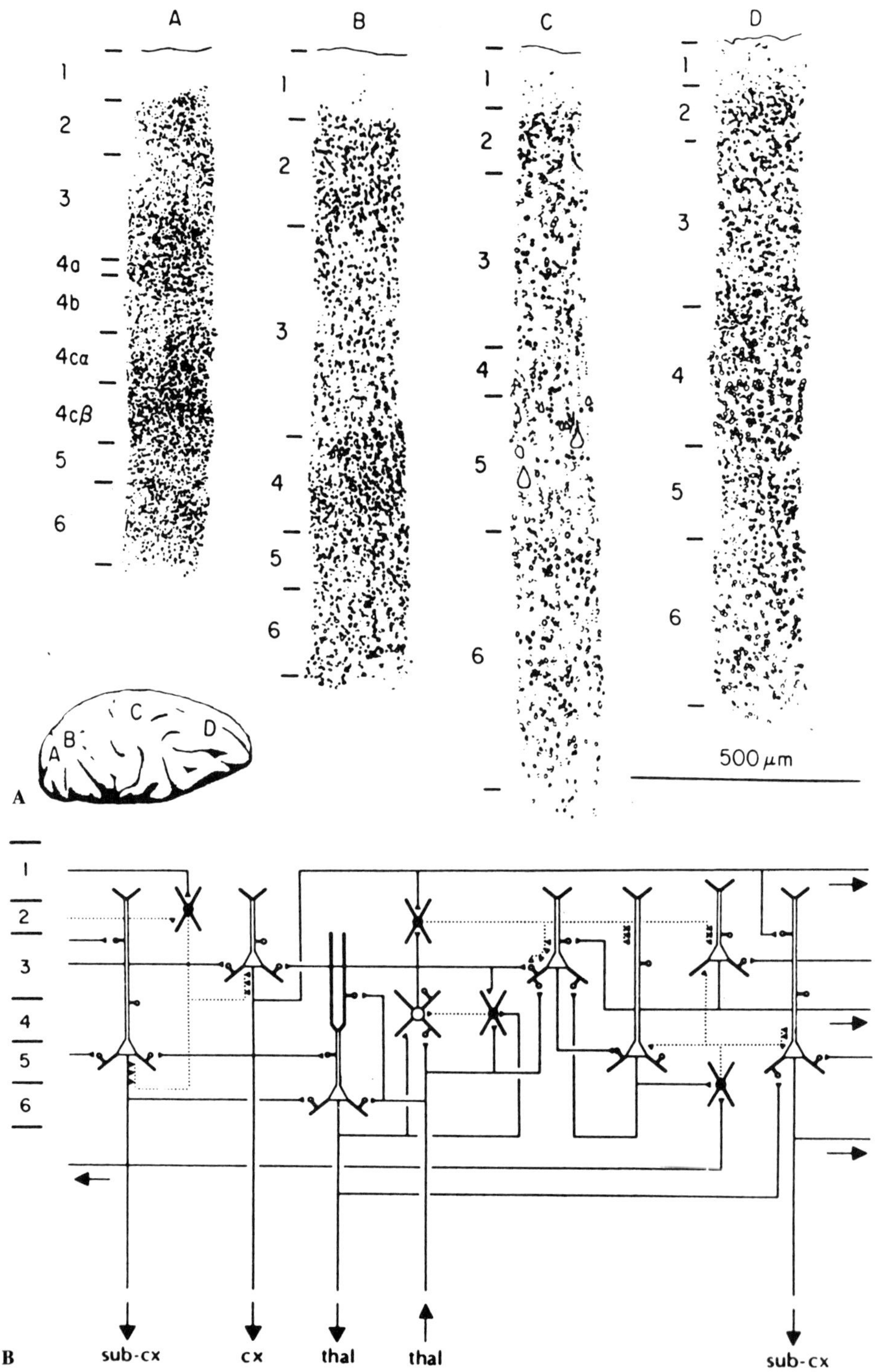
A
B
C
D
1
2
3
4a
4b
4cα
4cβ
5
6
4
500 μm
A
B
1
2
3
4
5
6
sub-cx
cx
thal
thal
sub-cx

Because any potential generated in the brain is due to changes across the cell membrane of neurons, an understanding of basic membrane physiology is necessary. All changes across the cell membrane are caused by changes in the partitioning of ionic concentrations between the extracellular and intracellular spaces. These changes generally occur as a result of ion-specific permeability changes in the membrane. Each ion has a very low leakage current through the lipid bilayer portion of the membrane (Figure 4-5). Thus the primary route through which ions are exchanged are protein channels that span the cell membrane. Most of these macromolecules have very complicated structures and act as enzymes with functional changes produced through allosteric interactions. For example, the occupation of a receptor site on an ion-specific protein produces a change in selective permeability for one or more ionic species. The protein responsible for such changes is an ionophore. The change in permeability may be the result of a change in the geometry (that is, increasing diameter), a change in the charge distribution in the channel, or both.

The receptors that reside on the ionophores discussed above are the primary sites of action of neurotransmitters and even neuropeptide neuromodulators. Some neurotransmitters act through chemical changes (second messenger) in the cell that eventually result in a change in cell metabolism or even a secondary membrane protein that changes ionic permeability. Neurotransmitters are generally excitatory or inhibitory, depending on what type of postsynaptic potential is generated, either EPSP or IPSP. The same neurotransmitter may have inhibitory or excitatory actions, depending primarily on the specific anatomic region being studied, although some general rules apply. For instance, the amino acid neurotransmitters glutamate and gamma-aminobutyric acid (GABA) are believed to be always excitatory and inhibitory, respectively; they are the primary neurotransmitters found in neocortex. Excitatory postsynaptic potentials usually arise from an increased permeability to sodium, calcium, or both. The stimulation of N-methyl-D-aspartate receptors by glutamate and other agonists produces an increased permeability to sodium and calcium. Generally sodium permeability changes are relatively brief (tens of milliseconds) and cause high-amplitude transmembrane potential changes, whereas increases in calcium permeability produces a lower amplitude and more

---

Figure 4-2. **A.** The cerebral neocortex shows a laminar organization with six distinct layers. Each specific anatomic site has a distinct pattern of cell density and size in each of these layers. Rather large pyramidal cells (Betz cells) are present in layer 5 of primary motor cortex, and a dramatic difference from primary visual cortex is evident. **B.** Local area network for segment of generalized visual cortex. GABAergic neurons are shown in black, with their axons depicted as dotted lines. Note their synapses on the axonal initial segment. Specific inputs are depicted, such as specific thalamic afferents (thal) and efferents terminating in other areas of neocortex (cx), subcortical cell groups in the brain and spinal cord (sub-cx), and reciprocal connections with thalamus (thal). (Reproduced with permission from Douglas and Martin, 1990.)

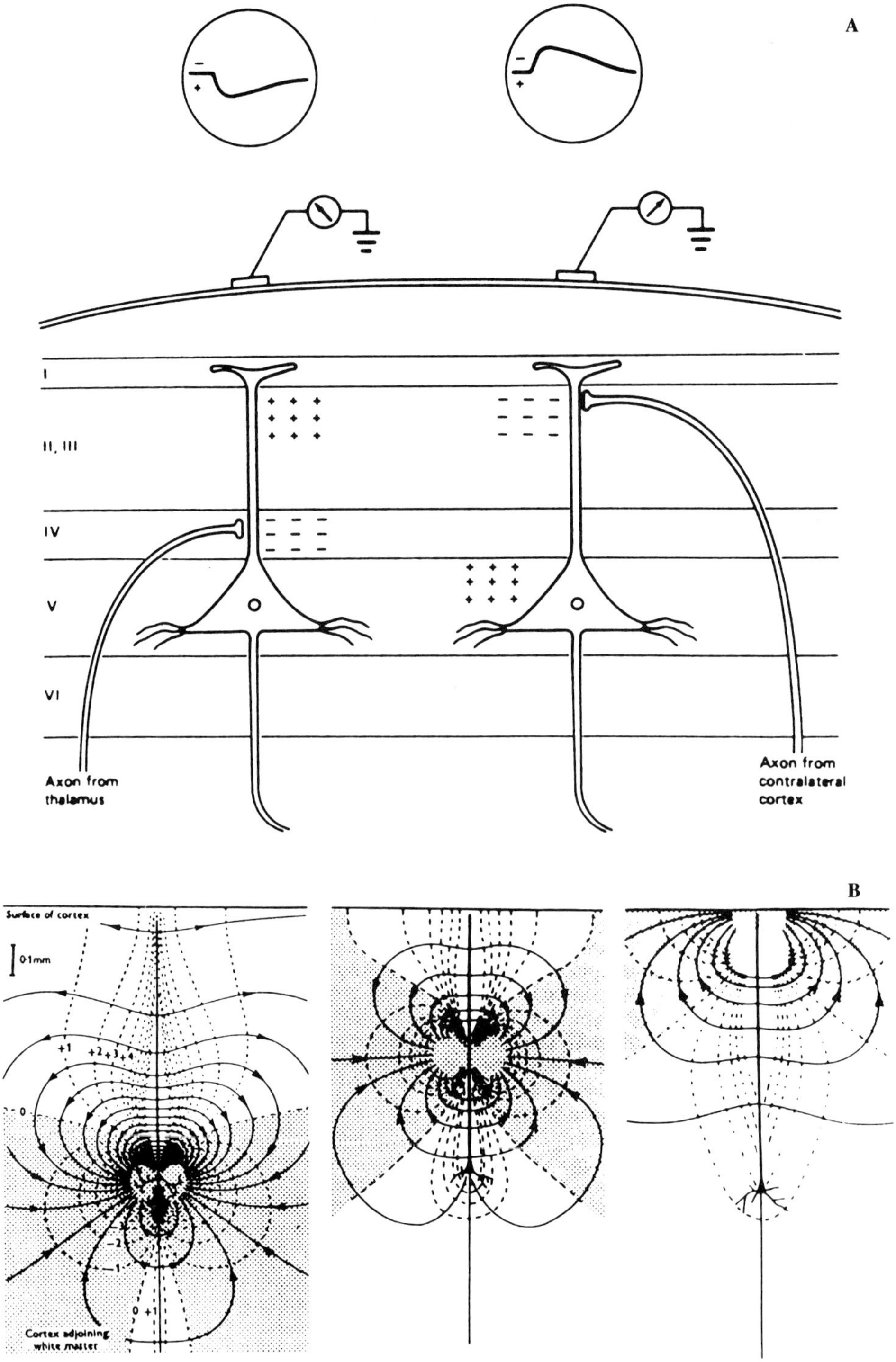
A
I
II, III
IV
V
VI
Axon from thalamus
Axon from contralateral cortex
B
Surface of cortex
0·1mm
+1
+2
+3
+4
0
−2
−1
0 +1
Cortex adjoining white matter

sustained potential change (hundreds of milliseconds). Inhibitory postsynaptic potentials may be generated from permeability changes in chloride, potassium, or both, with potassium producing the lower amplitude but sustained change and chloride a higher-amplitude, brief potential change. The best example of a neurotransmitter producing the latter is GABA, with two subtypes, $GABA_A$, which affects chloride through a direct interaction with the ionophore, and $GABA_B$, which affects potassium through a secondary messenger system (Cooper et al, 1991a). Maximum permeability changes will, of course, occur around the area of transmitter release and will decrease in magnitude in all directions away from this site. Even more sustained changes, inhibitory and excitatory, may occur in the presence of peptide neuromodulators (Cooper et al, 1991b).

Other ionophores may be triggered by modalities other than chemical mediation, such as transmembrane potential changes. These voltage-sensitive channels may be affected even by fields produced by other cells. The percentage of activated channels diminishes exponentially as we move away from the epicenter of the postsynaptic potential. These potentials also decay with time and may be assigned a time constant that is specific for that particular cell's membrane and the ion involved. Figure 4-6A shows an ideal cell membrane with partitioning of the most important ions in the resting state. This diagram shows that the direction of current flow follows a selective ion permeability change. Figure 4-6B shows how each conductance change affects transmembrane potential, with some details about receptor and neurotransmitter specificities and type of ionophore outlined in Table 4-2.

As noted previously, membrane potential changes may induce voltage-sensitive ionophore conformational change and trigger a cascade of increased ionic perme-

←

Figure 4-3. **A.** Scalp potential polarity is determined by the location on the cell and by which ion(s) has changes in permeability. There are opposite meter deflections for specific excitatory inputs from different anatomic sites. Thalamic afferents synapse near the soma in layer IV, producing a positive response, whereas inputs from contralateral cortex that synapse more distally on the same apical dendrite in layers II and III produce a negative change. **B.** The theoretical fields produced by depolarization at three different sites on a typical pyramidal cell are shown, with the first and last pattern corresponding to the first and second neurons in figure A, respectively. Current flow is indicated by the solid lines with arrows and isopotential contours are represented by dotted line, with positivity represented by the shaded areas and negativity by the clear areas. We can also consider that these three patterns could represent how a depolarization originating in the soma might transfer up the apical dendrite, with the propagation in the opposite direction ignored. (Reproduced with permission. (A) from Kandel, E.R. and Schortz, J.H. (Eds.). *Principals of Neural Science.* Amsterdam: Elsevier, 1990, p. 642. (B) from Crentzfeldt, O. and Houchin, J. Neuronal basis of EEG waves. In: *Handbook of Electroencephalography and Clinical Neurophysiology,* Vol. 2C (O. Creutzfeldt, Ed.). Amsterdam: Elsevier, 1974, pp. 5–55).

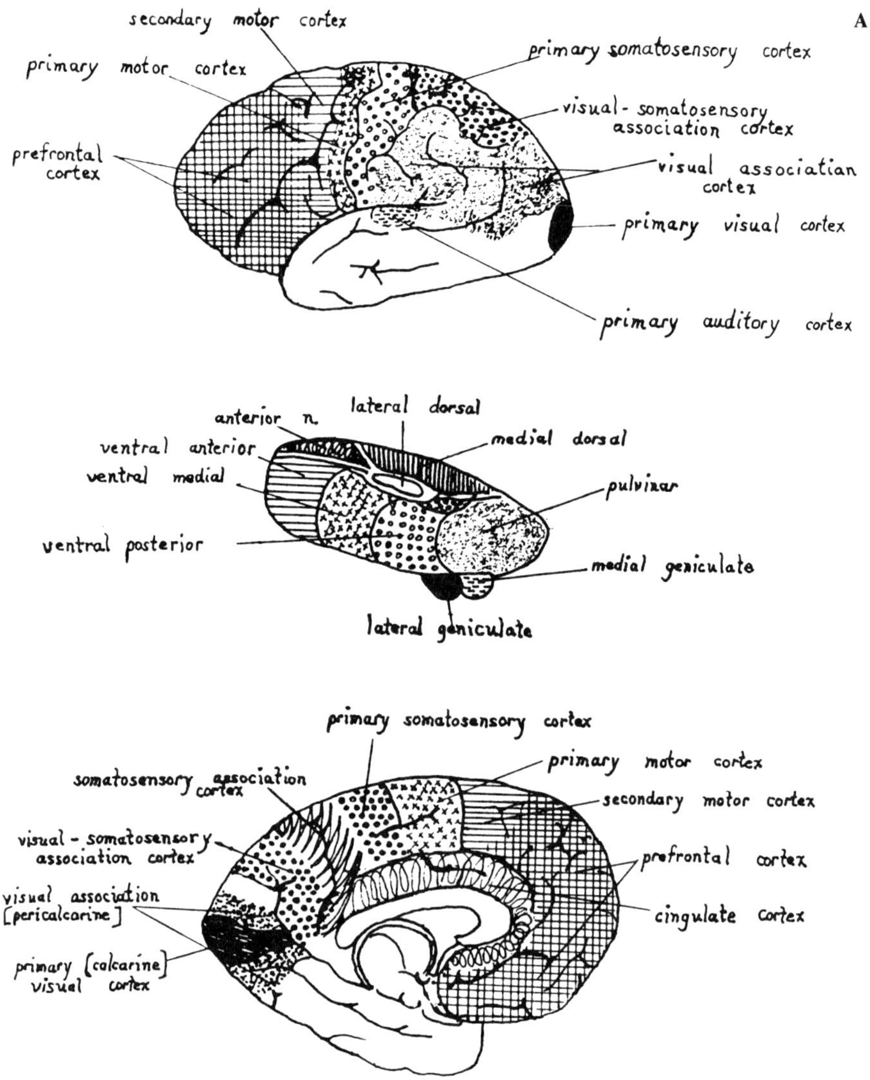

Figure 4-4. **A.** Medial and lateral views of left cerebrum and corresponding areas of the thalamus. Reciprocal connections occur between specific neocortical sites and thalamic nuclei (see Table 4-1). **B.** Thalamocortical local area network, with the reciprocal connections of specific thalamocortical relay neurons (TH-cx) with the thalamic reticular cells (RE). Ch 5 depicts an example of cholinergic projections from the brainstem to the thalamus, with other brainstem cholinergic nuclei contributing substantially. When these inputs are active, as in wakefulness, the RE are inhibited and the TH-cx are depolarized to the level of being sensitive to specific subcortical inputs. During sleep these brainstem cholinergic cell groups are quiescent, leaving the RE relatively depolarized and the TH-cx relatively hyperpolarized, setting up the resonant RE–Th-cx circuit that allows spindling. (Reproduced with permission from Steriade et al, 1990.) *Figure continues on the following page.*

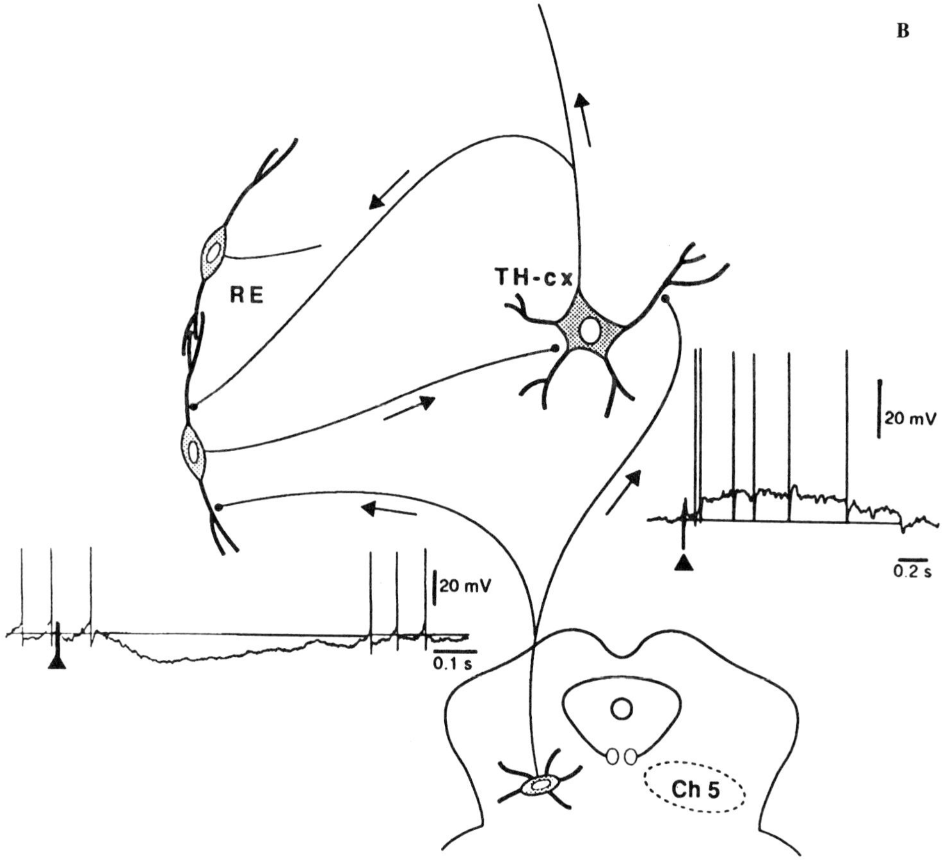

Figure 4-4. *(Continued)*

ability. A good example of the latter type are the voltage-sensitive potassium channels that also cause a relatively sustained hyperpolarization of the membrane. This latter sequence also occurs with action potentials in which an increase in sodium permeability is triggered if the potential at the initial segment of the axon is greater than a certain threshold value. The sodium channels stay open long enough for neighboring channels to be activated by the potential change. With myelinated axons in which membrane capacitance is high, there is less decay of depolarization and consequently greater activation of ionophores further down the axon. In these axons, ionophores are located only at locations devoid of myelin (nodes), with the distance between nodes (internodes) increasing for heavier myelination and consequently a more rapid conduction because there is less potential decay between nodes (Figure 4-1). This is why conduction block occurs with demyelination because potentials decay more rapidly, and therefore little or no activation of ionophores occurs at the next node. After some time the receptors

Table 4-1 Thalamic nuclei with their specific inputs (afferents) and outputs (efferents) with the latter usually neocortex

Nuclei	Afferents	Efferents
Specific		
Anterior	Mammillary body	Cingulate cortex
Ventral anterior	Globus pallidus	Premotor cortex, intralaminar
Ventral lateral	Cerebellar roof nuclei	Motor cortex
Ventral posterior	Medial lemniscus Spinothalamic tract Trigeminothalamic tract	Somesthetic cortex
Medial geniculate	Inferior colliculus	Auditory cortex
Lateral geniculate	Superior colliculus	Visual cortex
Nonspecific		
Intralaminar	Reticular formation	Widespread to cortex
Reticular	Thalamic efferents	Thalamic nuclei, reticular formation
Association		
Mediodorsal	Frontal cortex, amygdala, etc.	Frontal cortex, orbital cortex
Dorsal lateral	Ventral anterior, intralaminar	Parietal cortex
Dorsal posterior	Pulvinar, intralaminar	Parietal cortex
Pulvinar	Colliculi, intralaminar	Parietal, occipital, superior temporal cortex

From Fitzgerald, M. J. T. *Neuranatomy Basic and Applied*. E. Sussex: Baillière and Tindall, 1985.

disperse away from the nodal site, allowing limited signal propagation, but often new myelin forms at these sites with a diminished internodal distance. This facilitates a permanent slowing across this portion of the axon.

There is a wide variation in receptor type depending on the particular group of neurons examined. In neocortex, many different types have been elucidated, with others remaining ambiguous (McCormick, 1992). Glutamate and GABA receptors represent some of the most extensively studied types (Figure 4-5), found in abundance on the pyramidal cells of neocortex, but many others often have subtle effects. For any given pyramidal cell, the local extracellular potential is the result of the spatial and temporal summation of hundreds of EPSPs and IPSPs. The effect of a particular synapse also depends on its location on the cell—distal dendrite, proximal dendrite, cell body, axonal hillock, or distal axon. The latter is an example of an axo-axonal synapse, which is usually $GABA_A$ type (Figure 4-5A) and when active would have the greatest effect of any synapse, resulting in a decreased frequency of action potential firing. The increased chloride permeability produces a relative hyperpolarization and subsequently a decreased calcium influx that limits fusion of synaptic vesicles with the cell membrane. The examples

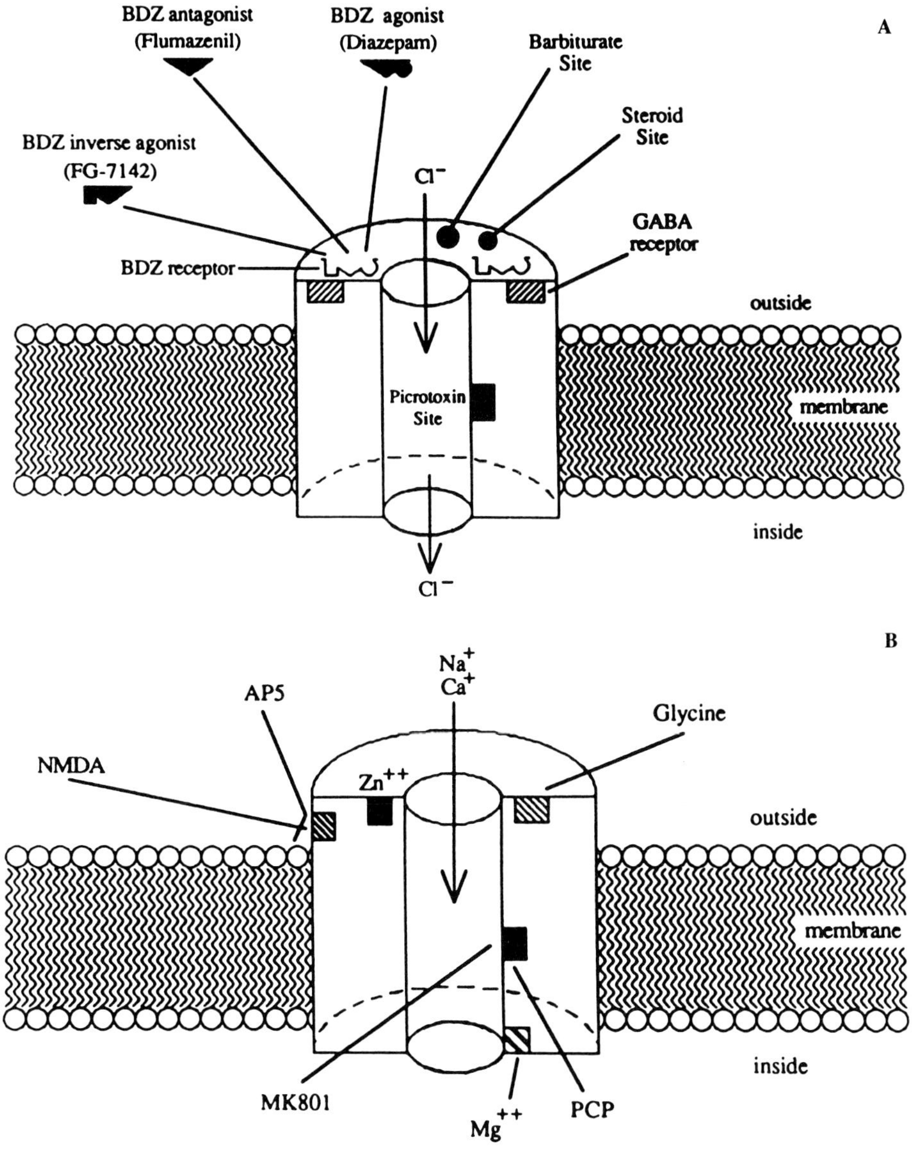

Figure 4-5. Two of the most common receptors in the neocortex. **A.** $GABA_A$ receptor with chloride ionophore, including multiple drug receptor sites. The $GABA_B$ receptor mediates increased potassium conductance or decreased calcium conductance through a second messenger system (see reference for details) and has a more sparse distribution in neocortex. **B.** N-methyl-D-aspartate receptor with the sodium and calcium ionophore shown, which also conducts potassium. Note the binding sites for zinc and magnesium, which are important in the regulation of ion flow as well as the receptor for two drugs, MK801 and phencyclidine ("angel dust"). (Figure and data reproduced with permission from Cooper et al, 1991a [Chapter 7].)

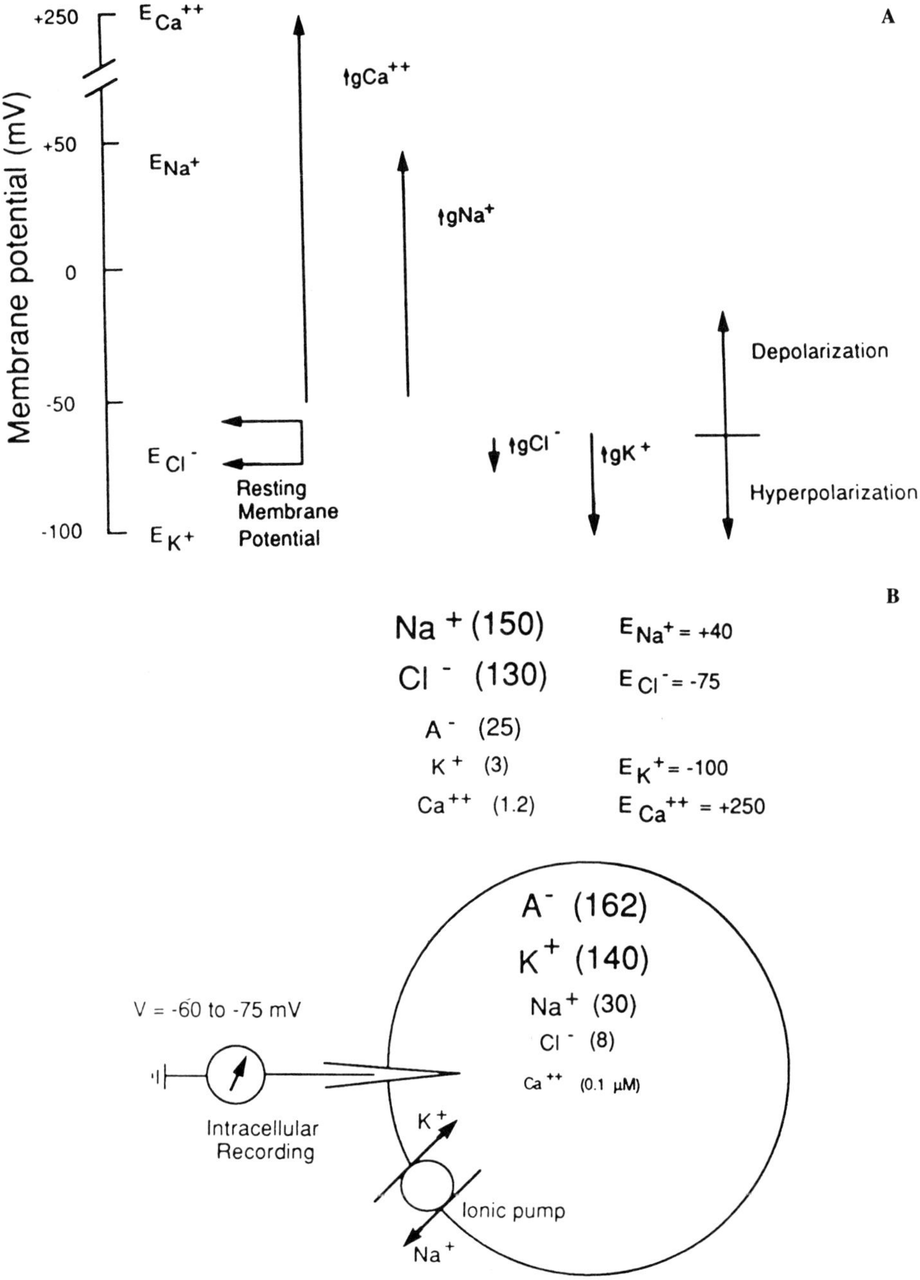

Figure 4-6. **A.** Distribution of ions across neuronal membranes (concentration measured in millimoles) and their equilibrium potentials (expressed in millivolts). At rest the cell membrane is permeable to potassium, sodium, and chloride and shows a voltage difference (inside vs. outside) of approximately -60 to -75 mV, as seen by an intracellular recording

Table 4-2 Neurotransmitters, Receptors and Associated Neuronal Ionic Current Changes

Response	Neurotransmitter	Receptor
$\uparrow I_{Na}, \uparrow I_K$	Glutamate	Quisqualate/Kainate
$\uparrow I_{Na}, \uparrow I_K, \uparrow I_{Ca}$	Glutamate	*N*-Methyl-D-aspartate
	Acetylcholine	Nicotinic
$\uparrow I_{Cl}$	Gamma-aminobutyric acid	$GABA_A$
$\uparrow I_{K,r}$	Acetylcholine	M_2
	Norepinephrine	$Alpha_2$
	Serotonin	$5\text{-}HT_{1A}$
	Gamma-aminobutyric acid	$GABA_B$
	Dopamine	D_2
	Adenosine	A_1
	Somatostatin	
	Enkephalins	mu, delta
$\downarrow I_{AHP}$	Acetylcholine	Muscarinic
	Norepinephrine	$Beta_1$
	Serotonin	(?)
	Histamine	H_2
$\downarrow I_M$	Acetylcholine	Muscarinic
$\downarrow I_{K,l}$	Acetylcholine	Muscarinic
	Norepinephrine	$Alpha_1$
	Serotonin	(?)
$\downarrow I_A$	Norephinephrine	$Alpha_1$
$\downarrow I_{Ca}$	Multiple transmitters	

From McCormick, P.A. Membrane properties and neurotransmitter actions. In: *Synaptic Organization of the Brain*, 3rd ed. G. Shepherd (Ed.). New York: Oxford University Press, 1990.

depicted in Figure 4-3 show two EPSPs arising from different anatomic areas and ending in two specific locations on the cell. The resulting extracellular potential distributions of these two excitatory inputs are of opposite polarity and would produce different signals at the scalp surface, which could be measured if sufficient neurons were "synchronous" (or simultaneously active).

On the spatial scale of scalp EEG, the potential is the result of thousands of simultaneous pyramidal cell discharges. Different spatial patterns of local pyramidal cells may vary, with different inputs producing a unique array of EPSPs

←

electrode. **B.** Effect of increasing membrane conductance (denoted as g) to calcium, sodium, chloride, or potassium. Increases in g-calcium or g-sodium bring the membrane potential toward more positive values (depolarization), whereas increases in g-chloride or g-potassium bring it toward more negative values (hyperpolarization). (Figure and caption reproduced with permission from McCormick, DA. Membrane properties and neurotransmitters. In: *The Synaptic Organization of the Brain*, 3rd ed. (G.M. Shepherd, Ed.). New York: Oxford University Press, 1990 [Chapter 2].)

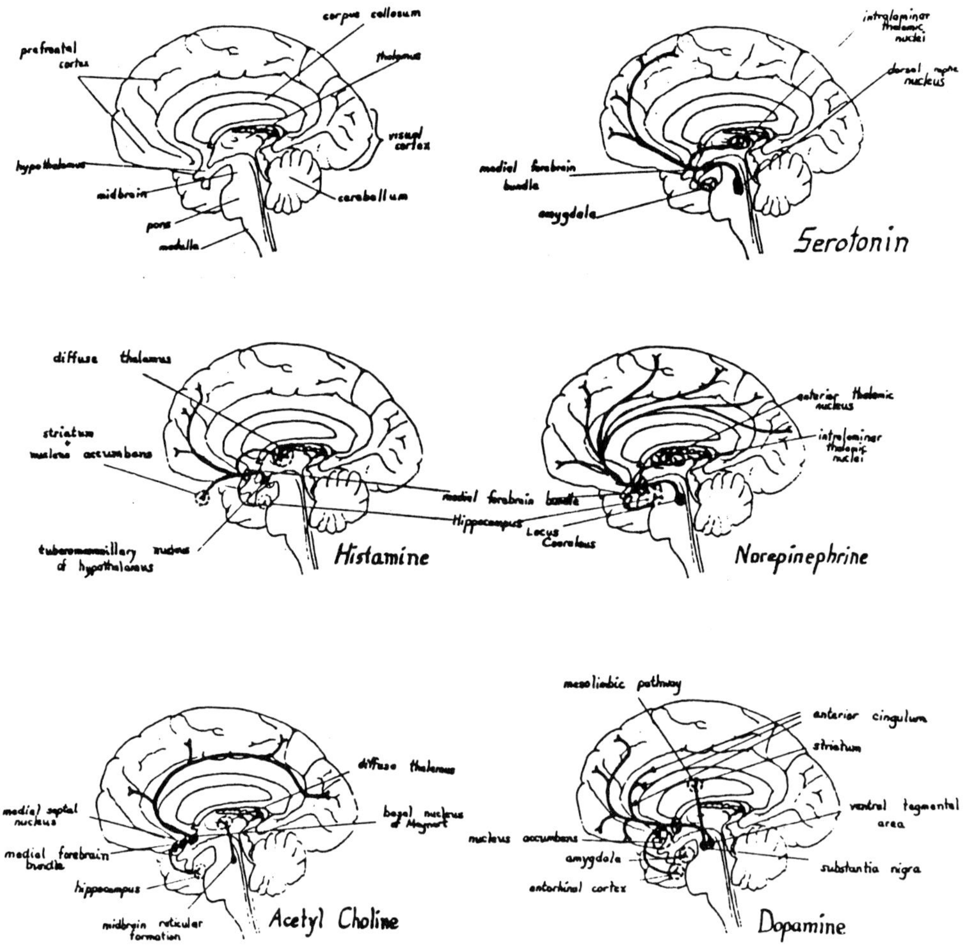

Figure 4-7. Brain diagrams depicting the approximate origins and terminations for five major neurotransmitter systems. Appropriate major anatomic areas are labeled in the first diagram for reference. These systems include brainstem inputs directly to neocortex but also as routed through the thalamus and forebrain structures.

and IPSPs. Despite this, the same scalp potential distribution at a particular instant may be produced from a variety of microscopic spatial patterns of neuronal activity, although different source distributions may produce different time courses of the scalp potential. Several simulation experiments have supported this idea (Nunez et al, 1991, Chapter 1).

Pyramidal cells are also influenced locally through dendrodendritic interactions from other pyramidal cells and at a distance from several brainstem nuclei and the anterior hypothalamus. The latter subcortical structures project to many neocortical pyramidal cells through different pathways providing diffuse, "nonspecific" inputs that collectively determine the "set point" (background state) of individual neurons. This effectively places constraints on which neuronal states are possible. Examples of this might be the bursting or tonic firing mode of a pyramidal cell or subcortical thalamic cortical relay and thalamic reticular cells (Figure 4-4B). The thalamocortical neurons, found in individual thalamic nuclei, represent the primary specific inputs arising from subcortical locations. These inputs are primarily glutaminergic and different regions of cortex tend to have specific thalamic thalamocortical relay cell groups; for example, prefrontal cortex receives input primarily from the dorsal medial thalamic nucleus and primary sensory cortex receives input from the ventral posterior nuclear thalamocortical relay neurons (Figure 4-4).

The origins of normal EEG rhythms (such as alpha rhythm, mu rhythm, and sleep spindles) and pathologic EEG manifestations have been sought since first described by Berger (1929). Our knowledge of the cellular and neurochemical bases of these patterns has advanced substantially. Almost all specific and many nonspecific cortical afferent connections are made through specific cell groups in the thalamus (Figure 4-4; Table 4-1). Diffuse cortical inputs also arise directly from the basilar nucleus of Meynert (cholinergic), locus coeruleus (noradrenergic), dorsal raphe nuclei (serotonergic), and ventral tegmental area (dopaminergic) and from other dopaminergic and cholinergic nuclei (Figure 4-7). Each of these diffuse projectional systems with different neurotransmitters affect particular areas of neurons and change the functional status of those cells. One of the best examples is the increased surround inhibition accompanying increased activity of the locus coeruleus, which increases the signal-to-noise ratio of sensory signals. Other examples of subcortical control of cortical state are discussed in several other chapters of this book. This input may change effective control parameters used in the theoretical studies of Chapters 5, 11, 13 and 14.

The alpha rhythm composes the most common component of the EEG "background." It is present when the participant is relaxed but alert, and is most prominent with the eyes closed. For many years this rhythm was thought to arise from thalamic pacemakers. Different thalamic nuclear groups are influential because they carry essentially all of the specific inputs to the cortex. The balanced influence or nonspecific inputs determines whether neocortical pyramidal cells are sensitive to these specific inputs. The frequency of the "alpha" background may be due primarily to cortical–cortical interactions with certain other well-recognized spatiotemporal patterns, such as sleep spindles arising from a resonant circuit involving the thalamus (Nunez, 1981a, 1981b; Steriade, 1989; Steriade et al, 1990). Work by Lopes da Silva and Storm van Leeuwen (1978) on canine alpha rhythms showed that thalamic input influences intracortical coherence minimally, with pulvinar activity having greater partial coherence with cortical rhythms than the lateral geniculate. This is noteworthy because the latter neural structure is usually thought to provide most specific occipital inputs. Specific thalamocortical relay neurons still have considerable influences on pyramidal cell activity and provide the inputs needed to produce activity such as vertex sharp waves and K complexes, which are believed to be responses to auditory stimuli (Niedermeyer,

1987c). This effect is much different than responses seen during wakefulness, when individual responses usually are not discernible from background EEG.

Sleep spindles and vertex sharp waves occur after a threshold change from loss of brainstem cholinergic inputs to specific thalamic nuclear groups. Spontaneous bursting of thalamic reticular cells takes place with diminution of normally inhibitory cholinergic inputs. This cholinergic activity is normally excitatory to thalamocortical relay cells, which become strongly hyperpolarized especially as a result of the increased GABA release through disinhibited thalamic reticular cells. Cortical projections arise from the thalamocortical cells with no direct projection from thalamic reticular cells, although these latter cells receive afferents from the neocortex. Cells of the anterior thalamic nuclear group that project to the limbic system do not receive inputs from the reticular nucleus. The frequency of reticular cell bursts correlates with the frequency of spindles, noting that the EEG manifestations are relayed through axons of the thalamocortical relay cells (Steriade et al, 1990). Because neurons of the reticular nucleus have influential dendrodendridic synapses, the cell group as a whole is synchronized, producing a similar phenomenon in the specific thalamic nuclear group. Figure 4-7 depicts the origin of specific diffuse projectional systems with their idealized cortical distribution. The details of the relation between developmental anatomy and the evolution of EEG rhythms, that is, in the neonate, are not known.

Measurement of EEG

For many years, analog EEG has been recorded using differential amplifiers and different types of display devices, such as the traditional strip chart recorder. Data recorded in this manner consist of continuous time series of electric potential for multiple channels of EEG displayed simultaneously. Digitization of analog data allows storage on different electronic media and subsequent analysis through computer, including reformatting and remontaging capability. "Montage" is a term used in clinical EEG that describes an optimal arrangement and presentation of input data channels corresponding to different electrode positions. Data may be collected with several montages designed to enhance certain features at specific scalp locations. Using the digital computer, we can view all the data with many enhancements. These may include those techniques that have been used traditionally in medicine and others that have caught on more slowly (such as surface Laplacians). Good discussion on bioelectrodes, amplifiers, and some basic physiology can be found in a recent book on medical instrumentation (Webster, 1992).

Digital EEG machines with 16 to 64 channels are available commercially from many vendors; most models are modestly priced ($20,000 to $100,000). Smaller laboratory computers also allow the convenient recording of evoked potentials. The potential generated in response to a single stimulus has an amplitude that is often 10 to 10,000 times smaller than the amplitude of continuous spontaneous activity. Epochs of EEG following a stimulus are averaged, a procedure which tends to yield activity that is time-locked to the stimulus. This method involves the implicit assumption that the desired evoked signal is uncorrelated to background EEG and that individual responses are stationary in time (show no jitter). Depending on the exact type of response that is sought and the state of the organism, these two assumptions may or may not be reasonable. The number of averages needed for a good final waveform depends on the level of the nervous system being examined. Examples include orders of 1,000 averages for brainstem EPs, 100 for visual EPs, and 10 for ERPs (such as P300). Sometimes the deviation from time stationarity may be an indication of disease and can be useful in diagnosing or tracking very subtle changes of therapy. A good introduction to digital and computer techniques in EEG can be found in Gotman (1990).

The application of spectral analysis in EEG has provided particular insights, and in many instances is the basis for further analyses. Every time an electroencephalographer "reads" a traditional 16- to 21-channel EEG he or she tries to perform a mental spectral analysis on all channels simultaneously. A dedicated microcomputer may be used to perform offline spectral analyses of each channel of EEG collected. Several epochs of EEG are usually averaged and spectra are calculated using a fast Fourier transform algorithm. Isopotential contour plots of scalp activity averaged for specific spectral bands, such as alpha 8 to 12 Hz and delta 0 to 4 Hz, are called "brain maps." Frequency analysis yields data that subsequently can be subjected to other methods for extracting information from the EEG, although such spatial maps are themselves interesting. For example, we use frequency data to calculate spatial coherence patterns, which are crude measures of dynamic interaction between different anatomic regions. Chapters 3, 7, and 8 contain further discussions of spectral analysis and coherence, and some exemplary applications are discussed later in this chapter.

Once scalp EEG has been collected, analyzed spectrally, and subjected to coherency analysis, serious problems with the spatial resolution of the data can still occur. Because of the inhomogeneous nature of the conducting medium, the calvarium, and its adjacent tissues, potentials generated by localized sources may be spread over large areas of the scalp by volume conduction (Nunez, 1981a; Chapter 1). Simply increasing the number of electrodes may be helpful but further transformations may dramatically improve resolution (Gevins, 1990; Nunez and Pilgreen, 1991). The surface Laplacian appears to be one such transformation that is especially robust based on mathematical simulations that are described in Chapter 1. The head inhomogeneities also produce a spatial low pass filter effect that causes loss of signal from the higher temporal frequency components of cerebral electrical signals. A possible physiologic basis for the observed connection between spatial and temporal frequencies is discussed in Chapters 3 and 11. This spatial–temporal filtering may cause a dramatic difference in the appearance of signals recorded from cortical and corresponding scalp locations and subcutaneous or intramuscular sites. Figure 4-8 shows discharging cortical neurons and the corresponding scalp EEG at one site. The high frequencies of the actual spike portion of he single unit activity are lost. These data suggest that much larger areas of synchronous neuronal discharges must occur for spikes to be visible in scalp recordings. In contrast, sinusoidal activity, such as the alpha rhythm or theta

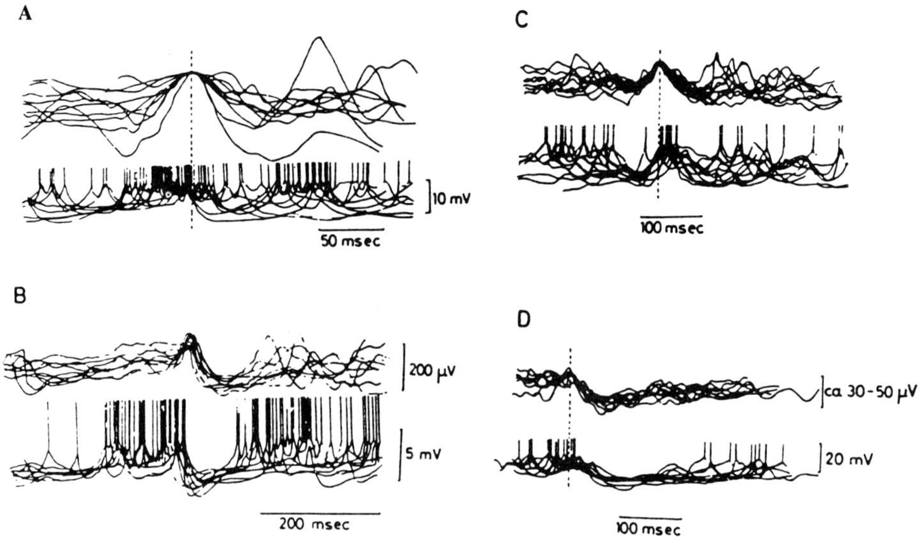

Figure 4-8. Correlation between EEG activity and synaptic events. Superimposed line drawings of EEG waves were collected according to their shape from two experiments (A and B and C and D); the cells were the same in A and B as in C and D, respectively. A and C: Mainly surface-negative waves of symmetrical shape. The surface waves correspond best with summated EPSPs and not with bursts of action potentials. B and D: Negative–positive waves. The surface-positive potential correlates best with synchronized IPSPs. The surface-negative potential corresponds to synchronized EPSPs. Individual synchronized action potentials are not reflected in the EEG. (Reproduced with permission from Creutzfeld, et al. Relations between EEG phenomenon and potentials of single cortical cells. II. Spontaneous and convulsive activity. *Electroencephalogr. Clin. Neurophysiol.* 20:19–37, 1966.)

activity, can be recorded at the scalp because they are synchronous over relatively large cortical areas.

Normal EEG

The EEG of any particular person has considerable temporal and spatial variability that depends on developmental age and physiologic state. "Behavioral state" is often used to describe the state of arousal of an organism (or human). This concept then refers to varied states of consciousness, including the different stages of sleep, but also refers to variation in the state of arousal based on different cognitive tasks that might depend on factors such as level of motivation. A person's affective state (mood) may have particular EEG correlates. As used here, this classification generally refers to personality traits of healthy persons, although pathologic examples exist, such as depressive and manic-depressive (or "bipolar") illnesses.

Combinations of physiologic monitors, such as electromyography (EMG) and electro-oculography (EOG), are used with EEG to determine stage of sleep

(Rechtschaffen and Kales, 1968). Figure 4-9A shows epochs of EEG during the stages of sleep and their associated physiologic attributes, which are also summarized in Table 4-3. This type of recording is a polysomnogram. Active cognitive tasks may show changes in the spontaneous EEG and may correlate with shifts in the peak power of background activity or shifts in coherence patterns. Pathologic conditions and pharmacologic agents may affect evoked or spontaneous EEG, often very selectively. These EEG effects may be caused by changes in specific neurotransmitters or associated receptors of neocortical neurons. Using the terminology of dynamic systems, we can say that EEG changes occur as the result of changes in neocortical control parameters, as discussed in Chapters 3 and 13.

Arousal threshold correlates substantially to different types of stimuli and level of slow wave (synchronous or non-rapid eye movement [REM]) sleep (Williams and Williams, 1966). As slow wave sleep deepens (in the transition from stages 1 to 4), alpha power in the EEG is lost progressively and the percentage of delta activity increases. The qualitative term "synchronous" is often used in EEG to denote the observation that different channels of scalp data do approximately the same thing at the same time, although amplitudes may differ. The coherency function is one quantitative measure of this synchrony and depends on EEG frequency. The presence of dominant delta activity (1 to 4 Hz) is the reason this stage of sleep is called "slow wave sleep." This is the lowest EEG frequency range routinely recorded in healthy persons. Figure 4-9B shows a typical spectral analysis of EEG during the different stages of sleep. As this progression to deeper sleep occurs, the threshold to arousal increases and simultaneously cognitive capability decreases.

During REM sleep, the arousal threshold may fluctuate from being greater than any stage of non-REM sleep to being less than any other stage of sleep. Usually the anterior horn cells (motor neurons) in the spinal cord are hyperpolarized during this stage of sleep. As a result, these neurons become less excitable and muscle tissue receives less input, resulting in the least muscle tone that can be measured in a healthy person not under the influence of pharmacologic agents. At this time, the person is, for all intents and purposes, paralyzed. This state is characterized by almost no chin muscle activity (EMG) in polysomnographic recordings (Figure 4-9). Rapid eye movement sleep is usually a time for continuous dreaming, much of which is related to subconscious activity (which is also probably subcortical, that is, of the limbic system). Thus the person studied could physically perform the content of his dreams but for the paralyzed state.

There is a sleep disorder called "REM behavioral disorder" in which this paralyzing influence appears to be faulty. Persons with this disorder physically act out their dreams and may even become violent (Schenck et al, 1986). Persons with narcolepsy have inescapable sudden onsets of REM sleep but also may have cataplexic attacks in which the physiologic part of REM sleep suddenly occurs and there is paralysis but no sleep. The sudden onset of this loss of muscle tone is often precipitated by an emotional stimulus such as a good joke or sexually explicit material. Patients with cataplexy have EEG and EOG that are characteristic of the awake state during the attack, although there is minimal EMG, as

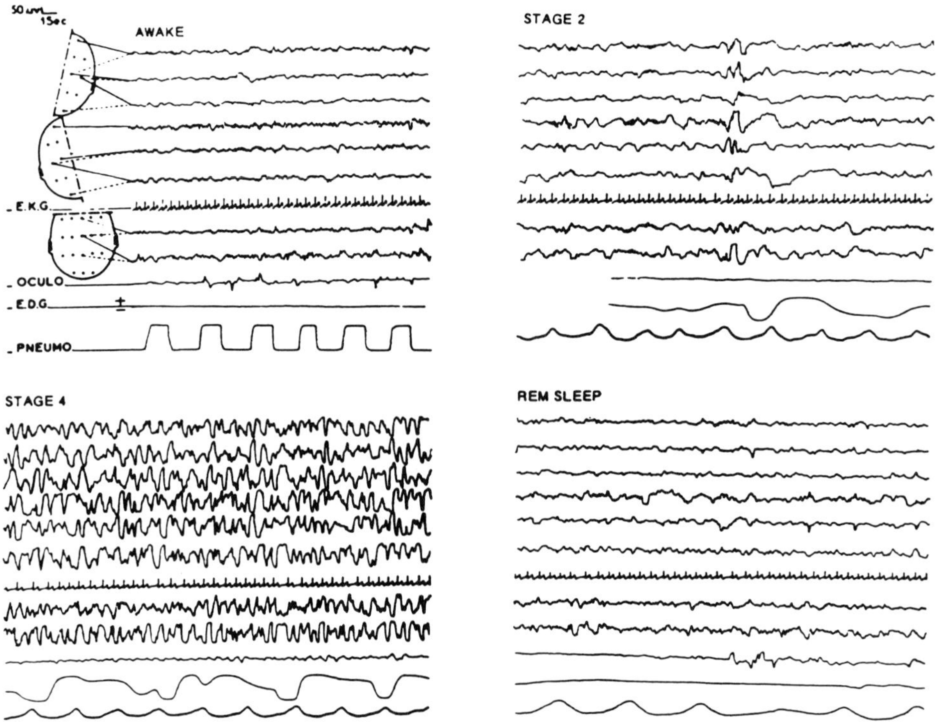
AWAKE
STAGE 2
STAGE 4
REM SLEEP
E.K.G.
OCULO
E.D.G.
PNEUMO

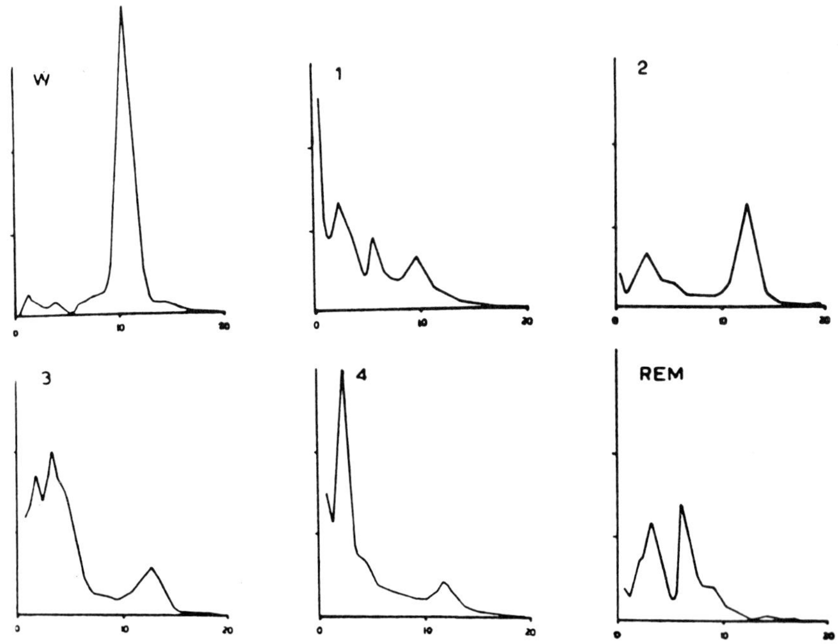
W
1
2
3
4
REM
0
10
20

Table 4.3 Psychological States and Their EEG, Conscious and Behavioral Correlates

Behavioral Continuum	Electroencephalogram Characteristics	State of Awareness	Efficiency
Strong, excited emotion; fear, rage, anxiety	Desynchronized: low to moderate amplitude; fast mixed frequencies	Restricted awareness; divided attention; diffuse, hazy; "confusion"	Poor: lack of control, freezing up, disorganized
Alert attentiveness	Partially synchronized: mainly fast low-amplitude waves	Selective attention, but may vary of shift; "concentration" anticipation; "set"	Good: efficient, selective, quick reactions; organized for serial responses
Relaxed wakefulness	Synchronized: optimal alpha rhythm	Attention wanders—not forced; favors free association	Good: routine reactions and creative thought
Drowsiness	Reduced alpha and occasional low-amplitude slow waves	Borderline partial awareness; imagery and reverie; dreamlike states	Poor: uncoordinated, sporadic, lacking sequential timing
Light sleep	Spindle bursts and slow waves (larger); loss of alphas	Markedly reduced consciousness (loss of consciousness); dream state	Absent
Deep sleep	Large and very slow waves (synchrony but on slow time bases); random irregular patterns	Complete loss of awareness (no memory of stimulation of dreams)	Absent
Coma	Isoelectric to irregular large slow waves	Complete loss of consciousness; little or no response to stimulation; amnesia	Absent
Death	Isoelectric: gradual and permanent disappearance of all electrical activity	Complete loss of awareness as death ensues	Absent

From Lindsley, D.B. Attention, consciousness, sleep and wakefulness. In: *Handbook of Physiology, Section I, Neurophysiology*. Vol. III. (J. Field, Magoun, H.W., and Hall, V.E., Eds.) Washington, DC: American Physiological Society, 1960.

←

Figure 4-9. A. A recording of EEG, eye movement (EOG), muscle activity (EMG), and respirations during four behavioral states. Note the progressive increase of slower frequencies as the person studied progresses to stage IV sleep and the marked similarity between EEG activity and wakefulness. Note the sudden appearance of activity in stage II sleep, which is the beginning of a K complex. B. Power spectra on one channel of EEG in wakefulness and the different stages of sleep. Note the progressive shift toward slower dominant frequencies with the dramatic decrease of activity in the 10-Hz range (background alpha rhythm) from awake to drowsy states (stage I).

occurs during REM sleep. During narcoleptic attacks, the EEG, EMG, and EOG are characteristic of actual REM sleep, dreaming occurs, and a feeling of refreshment is associated with waking. Chin EMG activity is absent during both of these types of attack because of the paralysis. The EEG of persons during REM sleep is desynchronysed and appears much like that for an awake activated person, with beta and theta activity most discernible in the unprocessed time series.

Coherency analysis has also been applied to the analysis of spontaneous EEG during sleep stages. In the study by Banquet (1983), spectral power for the four standard EEG bands plus interhemispheric and intrahemispheric coherency were calculated and further examined by principal components and correspondence analysis. A progressive decrease in interhemispheric coherence with stage of slow-wave sleep and a dramatic increase in interhemispheric coherence with onset of REM was observed. These effects were primarily observed for the delta and beta bands. This decreased coherence during non-REM sleep is not easily explained by a disabled thalamocortical relay system because the long- and short-range associations apparently are the important connections. Intrahemispheric coherence remained relatively low during all stages of non-REM sleep but was relatively high during wakefulness and REM sleep. Coherency during sleep stage IV of healthy persons was diminished to a level similar to that seen in epileptic patients after sectioning of the corpus callosum (the white matter structure connecting the two cerebral hemispheres) (Montplaisir et al, 1990; see Chapter 3). In this stage of sleep, cortical electrical activity appears synchronous when the functional connectedness between different cortical regions, as measured by coherence, is lowest.

Cognitive and Affective States: Spontaneous EEG and ERPs

Spontaneous waking EEG shows variation in spectral and spatial properties, depending on the cognitive load. This may be due in part to an increased level of arousal, which may produce a diffuse desynchronizing effect on much of the cortex. Thus broad-band rhythms occur predominantly because the usual alpha dominance is suppressed. Many studies have been done on the effects of mental tasks on ERPs; these are considered in Chapters 6 and 7. A summary of spontaneous EEG coherency reports can be found in French and Beaumont (1984), who note a large discrepancy between many studies during different tasks in a variety of subject groups. They also found large differences in relative and absolute coherency, depending on the reference location. Several studies have found similar differences between the sexes during a variety of cognitive tasks (Beaumont et al, 1978; Corsi-Cabrera et al, 1989; Flor-Henry and Koles, 1982). Women tend to have a higher EEG interhemispheric coherence than men at rest and for different cognitive tasks. Both sexes tend to have increased right intrahemispheric coherency during spatial tasks, with more variability during verbal tasks. Some studies also found increased left intrahemispheric coherence. These results may imply less hemispheric specialization in women than in men. We would expect the increased intrahemispheric coherency during spatial processing to be lower if this were true. These findings support the simplistic model of the left hemisphere as a sequential processor, in which we would not expect a high intrahemispheric coherency, and a model of the right hemisphere as a global processor, in which we would expect high intrahemispheric coherency associated with parallel processing. This can be explained by recalling that the many neurons simultaneously active for parallel processing produce a measurable scalp potential change, whereas in the sequential mode insufficient neurons would be active at any one time to produce a measurable potential change. Local extracellular electrodes or more spatially resolved surface EEG might show these and other changes, which are difficult to measure.

Specific EEG patterns have been associated with mood and affective state using steady-state evoked potential correlates of intelligence. The frontal lobes tend to show lateralization with left activation for positive and right activation for negative emotional stimuli, the right parietal area also shows some activation, as indicated by loss of alpha power for positive or negative emotional stimulus (Ahern and Schwartz, 1985; Davidson, 1988). Increased neuronal activity in the right parietal area for emotional stimuli is further evidence that this is the anatomic area responsible for the perception and at least partial processing of those stimuli. This has been recognized clinically for some time, and a scheme of emotional processing deficits has been described, called "aprosodia," that parallels the descriptions for aphasia (loss of language function) (Ross, 1981). The extremes of positive and negative emotional states are seen in the affective disorders, specifically bipolar illness and depression.

A study by Robinson (1989) explores the correlates of the frequency following response with intelligence. Participants were stimulated with sine wave modulated light at constant amplitude. The EEG response versus the stimulus frequency is examined as in Figure 4-10. The damping ratio may be estimated by the ratio of peak EEG amplitude to baseline over the entire stimulus frequency range. One, basically assumes the brain functions as a parallel RLC circuit with L and C analogous to equivalent excitatory and inhibitory ensembles, respectively. The natural frequency of the RLC circuit is

$$\omega_0 = 1/\sqrt{LC} \tag{4-1}$$

with damping ratio

$$\zeta = R/2\sqrt{L/C} \tag{4-2}$$

The damping ratio is one half of the standard quality factor, Q_0, which occurs at the natural frequency. In Robinson's paper there are various types of plots, revealing that individuals tend to cluster in specific regions which select for specific values of R, L, and C and show particular values for the natural frequency and damping ratio. These values reveal that high IQ tends to cluster in two regions, those with high natural frequencies which may reflect speed of information transfer and another group with lower values of natural frequency. This latter group has intermediate values of the damping ratio and termed "middling arousability." This

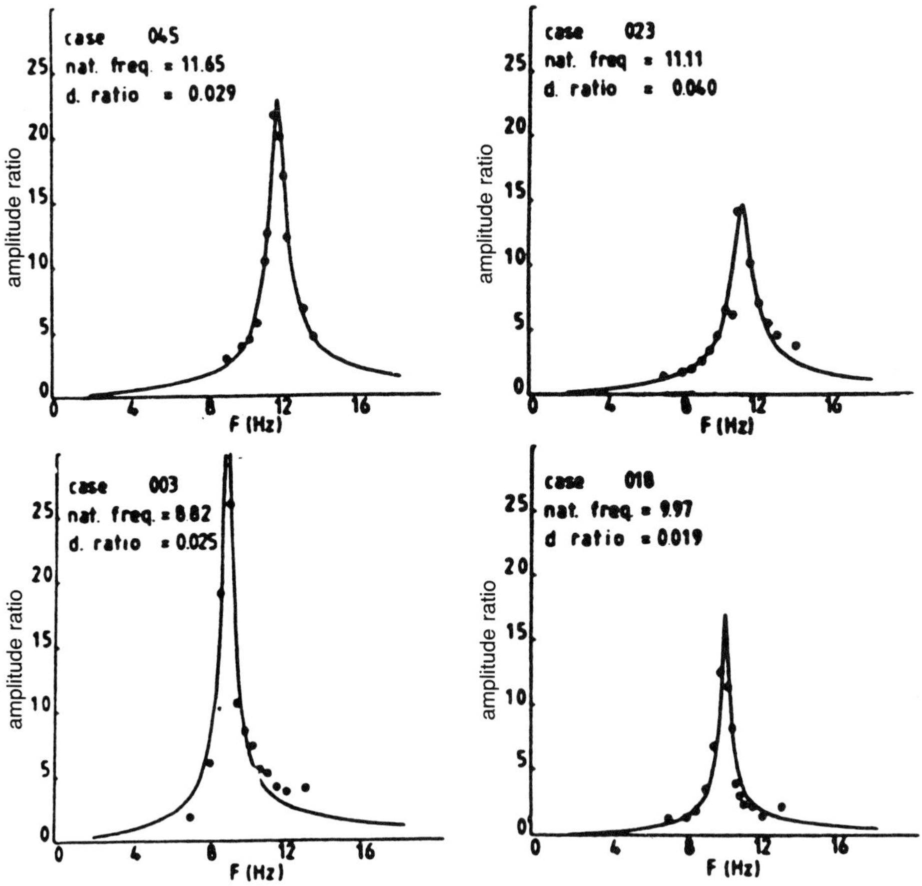

Figure 4-10. Amplitude ratios collected from a single channel of EEG at midline parietal position, whereas a dark-adapted participant is stimulated by specific frequencies of sine wave-modulated light. This curve is similar to that seen for a filter with a particular resonant frequency. (Reproduced with permission from Robinson, 1989.)

appears to reflect a system sensitive enough to detect signals of significance, both internal and external, but to not be easily saturated.

The presence of increased power of higher frequency components of visual evoked potential spectra has been reported to correlate with higher IQ scores (Flinn et al, 1977) and may relate to the higher natural frequencies described by Robinson (1989). Other investigations have been ongoing, with sine wave photic driving in the "background" while the participant is simultaneously presented with other stimuli in the same or different sensory domain, as discussed in Chapter 6.

Event-related potential research has been popular during the past 25 years. Specifically the "P300" has been the subject of many articles. These endogenous potentials are most often obtained using the "odd-ball paradigm," with potential data collected from 1 to 128 sites on the scalp using a variety of references. The P300 peak has been reported to arise from several locations, particularly the dorsomedial nucleus of thalamus, hippocampus, temporal neocortex, and prefrontal neocortex (Nunez and Pilgreen, 1991; Okada et al, 1983; Smith et al, 1990). It has been correlated with many psychophysiologic variables, including stimulus evaluation time, movement readiness, and stimulus updating. Its dependence on endogenous state and stimulus characteristics are varied and include stimulus frequency (especially spatial frequency for visual or temporal frequency for auditory stimuli), percentage of rare tones presented to the subject, novelty of rare tones, sequence of tones, regardless of whether motor responses are required,

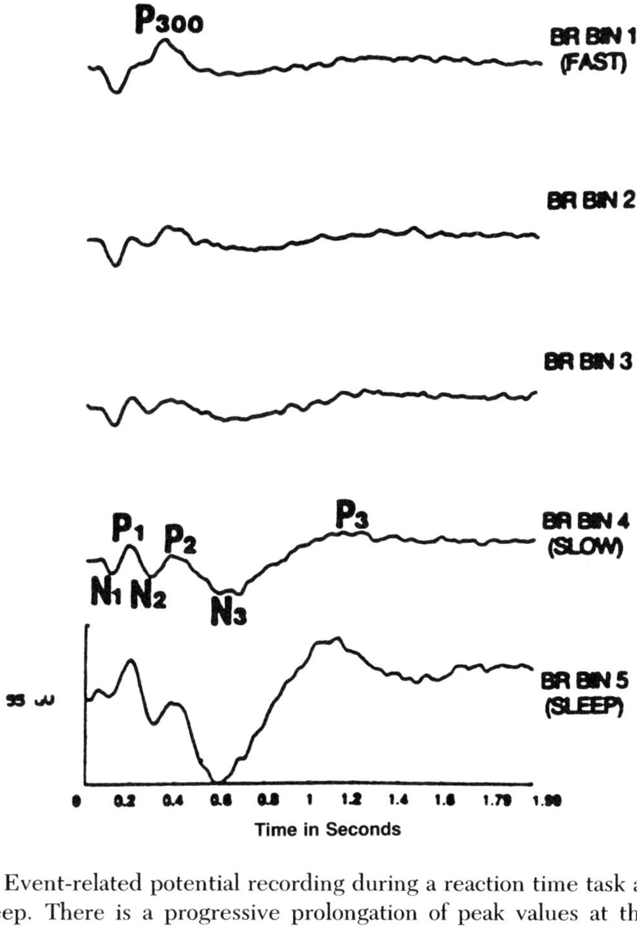

Figure 4-11. Event-related potential recording during a reaction time task as the participant falls asleep. There is a progressive prolongation of peak values at that time that correlates with loss of cognitive capacity. The BR BIN refer to different epochs of EEG data averaged for a specific range of reaction times. BIN 5 indicates no reaction. (Reproduced with permission from Ogilvie et al, 1991.)

and even the subject's level of motivation (Begleiter et al, 1983; Goodin et al, 1983; Pfefferbaum et al, 1983; Polich, 1986; Polich and Donchin, 1988).

Some studies have implied that novel stimuli occurring early in the sequence elicit more prefrontal sources, whereas the average of 10 or more poststimulus epochs usually show a central midline to parietal midline maximum (Knight, 1984; Wood and Wolpaw, 1982). Based on neocortical dynamics, this might be viewed as the high-level control processes of the frontal lobes that occur as a person acclimates to a new stimulus; later processing of the same or a very similar stimulus may be processed primarily in the parietal lobes. Many standard odd-ball stimuli may not be sufficiently "novel" to elicit this effect. Intracranial recordings of P300s during monitoring for possible epilepsy surgery have shown very active sources in the inferior parietal lobes and hippocampi during odd-ball experiments (Smith et al, 1990). These brain structures are intricately connected and related to learning and memory functions (Mesulam, 1985). Event-related potentials have broad use in behavioral research, with evidence of large amplitude changes at sleep onset (Ogilvie et al, 1991). Figure 4-11 shows ERP tracings obtained from an average over subjects, with behavioral state ranging from wakefulness to sleep onset. The results of a reaction time task reveal an increasing response latency as level of consciousness decreases (BIN 1-4) and no response (BIN 5) at sleep onset. Also in this study, FFTs were performed on 3 seconds of prestimulus EEG and showed a successive increase in power for theta and delta and simultaneous decreases in beta and alpha power. The significant change in delta occurred simultaneously with BIN 5. Thus many and varied neurophysiologic tools are available to analyze brain states that vary with respect to level of consciousness and other physiologic control parameters that may change across these states.

Developmental Perspectives—EEG From Prematurity to Senescence

Electroencephalographic rhythms show dynamic changes in many perspectives, especially for developmental. The most dramatic changes occur during the first few weeks of life, especially in premature neonates. Only in the last 10 to 15 years have enough of these infants survived to allow systematic studies to be performed. Of course, we should question the normalcy of infants this age, especially when an EEG has been requested, which implies that signs of some disorder have been noted. Only after an infant achieves appropriate developmental milestones and the EEG evolves into a clearly recognizable "normal" state can the proper correlations be made between brain state and the EEG. A succinct review of EEG ontogeny can be found in Niedermeyer (1987b).

The EEG evolves from a state of disorganization, "discontinuity," and incoherence toward a more organized, continuous, and coherent form. In this context, the term discontinuity refers to an EEG pattern of very low-amplitude periods lasting from 1 to several seconds interrupted by high-amplitude complex activity. It is useful to define the age of a neonate in terms of conceptual age (CA), the age measured in weeks from conception. Conceptual age correlates best with the

EEG and allows for a uniform comparison between premature and full-term neonates. Very premature infants (less than 28 weeks) have very undifferentiated EEGs, showing a burst–suppression pattern that does not vary between wakefulness and sleep and may be considered the extreme case of discontinuity. Periods of undetectable scalp potential lasting as long as 2 to 3 minutes and interrupted by high-voltage sharp and slow waves may be observed. Electroencephalographic activity such as this would be considered very abnormal in any other age group. Neonates who are 28 to 31 weeks from conception continue to have no differentiation of states of consciousness, but less discontinuity occurs, with new waveforms appearing like "ripples of prematurity," also called "delta brushes" because of the fast activity (16 Hz) superimposed on a delta (less than 0.5 Hz) oscillation (Lombroso, 1987). The delta brush is one of the hallmarks of a normally developing EEG and usually persists into the 40th week. Diffuse, relatively low-amplitude delta activity (usually less than 1 Hz) can be observed at this time. Differentiation between wakefulness, active sleep (REM), and quiet sleep (non-REM) begins between 32 and 35 weeks from conception. Wakefulness and active sleep EEG are very similar, with waves consisting of diffuse delta activity and occasional bursts of faster superimposed frequencies, but REM shows the usual eye movements characteristic of adult REM. Neonates of this age have a very poorly developed EOG because the retinal potentials have not yet developed, but eye movements may be observed easily by visual inspection. The quiet sleep state (non-REM) is particularly striking in these neonates, in whom bursts of high-amplitude and intermixed spike activity appear on a background of fairly marked amplitude suppression. Full-term neonates tend to spend about 60% of their time in active (REM) sleep, with the percentage of REM (that is, "REM density") diminishing throughout the rest of their lives.

Changes that usually take place in EEG patterns during the rest of the life of humans is minimal compared with what occurs until that time. The neonatal patterns described above usually disappear by 6 weeks from birth in a full-term infant. A posterior rhythm of approximately 4 Hz develops in the first 3 months, which accentuates with eye closure, and is believed to be the precursor to the alpha rhythm (Niedermeyer, 1987b). As the child ages, delta activity gradually disappears, although it may accentuate at some time in development perhaps because of dysynchrony between the development of the cortex and other grey matter. The occasional frontotemporal spikes and sharp waves disappear from the normal record. The frequency of the dominant background (or alpha) rhythm gradually increases until it attains its maximum value at about age 10 years, with a mean frequency of 10 Hz. Some fairly prominent 8-Hz activity is usually present by age 2 years. Slow activity gradually decreases until ages 25 to 30 years, when the "normal" adult EEG pattern is established. This age coincides with the final state of myelination (Courchesne, 1990). The implications of this anatomic and electrophysiologic data for EEG theories are considered in Chapters 2, 3, 11, and 12.

The normal EEG pattern persists into senescence (more than 70 years old), when episodic theta and delta activity may be seen in the temporal electrodes,

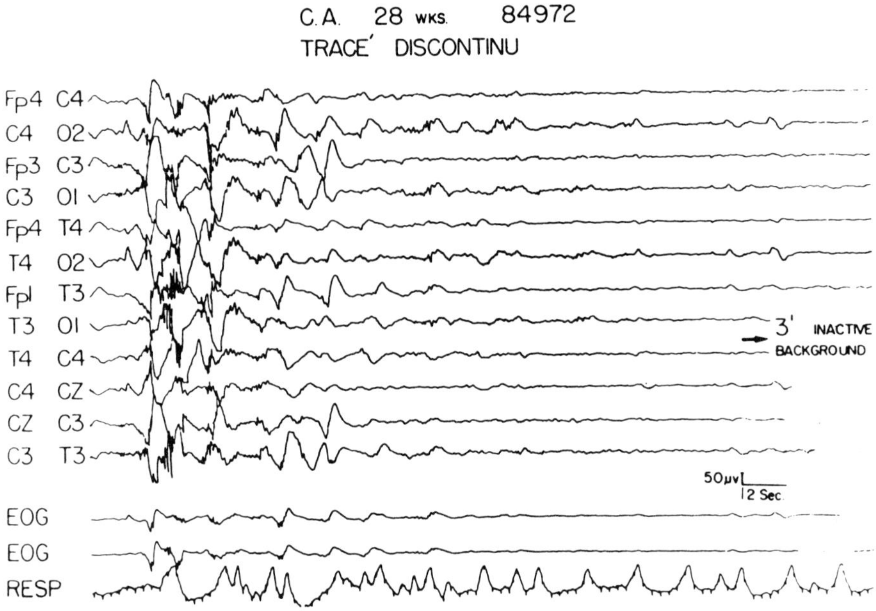

A

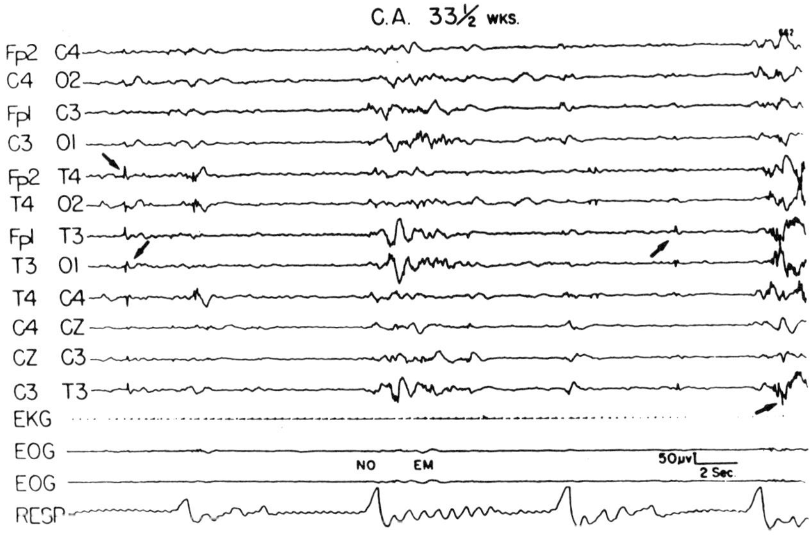

B

Figure 4-12. Development of EEG from prematurity to adulthood. **A.** Extreme case of tracé discontinu in 28-week-old neonate showing a period of very inactive background that lasts for approximately 3 minutes. There is relatively little differentiation among behavioral states at this point. **B.** Same child as in figure A but at 33.5 weeks, with shorter periods of relative inactivity. Spike discharges (normal at this age) are indicated by arrows.

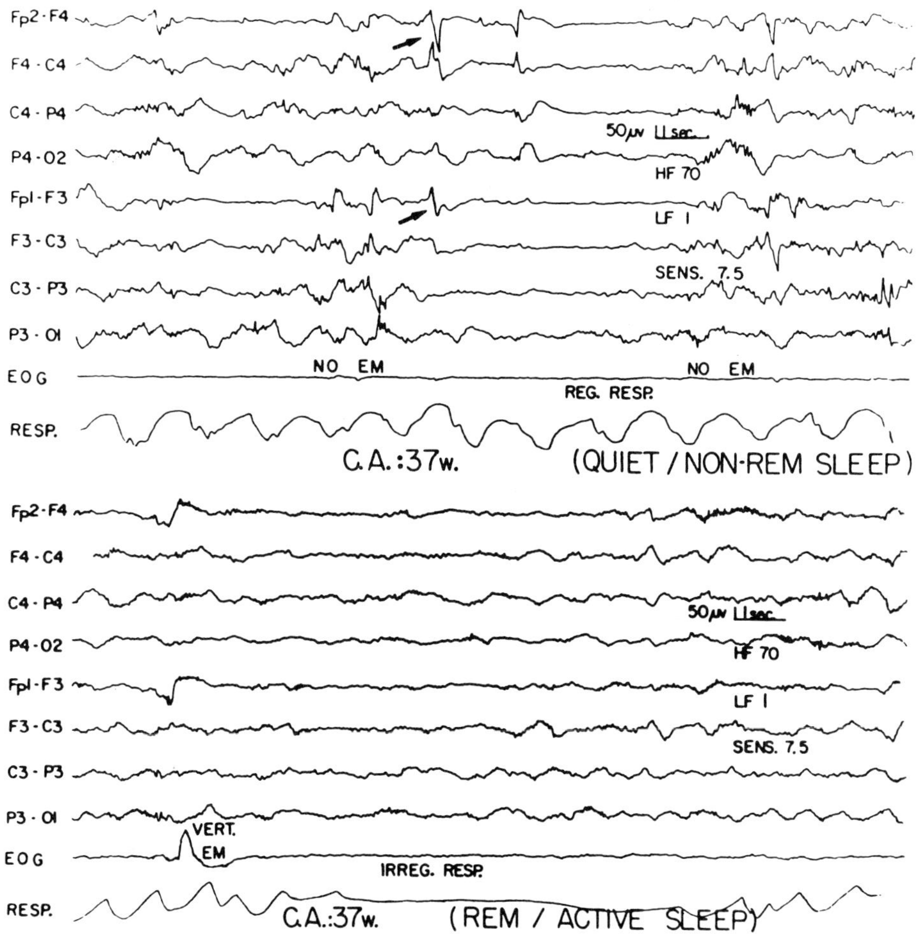

C

Figure 4-12. (*Continued*)

C. EEG of same infant as in figures A and B, now at 37 weeks, almost at full-term conceptual age, during well-differentiated behavioral states. Active (REM) sleep appears much as wakefulness and quiet (non-REM) sleep. Note the sharp discharges (normal) in the frontal regions, F3 and F4 (arrows). **D.** Two EEG tracings during light non-REM sleep, 10 months above showing typical pattern of spindles, and so on, and 9 months below showing more primitive pattern of spindles, which are dysnchronous between the two hemispheres. **E.** Three-year-old child during drowsiness with the very characteristic "hypnogogic hypersynchrony," consisting of high-amplitude rhythmic theta activity. **F.** 13-year-old during wakefulness, with well-developed alpha rhythm, mu rhythm (which disappears during clenched fist), and typical eye movement artifacts seen in the frontal leads. Although not very apparent in the figure, continued theta activity is superimposed on the alpha in the posterior channels. **G.** Typical adult pattern during wakefulness. (All figures reproduced with permission from Niedermeyer and Lopes da Silva, 1993.) *Figure continued on following page.*

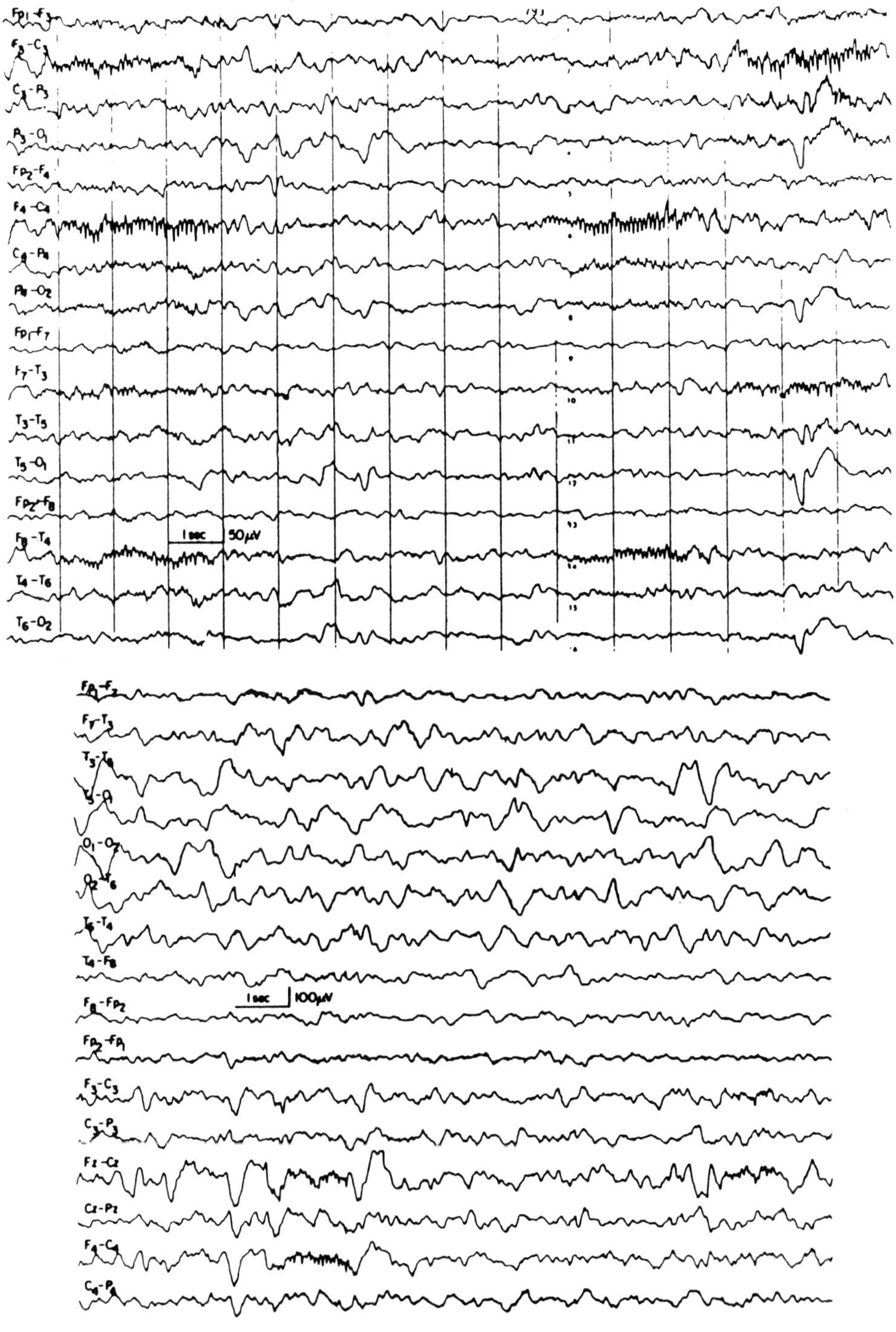

D

Figure 4-12. (*Continued*)

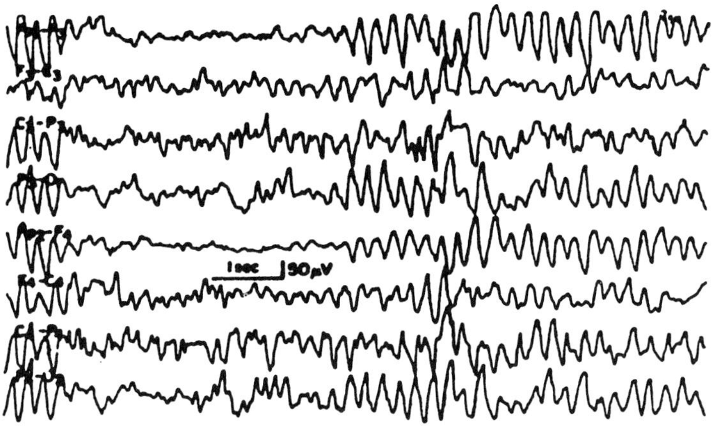

E

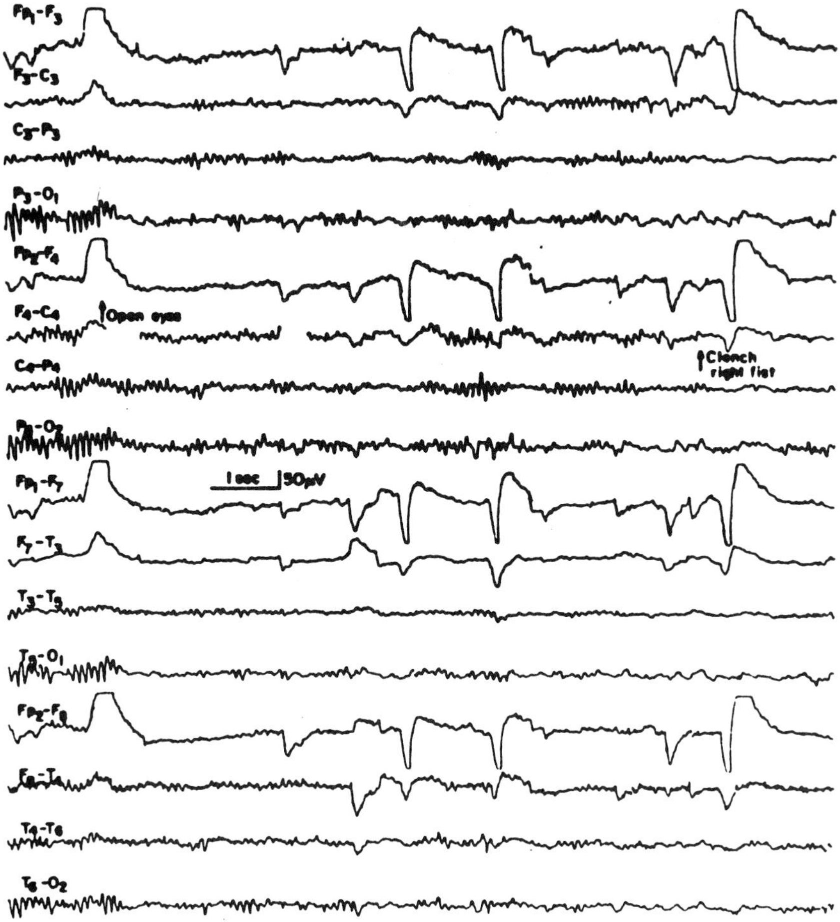

F

Figure 4-12. (*Continued*)

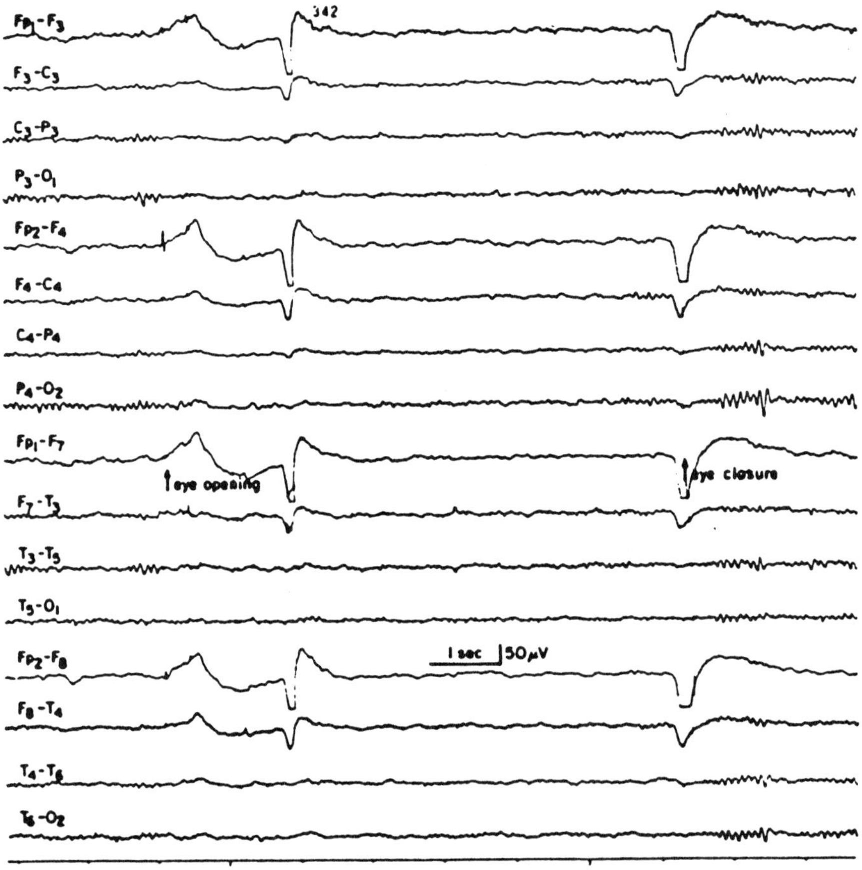

G

Figure 4-12. *(Continued)*

primarily on the left side, and is considered normal as long as it is present in less than 20% of the record and is accompanied by a normal background alpha rhythm. Figure 4-12 illustrates representative EEGs from different ages, ranging from prematurity to adulthood. Many special EEG patterns are observed in a small percentage of persons. Such patterns may be labeled normal or abnormal, depending on how closely they correlate with distinct clinical states. Table 4-4 chronicles that development of EEG using a logarithmically compressed time scale.

Use of spectral analysis has added new dimensions in EEG behavioral correlates. Interesting investigations have been performed in hemispheric activation and personality features of children and adults. We can predict which infants will cry in response to maternal separation based on which cerebral hemisphere is the most "activated," as measured by diminished alpha and slower EEG frequencies (Davidson and Fox, 1989). In the preseparation phase, infants who cry appear to have a relative activation of the right frontal lobe, with a trend toward left parietal activation that does not reach statistical significance. Infants who do not cry have relatively left frontal activation and no asymmetry of EEG power in the parietal recording sites in the preseparation phase. Figure 4-13 shows this using a histogram of the log of the relative power recorded from homologous locations in the frontal (F3, F4) and parietal (P3, P4) lobes.

A similar response has been observed with "stranger anxiety" (that is, crying when a stranger approaches) with EEG recorded in the baseline state. Infants

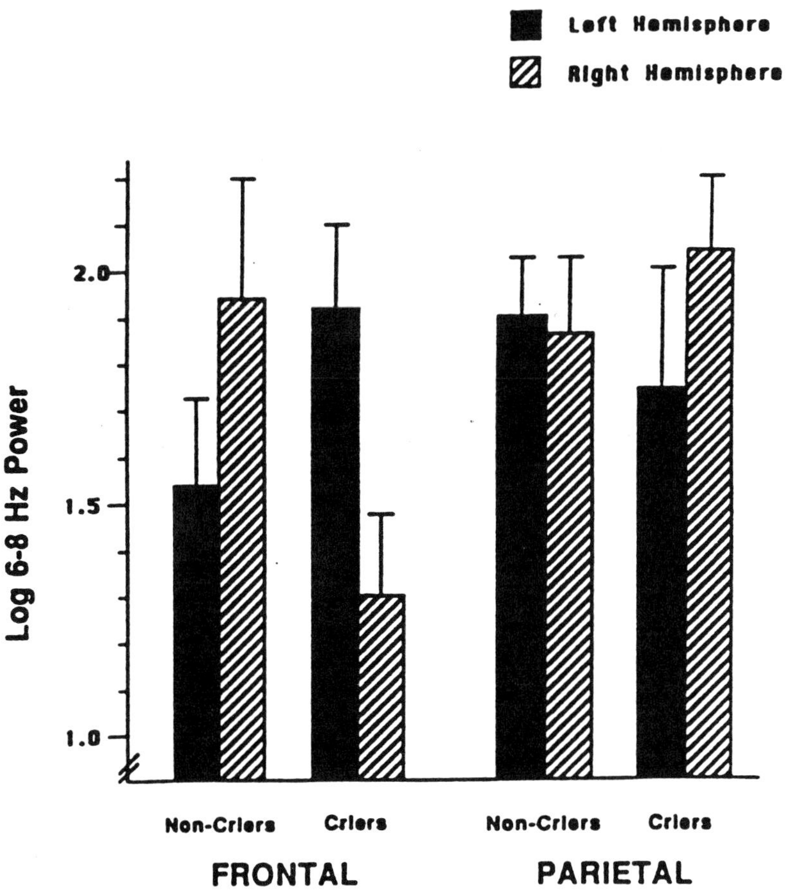

Figure 4-13. Histogram of log 6 to 8-Hz power for homologous (right and left) regions of the frontal and parietal areas for 10-month-old infants during quiet wakefulness. Infants who responded to maternal separation by crying and not crying are shown. Infants who do not cry have less left frontal activity and those who do cry have less right frontal activity, implying relative "activation" of those respective regions. (Reproduced with permission from Ahern and Schwartz, 1985.)

Table 4.4A Development of EEG Patterns in Premature and Full-term Infants

Chronologic age					0	4 weeks
Conceptional age	24	28	32	36	40	44 weeks
Awake				Pattern 3 Diffuse low voltage irregular activity →	Pattern 3 ('active moyenne') Diffuse low-voltage irregular theta and delta	
Active sleep (later REM sleep) 1. Irregular breathing 2. Frequent eye and limb movements 3. No tonic neck EMG			Pattern 2 Continuous slow waves 1 to 2 Hz	Continuous theta and delta →	Pattern 2 Mixed low-voltage irregular and 2 to 4-Hz slow waves	

Table 4.4A Development of EEG Patterns in Premature and Full-term Infants *(Continued)*

Chronologic Age				0 — 4 weeks
Conceptional age	24	28 — 32 — 36		40 — 44 weeks
Quiet sleep (later non-REM sleep) 1. Regular breathing 2. No eye and limb movement 3. Tonic neck EMG	Pattern 1 ('Discontinuous') a. Bursts ≤ 20 sec, delta ≥ theta ≥ alpha	1 to 2 sec / 4 to 6 Hz →	1 to 2 Hz →	Pattern 1 ('trace alternant') a. Bursts of 4 to 5 seconds 1 to 3 Hz
	b. Pauses: No activity ≤ 3 min	→	Shorter pauses low voltage may apear →	b. Low-voltage activity, 4 to 5 seconds
				Pattern 4 Continuous high-amplitude slow waves
			Frontal sharp transients and sporadic spikes	
		Delta brushes 10 to 20 Hz on 0.3 to 1 Hz		

EMG = electromyelogram; REM = rapid eye movement.

Table 4.4B The EEG from the Age of 1 Month to Adult Age

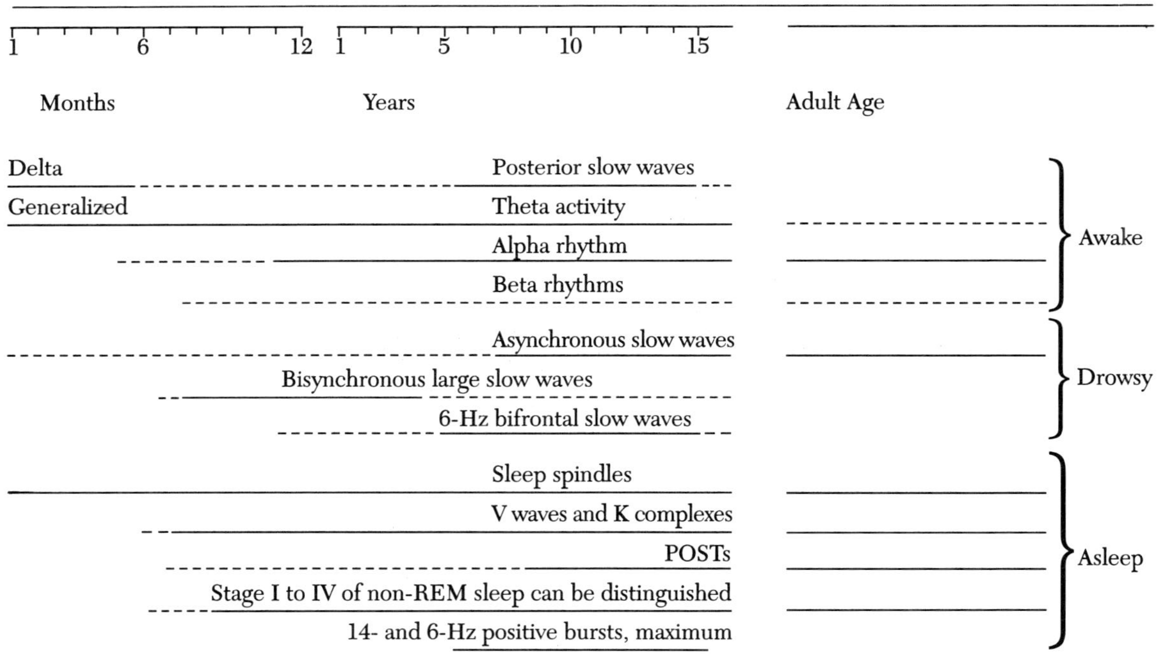

POST = Posterior occipital sharp transfer of sleep.
From Spehlmann, R. *EEG Primer.* Amsterdam: Elsevier, 1981.

who cried in response to an approaching stranger had relative right frontal activation (Davidson and Fox, 1989). The same authors (Fox and Davidson, 1986) completed a similar study earlier in which they examined infant facial response and spectral EEG in response to several tastes. That work suggested a relation between decreased power in the 3- to 6-Hz and 6- to 12-Hz bands in the left hemisphere and "interest" with sucrose water, along with a connection between the same EEG effects in right hemisphere and "disgust" with plain water. This effect was seen in the frontal and parietal regions of this group using methods that are different from the other paradigms. There were also some inconsistencies with this latter experiment; for example, the citric acid solution produced facial signs of "disgust" but no substantial asymmetry in EEG power. They concluded that in these 2- to 3-day-old full-term neonates, dysmaturity of this relatively "higher" cortical function is present much as poor correlation between sleep behavior and the EEG occurs in premature neonates.

Continued studies correlating EEG and emotional states in early development are important in medicine, because they may provide insight into anatomic functional correlations with respect to specific behaviors and could change some of our approaches to preschool and classroom settings. For instance, we could begin with a large cohort of children, follow them for a long period of time (such as 10 to 15 years), and collect EEG obtained according to specific emotional and cognitive paradigms. Standardized test scores and overall behavioral ratings would be performed concomitantly and correlated with different EEG measures. This procedure would provide ongoing correlates at particular stages of development. Participant dropout would then have little effect on statistical validity. Protocols similar to this are underway at some locations (Valdés et al, 1992).

Pharmacologic Effects on Brain State and EEG

Many pharmacologic agents have important effects on brain state, with many of these also producing consistent effects on EEG. Neurophysiologic effects may be manifest in the spontaneous EEG and evoked potentials, either of which may require intricate experimental paradigms combined with extensive post hoc analysis to show a pharmacologic effect. Many drugs cause drowsiness, a result that may be expected to produce EEG changes indicative of that physiologic state, including the different stages of sleep. Some experimental medications are studied using EPs, such as studies of P300 amplitude and latency correlates of cognitive change. Many of these changes are due to the interactions of neurotransmitters at a specific brain receptor site and anatomic location. The selectivity of most of these interactions is not well understood, and thus the mechanisms of most drugs that affect the neocortex and other brain structures are unknown (Gilman et al, 1990). Although we may understand which types of receptors are activated by different chemical agents, with many of these agents affecting many types of receptors, the importance of each interaction typically is not understood. Further discussion of this topic is provided in Chapter 13.

Despite our ignorance of detailed pharmacologic mechanisms, EEG effects of many of these agents can be generalized to a surprising degree. Spontaneous EEG generally stabilizes with pharmacologic influence, that is, less temporal variability of component waveforms occurs. The same drug also may stabilize certain arousal states and inhibit the transition to others. The EEG effects of some chemical agents were elaborated by Stumpf and Gogolak (1987). They provide a general summary of EEG observations. Overall, centrally acting agents may synchronize the EEG, desynchronize the EEG, or produce epileptiform changes (such as interictal spikes). Generally slower frequencies increase and faster frequencies decrease with synchronization. This state is commonly called "de-activation" in the medical literature. Desynchronization is accompanied by an increase of faster frequencies. Convulsants tend to produce spikes, sharp waves, spike and wave, and focal seizures and are thought to represent a distinct class of agents active in the central nervous system. We will discuss several chemical agents to illustrate the spectrum of effects on EEG and behavioral state.

A host of chemical agents produce excessive amounts of beta activity in the EEG. All of these drugs are sedatives/hypnotics. Barbiturates such as phenobarbital and benzodiazepines such as diazepam (Valium) are the most common examples that produce this effect. Drugs may have different effects on the EEG, depending on whether doses are therapeutic or toxic. This is especially true for barbiturates because very high doses produce an isoelectric EEG that is reversible as long as hypoxic brain damage due to respiratory suppression has not occurred. Of course, a continuum exists between the production of excessively high-amplitude beta activity and electrocerebral silence. As the dose of a barbiturate is increased, the background frequency may diminish and superimposed slower frequencies in the theta and delta range may appear until finally no normal rhythms remain. At some point the amplitude of these slower frequencies will begin to diminish until the onset of burst suppression, for which periods of absent EEG are separated by bursts of delta activity and finally electrocerebral silence. Figure 4-14 shows some of these early changes in the EEG during general anesthesia induction using thiopental (a very short-acting barbiturate that can be regulated precisely). Benzodiazepines do not appear to be able to suppress the EEG to this extent. The primary effect of both barbiturates and benzodiazepines appears to be at the level of the inhibitory chloride ionophore, each with its own specific binding site on the GABA receptor. The specific actions of GABA were discussed previously. Benzodiazepine receptor stimulation produces an increased frequency of inophore opening, and barbiturates prolong the length of time it stays open, both resulting in an increased chloride current (MacDonald, 1989). Spindle-like activity ranging from 15 to 30 Hz, depending on how long patients have been taking the drug, is seen primarily in the frontal regions but also spreading to the entire neocortex (Bauer, 1987). Drug-induced spindles tend to have a wide spatial distribution and increased persistence when compared with sleep spindles, which tend to be more confined to frontocentral neocortex. The effects of GABA augmentation, however, occur over the entire neocortex because the affected interneurons always occur in local circuits with pyramidal cells.

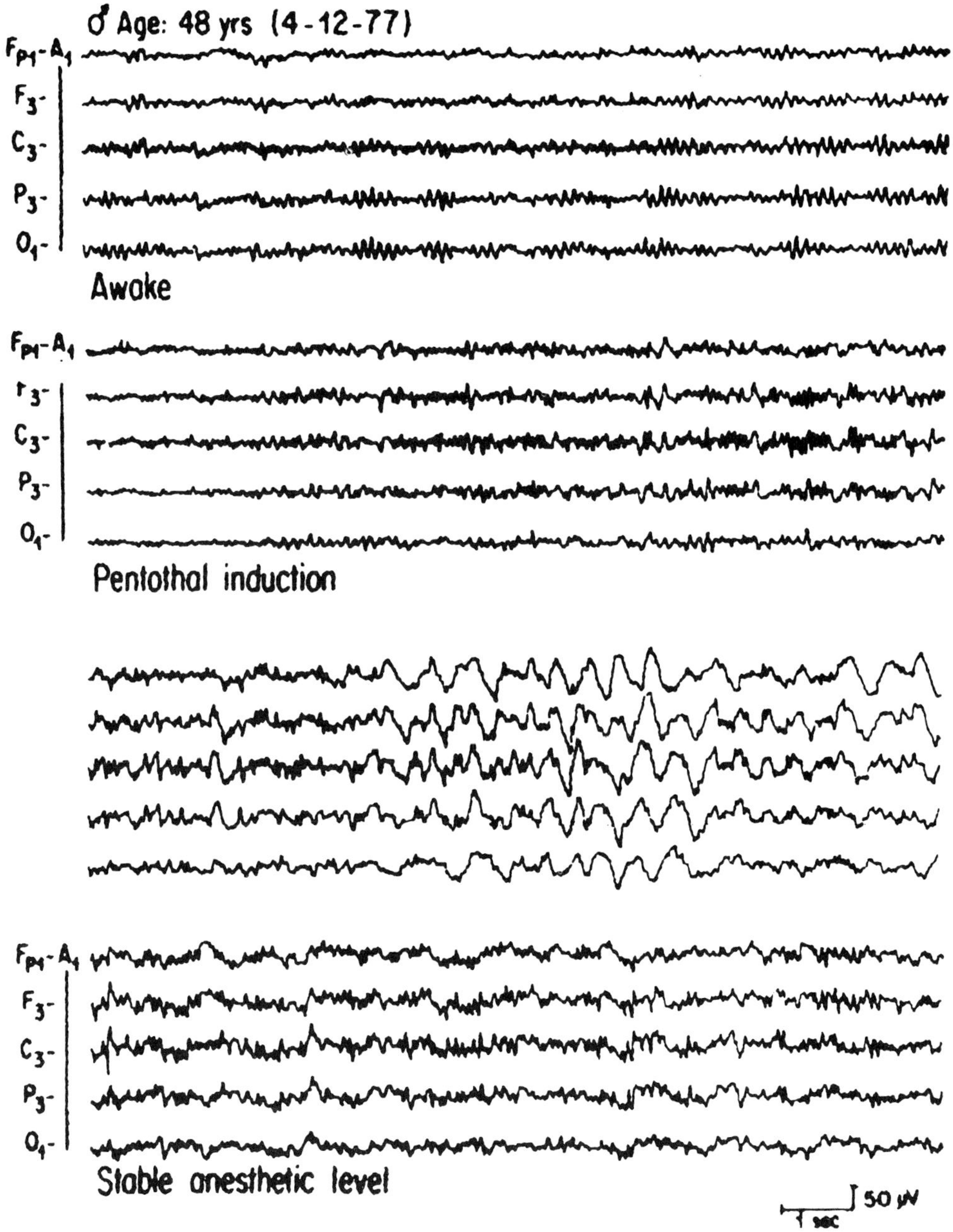

Figure 4-14. General anesthesia induction using thiopentol, a short acting barbiturate. Higher concentrations would result in a burst suppression pattern and finally at very high concentrations, no cerebral electrical activity. (Reproduced with permission from Sharbrough, F.W. Nonspecific abnormal eeg patterns. In: *Electroencephalography: Basic Principles, Clinical Applications, and Related Fields*, 3rd edition. (E. Niedermeyer and F. Lopes da Silva, eds.). Baltimore: Williams and Wilkins, 1993 [chapter 13].)

The presence of excess slow activity in the EEG has long been correlated with brain dysfunction. When it occurs focally (that is, confined to a specific neocortical location), it is associated with very specific neural dysfunction, whereas when it occurs over the entire neocortical surface a more generalized neurologic disorder is indicated. The latter condition is frequently called "encephalopathy." Generally, the slower the frequency content of the EEG, the greater the neurologic dysfunction. This occurs with increased dosages of phenobarbital, which produces a continuous slowing of background frequency and increasing depth of coma. An excess of slower frequencies is even seen in patients taking therapeutic doses of sedatives/hypnotics, although spectral analysis may be necessary for observation of these more subtle EEG changes. Thus therapeutic doses of these medications sometimes may produce neurologic dysfunction. For example, attention span and speed of information processing may be impaired in these patients.

Many pharmaceutical agents induce substantial changes in sleep characteristics, as evidenced by the monitoring of EEG and other physiologic variables. The sedative/hypnotic class of drugs provides one of the best examples. These agents generally produce a synchronization of all EEG rhythms. We can envision this as a tendency to force the brain state of the patient toward stage II sleep away from alertness and deeper stages of non-REM sleep. With diazepam and other benzodiazepines, REM sleep is well preserved, but the density of stages III and IV sleep diminishes. Phenobarbital and other barbiturates inhibit all brain states except stage II sleep, which, not surprisingly, is usually the stage of sleep in which spindle activity occurs. This might be described as a local energy minimum created by increased chloride ion currents in pyramidal cells, which are all induced by some of the most commonly prescribed drugs. It is immediately obvious why neuropsychologic impairment occurs in the central nervous system with these "demon drugs." Sedative/hypnotic agents produce irritability and hyperactivity in children, which is a "subcortical release" phenomenon in which the neocortex is disabled and behavior is dominated by limbic and brainstem control. These drugs may affect adults by increasing aggression and creating a tendency toward violence; this effect has been observed with some drugs more than others (Bond and Lader, 1988). Stimulants tend to produce the opposite effect, with desynchronization of activity and decreased amplitudes of all EEG frequencies, although beta and alpha activity may be enhanced. Such a desynchronized EEG is characteristic of persons with anxiety, in whom there may be excessive cortical activity, and thus the effect of sedatives/hypnotics may be useful.

Many other medications produce important effects on the EEG and behavior and may provide some insight into basic biophysical function. For example, anticholinergic agents, or at least drugs with antimuscurinic properties, produce amnesia and slowing and synchronization of the EEG (Bauer, 1987; Stumpf and Gogolak, 1987). These EEG characteristics are similar to those observed in non-REM sleep, especially stages III and IV in which spindle activity is less predominant. The EEG effects of antidepressants include synchronization, slowing of the background alpha rhythm, and increased production of fast and slower frequencies superimposed on the dominant background alpha. This latter effect is seen primarily with medications that enhance serotonin, such as imipramine or amitriptyline. More noradrenergic agents, such as desipramine and nortriptyline, tend to enhance the background alpha activity, produce desynchronization, or both. The synchronizing antidepressants also tend to have strong anticholinergic and antihistaminic properties, so some of their effects may be due to either or both of these mechanisms. Indeed, some authors have implicated a strong role for muscurinic mechanisms in depression and REM sleep latency (Ansseau et al, 1985). The newer antidepressants, such as fluoxetine (Prozac), which enhances serotonin selectively, produces a desynchronizing effect on the EEG (Lilly Research Centre Ltd., 1992). This effect contrasts with tricyclic antidepressants with strong serotonin-enhancing properties, described above, that tend to have a synchronizing effect. Thus histaminergic and cholinergic mechanisms may play an important role in physiologic changes and EEG manifestations. This is not surprising given the roles histaminergic projections from the hypothalmus and cholinergic projections from the midbrain and basal forebrain are thought to play in arousal mechanisms and their associated control parameters.

Pathologic Effects on EEG and Brain State

Brain function and EEG are affected by many variables. To name all the conditions and list the corresponding effects is useful, but such catalogs do not provide direct information on underlying physiologic mechanisms. Pathologic states can occur at almost any level, from the molecular to global anatomic scales. In many cases, very specific tracts may degenerate, often in response to the loss of a specific group of cells. The epilepsies are diseases that subsume all aspects of brain function. Alzheimer's disease affects several of the neuroanatomic and neurochemical systems previously discussed and deserves mention for itself and for its relation to affective states. Staggering social and economic effects are associated with these conditions, but Alzheimer's disease is especially costly in this context. These problems demand vigorous attack by qualified persons from all areas of biomedical science, including relevant physical science and engineering disciplines.

With epilepsy, almost every conceivable alteration of brain function and awareness occurs because of the presence of abnormal networks of synchronously discharging neurons. Often several characteristic interictal EEG patterns are associated with any specific epileptic syndrome, but the ictal EEG (recorded during the attack) correlates more with individual seizures. That is, several specific interictal EEG correlates may occur in patients who appear to have similar clinical seizures. Many epileptic syndromes have multiple seizure types associated with fairly typical interictal patterns, such as the "slow" spike and wave that occurs in the Lennox-Gastaut syndrome. These patients may have mixtures of atonic (sudden loss of muscle tone), tonic (stiffening), clonic (rhythmic jerking), tonic–clonic, and atypical absences that are similar to petit-mal seizures but may be more prolonged and have excessive psychomotor activity. With focal-onset seizures, our under-

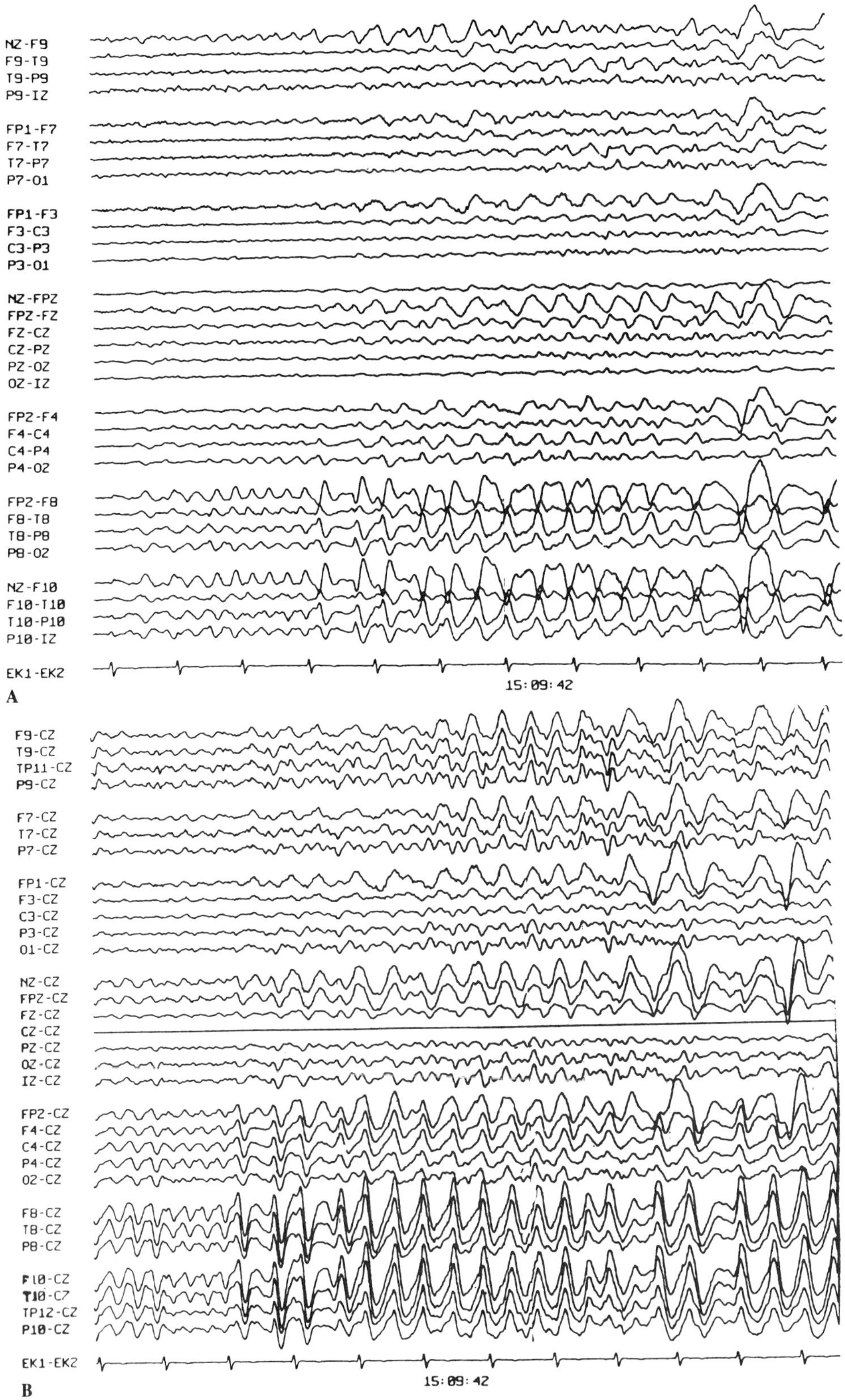
NZ-F9
F9-T9
T9-P9
P9-IZ
FP1-F7
F7-T7
T7-P7
P7-O1
FP1-F3
F3-C3
C3-P3
P3-O1
NZ-FPZ
FPZ-FZ
FZ-CZ
CZ-PZ
PZ-OZ
OZ-IZ
FP2-F4
F4-C4
C4-P4
P4-O2
FP2-F8
F8-T8
T8-P8
P8-O2
NZ-F10
F10-T10
T10-P10
P10-IZ
EK1-EK2
15:09:42
A
F9-CZ
T9-CZ
TP11-CZ
P9-CZ
F7-CZ
T7-CZ
P7-CZ
FP1-CZ
F3-CZ
C3-CZ
P3-CZ
O1-CZ
NZ-CZ
FPZ-CZ
FZ-CZ
CZ-CZ
PZ-CZ
OZ-CZ
IZ-CZ
FP2-CZ
F4-CZ
C4-CZ
P4-CZ
O2-CZ
F8-CZ
T8-CZ
P8-CZ
F10-CZ
T10-CZ
TP12-CZ
P10-CZ
EK1-EK2
15:09:42
B

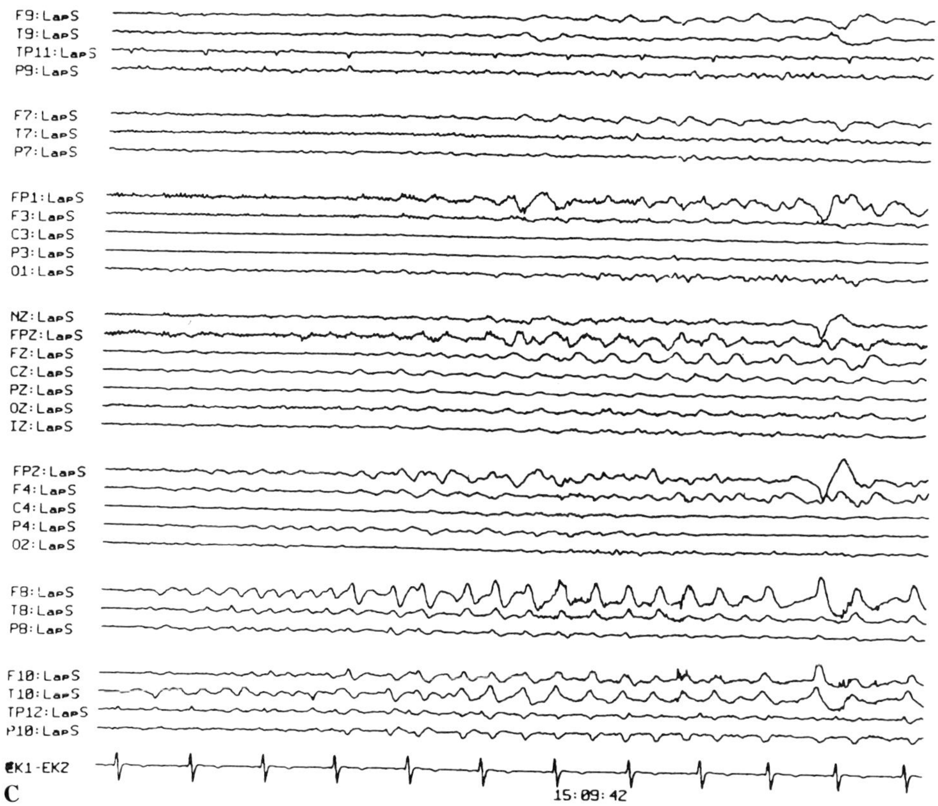

C

Figure 4-15. One epoch of EEG shown for the onset of a seizure. The digital data using 32 channels of EEG has been reformatted and printed out. **A.** Typical "referential" montage that from top to bottom are constituted by left temporal, left frontal–parietal, midline, then right frontal–parietal, and right temporal electrodes, respectively. Within each anatomic group, locations range from the front to the back of the head. Also shown are typical bipolar montage **B**, and Laplacian **C**, using similar anatomic grouping. The EKG artifact on the Laplacian appears in the same channels as at the beginning of the seizure. (Personal communication from F. Sharborough, Mayo Clinic, Rochester, Minnesota.)

standing of this EEG phenomenon is limited to a large extent because we cannot determine the exact site of origination using traditional scalp electrode placements.

The most widely known seizure type is a convulsion, which is also called a generalized tonic–clonic seizure. These seizures may arise as the consequence of an initial focal area of abnormally discharging neurons that eventually recruits sufficient new neurons to produce behavioral cognitive changes. In the physical sciences, this type of effect would be called a propagating instability. If the epileptogenic region is close enough to the scalp and the source distribution is oriented appropriately, changes in the scalp EEG may be observed. Of course, these physical limitations are common problems associated with EEG measurements. For example, there may be such a rapid spread of electrical activity involving the whole brain ("secondary generalization") that we cannot identify the underlying focus, which may be very deep in the brain. With some focal seizures, no ictal scalp EEG manifestation may be observed. These focal seizures include many complex partial seizures arising from frontal sources (Bancaud and Talairach, 1992). Seizures of this type often appear to be bizzare and are frequently thought to be hysterical because so many EEGs appear "normal" during the attack.

Because antiepileptic drugs frequently provide suboptimal seizure control, produce side effects that are often cognitive in nature, or both, surgical procedures to remove the offending epileptogenic tissue are common. Recent publication of several textbooks describing the surgical approach to epilepsy is evidence of this medical direction (Luders, 1992). EEG methods are essential to these surgeries, even in the operating room, where recordings from the surface of the brain (electrocorticography) may be used in preoperative evaluation and during resection to ensure surgical margins of nonepileptic tissue. Clinical results have been good, with many patients showing improved cognitive function. Thus a localized group of chronically discharging neurons appears to affect sufficient neurons throughout the neocortex to interfere with optimal information processing. Because scalp EEG alone often provides inadequate medical data, use of depth electrodes in the brain, subdural or epidural recordings from the neocortical surface, and other electrode placements have become an important prerequisite to removing epileptogenic tissue. New noninvasive techniques are being studied to identify patients who are not proper candidates for epilepsy surgery, although some invasive monitoring may always be necessary, such as for cases involving the intraoperative procedures noted above.

New approaches to scalp recordings are being used at some medical institutions (Sharbrough, 1990). The surface Laplacian clearly helps localize the beginning of ictal discharges, as noted in the data of Figure 4-15, obtained in Dr. Sharbrough's laboratory at the Mayo Clinic where we see that recordings confined to unprocessed potentials may not properly localize ictal discharges. Some of our work shows that interictal spike discharges have considerable spatial variability from spike to spike, as depicted in Figure 4-16 (Nunez and Pilgreen, 1988, 1991). Further advances may lead to techniques that localize deep epileptogenic zones from scalp-derived data but probably will require the concatenation of multiple algorithms using anatomic and physiologic information.

Alzheimer's disease poses one of the most imminent threats to the U.S. health care system. The acquired immunodeficiency disease syndrome is also an important threat, but patients with that disease do not require prolonged direct supervision and assistance with the activities of daily living. The manpower required to care for patients with Alzheimer's disease results in a local social system that consumes extensive resources and time of the patient's care givers. As the massive "baby boomer" population ages, the percentage of the U.S. population at risk for this disease will increase dramatically. Much EEG work on dementing conditions (of which Alzheimer's disease is the most common) has been done, with many reviews available for interested readers (Markand, 1990; Niedermeyer, 1987a). Many EEG changes have been described, such as loss or slowing of the normal

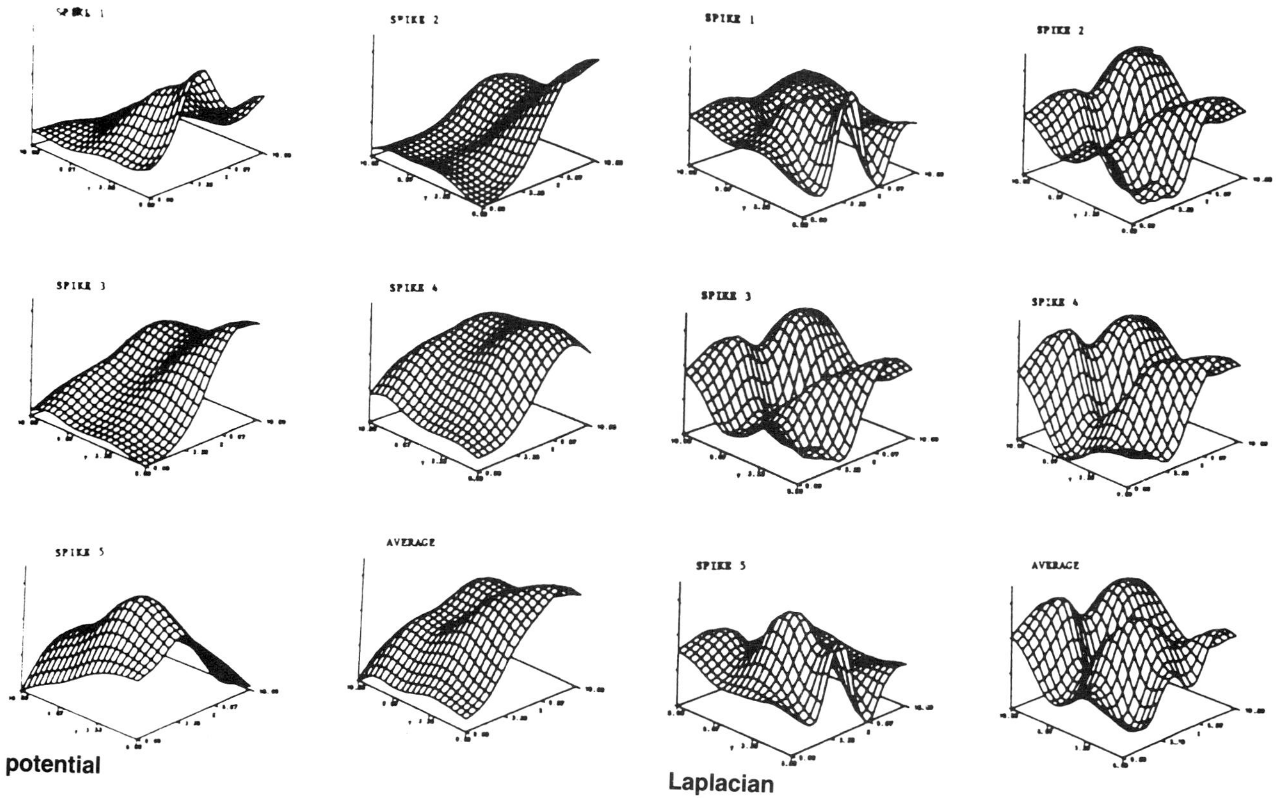

Figure 4-16. Data from five successive spike discharges using peak negative potential for plotting with respect to local spatial coordinates that correspond to an area of temporal neocortex. Note the rather dramatic spatial variability from one spike discharge to the next, which is better appreciated in the Laplacian. This range includes a horizontal dipole to a vertical dipole.

background alpha rhythm, excessive slowing in the theta and delta range, decreased K complexes, and even the absence or diminution of barbiturate-induced beta activity. All of these changes occur relatively late in the illness, when clinical signs are already obvious. It is common for substantial cognitive symptoms to be present (as measured by neuropsychologic scales) with a normal EEG. This latter finding may be due in part to the extreme redundancy of parallel neural systems; however, new methods to record EEG and analyze data should reveal more subtle EEG changes that are not observed by conventional methods. Now that pharmacologic treatments to reduce symptoms and slow the progression of the disease are being developed (one is now commercially available), early diagnosis is imperative.

Specific pathologic and anatomic changes occur in the brains of persons with Alzheimer's disease. Specifically the hippocampus and neocortical association areas degenerate (Figure 4-17). These are some of the primary structures responsible for the formation of new memory traces, the disturbance of which is the hallmark of Alzheimer's disease. Very specific microscopic changes occur (neurofibrillary

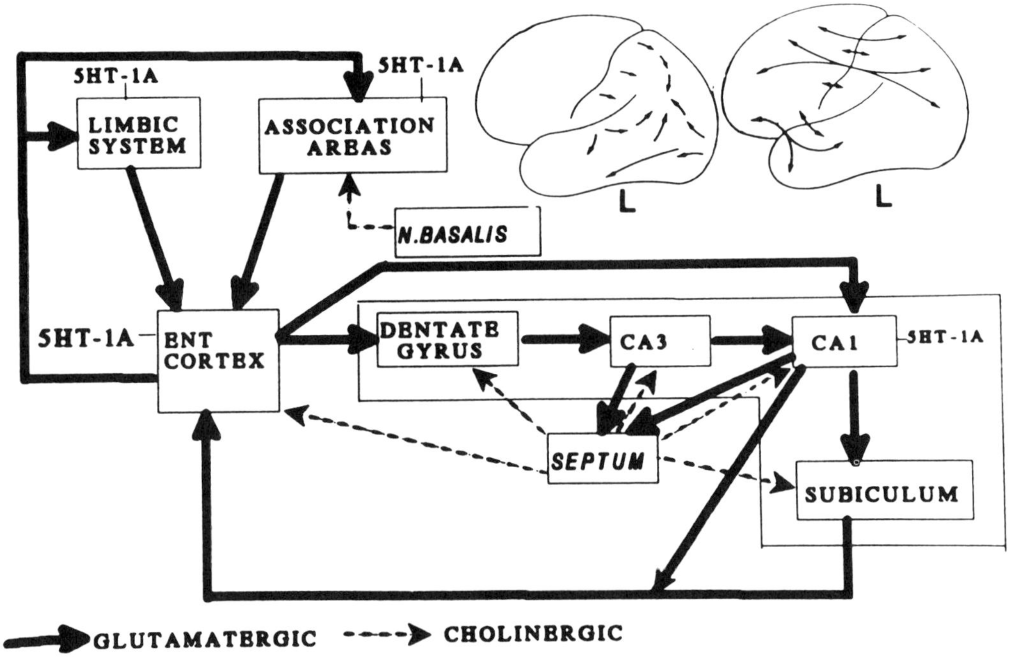

Figure 4-17. Known anatomic mediators of memory and other cognitive processes. In the left of the two lateral views of the left cerebral hemisphere, most arrows lead to the parietal heteromodal association area which is a major locus of degeneration of neocortex in Alzheimer's disease. Entorhinal cortex is affected early in the course of the illness and provides the major throughput to the hippocampus. (Reproduced with permission from Francis et al: Neurotransmitters and Neuropeptides, In: *Alzheimer's Disease* (R.D. Terry et al, eds). New York: Raven Press, 1994 [chapter 14].)

tangles and senile plaques) in the affected structures, possibly because of an abnormal expression of proteins (Katzman and Jackson, 1991). Many of these proteins have been described, and amyloid precursor protein is the protein most often mentioned. The number of plaques correlates with the degree of disturbed cognition (Blessed et al, 1968). The diffuse projectional systems described previously are involved to varying degrees, with the cholinergic system of the basal forebrain the most profoundly effected. These cholinergic structures are comprised primarily of the basilar nucleus of Meynert, diagonal band of Broca, and other systems in the same anatomic vicinity (Figure 4-7). The blockade of muscarinic receptors in neocortex produces EEG changes similar to those seen in Alzheimer's disease, along with impaired formation of new memory traces. The locus coeruleus and cells of the dorsal median raphe nuclei also degenerate in Alzheimer's disease, resulting in decreased noradrenergic and serotoninergic neocortical afferents. These latter changes are probably the cause of the sleep–wake disruption that is found so commonly in Alzheimer's disease and also may be responsible for other conditions, such as major endogeneous depression. Patients with Alzheimer's disease are often depressed, which may be the symptom that causes them to seek medical care. Later in the disease, patients lose insight and usually are seen only in a medical setting, when family members and friends physically escort them to the physician's office.

Recently more sophisticated analyses of EEG prompted the recognition of some early correlates of Alzheimer's disease. Because severe endogenous depression in the elderly can mimic dementia of Alzheimer's type, techniques to differentiate them early must be developed, especially because aggressive treatment of depression can have satisfactory results. Electroencephalographic spectra displayed topographically can differentiate most patients with Alzheimer's disease from those with similar conditions. With Alzheimer's disease subtle increases in slow activity occur, changes that are milder degrees of the more profound EEG changes described previously. Administration of medications to increase the availability of acetylcholine at the neocortical and hippocampal receptor sites improves these EEG parameters as objective measures of cognitive function (Leuchter et al, 1991). Spectral analysis of EEG during REM sleep may be a more sensitive discriminator between these groups. Event-related potentials were originally thought to hold great promise for this problem (Goodin et al, 1978), but because of the overlap of latency and amplitude measures between groups of normal, depressed, and Alzheimer's disease patients, individual discrimination is difficult (Blackwood et al, 1987; Muir et al, 1991; Pfefferbaum et al, 1984). Parallels can be drawn between the tendency toward synchronization in the EEG of Alzheimer's disease and that of slow-wave sleep, which both occur when cholinergic influence is diminished. Persons aroused from slow-wave sleep may deny that they were asleep but have complete amnesia for events that occurred, including such profound situations as sleepwalking and night terror. Thus slow-wave sleep is a form of physiologic dementia (Vanderwolf, 1992).

Depression is a common condition that affects about 10% of the U.S. population at some time in their lives. Recently investigators suggested that depression is more a neurologic than a psychologic disease because focal neurologic signs may appear and then disappear as the depression recedes, especially in adolescents (Brumback, 1993). The biochemical basis for this condition is complex, but physiologic observations include excessive firing of the locus coeruleus, down-regulation of beta receptors on neocortical cells, and augmented responsiveness to acetylcholine (Gold et al, 1988). Locus coeruleus activity is inhibited by the neurotransmitter GABA, which is reduced to the blood and spinal fluid of depressed patients. This firing rate is also decreased by tricyclic antidepressants and monamine oxidase inhibitors. A routine EEG in a depressed person may show nonspecific abnormalities, such as excess activity in the theta range, more frequently in patients without a family history of depression. When focal abnormalities occur, they tend to be in the right hemisphere (Small, 1987). More sophisticated EEG data analysis reveals changes that may provide insight into global and local pathophysiologic processes.

Spontaneous EEG coherence during specific cognitive paradigms and ERP measures have been used to analyze different pathologic states and to quantify drug action. Ford and colleagues showed that interhemispheric coherence was highest for unmedicated patients with schizophrenia compared with controls and decreased with use of antipsychotic medications such as haloperidol (Ford et al, 1986). Flor-Henry and Koles (1984) reported that right intrahemispheric coherence is increased for all psychotic states, with the greatest coherence values observed in schizophrenia. The smallest intrahemispheric coherences occur with major depression, with mania showing intermediate levels. That disturbances of physiology are confined to the right hemisphere is somewhat questionable. A more sophisticated study of coherence would use psychophysical paradigms designed to activate either hemisphere selectively, which is further subjected to a discriminant analysis. Healthy persons show an increased intrahemispheric coherence in the alpha band in the left frontal lobe that is not present in persons with schizophrenia, with other parts of the brain showing similar activation pattern in healthy persons and those with schizophrenia. This left frontal disturbance is partially normalized in patients with schizophrenia treated with appropriate medications (Morrison-Stewart et al, 1991). Many studies have shown an overall increased slowing in the delta and theta range in the frontal regions of persons with schizophrenia (Morihisa et al, 1983; Small, 1987). Studies using other methods have confirmed this finding and provided evidence that this may be secondary to decreased activity of the mesolimbic dopamine systems that project to the prefrontal areas, as sketched in Figure 4-6 (Weinberger et al, 1988). Depressed patients also have excessive activation of the right frontal areas as measured by EEG desynchronization (Schaffer et al. 1983).

Some congenital brain defects produce interesting EEGs. For example, agenesis of the corpus callosum occurs in a few persons and may be only partially missing with the splenium most commonly affected or complete with the entire structure missing. The anterior and posterior commissures remain intact in most cases and compensate for occipital interhemispheric information transfer, as suggested by EEG coherence studies (Nielsen et al, 1993). One of the more extreme examples of this anatomic disconnection occurs in the Acardi syndrome, in which complete agenesis of the corpus callosum, other associated anatomic brain anomalies, frequent mild mental retardation, and seizures occur. This condition has been observed only in females and is thought to be due to an X-linked recessive disorder that is lethal in males, with most dying while in utero (Naidu and Niedermeyer, 1993). The routine interictal EEG shows complete dysynchrony between the two cerebral hemispheres, which is especially dramatic in sleep, with sharp vertex and spindle activity. These persons are predisposed to develop a particularly severe form of seizure disorder called infantile spasms, with the frequent concomitant EEG pattern called hypsarrhythmia (Niedermeyer, 1993). The actual seizure attack often begins with flexion at the waist followed by rapid extension of legs, trunk, and arms; the symptoms are striking. The EEG during an infantile spasm consists of an almost complete loss of all background activity for a few seconds, which is commonly called an electrodecremental response. In Aicardi's syndrome, this may affect only one side of the body at a time, whereas it is bilateral for children with infantile spasms but no agenesis of the corpus callosum. The EEG in Figure 4-18 illustrates the marked differences each cerebral hemisphere may show for EEG activity such as seizure and sleep activity.

Many ERP studies have reported effects of depression and schizophrenia on the amplitude and latency of the P300. The amplitude of the P300 is reduced in

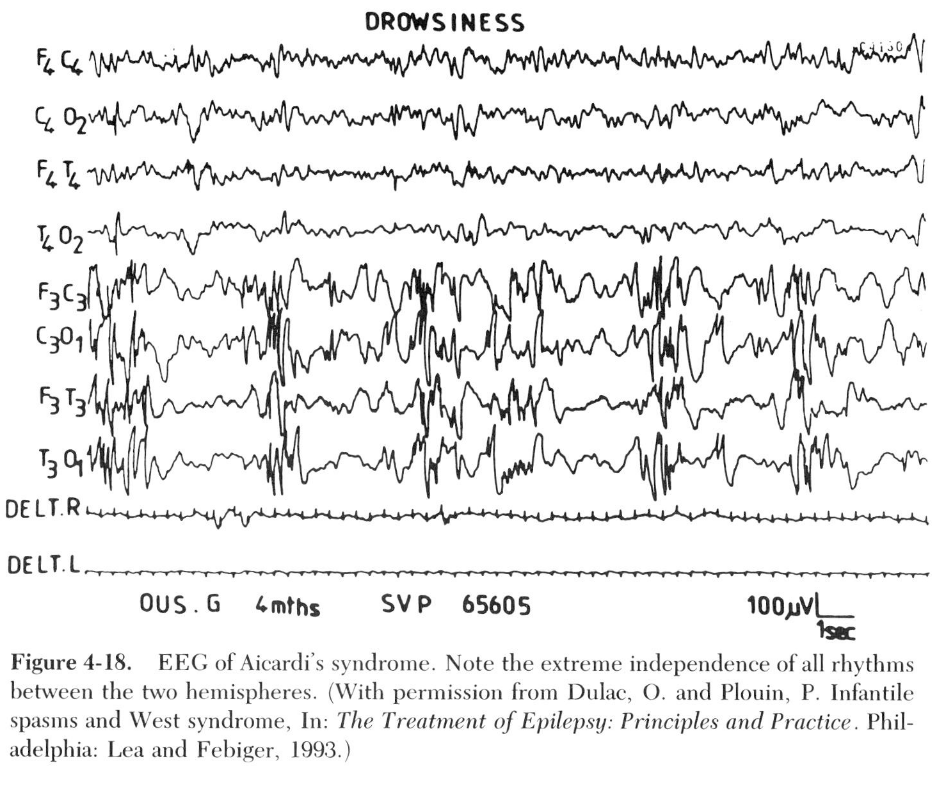

Figure 4-18. EEG of Aicardi's syndrome. Note the extreme independence of all rhythms between the two hemispheres. (With permission from Dulac, O. and Plouin, P. Infantile spasms and West syndrome, In: *The Treatment of Epilepsy: Principles and Practice*. Philadelphia: Lea and Febiger, 1993.)

both disorders, with a relative normalization after treatment. P300 latency is prolonged in schizophrenia, corresponding to an increase in memory scanning time, and does not improve with treatment (Blackwood et al, 1987). Muir and colleagues (1991) noted a prolonged latency of the P300 in patients with bipolar but not unipolar disease. Those with bipolar disease are often confused clinically with those with schizophrenia. Thus patients with schizophrenia and those with bipolar disease could also be confused based strictly on ERP data.

Summary

In this discussion of brain state and EEG, we considered several seemingly disparate topics. Basic anatomy of the brain was discussed, with emphasis on the diffuse projectional systems, the basic neurochemistry as it relates to EEG, EEG correlates of wide-ranging normal behavioral states, changes in the EEG over the human lifespan, and multiple causes of altered brain state as manifested in the EEG. This overview is superficial in its survey of individual topics, but we hope it provides some insight into how EEG studies can contribute to many areas of neuroscience. Future work regarding behavioral state and its disturbances should encompass newer techniques to analyze EEG and brain processes. Studies using surface Laplacians and cortical imaging to improve spatial resolution, coherence analysis, and other methods of time and space analysis combined with increased electrode density should provide much new information about brain function.

References

Ahern, G.L. and Schwartz, G.E. Differential lateralization for positive and negative emotion in the human brain: EEG spectral analysis. *Neuropsychologia*. 23:745–755, 1985.

Ansseau, M., Machowski, R., Georges, F., and Timsit-Berthier, M. REM sleep latency and contingent negative variation in endogenous depression: Suggestion for a common cholinergic mechanism. *Biol. Psychiatry*. 20:1303–1307, 1985.

Bancaud, J. and Talairach, J. Clinical semiology of frontal lobe seizures. In: *Frontal Lobe Seizures and Epilepsies*. (P. Chauvel, Delgado-Escueta, A. V., Halgren, E., Bancaud, J., Eds.) New York: Raven Press, p. 59–88, 1992.

Banquet, J.P. Inter- and intrahemispheric relationships of the EEG activity during sleep. *Electroencephalogr. Clin. Neurophysiol*. 55:51–59, 1983.

Bauer, G. EEG, drug effects, and central nervous system poisoning. In: *Electroencephalography, Basic Principles, Clinical Applications and Related Fields*. (E. Niedermeyer, Lopes da Silva, F., Eds.) Baltimore: Urban and Scharzenberg, 1987.

Beaumont, J.G., Mayes, A.R., and Rugg, M.D. Asymmetry in EEG alpha coherence and power: Effects of task and sex. *Electroencephalogr. Clin. Neurophysiol*. 45:393–401, 1978.

Begleiter, H., Porjesz, B., and Chou, C.L. P3 and stimulus incentive value. *Psychophysiology*. 20:95–101, 1983.

Berger, H. Uber das Elektrenkephalogramm des Menschen. *Archiv. für Psychiatrie*. 87:527, 1929.

Blackwood, D.H.R., Whalley, L.J., Christie, J.E., Blackburn, I.M., St. Clair, D.M., and

McInnes, A. Changes in auditory P3 event-related potential in schizophrenia and depression. *Br. J. Psychiatry.* 150:154–160, 1987.

Blessed, G., Tomlinson, E., and Roth, M. The association between quantitative measures of dementia and of senile change in the cerebral grey matter of elderly subjects. *Br. J. Psychiatry.* 114:797–811, 1968.

Bond, A. and Lader, M. Differential effects of oxazepam and lorazepam on aggressive responding. *Psychopharmacology.* 95:369–373, 1988.

Brumback, R.A. Is depression a neurologic disease. *Neurologic Clinics.* 11:79–104, 1993.

Cooper, J.R., Bloom, F.E., and Roth, H.R. Amino acid transmitters. In: *The Biochemical Basis of Neuropharmacology.* New York: Oxford University Press, 1991a.

Cooper, J.R., Bloom, F.E., and Roth, H.R. Neuroactive peptides. In: *The Biochemical Basis of Neuropharmacology.* New York: Oxford University Press, 1991b.

Corsi-Cabrera, M., Herrera, P., and Malvido, M. Correlation between EEG and cognitive abilities: Sex differences. *Int. J. Neuroscience.* 45:133–141, 1989.

Courchesne, E. Chronology of postnatal human brain development: Event related potential, positron emission tomography, myelinogenesis, and synaptogenesis studies. In: *Event-Related Brain Potentials.* (J.W. Rohrbaugh, Parasuraman, R., Johnson, R., Eds.) New York: Oxford, 1990.

Creutzfeldt, O.D. Generality of the functional structure of the neocortex. *Naturwissenschaften.* 64:507–517, 1977.

Davidson, R.J. EEG measures of cerebral asymmetry: Conceptual and methodological issues. *Int. J. Neuroscience.* 39:71–89, 1988.

Davidson, R.J., and Fox, N.A. Frontal brain asymmetry predicts infants' response to maternal separation. *Journal of Abnormal Psychology.* 98:127–131, 1989.

Douglas, R.J. and Martin, K.A.C. Neocortex. In: *The Synaptic Organization of the Brain.* (G.M. Sheperd, Ed.) New York: Oxford University Press, 1990.

Flinn, J.M., Kirsch, A.D., and Flinn, E.A. Correlations between intelligence and the frequency content of the evoked potential. *Physiological Psychology.* 5:11–15, 1977.

Flor-Henry, P. and Koles, Z.J. EEG characteristic of normal subjects: A comparison of men and women and of dextrals and sinistrals. *Research Communications in Psychology, Psychiatry and Behavior.* 7:21–37, 1982.

Flor-Henry, P. and Koles, Z.J. Statistical quantitative EEG studies of depression, mania, schizophrenia and normals. *Biol. Psychology.* 19:257–279, 1984.

Ford, M.R., Goethe, J.W., and Dekker, D.K. EEG coherence and power in the discrimination of psychiatric disorders and medication effects. *Biol. Psychiatry.* 21:1175–1188, 1986.

Fox, N.A. and Davidson, R.J. Taste-elicited changes in facial signs of emotion and the asymmetry of brain electrical activity in human newborns. *Neuropsychologica.* 24:417–422, 1986.

French, C.C. and Beaumont, J.G. A critical review of EEG coherence studies of hemisphere function. *Int. J. Psychophysiol.* 1:241–254, 1984.

Gevins, A.S. Analysis or multiple lead data. In: *Event-related brain potentials.* (J.W. Rohbraugh, Parasuraman, R., Johnson, J.R., Eds.) New York: Oxford University Press, 1990.

Gilman, A.G., Rall, T.W., Nies, A.S., and Taylor, P. *Goodman and Gilman's The Pharmacological Basis of Therapeutics.* New York: Pergamon Press, 1990.

Gold, P., Goodwin, F.K., and Chrousos, G.P. Clinical and biochemical manifestations of depression: Relation to the neurobiology of stress. *N. Engl. J. Med.* 319:348–353, 1988.

Goodin, D., Squires, K.C., and Starr, A. Long latency event-related components of the auditory evoked potential in dementia. *Electroencephalogr. Clin. Neurophysiol.* 101:447–458, 1978.

Goodin, D.S., Squires, K.C., and Starr, A. Variations in early and late event-related components of the auditory evoked potential with task difficulty. *Electroencephalogr. Clin. Neurophysiol.* 55:680–686, 1983.

Gotman, J. The use of computers in analysis and display of EEG and evoked potentials. In: *Current Practice of Clinical Electroencephalography.* (D.D. Daly, Pedley, T.A., Eds.) New York: Raven Press, 1990.

Katzman, R. and Jackson, J.E. Alzheimer disease: Basic and clinical advances. *J. Amer. Gerontol. Soc.* 39:516–525, 1991.

Knight, R.T. Decreased response to novel stimuli after prefrontal lesions in man. *Electroencephalogr. Clin. Neurophysiol.* 59:9–20, 1984.

Leuchter, A.F., Read, S.L., Shapira, J., Walter, D.O., and Smith, C. Stable bimodal response to cholinomimetic drugs in Alzheimer's disease: Brain mapping correlates. *Neuropsychopharmacology.* 4:165–173, 1991.

Lilly Research Centre Ltd., E.L.C. The human pharmacology of fluoxetine. *Int. J. Obes.* 16:49–54, 1992.

Lombroso, C. Neonatal electroencephalography. In: *Electroencephalography: Basic Principles, Clinical Applications and Related Fields.* (E. Niedermeyer, Lopes da Silva F., Eds.) Baltimore: Urban and Schwarzenberg, 1987.

Lopes da Silva, F.H. and Strom van Leeuwen, W. The cortical alpha rhythm in dog: The depth and surface profile of phase. In: *Architectonics of the Cerebral Cortex.* (M. A. B. Brazier, Petsche, H., Eds.) New York: Raven Press, 1978.

Luders, H.O. *Epilepsy Surgery.* New York: Raven Press, 1992.

MacDonald, R.L. Antiepileptic drug actions. *Epilepsia.* 30:S19–S28, 1989.

Markand, O.N. Organic brain syndromes and demenias. In: *Current Practice of Clinical Electroencephalography.* (D.D. Daly, Pedley, T.A., Eds.) New York: Raven Press, pp. 401–424, 1990.

McCormick, D.A. Neurotransmitter actions in the thalamus and cerebral cortex. *J. Clin. Neurophys.* 9:212–223, 1992.

Mesulam, M.-M. Patterns in behavioral neuroanatomy. In: *Principles of Behavioral Neurology.* (M.M. Mesulam, Ed.) Philadelphia: F.A. Davis, 1985.

Montplaisir, J., Nielsen, T., Cote, J., Boivin, D., Rouleau, I., and Lapierre, G. Interhemispheric EEG coherence before and after partial callosotomy. *Clin. Electroencephalogr.* 21:42–47, 1990.

Morihisa, J.M., Duffy, F.H., and Wyatt, R.J. Brain electrical activity mapping (BEAM) in schizophrenic patients. *Arch. Gen. Psychiatry.* 40:719–728, 1983.

Morrison-Stewart, S.L., Williamson, P.C., Corning, W.C., Kutcher, S.P., and Merskey, H. Coherence of electroencephalography and aberrant functional organisation of the brain in schizophrenic patients during activation tasks. *Br. J. Psychiatry.* 159:636–644, 1991.

Muir, W.J., St. Clair, D.M., and Blackwood, H.R. Long latency auditory event-related potentials in schizophrenia and in bipolar and unipolar affective disorder. *Psychol. Med.* 21:867–879, 1991.

Naidu, S., and Niedermeyer, E. Degenerative disorders of the central nervous system. In: *Electroencephalography: Basic Principles, Clinical Applications, and Related Fields.* (E. Niedermeyer, Lopes da Silva, F., Eds.) Baltimore: Williams and Wilkins, pp. 351–371, 1993.

Niedermeyer, E. EEG and dementia. In: *Electroencephalography: Basic Principles, Clin-*

ical Applications, and Related Fields. (E. Niedermeyer, Lopes da Silva, F., Eds.) Baltimore: Urban and Schwarzenberg, pp. 309–318, 1987.

Niedermeyer, E. Epileptic seizure disorders. In: *Electroencephalography: Basic Principles, Clinical Applications and Related Fields.* Baltimore: Williams and Wilkins, pp. 461–564, 1993.

Niedermeyer, E. Maturation and the EEG: Development of waking and sleep patterns. In: *Electroencephalography: Basic Principles, Clinical Applications and Related Fields.* Baltimore: Urban and Schwarzenberg, pp. 167–191, 1993.

Niedermeyer, E. Sleep and EEG. In: *Electroencephalography: Basic Principles, Clinical Applications and Related Fields.* Baltimore: Urban and Schwarzenberg, pp. 156–166, 1993.

Niedermeyer, E. and Lopes de Silva, F. *Electroencephalography: Basic Principles, Clinical Applications and Related Fields.* Baltimore: Williams & Wilkins, pp. 461–564, 1993.

Nielsen, T., Montplaisir, J., and Lassonde, M. Decreased interhemispheric EEG coherence during sleep in agenesis of the corpus collosum. *Eur. Neurol.* 33, 173–176, 1993.

Nunez, P.L. *Electric Fields of the Brain: The Neurophysics of EEG.* New York: Oxford University Press, 1981a.

Nunez, P.L. A study of the origins of the time dependencies of scalp EEG. II. Experimental support of theory. *IEEE Trans. Biomed. Eng.* 28:281–288, 1981b.

Nunez, P.L. and Pilgreen, K.L. Laplacian evaluation of epileptic spike foci. Presented at the American Electroencephalographic Society Annual Scientific Meeting, San Diego, California, 2–5 October, 1988.

Nunez, P.L. Towards a physics of neocortex. In: *Advanced Methods of Physiological Systems Modeling.* (V.Z. Marmarelis, Ed.) New York: Plenum Press, 1989.

Nunez, P.L. Physical principles and neurophysiological mechanisms underlying event related potentials. In: *Event Related Potentials of the Brain.* (J. Rohrbaugh, Johnson, R., Parasuraman, R., Eds.) New York: Oxford University Press, 1990.

Nunez, P.L. and Pilgreen, K.L. The spline Laplacian in clinical neurophysiology: A method to improve EEG spatial resolution. *J. Clin. Neurophys.* 8:397–413, 1991.

Nunez, P.L., Pilgreen, K.L., and Law, S.K. Mapping of evoked potentials. In: *Evoked Potentials Review.* (C. Barber, Taylor, M.J., Eds.) Nottingham, UK: IEPS Publications, 1991.

Ogilvie, N.D., Simons, I.A., Kuderian, R.H., MacDonald, T., and Rustenburg, J. Behavioral, event-related potential, and EEG/FFT changes at sleep onset. *Psychophysiology.* 28:54–64, 1991.

Okada, Y.C., Kaufman, L., and Williamson, S.J. The hippocampal formation as as source of the slow endogenous potentials. *Electroencephalogr. Clin. Neurophysiol.* 55:417–426, 1983.

Pfefferbaum, A., Ford, J., Johnson, J.R., Wenegrat, B., and Kopell, B.S. Manipulation of P300 latency: Speed vs. accuracy instructions. *Electroencephalogr. Clin. Neurophysiol.* 55:188–197, 1983.

Pfefferbaum, A., Wenegrat, B.G., Ford, J.M., Roth, W.T., and Kopell, B.S. Clinical application of the P3 component of event-related potentials. II. Dementia, depression and schizophrenia, *Electroencephalogr. Clin. Neurophysiol.* 59:104–124, 1984.

Polich, J. Attention, probability, and task demands as determinants of P300 latency from auditory stimuli. *Electroencephalogr. Clin. Neurophysiol.* 63:251–259, 1986.

Polich, J. and Donchin, E. P300 and the word frequency effect. *Electroencephalogr. Clin. Neurophysiol.* 70:33–45, 1988.

Rechtschaffen, A. and Kales, A. *A Manual of Standardized Terminology, Techniques, and*

Scoring System for Sleep Stages of Human Subjects. Washington, DC: U.S. Department of Health, Education and Welfare, Public Health Service, U.S. Government Printing Office, 1968.

Robinson, D.L. The neurophysiological bases of high IQ. *Int. J. Neuroscience.* 46:209–234, 1989.

Ross, E.D. The aprosodias: Functional-anatomic of the affective components of language in the right hemisphere. *Arch. Neurol.* 38:561, 1981.

Schaffer, C.E., Davidson, R.J., and Saron, C. Frontal and parietal electroencephalogram asymmetry in depressed and nondepressed subjects. *Biol. Psychiatry.* 18:753–762, 1983.

Schenck, C.H., Bundlie, S.R., Ettinger, M.G., and Mahowald, M.W. Chronic behavioral disorders of human REM sleep: A new category of parasomnia. *Sleep.* 9:293–308, 1986.

Sharbrough, F.W. Electrical fields and recording techniques. In: *Current Practice of Clinical Electroencephalography.* (D.D. Daly, Pedley, T.A., Eds.) New York: Raven Press, 1990.

Small, J.G. Psychiatric disorders and EEG. In: *Electroencephalography: Basic Principles, Clinical Applications and Related Fields.* (E. Niedermeyer, Lopes da Silva, F., Eds.) Baltimore: Urban and Scharzenberg, 1987.

Smith, M.E., Halgren, E., Sokolik, M., Baudena, P., Musolino, A., Liegeois-Chauvel, C., and Chauvel, P. The intracranial topography of the P3 event-related potential elicited during auditory oddball. *Electroencephalogr. Clin. Neurophysiol.* 76:235–248, 1990.

Speckmann, E.J. and Elger, C.E. Introduction to the neurophysiological of the EEG and DC potentials. In: *Electroencephalography: Basic Principles, Clinical Applications and Related Fields.* (E. Niedermeyer, Lopes da Silva, F., Eds.) Baltimore: Urban and Schwarzenberg, 1987.

Steriade, M. Brain electrical activity and sensory processing during waking and sleep states. In: *Principles and Practice of Sleep Medicine.* (M.H. Kryger, Roth, T., Dement, W.C., Eds.) Philadelphia: WB Saunders, 1989.

Steriade, M., Gloor, P., Llinas, R.R., Lopes da Silva, F.H., and Mesulam, M.-M. Basic mechanisms of cerebral rhythmic activities. *Electroencephalogr. Clin. Neurophysiol.* 76:481–508, 1990.

Stumpf, C. and Gogolak, G. EEG and neuropharmacology—An experimental approach. In: *Electroencephalography: Basic Principles, Clinical Applications and Related Fields.* (E. Niedermeyer, Lopes da Silva, F., Eds.) Baltimore: Urban and Scharzenberg, 1987.

Valdés, P., Valdés, M., Carballo, J.A., Alvarez, A., Diaz, G.F., Biscay, R., Pez, M.C., Szava, S., Virus, T., and Quesada, M.E. QEEG in a public health system. *Brain Topography.* 4:259–266, 1992.

Vanderwolf, C.H. The electrocorticogram in relation to physiology and behavior: A new analysis. *Electroencephalogr. Clin. Neurophysiol.* 82:165–175, 1992.

Webster, J.G. *Medical Instrumentation: Application and Design.* Boston: Houghton Mifflin Company, 1992.

Weinberger, D.R., Berman, K.F., and Illowsky, B.P. Physiological dysfunction of dorsolateral prefrontal cortex in schizophrenia: III. A new cohort and evidence for a monoaminergic mechanism. *Arch. Gen. Psychiatry.* 45:609–615, 1988.

Williams, H.L. and Williams, C.L. Nocturnal EEG profiles and performance. *Psychophysiology.* 3:164–175, 1966.

Wood, C.C. and Wolpaw, J.R. Scalp distribution of human auditory evoked potentials. II: Evidence for overlapping sources and involvement of auditory cortex. *Electroencephalogr. Clin. Neurophysiol.* 54:25–38, 1982.

5

Dynamics of Electrical Activity of the Brain, Local Networks, and Modulating Systems

FERNANDO H. LOPES DA SILVA

A detailed analysis of the anatomic and functional organization of the brain indicates that to understand the dynamics of electroencephalogram (EEG) (and magnetoencephalograph [MEG]) activity, we must consider not only the electric behavior of single neurons but also the properties of the local circuits, including the synaptic processes that are essential in neuronal interactions. This chapter is an overview of phenomena relevant to understanding the dynamics of the neocortical EEG, from the behavior of the single neuron membrane to the dynamics of large neuronal networks. Processes in neocortex are emphasized, but the activity of other structures are also considered, such as the thalamus, which is directly related to the neocortical EEG. In this respect, it is convenient to consider three questions that correspond to different levels of complexity:

1. Are the rhythmic characteristics of neocortical EEG signals determined by intrinsic membrane pacemaker activity of individual neurons?
2. Are local synaptic interactions responsible for the neuronal synchrony underlying cortical field potentials that form the EEG?
3. Do the complex dynamics of large neuronal networks lead to the emergence of novel properties, that is, those that are not apparent in neuronal elements but are revealed in neocortical EEG signals?

EEG Rhythms, Intrinsic Neuronal Pacemakers, and Synaptically Driven Initial Conditions

The idea that EEG rhythmic activity is determined primarily by neuronal pacemakers has been a constant assumption in neurophysiology (Andersen and Andersson, 1968). However, until recently there has been no experimental evidence to support such an assumption. An important step forward in this respect was the discovery by Jahnsen and Llinás (1984a, 1984b) that some types of thalamic neurons can display oscillatory behavior in vitro, even after synaptic transmission is blocked. Given the appropriate background state (control parameters) and initial conditions, such neurons can generate intrinsic membrane oscillations mainly in the frequency range of 6 to 10 Hz. In the context of this discussion, we must ask whether these oscillations are autonomous. We must emphasize that autonomy, in the context of the issue considered here (and in Chapter 3), means that the neuronal oscillatory behavior is intrinsic, that is, it is independent of inputs, as we would expect from a real "pacemaker," as found in some heart cells.

To reply to the autonomy issue, we must consider the main ionic conductances of these thalamic neurons. These neurons are usually called thalamocortical relay cells (TCR) because they form the relays between the extrathalamic inputs and the cortex. The TCR cells constitute an essential link in the local thalamic circuits. Studies of ionic conductances of these TCR cells (reviewed in Steriade and Llinás, 1988; Steriade et al, 1990) showed that they may oscillate preferentially at about 6 or 10 Hz, depending on initial conditions, that is, on the level of the initial membrane potential. Switching from one mode of oscillation to another is voltage dependent. In simple terms, the TCR cell tends to oscillate at 10 Hz when the initial state of membrane voltage is relatively more depolarized than the normal resting state, and at 6 Hz when it is relatively more hyperpolarized, as shown in Figure 5-1. Thus the initial conditions appropriate for the oscillatory behavior at the lower frequency range (6 Hz) are different from those necessary for the higher-frequency (10 Hz) oscillations.

Because these two types of oscillatory behavior are fundamentally important to understanding how different mechanisms interact to determine oscillatory behavior, we will consider them in more detail. The 6-Hz type of oscillation needs an initial hyperpolarized state that can be achieved by a combination of synaptic and intrinsic potentials, specifically by an inhibitory postsynaptic potential (IPSP) and through potassium currents (the A current and a Calcium [Ca^{2+}-dependent potassium [K$\pm$] current). The hyperpolarization is necessary for the de-inactivation of a low-threshold Ca^{2+} conductance that, thereafter, depolarizes the TCR cell and leads to generation of an action potential. This process can become repetitive, particularly if the action potential can activate an inhibitory neuron that causes the IPSP on the TCR cell through an inhibitory feedback loop (recurrent). The 10-Hz type of oscillation requires a shift in membrane voltage in the depolarizing direction, which under natural conditions depends on an appropriate synaptic input. In addition, depolarization activates a persistent sodium conductance that can lead to triggering fast sodium-mediated, high-threshold action potentials. The process can also become repetitive if sufficient depolarizing bias (about 10 mV) is present. An important contribution to this depolarization shift under natural conditions may be a cholinergic input that ensures decreased potassium conductance of the TCR cell (but see also the section Interaction Between Local Systems and Modulating Systems for the possible role of nitric oxide).

The neurons of the reticular nucleus also can generate two types of activity—

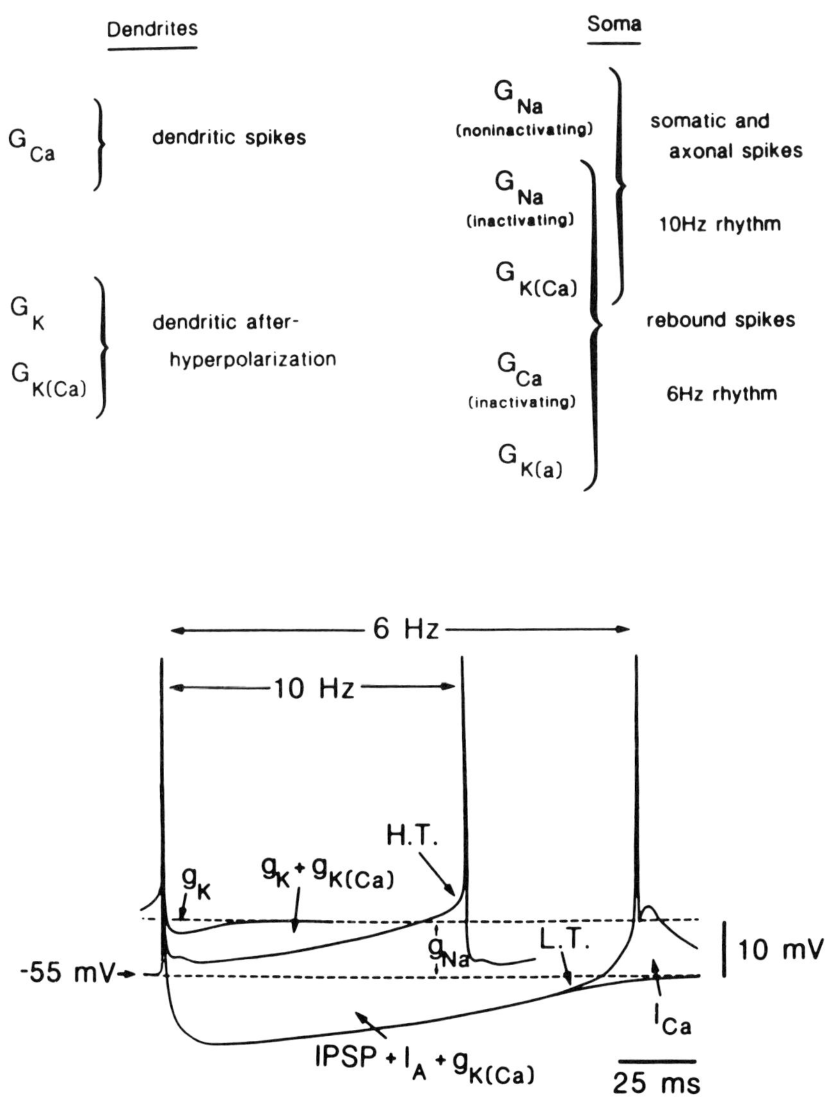

Figure 5-1. The main conductances (g) of thalamic neurons and their contribution to the generation of thalamic oscillations. g_K = potassium conductance; $g_{K(Ca)}$ = calcium-dependent potassium conductance; HT = high-threshold spike; LT = low-threshold spike; IPSP = inhibitory postsynaptic potential; I_A = potassium A current. (Adapted with permission from Steriade and Llinás, 1988).

rhythmic high-frequency bursts of action potentials or single-spike (tonic) activity. The former correspond to the EEG spindles seen in drowsiness and slow-wave sleep and the latter to the alert state. The transition between the two modes is voltage dependent and determined primarily by the presence of a low-threshold calcium current that is activated at membrane potentials more negative than −60 mV (Jahnsen and Llinás, 1984a, 1984b, Avanzini et al, 1989). Of course, in in vitro preparations the initial conditions and control parameters necessary for oscillatory behavior to occur can be created artificially by manipulating the membrane potential.

When the neurons under study are part of a functioning nervous system the mechanisms of external control are quite different. In this case initial conditions and control parameters are created by the action of synaptic inputs and thus depend on the activity of other neuronal elements of the local network, or even of elements from distant networks. Because of the dependence on such external input, the oscillatory behavior of TCR and reticular nucleus neurons cannot be considered autonomous. Indeed, Steriade and colleagues (1985) showed that the thalamic nuclei cannot generate spindle oscillations after disconnection from the reticular nucleus. Therefore an intact feedback circuit is needed for this type of activity. This implies that when discussing the mechanisms responsible for rhythmic behavior, we must emphasize the dynamics of the neuronal networks, considering (but not overemphasizing) the intrinsic activities of the different types of neurons (Lopes da Silva, 1991; Buzsáki, 1991). In this sense the thalamic neurons differ essentially from the heart cells of the sinoatrial node that can maintain oscillatory behavior, even in the absence of specific input other than energetic. Nevertheless, the reticular nucleus neurons can display oscillating spindles after disconnection from their inputs, but the origin of the oscillations probably depends on a change in driving forces (Steriade, 1993).

Freeman (1992) also addressed this issue of whether oscillations occur as a property of neurons that oscillate intrinsically as individuals or through synaptic interactions among neurons that may, or may not, oscillate individually. Based on his observations in paleocortex that 90° phase lags occur between the activity of closely situated neurons, Freeman concluded that interneuronal feedback is the basis for cortical oscillations rather than the intrinsic autonomous oscillations of individual neurons.

Until this point we have considered whether neuronal oscillations may be considered autonomous, focusing on the generation of thalamic rhythmic activities of low frequency. However, we should also consider whether the same principle applies to other forms of rhythmic activity. In this respect, we must discuss the cellular basis of the relatively high-frequency activity in the beta/gamma range of the neocortex, which recently prompted much interest because it is prominent in the awake state and it may play a role in perception (Gray et al, 1990, Eckhorn et al, 1988) and consciousness (Llinás and Ribary, 1993).

It is useful to consider first that neocortical cells can be classified in three groups according to physiologic and morphologic criteria (Connors et al, 1982; Connors and Gutnick, 1990; McCormick et al, 1985).

1. Fast spiking neurons: These have fast action potentials (0.5 milliseconds) and do not accommodate prolonged depolarization; morphologically they correspond to nonpyramidal neurons, probably inhibitory interneurons.

2. Regular spiking neurons: The action potentials have a duration of about 1.5 milliseconds and are usually followed by different types of after-potentials; they rapidly accommodate prolonged depolarization; morphologically they are classified as pyramidal cells of medium and small size.

3. Intrinsic bursters: At threshold they react by generating a burst of action potentials; in response to prolonged depolarization, they generate both bursts and single spikes with little adaptation; morphologically they have been identified as the large pyramidal cells of layer V.

Within the subgroup of neocortical interneurons, a division into two classes of "oscillations" has been proposed by Llinás and colleagues (1991)—"broad" and "narrow" frequency oscillators. The former respond to current pulses by the sequential activation of voltage-gated sodium and potassium conductances, leading to irregular oscillatory firing in the range of 10 to 40 Hz, depending on membrane potential. The latter show subthreshold oscillations that are independent of the membrane potential if a certain degree of depolarization is attained. The average frequency of the oscillations is 44.7 ± 4.64 Hz (at 37°C). Action potentials occur at the peak of the membrane oscillations. Based on these experimental findings, Llinás (1992) proposed the following hypothesis to account for the high-frequency (about 40 Hz) oscillation. The input from the thalamus that impinges on inhibitory interneurons of the cortical layer IV provides sufficient depolarizing input so that the membrane of these neurons are able to oscillate at about 40 Hz. In this way, IPSPs at this frequency would be generated in the pyramidal cells, as shown by Gray and coworkers (1989) and Ferster and Koch (1987). According to the same hypothesis, and because the cortical pyramidal cells project back to the thalamus, both to TCR and reticular nucleus (RE) cells, the latter would receive a rhythmic input at about 40 Hz.

The plausibility of this hypothesis is not very strong because Gray and coworkers (1989) did not find 40-Hz oscillations in the thalamus. This corroborates observations from our laboratory of rhythmic activity in the beta frequency range (18 to 40 Hz) over the visual cortex of the visually attentive dog, whereas no such rhythmicity was encountered in the lateral geniculate nucleus (Lopes da Silva et al, 1970). However, oscillations in the 40 Hz range have been recorded in the cat from the ventral mesencephalic tegmentum (Montaron et al, 1982), which represent a close relation to oscillations in the same frequency range over discrete cortical areas, specifically a frontal beta focus in motor areas 4 and 6 and a parietal focus in area 5, whereas no similar oscillations were recorded from the somatosensory cortex (areas 1, 2, and 3) (Bouyer et al, 1987). Furthermore, Steriade and associates (1991) reported the presence of fast oscillations (20 to 40 Hz) in some thalamocortical neurons and the potentiation of these oscillations in cortical EEG by brainstem cholinergic projections relayed in the thalamus. Our study in the awake dog, in which different subareas over the cortex displayed rhythmic activities within the beta range but at different dominant frequencies, and studies in the cat by Bouyer and colleagues (1987) indicate that a monorhythmic oscillation recordable directly over the whole neocortex was not found experimentally. Thus a uniform 40-Hz oscillatory system over the whole neocortex and thalamus is not likely.

Local Network Properties

Before considering the local network properties that play an essential role in the oscillatory behavior of TCR cells, we must address the role of synaptic processes in the activation and modulation of local neuronal activity. We will also consider the thalamic circuits as an example of a local network.

Synaptic Processes: Activators and Modulators

Extrinsic and intrinsic synaptic processes are distinguished by whether the corresponding axons belong to cells within the same brain structure or outside it. In relation to the TCR cells, the primary intrinsic circuit within the thalamus consists of two main cell types in addition to the TCR cells: the RE neurons and the intrinsic local neurons (IN), as shown in Figure 5-2. The RE forms a layer of neurons that surrounds the thalamic-specific and midline nuclei and receives collaterals from the axons of TCR cells. Their axons provide the inhibitory synaptic input to the TCR cells and also to the IN. Both the RE and IN cells are gamma-aminobutyric acid (GABA)-ergic, which means that the feedback from RE to TCR cells is inhibitory. This inhibitory feedback, and probably also that of the local INs, can be considered an intrinsic activator of the rhythmic behavior of the thalamic network, because it is required for at least some of the oscillatory modes to occur. In contrast, we may consider the other synaptic inputs as mainly modulators of the network activity. This means that they can help to change the mode of activity. The latter mainly provide extrinsic control over the network.

These extrinsic inputs consist of cholinergic pathways, noted above, noradrenergic and serotonergic pathways, regardless of whether they occur in combination with neuropeptidergic synapses. The cholinergic inputs can play an important role as modulators because they change the modes of activity of the thalamic circuits. As indicated above, the cholinergic synaptic input to the TCR cell decreases potassium conductance and thus induces a depolarization bias, whereas it increases potassium conductance in the RE neurons, leading to the hyperpolarization of these cells. In this way, the intrinsic inhibitory feedback loop between the TCR and RE neurons becomes inoperative and the lower-frequency range oscillations that depend on the contribution of the IPSP, mediated in this way, can no longer occur. Spindle types of rhythmic oscillations that occur in the thalamus and in the cortex are modulated critically by the state of the cholinergic inputs. The modulating role of the noradrenergic and serotonergic inputs can be considered in light of in vitro and in vivo studies, as discussed later in this chapter.

As noted previously, different types of oscillations can occur in the specific thalamic nuclei. Under anesthesia, particularly with barbiturates, the conditions for the occurrence of low-frequency rhythmic oscillations are met. However, under

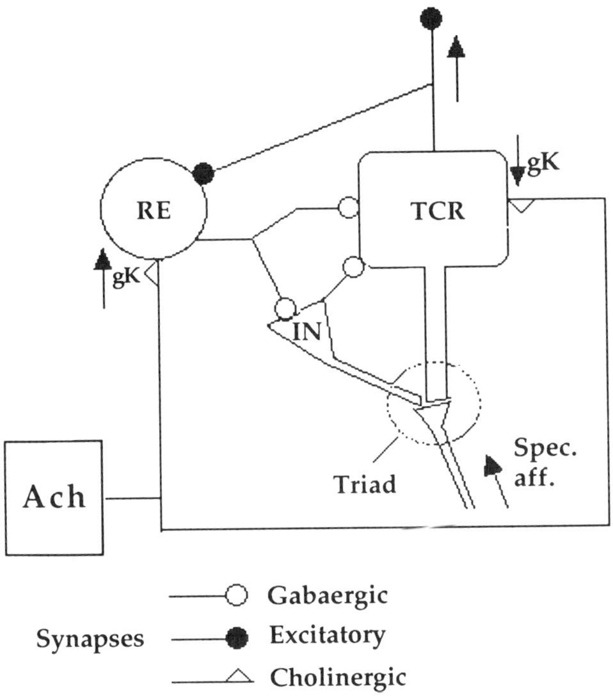

Figure 5-2. Simplified scheme of a thalamic neuronal network. The thalamocortical relay cell (TCR); the reticular thalamic neuron (RE), and the local interneurons (INs) are indicated along with projections from cholinergic (Ach) and other modulating inputs. The synaptic triad formed by the dendrites of TCR and IN neurons with the specific afferent (spec aff) fibers is also indicated. Three types of synapse are shown: excitatory, GABAergic (inhibitory), and cholinergic. The effect of the latter on RE neurons is assumed to be an increase in potassium conductance (g_K), whereas on TCR neurons the effect is the opposite. (Adapted with permission from Lopes da Silva, 1991).

normal conditions in the awake animal, specifically during eyes closure, in which alpha rhythm dominates (Lopes da Silva et al, 1973a), the state of depolarization of TCR cells and the amount of RE feedback are probably different from that under barbiturate anesthesia, because higher-frequency oscillations of the alpha frequency range usually occur. Indeed barbiturate spindles and alpha oscillatory bursts differ in frequency content and also in the degree of correlation between signals recorded from different brain areas (Lopes da Silva et al, 1973b). This means that we must also account for the network dynamics and the interarea relations when we consider the occurrence and distribution of rhythmic activities in the brain.

We have described the conditions necessary for relatively low-frequency oscillations to occur in thalamocortical circuits. But what about oscillations occurring at other frequency ranges? They appear also to depend on initial conditions and control parameters set by input activity. Indeed previously we indicated that the

40-Hz oscillation of the inhibitory interneurons of layer IV of neocortex also depends on a sufficient depolarizing bias provided by afferent synaptic inputs. We must always account for the initial conditions and external control that are essential for bringing individual neurons into oscillation. Generally these conditions are met as a consequence of the activity of specific and nonspecific inputs.

Feedforward and Feedback Loops

Until now, we have considered the thalamic circuits as a paradigm for local network interactions responsible for EEG rhythmic activity. However, not all structures are organized in the same way, although some general principles are apparently valid for most brain systems. Here we examine basic aspects of the organization of local networks of the neocortex. Generally a local network consists of a characteristic cell type, such as the TCR cells of the thalamus or the pyramidal cells of layer IV of the neocortex, and of populations of interneurons that provide inhibitory and excitatory feedback. Furthermore, the primary extrinsic input may not impinge directly on the main cell type but only through feedforward inhibitory, or excitatory, local pathways. These principles of organization are shown in Figure 5-2. Because here we are interested primarily in the dynamics of the neocortex, we will determine how such a general scheme is justified by considering current knowledge of the anatomy and physiology of neocortex.

The neocortex, in contrast to the thalamus, has many excitatory interconnec-

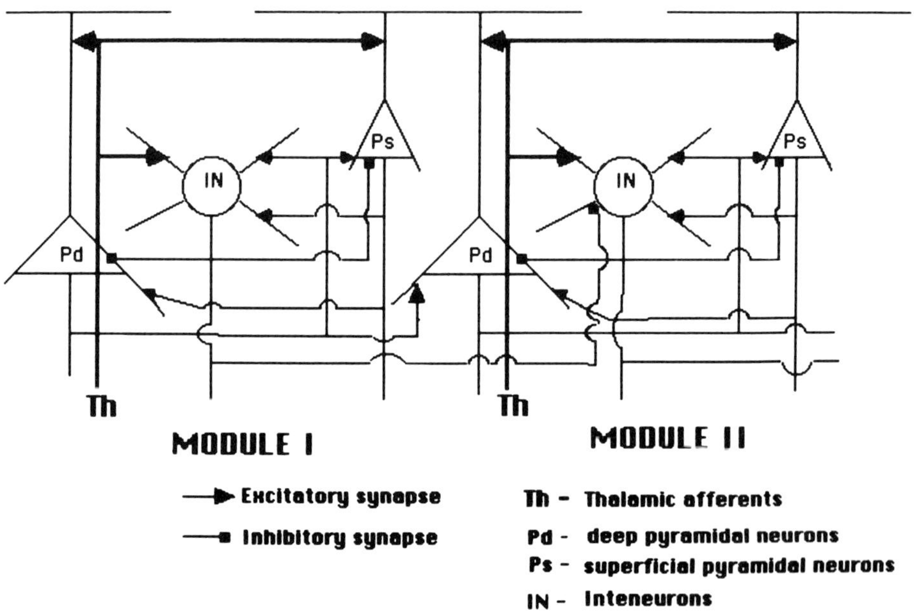

Figure 5-3. A chain of cortical neurons interconnected by excitatory and inhibitory synaptic contacts.

tions. Quantitative anatomy of the neocortex indicates that, at least in the mouse, probably 85% of the synapses are excitatory (type I) and only 15% are inhibitory (type II) (Braintenberg and Schüz, 1991; see also Chapter 2). An interesting feature of inhibitory synapses is that a few presumed inhibitory synapses are created on interneurons. Excitatory synapses are made on pyramidal cells and on interneurons, regardless of whether the latter are inhibitory or excitatory. In this way, the scheme of Figure 5-3 describes the different types of feedforward and feedback loops encountered in neocortex.

We noted that strong experimental evidence for the importance of feedback loops in neuronal networks as the basis for oscillatory behavior is based on the fact that phase lags of 90° have been encountered between the activity of inhibitory and excitatory neurons, with the former lagging the latter (Freeman, 1975; Eeckman and Freeman, 1990). This 90° degree phase shift can be explained by the dynamics of the network represented in Figure 5-3. Indeed, here we can distinguish four steps in the interneuronal dynamics: (1) activation of the excitatory neurons, (2) activation of the inhibitory neurons, (3) inhibition of the excitatory neurons, and (4) disexcitation of the inhibitory neurons and subsequent disinhibition of the excitatory neurons. Through these steps, a whole cycle (360°) can restart. According to this scheme, maximal excitatory activity is preceded by minimal inhibitory activity that occurs one quarter of a cycle earlier. In Freeman's study (1992), the mean passive time constant was 4.5 milliseconds in many cortical neurons. We may also assume that most excitatory synapses occur on the dendrites, that the mean dendritic cable delay is about 2.3 milliseconds, and that a spike delay of about 0.5 millisecond occurs. If all neurons of the feedback loop had identical properties, these values would result in a 25-millisecond cycle, which corresponds to a dominant frequency of about 40 Hz.

Synchrony and Spatial Propagation

First we will consider how synchrony occurs in neuronal populations, particularly in the cortex, and also how synchronous activity is organized in the spatial domain, that is, whether and how propagation of cortical activity occurs.

In general EEG signals and other types of local field potentials (LFPs) are manifestations of the synchronous activity of neuronal assemblies. This implies that cortical neurons can form active assemblies, or populations, that show a high degree of synchrony. Such synchrony can be shown using signal analysis techniques, specifically by computing auto- and cross-correlation functions of single or multiple spike trains (Abeles and Gerstein, 1988; Gerstein et al, 1983), spike-triggered averaging of local field potentials (or local EEG), or by calculating the probability of firing of populations of single units conditional on the LFPs (Freeman, 1987). Studies of this type were conducted extensively in the olfactory regions of the brain (Freeman, 1975), the entorhinal cortex (Eeckman and Freeman, 1990), the hippocampus (Horowitz, 1972), the auditory cortex (Abeles, 1982), and the motor cortex (Allum et al, 1982). Furthermore, synchronous activity of multiple neurons in the visual cortex was described (Eckhorn et al, 1988; Gray et al, 1989;

Engel et al, 1990). Of course we must consider whether synchrony between the firing of single neurons is determined by a common input, a question which is discussed below.

We note that the relation between the activity of neuronal assemblies and local EEG signals should not be reduced to a relation between spike trains and LFPs, because there are other aspects of neuronal activity that can directly contribute to the LFPs, specifically subthreshold soma-dendritic membrane potentials. In the context of this discussion, the quantitative aspects of the relation of neuronal activity and LFP should be emphasized. Regarding this issue, two studies are particularly relevant. Nunez (1981 and Chapter 1 of this volume) estimated that the relative contribution of synchronous generators (represented by M) to a given local EEG, to asynchronous neuronal generators (N), uniformly distributed in a cortical volume, can be expressed by $M/\sqrt{N}$. A numerical example of the application of this rule yields the following result: Assuming that the cortex can be subdivided into "square root compartments," as proposed by Braitenberg and Schüz (1991), each one containing 10^5 neurons and having a cross-section of 1 mm in humans, we can estimate the contribution to the LFP of 10% synchronous neurons among a population of 90% asynchronous neurons. This contribution of the 10% synchronous neurons would be 32 times greater than that contributed by the rest of the population.

This simple model clearly illustrates how strongly the amplitude of the local EEG depends on the synchrony of the underlying neurons. In fact, if this synchrony did not exist, it would be difficult to record any EEG signal at a distance from its sources. In addition, different aspects of the scalp EEG appear to have clearly different properties regarding the degree of synchrony of the underlying generators. In a recent study of the spatial variance of EEG/MEG signals in humans, de Munck and colleagues (1992) suggested that although alpha activity can be described by a statistical model consisting of clustered sources with a fixed position and varying amplitude, activity within the other frequency bands appears to be generated by randomly distributed sources that generate EEG signals with a covariance that depends only on interelectrode distance.

What is the anatomic and physiologic substrate responsible for the synchrony? The basic substrate for synchrony in neuronal populations is the existence of groups of neurons interconnected by mutual excitatory and inhibitory synaptic connections, as indicated in Figure 5-3. We are particularly interested in this organization of the cortex, because the cortical activity is of paramount importance for understanding EEG phenomena. Quantitative anatomy (Braitenberg and Schüz, 1991) shows that cortical pyramidal neurons contact, probably by excitatory synapses, about as many other pyramidal neurons as they have synapses, which accounts for about 8000 in a compartment of 1 mm cross-section in the mouse. These form the short-range intracortical connections. At this level divergence of the outputs of one neuron to many other neurons is strong, as is convergence of inputs from many cells onto a given pyramidal neuron. Regarding the synaptic contacts of the other types of cortical neurons, specifically the stellate cells, or interneurons, no quantitative data are available, but inhibitory synapses probably are not as diffusely spread over the dendritic trees of other neurons as are excitatory synapses. Therefore they may be more effective than their relatively small number would suggest, because they tend to be concentrated on specific sites of the soma/axon hillock and on dendrites of pyramidal neurons. Sometimes these synapses may be particularly effective, as in the example of chandelier cells that synapse at the axon hillock of the target cells (Somogyi et al, 1983).

In addition to the short-range system of intracortical connections, the pyramidal neurons also have axon collaterals that leave the cortex for the white matter and re-enter another distant cortical area. These corticocortical connections constitute the long-range system. The short-range system terminates mainly on the deep layers of the cortex, that is, on the basal dendrites of pyramidal neurons, whereas the long-range connections terminate in the upper cortical layers—on the apical ramifications of these neurons. When considering these characteristics of the anatomic substrate of the cortical organization, we must examine corresponding physiologic properties. The most relevant aspect of the latter is revealed by studying the correlations between cortical neurons. In the visual cortex of the cat, Toyama and associates (1981) found two main types of correlation between neurons. According to one type, the action potential of one neuron is followed by excitation of another cell with a time delay of 1 millisecond and lasting 5 to 15 milliseconds. In another case, an action potential is followed by inhibition of the other cell lasting 40 to 80 milliseconds. Nelson and coworkers (1992) computed cross-correlations between pairs of neuronal spike trains. They found essentially a slow type of cross-correlogram with a half-peak width of 100 to 1,000 milliseconds (mean, 400 milliseconds) and faster types with means of 3 or 30 milliseconds.

Similar results were obtained by Vijn (1992) using a "synchrony" measure (that is, a normalized correlation value); he reported correlations between a single spike and the local field potentials over at least 2 seconds that had a broad spatial extent sometimes covering one visual area in the cat. This study showed clearly that the EEG frequency bands that showed synchrony with single action potentials were not limited to the high-frequency range but also included relatively low frequencies. These results were obtained with no stimulation. During visual stimulation, this rather widespread form of synchrony decreased. In addition, Nelson and coworkers (1992) reported that the low-frequency type of cross-correlogram was found primarily with no stimulation, whereas high-frequency synchronous oscillations were encountered in the stimulated state.

In several studies, high-frequency synchrony between series of spikes of cortical neurons was evident during specific forms of stimulation (Eckhorn et al, 1988; Gray et al, 1989; Gray and Singer, 1987, 1989). These authors found clear synchronous firing of small populations of cortical neurons, even in anaesthetized animals, with visual stimulation. The discharge pattern of these neurons was typically oscillatory in the high-frequency range (20 to 70 Hz, called beta or gamma ranges). Synchronous discharges were usually recorded between neurons within the same or adjacent cortical areas. In most other studies, substantial cross-correlations of spike trains were found only to distances of 2 mm between recording sites (Toyama et al, 1981; Michalski et al, 1983; Ts'o et al, 1986). More recently, phase locking of oscillatory responses at a distance as great as 7 mm over the cortical surface were reported (Gray et al, 1989; Gray et al, 1992; Engel et al, 1990), even between symmetric areas over the two hemispheres (Engel et al, 1990). The correlations of spindles recorded from several cortical sites were stronger the nearer the corresponding receptive fields were positioned. In addition, correlations between oscillatory spindles of the LFPs and single-cell spike trains were found. Cortical oscillations in the beta/gamma frequency range at the single-cell level are matched by LFPs (or local EEG) and have rhythmic activities within the same frequency range, particularly during visual attentive states, as recorded in dogs (Lopes da Silva et al, 1970), cats (Bouyer et al, 1981; Rougeul-Buser et al, 1979), and humans (Sheer, 1976).

An important issue in the context of this discussion is whether evidence exists for propagated activity over the cortical surface. The data on cross-correlation functions, whether of single-cell spike trains for LFPs, is not very consistent in this respect. Eckhorn and associates (1992) reported that phase differences between correlated beta/gamma oscillations recorded from several cortical sites could be recorded up to 180°, but they did not find a systematic phase shift with distance along the cortical surface. Indeed they concluded, as Engel and colleagues (1991) did, that the average phase difference between most recording positions was zero. Nevertheless Gray and associates (1992) reported that consistent time delays in the cross-correlograms of 5 milliseconds between two spike trains, oscillating with a period of 22 milliseconds, could be observed. This is particularly interesting because this time lag corresponds to a phase difference of about 82°, which indicates that the two cells may be connected by an inhibitory feedback loop. Accordingly, this experimental evidence supports the idea that the cortical network subserving this type of rhythmic activity consists of excitatory and inhibitory neurons connected by feedback loops, as the scheme of Figure 5-3 indicates.

In contrast to the lack of clear evidence for a consistent pattern of propagation over the cortical surface of the beta/gamma oscillations, experimental evidence shows such propagation of the lower frequency rhythmic activity in the alpha range. Using the dog for an experimental model, the local generation of alpha rhythms within layer IV/V of the cortex (Lopes da Silva and Storm van Leeuwen, 1977) was shown, and phase shifts corresponding to propagation velocities over the cortical surface of 0.3 m/second were measured (Lopes da Silva and Storm van Leeuwen, 1978). In addition, Wright and Sergejew (1991) estimated that the velocity of waves propagating over the occipital-parietal cortex of the cat in the 1- to 30-Hz frequency range was 0.1 to 0.3 m/second.

A theoretical study of the behavior of a chain of cortical neurons, with random input, showed that these experimental findings were compatible with the following model of the cortical neuronal network responsible for the alpha rhythmic activity (van Rotterdam et al, 1982):

1. The relation between input and output spike densities can be described approximately by second-order transfer functions, in which the inhibition has a longer time constant than the excitation.

2. The strength of the interconnectivity decreases exponentially with distance.
3. The characteristic length of the spatial decay of the inhibition and of the excitation was about 160 to 330 μm. The quantitative data used in this model to obtain a good fit to the experimental results were in the same range as the dimensions of the basic cortical space module, that is, a corticocortical column of 200 to 300 μm diameter (Szentágothai, 1978).

In formal terms, the behavior of a chain of neurons responsible for the generation and propagation of rhythmic activity over cortical tissue can be described by a non-linear partial differential equation, as discussed in van Rotterdam and associates (1982). Excellent reviews of similar theories and models of the generation of EEG rhythmic activities are by Lagerlund and Sharbrough (1988); Wright and Kydd (1992), who tried to integrate different theoretical approaches; and Jansen and coworkers (1992), who developed a model to explain the relation between "spontaneous" EEG and evoked potential activity. It is, of course, of particular interest to relate the finding of short waves at the milimmetric scale over the cortex to long-wavelength activity at the global brain level, noted by Nunez (1989). The global approach is discussed in Chapter 2 and treated in detail in Chapter 11. Possible relations between small- and large-scale EEG are summarized in Figure 3-26.

Interaction Between Local Systems and Modulating Systems

Previously we addressed local neuronal networks responsible for oscillatory, synchronous activity in the cortex. We emphasized that the shift in mode of activity of the thalamic and cortical neurons under natural conditions depends on the state of afferent activity. Accordingly, these inputs should be considered the modulators of the thalamocortical circuits, as indicated in Figure 3-8. They are responsible for setting the initial conditions and control parameters that determine the mode of activity of the neuronal elements within the neuronal networks.

Next we will consider how this local cortical activity is influenced by modulating systems involving subcortical structures and how this interaction is important in explaining some general properties of EEG phenomena. Specifically we discuss the influence of chemical systems arising from subcortical structures on thalamocortical circuits.

Three main chemical systems can be distinguished in this respect: the cholinergic, the noradrenergic, and the serotonergic. Without becoming too specific (for details see Steriade et al, 1990), we know that the main action of the inputs mediated by these neurotransmitters on the thalamocortical circuits is to shift the operating point of these circuits from the "burst firing mode" that corresponds to a state characterized by decreased transfer of information from the periphery to the cortex, as seen during drowsiness, into a "single-spike firing mode" (tonic activity) associated with increased responsiveness to different inputs, which occurs during alert states.

The biophysical substrate of these actions was clarified in the last decade.

Acetylcholine (Ach) has several rather complex actions on thalamocortical relay and on reticular nucleus neurons. Local application of Ach on TCR, and also on neocortical cells, induces fast depolarization associated with increased membrane conductance (mediated through nicotinic receptors), followed by slow hyperpolarization (muscarinic receptors) associated with decreased potassium conductance (McCormick and Prince, 1987). Stimulation of brainstem cholinergic systems causes a depolarized state associated with blocked potassium currents (McCormick, 1990), corresponding to an EEG state characterized by the absence of well-defined rhythmic activity, that is, by the "desynchronized state." On reticular nucleus neurons, the application of Ach causes hyperpolarization mediated by muscarinic receptors (M2 subtype; McCormick and Prince, 1986). This hyperpolarization of the reticular nucleus neurons on the one hand, and the depolarization of the thalamocortical neurons on the other, decreases the inhibitory feedback in the thalamic circuit and thus causes the disappearance of the conditions necessary for rhythmic activity to occur. Several assemblies of cholinergic neurons exist in the forebrain and brainstem; the most rostral assemblies located in the nucleus basalis project directly to the neocortex, and those situated in the pontomesencephalic reticular formation project to thalamic nuclei (for more detail see Mesulam, 1988). Activation of the cholinergic system arising in the nucleus basalis can directly modulate the neocortical circuits, block neurons of the reticular nucleus, and suppress the oscillations generated in the thalamocortical feedback neuronal networks (Buzsáki et al, 1988).

Related to actions of the cholinergic system, the possibility that the diffusible messenger nitric oxide may also play a role in regulating oscillatory activity in TCR cells was suggested recently by Pape and Mager (1992). The enzyme responsible for nitric oxide synthesis, nitric oxide synthase is localized specifically in the cholinergic brainstem–thalamic fibers. Activation of these fibers can lead to release of nitric oxide onto TCR cells and can evoke a voltage-dependent inward current that increases with the level of hyperpolarization. This indicates that nitric oxide modulates the hyperpolarization-activated cation current (I_h) (McCormick and Pape, 1990). In this way the Ca^{2+}-mediated burst activity that is essential for the oscillatory mode is greatly reduced. Activation of the cholinergic fibers probably can release nitric oxide and Ach. Because nitric oxide is readily diffused, this activation may control the functional state of the entire thalamocortical neuronal network.

Noradrenaline (mediated through alpha$_1$ receptors) and serotonin (through 5-HT$_2$ and possibly 5-HT$_{1c}$) cause, on the one hand, a mixed Na^+/K^+ current in thalamocortical neurons, reducing the ability of these neurons to fire rhythmic bursts (Pape and McCormick 1989). On the other hand, they induce in the neurons of the thalamic reticular nucleus a slow depolarization with a decrease in input conductance that is mediated by a decrease in "leak" potassium conductance (McCormick and Wang, 1991). This slow depolarization biases the membrane potential of these neurons in such a way that burst firing is inhibited, whereas single-spike activity is promoted. However, the action of noradrenaline on thalamocortical neurons may be rather complex because the application of this drug may block thalamic bursting through $alpha_1$ while promoting it through $alpha_2$ receptors (Buzsáki et al, 1990). The end result will depend on a balance between the two subsystems that is not clear.

In addition, a particular type of cortical oscillatory state, characterized by beta/gamma activity (35 to 40 Hz) recorded from the motor and parietal cortex of the cat (Bouyer et al, 1987) during attentive behavior, appears to depend on an integral dopaminergic system because it is suppressed by lesions of the ventral tegmental area (Montaron et al, 1982). The state of cortical networks characterized by the beta/gamma mode of activity may correspond to an optimum for synaptic transfer (Sheer, 1976; Steriade et al, 1990).

Experimental evidence, based mainly on investigations of the effects of pharmacologic manipulation of the cholinergic and the serotoninergic systems, both on behavior and on the EEG, shows that neocortical EEG activity in the fast frequency range (beta/gamma) is regulated primarily by direct ascending cholinergic and serotonergic inputs on the neocortex that bypass the thalamus (Vanderwolf and Stewart, 1988; Vanderwolf, 1992).

Complex Nonlinear Dynamics and Bifurcations: Transition to Epileptic Behavior

Our knowledge of the intrinsic properties of the neurons responsible for the EEG phenomena, as described above, allows us to conclude that these act as essential nonlinear elements that possess not only static, such as threshold and saturation, but also dynamic nonlinearities that are voltage dependent. The neuronal networks considered here must be regarded as dynamic nonlinear systems. Furthermore, the existence of feedforward and feedback connections with distributed time delays make the behavior of these networks complex. This complexity is accentuated by the existence of intricate modulating inputs that can affect these networks at several sites and in different ways, depending on multiple regulating factors. Therefore it is not surprising that several researchers have applied, in the last decade, the relatively new mathematical notions and techniques of "complex dynamic nonlinear systems" to the study of neuronal processes.

In the section Synchrony and Spatial Propagation we suggested that activity in a chain of neurons can be described formally by a nonlinear partial differential equation that was linearized to obtain an analytical solution (van Rotterdam et al, 1982). The linearized equations yielded the following dispersion relation relating frequency (ω) to wave number (k):

$$D_L(k, \omega) = \frac{(j\omega + b)^2(j\omega + a)^2(k^2 + c^2)(k^2 + d^2) + Q(abcd)^2}{(j\omega + b)^2(k^2 + c^2)(k^2 + d^2)(1 + Q)a^2} = 0 \quad (5.1)$$

Here, a^{-1} and b^{-1} are excitatory and inhibitory postsynaptic potential rise times, respectively. Also excitatory and inhibitory intracortical connections were assumed to decrease exponentially with characteristic distances c^{-1} and d^{-1}, respectively. Q is a nondimensional control parameter characterizing the strength of coupling between excitatory and inhibitory neurons. The notation has been altered from the original paper to be consistent with theoretical studies presented in Chapter 11.

Equation (5.1) yields two pairs of roots, $\omega_i(k)$, representing two branches of the dispersion relation (two separate kinds of wave phenomena). Traveling waves are predicted with phase velocities ω_{Ri}/k, depending on the characteristic lengths for the fall-off of numbers of excitatory and inhibitory intracortical synaptic contacts and PSP rise times. Phase velocities observed with "micro-EEG" electrodes in recording of canine alpha rhythm have been reported to be in the 0.3 to 1.2 m/second range (Lopes da Silva and Storm van Leeuwen, 1978). Uncertainty in cortical histology and physiology makes precise comparisons impossible, but observed and predicted phase velocities appear to have the same order of magnitude. This description of alpha waves of short wavelength propagating away from various cortical epicenters (similar to waves caused by rain drops on a pond) contrasts with the more macroscopic view of scalp EEG as composed of standing and traveling waves of spatial wavelength comparable to head size, as described in Chapter 11. However, these two views are not mutually exclusive, as discussed in Chapters 2, 3, 11, 13, and 14.

The intracortical parameters c and d apparently are in the general range of 30 to 500 cm^{-1}. The poorly conducting skull and other volume-conductive effects limit scalp recordings to wave numbers with k less than 0.5 to 1.0 cm^{-1} (Nunez, 1981; Chapter 1). Thus, for purposes of comparison with scalp EEG (or cortical recordings using electrodes of diameters that are several millimeters larger), we can set $k = 0$ in (5.1). For Q less than but of the order of the threshold value

$$Q_{TH} = \frac{(a + b)^2}{ab} \tag{5.2}$$

(5.1) yields two pairs of complex roots $\omega_i = \omega_{Ri} - j\gamma_i$, of which one pair is "overdamped," $|\gamma/\omega_R| > 0.5$. The other pair becomes more weakly damped as the coupling constant (control parameter) Q approaches the threshold. For $Q > Q_{TH}$, this pair of roots becomes unstable. The frequencies of the pair of modes for Q near Q_{TH} are

$$\omega_R = \pm\sqrt{ab} \tag{5.3}$$

In the examples discussed by van Rotterdam and associates (1982), EPSP and IPSP rise times of $a^{-1} \sim 10$ milliseconds and $b^{-1} \sim 20$ milliseconds, respectively, were assumed so that with these parameters frequencies in the alpha range would predominate, that is

$$|\omega_R| = 71 \text{ rad/sec or } f \approx 11 \text{ Hz} \tag{5.4}$$

We must realize that the linearization above represents a large simplification. Indeed, the behavior of these neuronal networks can be described better by a set of coupled nonlinear differential equations both in space and time. An important property of such neuronal networks and the corresponding equations (those with more than two degrees of freedom) is that they can display unpredictable behavior over long time scales. In the mathematical language of nonlinear dynamics, this means that they can display chaotic behavior. We can then state that the system has a strange, or chaotic, attractor. Indeed, such systems can have multiple stable states that can be characterized by the type of attractor. The idea of an attractor, in the sense used here, should be clarified. A dynamic system can be described by plotting the evolution of the time variables $\{X_1(t), \ldots X_n(t)\}$ in n-dimensional space; the system's dynamics can then be given by trajectories representing the evolution of the system with time. The set of trajectories that correspond to the state of dynamic equilibrium, that is, the state reached after transients disappear, is called an attractor of the system. Three main types of attractors can be distinguished: the point attractor, which occurs when the system has a steady output; the limit cycle attractor, which occurs with periodic oscillations; and the strange, or chaotic, attractor, which occurs when the system exhibits aperiodic or quasi-periodic, broad-spectrum activity (for more detail see Thompson and Stewart, 1986 or Chapter 10 of this book). Complex dynamic systems may exhibit different states characterized by the corresponding type of attractor, depending on initial conditions and on the system's control parameters. Thus they can exhibit bifurcations (radical changes in dynamic properties resulting from parameter changes) between different states of the same system.

An interesting theoretical issue is whether the neuronal networks responsible for the EEG phenomena discussed here exhibit chaotic oscillations. A practical question is how to determine this, given a sample of EEG signal. The answer is not simple. Several researchers approached this question by computing parameters that describe the behavior of the attractor, such as the Lyapunov exponents and the correlation dimension (Schuster, 1984). A practical limitation of these computations is that, in general, just a relatively short time sample of the characteristic, usually noisy, EEG signal is disposed. Furthermore, these signals are generated by systems with several inputs that can also be noisy. Therefore, it may be difficult or impossible to distinguish "noise" from "chaos" under these circumstances. Thus several analyses of EEG reported in the literature do not give a clear answer to this question.

Recently Pijn and coworkers (1991) calculated the correlation dimension of EEG signals recorded under different behavioral conditions, using surrogate signals to control for false-positive conclusions about the existence of a chaotic state. They concluded that EEG states characteristic of a restful awake state or an active exploratory state in the rat could not be distinguished from complex filtered noise, whereas the EEG typical of epileptiform seizure activity behaved as a chaotic signal of relatively low dimension (between 2 and 4). A similar result was found for human EEG recorded from the temporal and frontal cortex using subdural and depth electrodes (Pijn, personal communication).

Another limitation on these kinds of studies is that application of mathematical tools used to characterize the dynamics of complex systems implies that these systems are autonomous (Grassberger and Procaccia, 1983). This is not the case for brain signals under usual conditions (Freeman 1992). Because a low correlation dimension was found during epileptiform seizures suggests that the neuronal networks behave quasi-autonomously in this state. This is a reasonable assumption because the brain is unresponsive to environmental inputs during most types of seizures. Although not using surrogate signals for control, Babloyantz and Destexhe (1986) also found a low dimension (about 2) during a petit mal seizure recorded from a patient's scalp. Freeman (1988) reported a low correlation dimension for EEG signals recorded from the olfactory system in animals during a state of relaxed and unmotivated waking and during a form of partial complex seizure that resembles petit mal seizure in humans. A recent survey of the relevant literature on the topic of the interpretation of EEG signals as manifestations of chaotic behavior in complex dynamic neuronal networks was completed by Basar and colleagues (1989).

Summary

Our understanding of the processes responsible for the generation of EEG and MEG phenomena recently has advanced considerably. Several advances should be mentioned in conclusion because they have made the most important contributions to our new insights.

First, experimental knowledge has accumulated in the last decade on intrinsic membrane properties of single neurons that comprise part of the neuronal networks underlying EEG phenomena.

Second, new data has been developed on the microscopic structure of these networks, including the pattern of interconnections between different types of neurons and the functional organization of the chemical systems that regulate and modulate their behavior.

Third, the construction of computer models and the performance of simulation studies has clarified the behavior of these networks in terms of elementary and global properties.

Fourth, recently developed mathematical tools, derived from the theory of complex dynamic systems provide a new approach for the analysis of such complex nonlinear systems and may allow us to bridge the gap between the microscopic level of the neuron and the more macroscopic level of the local cortical and subcortical fields, as revealed by EEG signals.

A combination of research along these different lines, in a multidisciplinary setting and performed as a cooperative effort, is necessary to increase our understanding of the functional organization of complex neuronal networks and of the physiologic importance of the electrophysiologic signals that they generate. Multidisciplinary issues are discussed in many different contexts in other parts of this book.

Acknowledgments

The expert secretarial help of Truc Ngo-Ha and Cristine Knaap-Cabi is gratefully acknowledged.

References

Abeles, M. Studies of brain function. In: *Local Cortical Circuits: An Electrophysiological Study*. Berlin: Springer-Verlag, pp. 28–30, 1982.

Abeles, M. and Gerstein, G.L. Detecting spatiotemporal firing patterns among simultaneously recorded single neurons. *J. Neurophysiol.* 60:909–924, 1988.

Allum, J.H.J., Hepp-Raymond, M.C., and Gysin, R. Cross-correlation analysis of interneuronal connectivity in the motor cortex of the monkey. *Brain Res.* 231:325–334, 1982.

Andersen, P. and Andersson, S.A. *Physiological Basis of the Alpha Rhythm*. New York: Appleton-Century-Crofts, 1968.

Avanzini, G., de Curtis, M., Panzica, F., and Spreafico, R. Intrinsic properties of nucleus reticularis thalami neurones in the rat studied in vitro. *J. Physiol.* (London). 416:111–112, 1989.

Babloyantz, A. and Destexhe, A. Low-dimensional chaos in an instance of epilepsy. *Proc. Nat. Acad. Sci. USA*. 83:3513–3517, 1986.

Basar, E., Basar-Eroglu, C., Röschke, J., and Schütt, A. The EEG is a quasi-deterministic signal anticipating sensory-cognitive tasks. In: *Brain Dynamics*. (E. Basar and Bullock, T.H., Eds.) Berlin: Springer-Verlag, pp. 43–71, 1989.

Bouyer, J.J., Montaron, M.F., and Rougeul, A. Fast fronto-parietal rhythms during combined focused attentive behavior and immobility in cat: Cortical and thalamic localizations. *Electroencephogr. Clin. Neurophysiol.* 51:244–252, 1981.

Bouyer, J.J., Montaron, M.F., Vahneé, J.M., Albert, M.P., and Rougeul, A. Anatomical localization of cortical beta rhythms in cat. *Neuroscience*, 22:863–869, 1987.

Braintenberg, V. and Schüz, A. *Anatomy of the Cortex. Statistics and Geometry*. Berlin: Springer-Verlag, 1991.

Buzsáki, G. The thalamic clock: Emergent network properties. *Neuroscience*. 41:351–364, 1991.

Buzsáki, G., Bickford, R.G., Ponomareff, G., Thal, L.J., Mandel, R., and Gage, F.H. Nucleus basalis and thalamic control of neocortical activity in the freely moving rat. *J. Neuroscience*. 8:4007–4026, 1988.

Buzsáki, G., Laszlovszky, I., Lajtha, A., and Vadasz, C. Spike-and-wave neocortical patterns in rats: Genetic and aminergic control. *Neuroscience*. 38:323–333, 1990.

Connors, B.W. and Gutnick, M.J. Intrinsic firing patterns of diverse neocortical neurons. *Trends in Neuroscience*. 13:99–104, 1990.

Connors, B.W., Gutnick, M.J., and Prince, D.A. Electrophysiological properties of neocortical neurons in vitro. *J. Neurophysiology*. 48:1302–1320, 1982.

de Munck, J.C., Vijn, P.C.M., and Lopes da Silva, F.H. A random dipole model for spontaneous activity. *IEEE Trans. Biomed. Eng.* 39:791–804, 1992.

Eckhorn, R., Bauer, R., Jordan, W., Brosch, M., Kruse, W., Munk, M., and Reitboeck, H.J. Coherent oscillations: A mechanism of feature linking in the visual cortex? Multiple electrode and correlation analysis in the cat. *Biol. Cybern.* 60:121–130, 1988.

Eckhorn, R., Schanze, T., Brosch, M., Salem, W., and Bauer, R. Stimulus-specific synchronizations in cat visual cortex: Multiple microelectrode and correlation studies from several cortical areas. In: *Induced Rhythms in the Brain*. (E. Basar and Bullock, T.H., Eds.) Boston: Birkhäuser, pp. 47–80, 1992.

Eeckman, F.H. and Freeman, W.J. Correlations between unit firing and EEG in the rat olfactory system. *Brain Res.* 528:238–244, 1990.

Engel, A.K., König, P., Gray, C.M., and Singer, W. Stimulus-dependent neuronal in cat visual cortex: Inter-columnar interaction as indicated by cross-correlation analysis. *Exp. Neurol.* 6:12–29, 1990.

Engel, A.K., König, P., Kreiter, A.K., and Singer, W. Interhemispheric synchronization of oscillatory neuronal responses in cat visual cortex. *Science.* 252:1177–1179, 1991.

Ferster, D. and Koch, C. Neuronal connections underlying orientation selectivity in cat visual cortex. *Trends in Neuroscience.* 10: 487–492, 1987.

Freeman, W.J. *Mass Action in the Nervous System.* New York: Academic Press, 1975.

Freeman, W.J. Techniques used in the search for the physiological basis of the EEG. In: *Handbook of Electroencephalography and Clinical Neurophysiology.* Vol. 3A. Part 2. (A.S. Gevins and Remond, A., Eds.) Amsterdam: Elsevier, pp. 583–664, 1987.

Freeman, W.J. Strange attractors that govern mammalian brain dynamics shown by trajectories of electroencephalographic (EEG) potential. *IEEE Trans. Circ. Syst.* 35:781–783, 1988.

Freeman, W.J. Predictions on neocortical dynamics derived from studies in paleocortex. In: *Induced Rhythms in the Brain.* (E. Basar and Bullock, T.H., Eds.) Boston: Birhäuser, pp. 183–201, 1992.

Gerstein, G.L., Bloom, M.J., Espinosa, I.E., Evanzuk, I.E., and Turner, M.R. Design of a laboratory for multineuron studies. *IEEE Trans. Syst. Man. Cyber.* SMC-13: 668–676, 1983.

Grassberger, P. and Procaccia, I. Measuring the strangeness of strange attractors. *Physica.* 9D:189–205, 1983.

Gray, C.M., Engel, A.K., König, P., and Singer, W. Mechanisms underlying the generation of neuronal oscillations in cat visual cortex. In: *Induced Rhythms in the Brain.* (E. Basar and Bullock, T.H., Eds.) Boston: Birkhäuser, pp. 29–45, 1992.

Gray, C.M., König, P., Engel, A.K., and Singer, W. Oscillatory responses in cat visual cortex exhibit inter-columnar synchronization which reflects global stimulus properties. *Nature.* 338:334–337, 1989.

Gray, C.M., Engel, A.K., König, P., and Singer, W. Stimulus-dependent neuronal oscillations in cat visual cortex: Receptive field properties and feature dependence. *Eur. J. Neurosci.* 2:607–619, 1990.

Gray, C.M. and Singer, W. Stimulus-specific neuronal oscillations in orientation columns of cat visual cortex. *Proc. Natl. Acad. Sci.* USA, 86:1698–1702, 1989.

Gray, C.M. and Singer, W. Stimulus specific neuronal oscillations in the cat visual cortex: A cortical functional unit. 2nd IBRO Congress, *Neuroscience* (Suppl.), p. 1301, 1987.

Horowitz, J.M. Evoked activity of single units and neural populations in the hippocampus of the cat. *Electroencephogr. Clin. Neurophysiol.* 32:227–240, 1972.

Jahnsen, H. and Llinás, R. Electrophysiological properties of guinea-pig thalamic neurons: An in vitro study. *J. Physiol.* (London). 349:205–226, 1984a.

Jahnsen, H. and Llinás, R. Ionic basis for the electroresponsiveness and oscillatory properties of guinea-pig thalamic neurones in vitro. *J. Physiol.* (London). 349:227–247, 1984b.

Jansen, B.H.J., Zouridakis, G., and Brandt, M.E. A neurophysiologically-based mathematical model of flash visual evoked potentials. *Biol. Cybern.* 68:275–283, 1993.

Lagerlund,T.D. and Sharbrough, F.W. Computer simulation of neuronal circuit models of rhythmic behavior in the electroencephalogram. *Comput. Biol. Med.* 18:267–304, 1988.

Llinás, R. Oscillations in CNS neurons: A possible role for cortical interneurons in the generation of 40-Hz oscillations. In: *Induced Rhythms in the Brain.* (E. Basar and Bullock, T.H., Eds.) Boston: Birkhäuser, pp. 269–286, 1992.

Llinás, R.R., Grace, A.A., and Yarom, Y. In vitro neurons in mammalian cortical layer 4 exhibit intrinsic oscillatory activity in the 10- to 50-Hz frequency range. *Proc. Natl. Acad. Sci.* USA. 88:897–901, 1991.

Llinás, R. and Ribary, U. Coherent 40-Hz oscillation characterizes dream state in humans. *Proc. Natl. Acad. Sci.* USA. 90:2078–2081, 1993.

Lopes da Silva, F.H. Neural mechanisms underlying brainwaves: From neural membranes to networks. *Electroencephogr. Clin. Neurophysiol.* 79:81–93, 1991.

Lopes da Silva, F.H., Van Rotterdam, A., Storm van Leeuwen, S., and Tielen, A.M. Dynamic characteristics of visual evoked potentials in the dog. II. Beta frequency selectivity in evoked potentials and background activity. *Electroencephogr. Clin. Neurophysiol.* 29:260–268, 1970.

Lopes da Silva, F.H., Van Lierop, T.H.M.T., Schrijer, C.F., and Storm van Leeuwen, W. Organization of thalamic and cortical alpha rhythms: Spectra and coherences. *Electroencephogr. Clin. Neurophysiol.* 35:627–639, 1973a.

Lopes da Silva, F.H., Van Lierop, T.H.M.T., Schrijer, C.F., and Storm van Leeuwen, W. Essential differences between alpha rhythms and barbiturate spindles: Spectra and thalamo-cortical coherences. *Electroencephogr. Clin. Neurophysiol.* 35:641–645, 1973b.

Lopes da Silva, F.H. and Storm van Leeuwen, W. The cortical source of the alpha rhythm. *Neurosci. Lett.* 6:237–241, 1977.

Lopes da Silva, F.H. and Storm van Leeuwen, W. The cortical alpha rhythm in dog: The depth and surface profile of phase. In: *Architecture of the Cortical Cortex.* (M.A. Brazier and Petsche M., Eds.) New York: Raven Press, pp. 319–333, 1978.

McCormick, D.A. Cellular mechanisms of cholinergic control of neocortical and thalamic neurons. In: *Brain Cholinergic Systems.* (M. Steriade and Biesold, D., Eds.) Oxford: Oxford University Press, pp. 236–264, 1990.

McCormick, D.A., Connors, B.W., Lighthall, J.W., and Prince, D.A. Comparative electrophysiology of pyramidal and sparsely spiny stellate neurons of the neocortex. *J. Neurophysiol.* 54:782–806, 1985.

McCormick, D.A. and Prince, D.A. Acethylcholine induces burst firing by activating a potassium conductance. *Nature.* 319:402–405, 1986.

McCormick, D.A. and Prince, D.A. Actions of acethylcholine in the guinea-pig and cat medial and lateral geniculate nuclei in vitro. *J. Physiol.* (London). 392:147–165, 1987.

McCormick, D.A. and Pape, H.-C. Properties of a hyperpolarization-activated cation current and its role in rhythmic oscillation in thalamic relay neurons. *J. Physiol.* 431:291–318, 1990.

McCormick, D.A. and Wang, Z. Serotonin and noradrealine excite GABAergic neurones of the guinea-pig nucleus reticularis thalami. *J. Physiol.* (London). 442:235–155, 1991.

Mesulam, M.-M. Central cholinergic pathways: Neuroanatomy and some behavioral implications. In: *Neurotransmitters and Cortical Function.* (M. Avoli, Reader, T.A., Dykes, R.W., and Gloor, P., Eds.). New York: Plenum, 237–260, 1988.

Michalski, A., Gerstein, G.L., Czarkowska, J., and Tarnecki, R. Interactions between cat striate cortex neurons. *Exp. Brain Res.* 51:97–107, 1983.

Montaron, M.-F., Bouyer, J.-J., Rougeul, A., and Buser, P. Ventral mesencephalic tegmentum (VMT) controls electrocortical beta rhythms and associated attentice behaviour in the cat. *Behav. Brain Res.* 6:129–145, 1982.

Nelson, J.I., Salin, P.A., Munk, M.H.J., Arzi, M., and Bullier, J. Spatial and temporal coherence in cortico-cortical connections: A cross-correlation study in areas 17 and 18 in the cat. *Visual Neuroscience.* 9:21–37, 1992.

Nunez, P.L. *Electric Fields of the Brain.* New York: Oxford University Press, 1981.

Nunez, P.L. Generation of human EEG by a combination of long and short range neocortical interactions. *Brain Topography.* 1:199–215, 1989.

Pape, H.-C. and Mager, R. Nitric oxide controls oscillatory activity in thalamocortical neurons. *Neuron.* 9:441–448, 1992.

Pape, H.C. and McCormick, D.A. Noradrenaline and serotonin selectively modulate thalamic burst firing by enhancing a hyperpolarization–activated cation current. *Nature* 340:175–178, 1989.

Pijn, J.-P., Van Neerven, J., Noest, A., and Lopes da Silva, F.H. Chaos or noise in EEG signals; dependence on state and brain site. *Electroencephogr. Clin. Neurophysiol.* 79:371–381, 1991.

Rougeul-Buser, A., Bouyer, J.J., Dedet, L., and Debray, O. Fast somatoparietal rhythms during combined focal attention and immobility in baboon and squirrel monkey. *Electroencephogr. Clin. Neurophysiol.* 46:310–319, 1979.

Schuster, G.H. *Deterministic Chaos, An Introduction.* Weinheim: Physik-Verlag, 1984.

Sheer, D.E. Focused arousal and 40-Hz EEG. In: *The Neurophysiology of Learning Disorders.* (R.M. Knights and Bakker, D.J., Eds.) Baltimore: University Park Press, pp. 71–78, 1976.

Somogyi, P., Kisvarday, Z.F., Martin, K.A.C., and Whitteridge, D. Synaptic connections or morphologically identified and physiologically characterized large basket cells in the striate cortex of cat. *Neuroscience.* 10:261–294, 1983.

Somogyi, P., Nunzi, M.G., Gorio, A., and Smith, A.D. A new type of specific interneuron in the monkey hippocampus forming synapses exclusively with the axon initial segments of pyramidal cells. *Brain Res.* 259:137–142, 1983.

Steriade, M. Cellular substrates of brain rhythms. In: *Electroencephalography: Basic Principles, Clinical Applications and Related Fields.* (E. Niedermeyer, and Lopes da Silva, F.H., Eds.) Baltimore: Williams and Wilkins, pp. 27–62, 1993.

Steriade, M. and Llinás, R.R. The functional states of the thalamus and the associated neuronal interplay. *Physiological Reviews.* 68:649–742, 1988.

Steriade, M., Deschênes, M., Domich, L., and Mulle, C. Abolition of spindle oscillations in thalamic neurons disconnected from nucleus reticularis thalami. *J. Neurophysiol.* 54:1473–1497, 1985.

Steriade, M., CurroDossi, T., Pare, D., and Oakson, G. Fast oscillations (20–40 Hz) in the thalamo-cortical systems and their potentration by mesopontine cholinergic nuclei in the cat. *Proc. Natl. Acad. Sci.* USA. 88:4396–4400, 1991.

Steriade, M., Gloor, P., Llinás, R.R., Lopes da Silva, F.H., and Mesulam, M.M. Basic mechanisms of cerebral rhythmic activities. *Electroencephogr. Clin. Neurophysiol.* 76:481–508, 1990.

Szentágothai, J. The local neuronal apparatus of the cerebral cortex. In: *Cerebral Correlates of Conscious Experience.* Inserm Symposium No. 6. (P. Buser and Rougeul-Buser, A., Eds.) Amsterdam: Elsevier, pp. 131–138, 1978.

Thompson, J.M.T. and Stewart, H.B. *Nonlinear Dynamics and Chaos*. New York: Wiley, 1986.

Toyama, K., Kimura, M., and Tanaka, K. Cross-correlation analysis of interneuronal connectivity in cat visual cortex. *J. Neurophysiology*. 46:191–201, 1981.

Ts'o, D.Y., Gilbert, C.D., and Wiesel, T.N. Relationships between horizontal interactions and functional architecture in cat striate cortex as revealed by cross-correlation analysis. *J. Neurosci.* 6:1160–1170, 1986.

Vanderwolf, C.H. The electrocorticogram in relation to physiology and behavior: A new analysis. *Electroencephogr. Clin. Neurophysiol.* 82:165–175, 1992.

Vanderwolf, C.H. and Stewart, D.J. Thalamic control of neocortical activation: A critical re-evaluation. *Brain Res. Bull.* 20:529–538, 1988.

van Rotterdam, A., Lopes da Silva, F.H., van den Ende, J., Viergever, M.A., and Hermans, A.J. A model of the spatial-temporal characteristics of the alpha rhythm. *Bull. Math. Biol.* 44:283–305, 1982.

Vijn, P.C.M. Coherent Neuronal Activity Underlying the EEG. Ph.D. thesis. The Netherlands: University of Amsterdam, 1992.

Wright, J.J. and Kydd, R.R. The electroencephalogram and cortical neural networks. *Network*. 3:341–362, 1992.

Wright, J.J. and Sergejew, A.A. Radial coherence, wave velocity and damping of electrocortical waves. *Electroencephogr. Clin. Neurophysiol.* 79:403–412, 1991.

6

Steady-State Visually Evoked Potentials, Brain Resonances, and Cognitive Processes

RICHARD B. SILBERSTEIN

A rapid change in a sensory stimulus evokes a transient evoked potential (EP) and, if this stimulus occurs repetitively at a rate high enough to prevent the EP from returning to a baseline state, the elicited response is called a steady-state evoked potential (Regan, 1966, 1989). This chapter begins with a discussion of the steady-state evoked potentials elicited by visual stimuli, in the context of the brain mechanisms responsible for the generation of driven rhythmic activity. This is followed by a consideration of the steady-state visually evoked potential (SSVEP) as a core component of a method to study brain electrophysiologic correlates of cognitive processes. Readers interested in pursuing the broader topic of steady-state potentials are referred to Regan's monograph on this subject (Regan, 1989).

The Steady-State Visually Evoked Potential

A distinctive feature of the SSVEP is that it comprises sinusoidal components at the stimulus frequency and its harmonics; thus any specific harmonic of the SSVEP is completely specified when the amplitude and the phase difference between the stimulus and response are known (Speckreijse et al, 1977, Regan, 1989). For brevity, and unless otherwise stated, the phase difference between stimulus and response will simply be called the SSVEP "phase." This spectral purity can be exploited to yield high signal-to-noise ratios and thus make the SSVEP a useful tool to study the neural processes underlying brain rhythmic activity.

The amplitude and phase of the SSVEP are a function of the frequency, modulation depth, and spatial structure of the driving stimulus (Regan, 1989; Speckreijse and Reits, 1982; Tyler et al, 1978; Van Der Tweel and Verduyn Lunel, 1965). An unstructured sinusoidal visual flicker will elicit a sinusoidal SSVEP

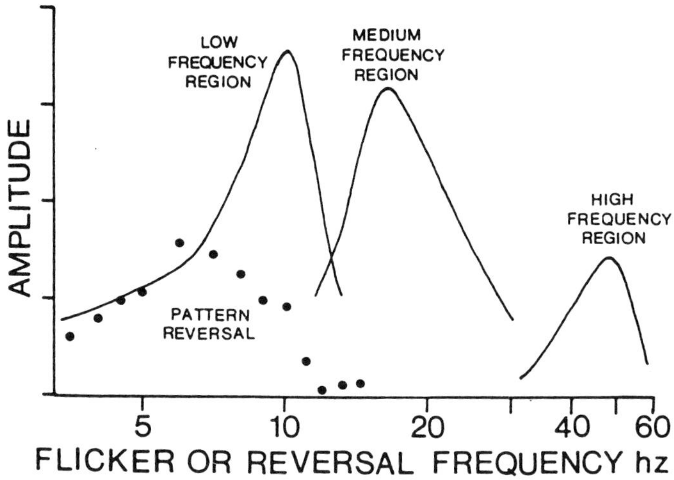

Figure 6-1. Amplitude spectrum of SSVEP for unstructured and structured stimuli. The amplitude of the SSVEP elicited by an unstructured flicker is indicated by solid lines. The dotted line represents the amplitude of the SSVEP produced by an alternating checkerboard. The checkerboard response occurs at twice the reversal frequency, that is, at the alternation frequency. (Modified with permission from Regan, 1989.)

characterized by a frequency tuning curve with three peaks. These are illustrated in Figure 6-1, in which the amplitude peaks occur at frequencies of approximately 10 Hz, 20 Hz, and 40 Hz. Each of these peaks is thought to be associated with a distinct "frequency channel" (Regan, 1989) having a characteristic latency. This apparent latency of the SSVEP can be determined from the variations of SSVEP phase with reference to the stimulus frequency. With the SSVEP, elicited by an unstructured flicker, the latency of the response elicited by stimuli in the frequency range of 4 to 15 Hz is approximately 200 to 275 milliseconds, whereas those elicited between 18 and 30 Hz are associated with a latency of approximately 85 to 120 milliseconds; those elicited above 40 Hz have a latency of approximately 30 to 60 milliseconds.

In contrast to the three peaks of the SSVEP tuning curve elicited by an unstructured flicker, an alternating checkerboard elicits an SSVEP at the alternation rate, with only one amplitude maximum at approximately 10 Hz and an associated latency of approximately 270 milliseconds (Regan, 1972, 1989).

Visual Pathways

Some brief comments on visual pathways and neurophysiology are needed before considering the cortical mechanisms that may underlie some features of the SSVEP. Considerable evidence exists for at least two parallel and complementary visual processing pathways. One originates predominantly in the smaller retinal ganglion cells concentrated in the foveal or central region of the retina and is called P cells

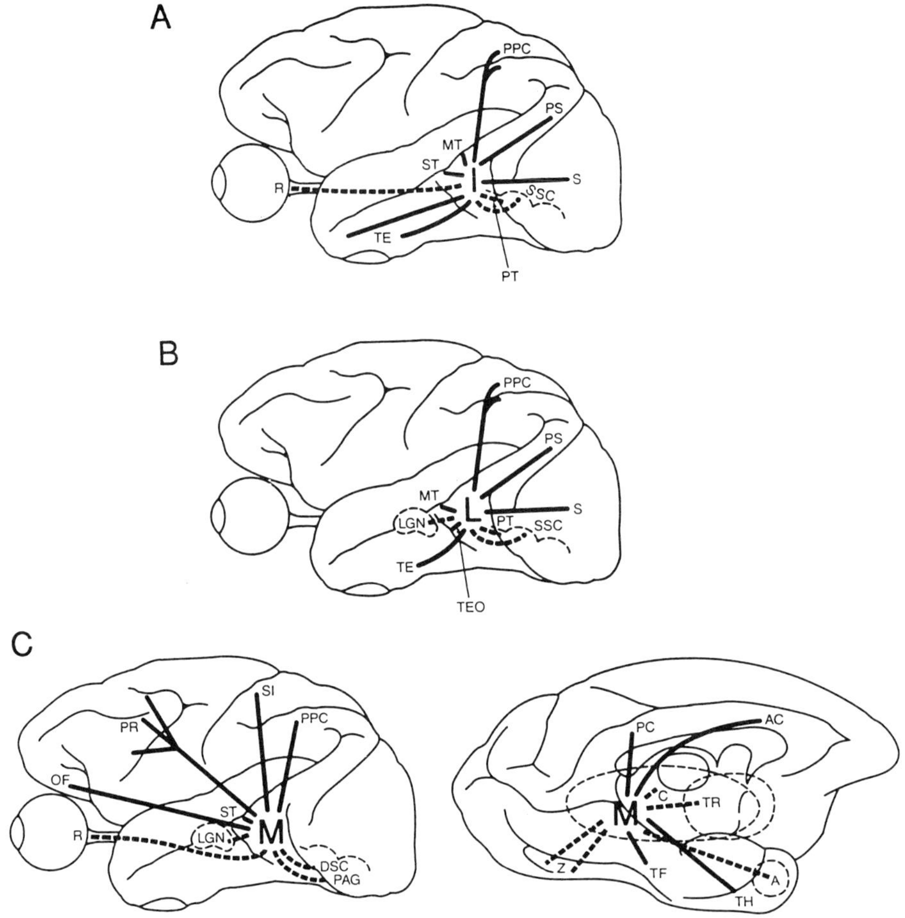

Figure 6-2. Anatomic connections of subdivisions of the pulvinar. **A**. The cortical and subcortical pathways of the cytoarchitectonically defined inferior pulvinar (I). **B**. The relation of the cytoarchitectonic lateral pulvinar (L) with other parts of the brain. **C**. Lateral and medial surfaces of the brain showing pathways of the cytoarchitectonically defined medial subdivision of the pulvinar (M). Because most cortical connections are reciprocal, directions are not specified. Dashed lines indicate subcortical structures and pathways. A = amygdala; AC = anterior cingulate cortex; C = claustrum; DSC = deep layers of superior colliculus; LGN = lateral geniculate nucleus; MT = middle temporal cortex; OF = orbitofrontal cortex; PAG = periaqueductal gray; PC = posterior cingulate cortex; PPC = posterior parietal cortex; PR = prefrontal cortex; PS = prestriate cortex; PT = pretectum; R = retina; S = striate cortex; SI = primary somatosensory cortex; SSC = superficial layers of superior colliculus; ST = superior temporal cortex; TE, TEO, TF, and TH = von Bonin and Bailey subdivisions of temporal cortex; TR = thalamic reticular nucleus; "Z" = brainstem sites including locus coeruleus, abducens, pedunculo-pontine tegmental, and dorsal raphe nuclei. (Reproduced with permission from Robinson and Petersen, 1992.)

(Bodis-Wollner et al, 1990). The P-retinal ganglion cells are characterized by moderate conduction velocities, small receptive fields, strong center surround inhibition, high-contrast sensitivity, and a tendency to adapt slowly to a stationary stimuli. Such features make this system ideal for conveying information about contrast and spatial structure of slowly changing visual stimuli (Merigan, 1991; Van Essen et al, 1992).

In addition to the P cells, another retinal ganglion cell population comprising larger cells has been called M cells. The M cells are distributed more widely throughout the retina and are characterized by high conductions velocities, larger receptive fields, lower-contrast sensitivity, and rapid adaptation to a stationary stimulus. These features are optimal for rapidly conveying information about changes in the visual environment. The populations also differ in terms of their response to a sinusoidal stimulus. The P system of cells appears to respond best over a range of frequencies from 1 to 20 Hz, whereas the M system can respond over a wider range of 5 to 40 Hz (Derrington and Lennie, 1984; Van Essen et al, 1992). The differences in temporal response are apparent in the electroretinogram (ERG), in which pattern-contrast reversal is undetectable beyond 20 Hz, whereas the ERG elicited by a uniform field flicker is apparent at 40 Hz (Baker and Hess, 1984).

Differences at the retinal level are preserved throughout the later stages of cortical and subcortical processing of visual information (see Figure 6-2). The P system projects primarily to the parvocellular layer of the lateral geniculate nucleus (LGN), whereas the M system projects primarily to the magnocellular layer of the LGN, the pulvinar nucleus of the thalamus, and the superficial layers of the superior colliculus (SC). The pulvinar nucleus is especially prominent in primates (Bender, 1988; Robinson and Petersen, 1992). The cortical projection patterns of both systems remain segregated in the striate and visual association areas. One of the largest differences between these systems is apparent from the projections of the SC and pulvinar nucleus. These nuclei do not process information conveyed by the P system but only the M system. In addition to the M projections of the LGN, there are also the M projections of the pulvinar and SC, which include several cortical areas such as the striate cortex, visual association cortex, temporal cortex, primary somatosensory cortex, and prefrontal cortex (Robinson and Petersen, 1992; Schiller, 1985; Van Essen et al, 1992).

These neuroanatomic differences are also complemented by a range of functional differences. The M system responds best to rapid, low-contrast, or diffuse changes in luminance, whereas the P system appears optimized for high contrast and high spatial frequency. The differences in spatial sensitivity between the M and P systems are also reflected in differences in temporal sensitivity, with the M system responding to higher temporal frequencies. The P system therefore responds most effectively to visual stimuli characterized by low temporal frequencies and rapid spatial variations in luminance, whereas the M system is optimized for higher temporal frequencies and lower spatial variations in luminance.

Spatial variation in luminance is frequently characterized in terms of spatial frequency, with units of cycles per degree. If the stimulus repeats itself spatially, as in a sinusoidal grating, the number of repetitions per degree subtended at the observer is the spatial frequency. Strictly speaking, this definition is only true for sinusoidal gratings, although two-dimensional Fourier transforms allow us to apply the concept to any two-dimensional visual structure (see Figure 1-15). Restating the differences between the M and P systems in terms of the temporal and spatial characteristics of the optimum visual stimuli, the M system is optimized for high temporal and low spatial frequencies, whereas the P system is optimized for low temporal and high spatial frequency. These differences are also reflected in the latency of the SSVEP elicited by visual stimuli preferentially activating the M or P system. Repetitive visual stimuli possessing high temporal frequencies, low spatial frequencies, or both preferentially activate the M system with its higher conduction speeds and thus give rise to shorter SSVEP latencies (Tyler et al, 1978). These findings were confirmed with magnetic recordings by Williamson and colleagues (1978), who showed that the steady-state visually evoked field latency decreased with decreasing spatial frequency of the visual stimulus.

The differences between the M and P systems also may account for the observation that the SSVEP elicited by a checkerboard (high spatial frequency) has a single maximum at approximately 10 Hz, whereas the SSVEP elicited by an unstructured flicker (low spatial frequency) possesses maxima at 10, 20, and 40 Hz. With small checks, the checkerboard stimulus would preferentially activate the P system, which operates over a lower range of temporal frequencies than the M system. This implies that activity evoked by alternating visual stimuli, with a high spatial frequency composition, is more strongly low pass filtered than the activity evoked by unstructured stimuli, which preferentially activate the M system. The M system therefore is more likely to stimulate the cortex at higher temporal frequencies than is the P system. If the 10-, 20-, and 40-Hz peaks reflect global or local cortical resonance properties (Nunez, 1989; Chapters 2 and 3), the M system, with its wider temporal bandwidth, is more likely to activate the 20-Hz and 40-Hz peaks, whereas the P system, with its smaller bandwidth, can only activate the 10-Hz frequency resonant mode.

A report of SSVEPs in the 20-Hz range, which are evoked by isoluminance color stimuli (Regan, 1970) is an apparent inconsistency with this explanation. These stimuli are organized to present a rapid variation in color with constant luminance or subjective brightness. Because color information is processed almost exclusively by the P system (Eskin and Merigan, 1986), the above model would predict that such stimuli could only elicit a low-frequency SSVEP peak, similar to the checkerboard SSVEP.

Reconciliation of this model with the existence of 20-Hz isoluminance SSVEPs can be achieved by recognizing the practical difficulty of achieving a completely isoluminant stimulus with color variation (Le Grand, 1972). The color balance required to achieve isoluminance varies slightly with retinal location. A restricted color-varying stimulus that is isoluminant in the central retina might not be so in the peripheral retina (Regan, 1989, p. 450). This would yield a luminance variation that may be able to activate the M system. The experimental problem is compounded further by trying to generate isoluminant stimuli with high spatial frequencies, such as checkerboards. Such stimuli are likely to give rise to chromatic aberrations that, in turn, deviate from the isoluminant condition and thus allow luminance variations.

Signal Processing

Most signal-processing techniques that exploit the spectral characteristics of the SSVEP use an analog or digital variant of Fourier analysis. This entails integrating the product of the EEG signal with sine and cosine waveforms phase locked to the sinusoidal stimulus waveform, yielding the sine and cosine Fourier coefficients of the EEG signal. This is equivalent to narrow band filtering of the EEG, with a filter centered precisely at the stimulus frequency. The bandwidth of this filter is determined largely by the duration of the integration period, in which longer integration periods yield more narrow bandwidths of the filter.

Is there an optimal integration period? The answer depends on the temporal variations of the SSVEP. If the SSVEP amplitude is unchanging over an interval T, all the signal power at the stimulus frequency is concentrated in a bandwidth 1/T, and it is appropriate to set the integration period to T. If, on the other hand, the SSVEP amplitude is changing, then the bandwidth of the SSVEP will be proportional to the bandwidth of the signal controlling the SSVEP amplitude. Under these circumstances, the integration period is a tradeoff between noise reduction and bias. A longer integration period will yield a more narrow bandwidth and thus lower noise. This lower noise is purchased at the price of a reduced capacity to follow temporal changes in the SSVEP. If we are prepared to discard the time-varying component of the SSVEP, we can increase the integration duration to yield a frequency resolution limited only by the recording duration.

A specific advantage of using Fourier analysis to estimate the SSVEP is the relative noise and artifact insensitivity of this technique (Regan, 1989; Silberstein et al, 1992). This is a consequence of the fact that most common artifacts, such as electro-oculograph (EOG) and electromyelography (EMG), have their power distributed over a range of frequencies. In contrast, all of the SSVEP signal power is concentrated at the stimulus frequency or its harmonics. Considering the Fourier analyzer as a narrow band filter, its artifact sensitivity is estimated by determining the ratio of the artifact variance before Fourier analysis to the artifact variance after Fourier analysis. The larger this ratio, the larger the attenuation and therefore the lower the sensitivity to this artifact. This ratio has been evaluated for EMG, eye-blink artifacts, and EOG. With the integration period set to 10 seconds (Silberstein et al, 1992b) the ratio is 1.0 for the SSVEP at the stimulus frequency (indicating no attenuation) is 4,300 for EMG, 11,000 for EOG, and 19,000 for eye-blink artifacts. Knowing the level of attenuation applied to the artifacts enables us to determine appropriate thresholds for the rejection of artifact-contaminated EEG epochs. The issue of artifact sensitivity is critically important when considering the electrophysiologic correlates of cognitive processes. Some findings have been invalidated by the subsequent discovery that electrophysiologic artifacts have contaminated the results (Karson et al, 1987).

Two aspects of the SSVEP are considered in subsequent sections. In the next section, high-frequency resolution techniques examine the amplitude and phase topography of the SSVEP. The major context for this discussion is the possible contribution of traveling and standing waves to the scalp and cortical topography. In a subsequent section, frequency resolution is reduced to increase temporal resolution for an examination of changes in the SSVEP topography associated with cognitive processes.

Phase and Amplitude Topography of the SSVEP

Unlike the high- and intermediate-frequency components of the SSVEP, the low-frequency SSVEP appears to originate over a wider area than the visual cortex (Speckreijse et al, 1977). As such, the mechanisms responsible for the low-frequency SSVEP are more likely to provide information about general mechanisms underlying both driven and spontaneous rhythmic activity. In this section, we consider certain features of the low-frequency SSVEP amplitude and phase distribution in light of the possible contribution of cortical wave-like processes to the genesis of the SSVEP.

The topography of the low-frequency SSVEP is generally characterized by an amplitude maximum in the occipitoparietal region. Sometimes this occipitoparietal amplitude maximum is accompanied by a smaller amplitude maximum in the frontal region. The phase topography of the SSVEP shows considerable intersubject variability, with some participants exhibiting little variation in phase over the scalp, others showing a larger smooth variation in phase, whereas a third group may have one or more sharp 180° phase discontinuities. In a study of 40 subjects, we noted that approximately 40% showed a continuous variation in phase along the midline, whereas approximately 30% showed a sharp 180° phase change between electrodes Cz and Pz (Silberstein et al, 1992a). Those scalp SSVEP topographies with a sharp 180° phase change also exhibited a sharp minimum in amplitude in the vicinity of the phase change. Figure 6-3 illustrates two typical examples of the smooth and discontinuous phase variations. Before commenting on the significance of the smooth phase variations, we should briefly consider the mechanisms that may contribute to the phase discontinuity.

We suggest that at least two possible mechanisms could account for the sharp phase change and the associated amplitude minimum. The most simple explanation assumes the existence of a driven tangential dipole oriented parallel to the midline and located in the vicinity of the Rolandic fissure of each hemisphere. Such an interpretation is consistent with the conclusions of Kaufman and Williamson, who examined the brain magnetic field elicited by a visual stimulus comprising a vertical grating, the velocity of which was changed sinusoidally at a frequency of 7 Hz. They suggested that the evoked magnetic fields could be accounted for by two sets of generators in each hemisphere, a pair of occipital dipoles and a pair of

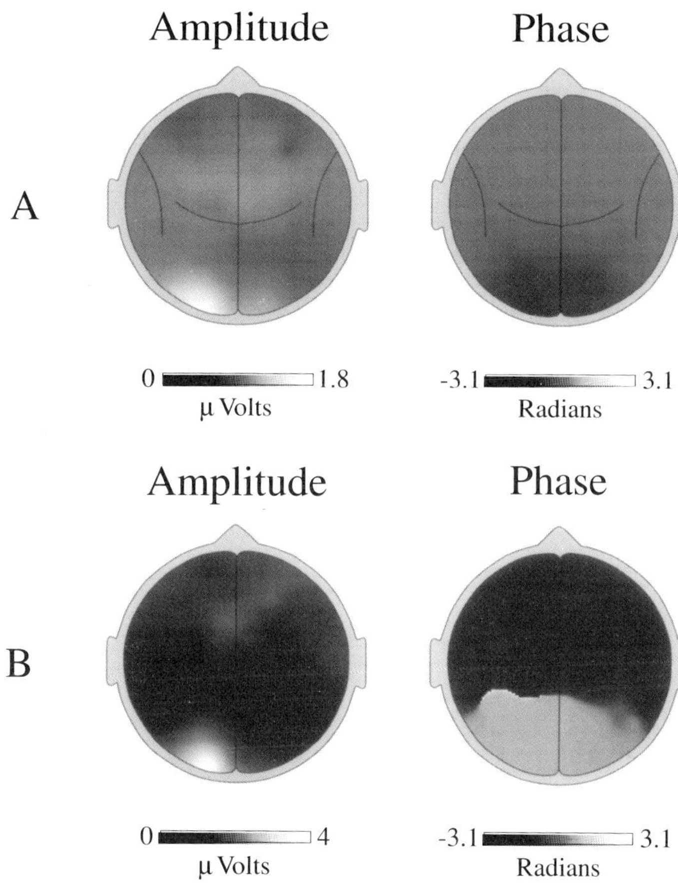

Figure 6-3. Topography of the SSVEP evoked by an unstructured 13-Hz visual flicker in two subjects. Participant A showed continuous variation in phase along the midline, whereas subject B showed a 180° discontinuity in phase along the midline. The amplitude minimum coincides with the region of most rapid phase change.

deep tangential dipoles located in the Rolandic fissure (Kaufman and Williamson, 1990; Lounasmaa et al, 1985).

Another explanation for the sharp phase change and amplitude minimum presupposes the existence of two radial dipole layers, with a 180° phase difference in each hemisphere. In each hemisphere, one such dipole layer would be situated in the frontal region whereas the other would be located in the parietal region. Radial dipole layers with such characteristics would be consistent with standing wave patterns in which the responses on either side of a nodal line have a phase difference of exactly 180°. One way to distinguish between these two possibilities is to examine the temporal correlation between anterior and posterior maxima or poles. A single tangential dipole of time-varying amplitude in each hemisphere should yield a high correlation between the amplitudes at each of the two poles.

If, on the other hand, the topography is the result of a pair of radial dipole layers in each hemisphere, the correlation should vary widely, depending on the extent to which a common mechanism, such as arousal, modulates both radial dipole layers. Preliminary studies indicate that some subjects with the sharp 180° phase change show a low correlation (less than 0.26) that does not appear to be accounted for by the contribution of uncorrelated noise (Silberstein et al, 1992a). This suggests that the radial dipole layer pair explanation probably better accounts for some aspects of the observed topography.

Traveling Waves and Continuous Variations in Phase

In approximately 40% of participants, the SSVEP shows not a sharp change but rather a smooth variation in phase along the midline. A typical example of the smooth phase distribution is illustrated in Figure 6-3B. A single dipole cannot account for such a distribution. This spatial variation in phase is consistent with several possible models, including traveling waves at the stimulus frequency moving roughly parallel to the midline. Nunez (1981, 1989) brought attention to the possibility of traveling and standing waves mediated by the long corticocortico fibers. The possibility that the frontoparietal association fiber system could sustain such a phenomenon is consistent with the findings of high parietofrontal coherence in the ongoing EEG at alpha frequencies (Thatcher et al, 1986). More recently, Hughes and associates (1992) presented transient event-related potential (ERP) data supporting the hypothesis of cortical traveling waves having speeds of 4 to 7 m/second.

In our study, monopolar electrical measurements referenced to linked earlobes yielded a range of velocities from 10 to 18 m/second, with a mean velocity of 14.7 m/second after applying a folding factor of 2.1 (Burkitt et al, 1992; Burkitt et al, 1993). This factor is needed to account for the effects of cortical folding on the scalp velocity estimate (Nunez, 1981). By applying the same cortical folding factor with magnetic measurements, we obtained a velocity range of 5.8 to 8.0 m/second (mean 6.6 m/second). The disparity between the magnetic and electrical velocity estimates is due in part to reference electrode and volume conduction effects. An active electrode adds a common signal to each recorded site and thus reduces the apparent phase difference between the scalp sites. This reduction will be associated with a more shallow phase gradient and therefore greater apparent velocity. Volume conduction effects also tend to reduce the cortical phase differences when recorded on the scalp.

Bipolar recording techniques remove reference electrode effects, and closely spaced bipolar recordings act as a spatial high pass filter that partially compensates for the volume conduction effects. This was described in more detail in Chapter 1. When applying bipolar recordings to determine the midline scalp phase gradient, the estimated velocities are reduced and are more consistent with the magnetic measurements (Burkitt et al, 1992). Figure 6-4 illustrates the midline SSVEP velocity histogram derived from monopolar electrical, bipolar electrical,

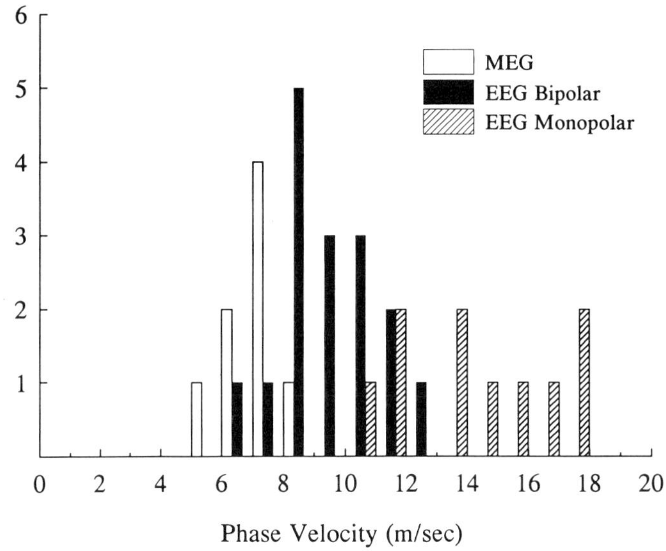

Figure 6-4. Histogram of estimated SSVEP phase velocities using three measurement methods. The open bars represent the result for a series of magnetic recording locations along the midline. The cross-hatched bars represent the velocities estimated from monopolar recording sites on the midline, whereas the solid bars represent the velocities for bipolar recordings derived from the same recording sites used with the monopolar recordings. Monopolar recordings were referenced to linked earlobe. The SSVEP was elicited by an unstructured 10-Hz flicker.

and magnetic recordings. The bipolar electrical and magnetic estimates of velocity are close to the 6 to 9 m/second predicted by the Nunez model of the EEG (Nunez, 1981, 1989).

Stimulus Structure and SSVEP Phase Topography

The Nunez model of the EEG suggests the existence of traveling and standing waves mediated by corticocortico fibers. In this model, a sinusoidal drive may give rise to traveling or standing waves on a closed surface. As outlined in Chapters 11 and 12, if the waves are weakly damped, they may interfere and form standing waves. Standing waves also occur more often in a weakly damped environment with two or more widely separated sources. The converse case of strong damping reduces the possibility of waves interfering and is therefore more likely to give rise to traveling waves.

This model suggests that a sinusoidal drive may permit standing or traveling waves, depending on the specific features of cortical neuroanatomy and damping. Specifically, a structured sinusoidal visual stimulus, with its more restricted projection to the striate cortex, is more likely to yield traveling waves. In contrast, an unstructured sinusoidal stimulus, with its more extensive cortical projections (see Visual Pathways) is more likely to allow interference and thus standing waves. These predictions appear to be supported by the results of a study in which the midline phase topography was measured in 18 male subjects viewing an alternating checkerboard and an unstructured flicker (Burkitt et al, 1992, 1993). During the checkerboard stimulation, 15 subjects exhibited a smooth phase change with distance, 2 had a sharp π phase change, whereas 1 could not be classified. During the unstructured stimulus, 8 participants showed a smooth phase change, 9 had a sharp phase change of approximately π radians, and the remaining 1 could not be classified. Results for one subject are illustrated in Figure 6-5.

In all, phase topography for 11 participants did not change, whereas the remaining 7 showed a phase topography suggestive of traveling waves during the checkerboard stimulus and standing waves during the unstructured flicker. No participant exhibited a change in the reverse direction.

These findings, although still considered preliminary, are consistent with the idea of cortical traveling and standing waves sustained by the rapidly conducting corticocortico fibers. It could be argued that subjects showing a change in topography with stimulus parameter may have levels of cortical damping or connectivity that could yield a standing or traveling wave mode depending on the spatial distribution and strength of the sinusoidal cortical drive. That is, for a specific level of cortical damping, the more restricted striate cortex activation elicited by the checkerboard stimulus yields traveling waves with amplitudes that decrease to a low level before interfering with other waves. This yields a traveling wave process and a consequent smooth change in midline phase with distance. By contrast, the unstructured stimulus projects to the occipital and frontal cortices, thereby increasing the possibility of interference between waves traveling in the anterior and posterior directions. By the same argument, the eight participants who consistently exhibited smooth phase changes may have been characterized by a higher level of cortical damping that prevented the interference of traveling waves under both stimulation arrangements. Conversely, the two participants who consistently exhibited sharp phase changes suggesting standing waves may have showed a lower level of cortical damping that permitted interference to occur with both stimulation arrangements.

Deblurring the SSVEP

As noted in Chapters 1 and 7, the electrical activity recorded on the scalp is a spatial low pass representation of the signal generated on the cortical surface. Several high resolution techniques are available to compensate for this spatial blurring. These range from the model-independent techniques based on local and global Laplacians (Hjorth, 1975; Nunez and Pilgreen, 1991) to a variety of model-dependent techniques described in Chapters 1 and 7. We have implemented a deblurring technique based on smoothing spherical splines (Wahba, 1981) called cortical imaging (CI) (Cadusch et al, 1992; Nunez et al, 1994). Cortical imaging

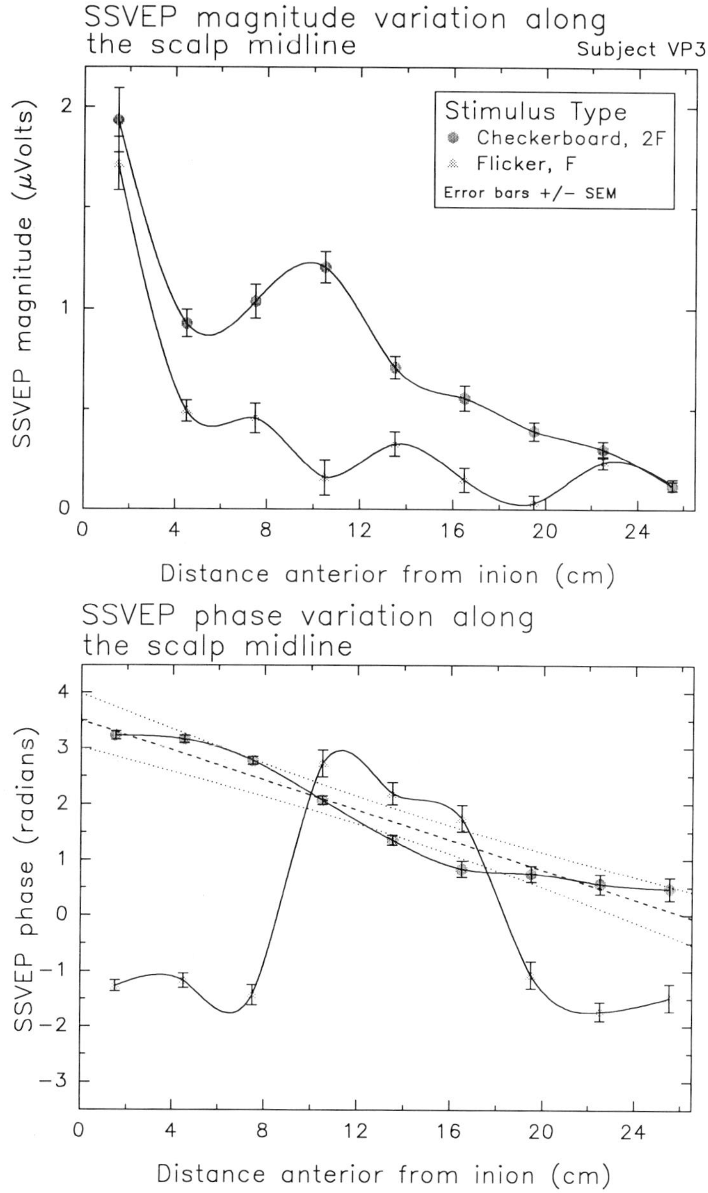

Figure 6-5. Illustration of SSVEP midline magnitude and phase associated with a 10-Hz unstructured flicker and a checkerboard stimulus alternating at 10 Hz. The upper panel illustrates variation of SSVEP magnitude with distance, whereas the lower panel illustrates changes in phase. The flicker stimulus is associated with a rapid phase change of approximately π radians between 14 and 16 cm anterior of the inion. The checkerboard stimulus in the same subject yields a smoother phase change and an associated uncorrected phase velocity of 3.4 m/second. A smooth phase change is assumed if a linear regression yields a correlation coefficient with a magnitude of more than 0.9.

is based on a three- or four-layer conducting sphere model and incorporates the capacity to select the optimal tradeoff between the smoothness of fit and spatial noise. Although smoothing spherical splines are used to interpolate the scalp potential, the explicit relation between cortical potentials and scalp potentials also permits an estimation of the smoothing spline approximation for the cortical potential (on a spherical surface). Cortical imaging has been tested with simulated and recorded 64-channel data and yields results consistent with the spline–Laplacian technique developed by Nunez and colleagues (Nunez et al, 1993, 1994).

The application of CI to the SSVEP reveals a more complex topography than that observed on the scalp. Figure 6-6 shows the scalp and corresponding CI topographies for the SSVEP. The scalp maxima in the frontal and occipital regions are replaced with at least three clear maxima in the occipital region and a less-defined set of frontal maxima in the CI topography. The sharp phase changes of approximately 180° between the various maxima are noteworthy. This pattern appears to be a consistent finding with the SSVEP and is probably not an artifact of the CI algorithm for two reasons. First, both the spline–Laplacian and CI yield similar results (Nunez et al, 1993, 1994). Second, when CI is applied to the scalp topography derived from an average of 40 persons, the sharp 180° discontinuities in phase are not apparent (Schier et al, 1992). This is probably a reflection of the intersubject variability in the position of the amplitude maxima and phase changes. Had the phase changes apparent in Figure 6-6 (cortex) resulted from CI artifacts, they should have been as prominent in the averaged data as in the individual maps.

The mechanism responsible for the sharp phase changes is unclear at this stage. Several mechanisms have been proposed, and more than one may be involved. One suggested mechanism for the 180° phase changes posits the existence of dipole projections from different cortical regions. In regions where two opposing cortical dipole sheets do not cancel each other, such as on either side of a sulcus, a "resultant" source will be apparent. If the two dipole sheets yield signals that are close to cancellation, regional variations in the resultant source could mimic tangential dipoles and thus exhibit the sharp 180° phase changes.

Another explanation for the sharp 180° phase changes is interference patterns caused by traveling waves emerging from multiple cortical sources. For this mechanism to operate, two conditions must apply. The stimulus must create traveling waves and there must be multiple, spatially restricted sources separated by more than one half a wavelength.

The neuroanatomy of the visual system, especially the M system, suggests that the condition of multiple sources may be satisfied. The second condition implies a requirement for wavelengths of approximately 10 cm or less at a stimulus frequency of 13 Hz. For nondispersive waves, this parameter requires wave velocities of less than 1.3 m/second. Several groups of investigators have reported evidence of intracortical propagation velocities of 0.1 to 0.5 m/second in mammalian brains (Lopes da Silva et al, 1978; Wright and Sergejew, 1991). At a stimulus frequency of 13 Hz, a conduction velocity of 0.5 m/second yields a wavelength of 6.5 cm, a distance comparable to the separation of the different cortical regions responding

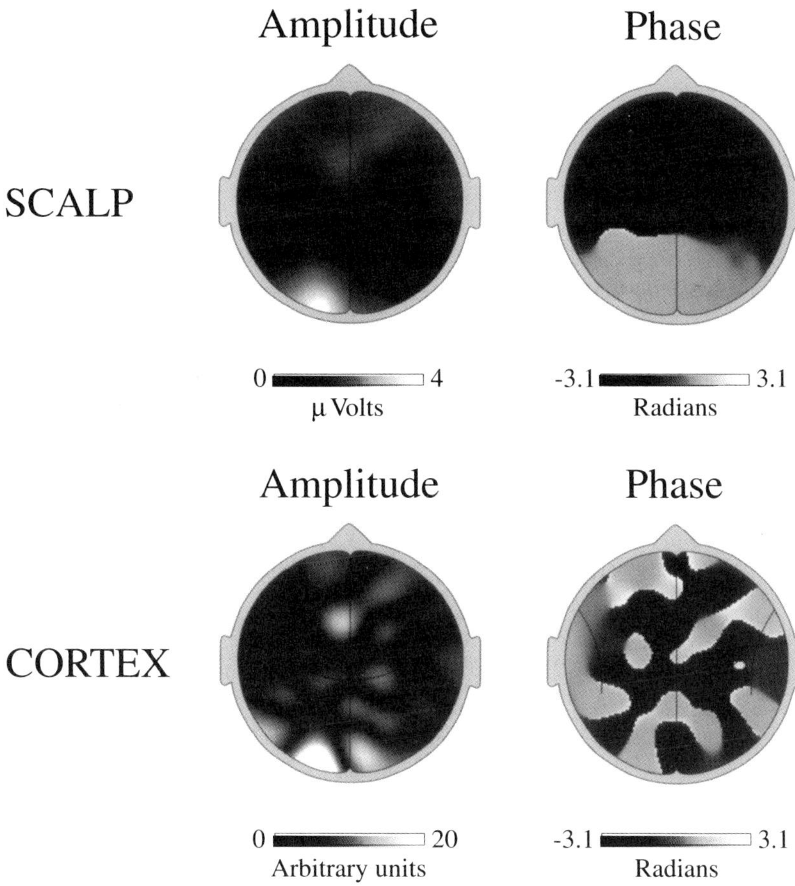

Figure 6-6. Top row, labeled "scalp," illustrates scalp SSVEP amplitude and phase distribution evoked by an unstructured 13-Hz flicker. The bottom row, labeled "cortex," illustrates the SSVEP amplitude and phase after the application of cortical imaging. The relatively uncomplicated scalp topography characterized by two local amplitude maxima and one sharp phase change is replaced by a more complex distribution of maxima with sharp 180° phase changes separating regions of constant phase. This type of cortical imaging pattern of sharp phase changes is observed in all subjects, regardless of whether the scalp distribution of phase is characterized by a smooth or sharp change illustrated in Figure 6-3.

to the visual stimulus. As both conditions appear to be satisfied, the standing wave interference mediated by the slow intracortical fibers could be the origin of the distinctive phase signature observed with CI.

A third possible mechanism for the amplitude and phase patterns seen in CI topographies concern an intriguing finding described in Chapter 11. Simulations of dispersive brain waves on a spherical surface indicate the possibility that high spatial modes, analogous to higher spatial frequencies, are associated with low temporal frequencies. These lower temporal frequencies occur with higher levels of the cortical control parameter B and are thought to represent limit cycle oscillations. The complex CI topographies, suggestive of higher spatial modes, therefore could be the result of such limit cycle oscillations.

These data suggest three possible mechanisms capable of sustaining traveling and standing waves. The high spatial frequency phase topography observed with CI could be mediated by a low-velocity, millimetric scale, local mechanism, or a high-velocity centimetric scale mechanism associated with limit cycle oscillations. In contrast, the low spatial frequency features observed in the scalp topography are mediated solely by a high-velocity, centimetric scale mechanism sustained by long-range association fibers. The high spatial detail or high spatial frequencies apparent with CI are eliminated by the low pass filtering characteristics of the cortex–skull interface. Scalp recordings therefore tend to emphasize the high-velocity, long wavelength centimetric scale phenomena, whereas CI deblurred scalp recordings make the high spatial frequency, short wavelength scale phenomena more apparent (see Figures 1-28, 3-13, and 3-14).

Magnetic measurements of phase variation with distance suggest that cortical traveling waves have a velocity of approximately 6 m/second, an observation consistent with the contribution of the long-range or centimetric scale fibers. This may appear inconsistent with the fact that magnetoencephalographic (MEG) recordings are unaffected by the potential smearing resulting from cortex–skull resistivity differences and therefore should yield a phase topography similar to CI. However, the spatial resolution of the MEG is compromised because the MEG-sensing coil is frequently at least 2 cm from the cortical surface. In contrast, scalp electrodes are placed approximately 1.0 to 1.2 cm from the cortical surface. Thus the increased spatial resolution of the MEG resulting from the absence of potential smearing is partly lost by the greater distance of the sensing coil from the cortical surface. If the effects of distance are not compensated for, the resultant spatial low pass filtering characteristics of the MEG recording tend to emphasize the long wavelength characteristics of the SSVEP phase profile.

It is possible that several of the mechanisms described above operate simultaneously, with the CI topography accounted for by a combination of low-velocity millimetric scale local interference effects, and high-velocity centimetric scale global effects. While the tangential dipole explanation may be correct in some cases it does not appear to be consistent with the observation that SSVEP spatial patterns are frequency-dependent as discussed in Chapter 12. However, the issue will be resolved only with higher resolution recordings and more extensive recordings from the primate cortical surface.

Steady-State Potentials and Cognition

This chapter is concluded with a discussion of the relation between SSVEP and cognitive processes. The rationale for including this segment is twofold. First, it gives an overview of the manner by which driven activity can be used to examine time-varying brain electrical activity associated with cognitive processes. Second, the SSVEP changes associated with cognitive processes provide more information on the mechanisms responsible for SSVEP.

Most studies investigating the relation between cognitive processes and electrophysiologic parameters have used the EEG or transient EPs (Gevins and Cutillo, 1986; Chapter 7). Relatively few studies have examined the relation between cognitive processes and steady-state potentials. Of the studies considering this topic, most have investigated the effects of cognitive and attentional processes on the 40-Hz auditory steady-state potential elicited by repetitive clicks with a frequency of 40 Hz (Galambos, 1982). These studies report mixed findings. Galambos and Makeig (1988) drew attention to the fluctuations in the 40-Hz auditory steady-state evoked potential and considered the relation between these and cognitive processes. Although the fluctuations were originally thought to index "shifts in arousal," subsequent studies failed to confirm this hypothesis (Galambos and Makeig, 1988). The authors also reported no obvious relation between the auditory steady-state evoked potential and performance or perception. In an extensive study, Linden and associates (1987) could not find any effects of selective attention on the auditory steady-state potential, although the same participants showed strong selective attention effects in the late components of the transient ERP. Although no clear relation between shifts in attention and the auditory steady-state potential was found, a change in the pitch of the 40-Hz tone bursts was associated with a consistent, transient-phase deviation corresponding to reduced latency of approximately 2 to 5 milliseconds. These phase changes were associated with a transient reduction in auditory somatosensory evoked potential (SSEP) amplitude (Galambos and Makeig, 1988; Makeig and Galambos, 1989). These observations were confirmed and extended in two studies reported by Rohbraugh and coworkers (1989, 1990). The effects of salient auditory and visual "foreground" stimuli on the auditory SSEP elicited by "background" 40-Hz tone bursts comprised a similar transient-phase deviation.

The few reported studies of the relation between cognitive processes and the SSVEP can be grouped into two categories, depending on whether the cognitive measure and the SSVEP were determined simultaneously. Nonsimultaneous measurements could be considered to tap relatively stable features of the correlation between the SSVEP and cognitive processes (such as ability or cognitive style), whereas simultaneous measurements may provide additional information about the dynamic relation between cognitive processes and the SSVEP.

SSVEP and Performance

One of the first studies to show a relation between an SSVEP parameter and task capability was reported by Wilson and O'Donnell (1986). In this study, subjects performed a memory task that required them to classify a set of presented objects as "target" or "nontargets." In this protocol, the reaction time for the identification of a target was proportional to the number of targets held in the memory set. In plotting reaction time against the number of targets, two measures were derived: the gradient of the line, indexing the additional time required to compare a stimulus with each item in the memory set, and the intercept, interpreted as the processing time needed to encode the stimulus information and execute the response.

The latency of the SSVEP elicited by a diffuse flicker was also estimated in the same participants. Steady-state visually evoked potentials in the 15- to 23-Hz intermediate-frequency range yielded apparent latencies of 82 to 125 milliseconds, and the 40- to 59-Hz high-frequency range yielded apparent latencies of 36 to 98 milliseconds. These latencies were correlated with specific performance measures in the memory task. The high-frequency SSVEP latency was correlated with the intercept or "encoding time," whereas the intermediate-frequency SSVEP latency was correlated with the gradient of reaction time versus memory set size. These results suggest that the different stimulus frequencies gauge different aspects of the memory-scanning task. The high-frequency components are hypothesized to index the sensory–motor aspects of the task, whereas the low-frequency components are hypothesized to index the neural processes involved in accessing the contents of working memory.

Another approach to the relation between the SSVEP and cognitive processes has been described by Robinson (1985, 1989). In a series of studies, Robinson reported a relation between SSVEP parameters and IQ scores as measured by the Wechsler Adult Intelligence Scale. The SSVEP elicited by an unstructured flicker was parametrized in terms of a damped simple harmonic oscillator. Robinson claimed a negative correlation between IQ score and damping ratio when the natural frequency is less than 10.2 Hz and a positive correlation when the natural frequency is greater than 10.2 Hz. These correlations were interpreted in terms an inverted U relation between arousal and performance. Although these results suggest a relation between the SSVEP and intelligence, they have not been accepted without criticism (Robinson, 1990; Stowell, 1990). More recent studies suggest that scores on psychological tests are, in fact, correlated with shorter latency of evoked potentials (Duffy et al, 1993).

SSVEPs and Time Varying Cognitive Processes

The capacity to assess SSVEP phase and amplitude in as few as 1 to 10 seconds of recorded activity allows possible study of the temporal variations of these SSVEP parameters, which may be associated with cognitive processes. As previously noted, the Fourier integration period, in large part, determines the bandwidth of SSVEP variations in amplitude and phase that can be estimated. An analogous constraint applies to averaged transient ERPs. This is a consequence of the assumption underpinning averaging, specifically that signal and noise are stationary over the time required to record the responses. In many cognitive experiments, averaging periods vary from as little as 60 seconds to as much as 8 hours. Such intervals impose severe constraints when it is necessary to examine changes in ERP components, which may occur during a period of 1 to 30 seconds.

A technique based on the SSVEP, which appears to combine sensitivity to cognitive processes and resistance to artifacts with short data acquisition periods, is the steady-state probe topography (SSPT) (Silberstein et al, 1990; Silberstein, 1992). It is characterized by the following three features

1. The stimulus eliciting the SSVEP is a uniform flicker irrelevant to the cognitive tasks performed by the persons studied.
2. The integration duration of the Fourier analyzer used to estimate the response is variable but generally exceeds 1 second.
3. Brain electrical activity is recorded from either 64 or 128 scalp sites.

Applications of SSPT are illustrated with two cognitive tasks—a visual vigilance task and the Wisconsin Card Sort Test (WCST), a neuropsychological task that probes prefrontal function. The vigilance task is based on an analysis with a temporal resolution of 10 seconds, whereas the WCST is analyzed with a resolution of 1 second.

SSPT in a Visual Vigilance Task

With the vigilance task, 13 male participants were required to fixate on the center of a video monitor and observe a sequence of 180 shapes—60 squares followed by 60 circles followed by another 60 squares. Circles and squares were presented at a rate of 1 per second. Participants were required to view the 180 shapes three times, with each of the three viewings constituting a trial. During the first and second trials, the subjects were requested to fixate on the center of the monitor and observe the sequence of shapes. Visual vigilance was increased in the third trial by asking subjects to identify a modified circle that was to appear in the trial. Before the appearance of the modified circle, subjects did not know which circle had been modified or the nature of the modification.

The results have been described in detail previously (Silberstein et al, 1990). When trials 3 and 2 were compared at equivalent points in time, the heightened vigilance in trial 3 was associated with reduced SSVEP amplitude and increased phase lag. The time course of these changes at a right parietal site (electrode 42) is illustrated in Figure 6-7. The topography of these changes when the circles appeared is illustrated in Figure 6-8 with the distribution of the square root of Hotelling's T^2 parameter (Hotelling's T). This parameter can be considered a multidimensional extension of the Student's t-test (Picton et al, 1987).

Compared with trial 2, the appearance of the circles in trial 3 was associated with a transient occipital SSVEP attenuation and an increased phase lag. In the frontal region, the amplitude was also reduced but the phase was advanced. This is illustrated in Figure 6-9. During 20 of the following 60 seconds, while participants waited for the modified circle to appear, the dominant effect on the SSVEP was an amplitude reduction in the right parietotemporal region. These task-related

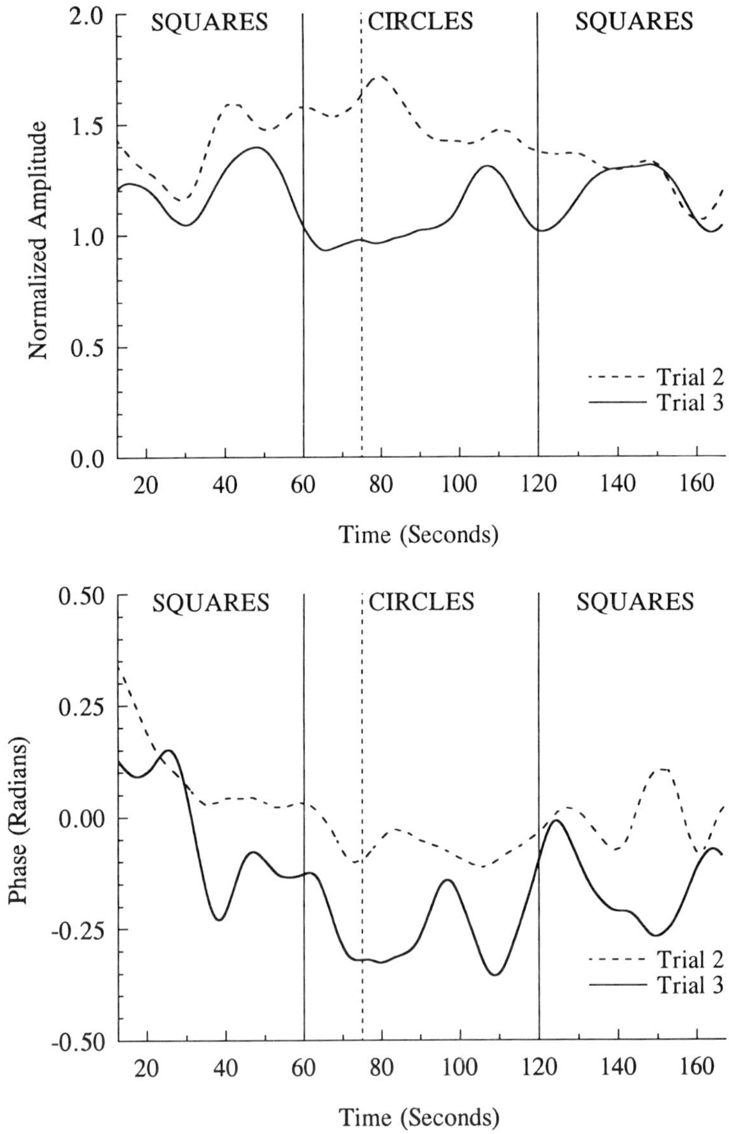

Figure 6-7. Time course of the amplitude and phase of the 13-Hz pooled SSVEP elicited by a flicker superimposed over a visual vigilance task consisting of 180 shapes (60 squares, 60 circles, and 60 squares) presented at a rate of one per second. The effects of increased vigilance in trial 3 on the amplitude of the SSVEP are illustrated in the top set of graphs. The top graph corresponds to the SSVEP amplitude estimated with a 10-second integration window. The dotted line represents trial 2, the reference trial, whereas the solid line represents trial 3. The bottom graphs illustrate the equivalent time series for SSVEP phase. Recording site is electrode 42, located in the right parietotemporal region.

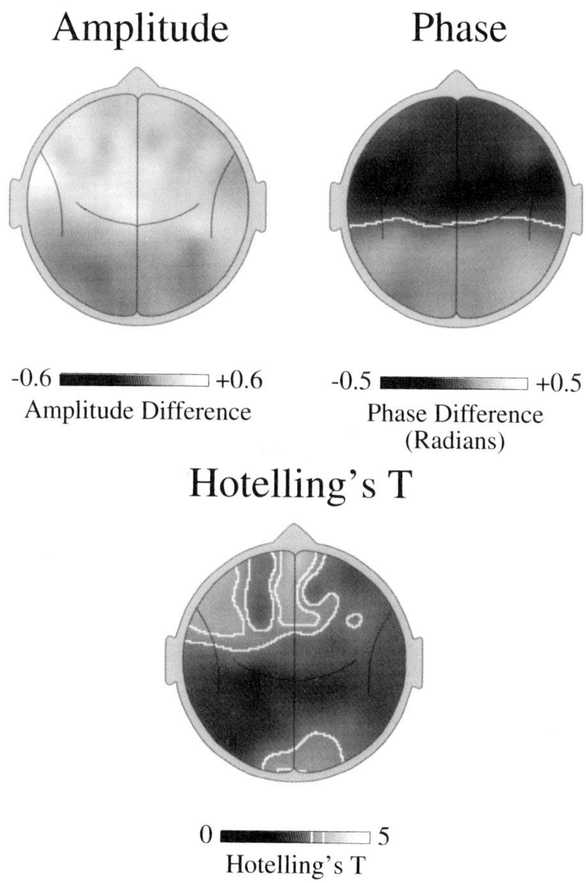

Figure 6-8. Topographic distribution of the differences in amplitude and phase between trials 2 and 3 when the circles appeared. In the map labeled "amplitude," lighter shades indicate areas in which the amplitude was smaller in trial 3 compared with trial 2. In the map labeled "phase," lighter shades correspond to areas in which the phase in trial 3 was smaller than in trial 2. For the phase maps, the lighter shades indicate increased SSVEP latency, whereas the darker shades regions indicate decreased SSVEP latency. The parietal, temporal, and occipital areas show a latency increase, whereas the frontal region shows a latency decrease at this time. The white contour lines in the "phase" and "amplitude" maps indicate the regions of zero difference. The map labeled "Hotelling's T" illustrates the topographic distribution of the square root of the Hotelling's T2 parameter based on a paired comparison between trials 3 and 2. Iso-T values of 4.31, 3.43, and 3.05, corresponding to single comparison P values of 1.0%, 0.5%, and 0.1%, respectively, are indicated by white contour lines. The Hotelling's T map shows that the most consistent differences between trials 3 and 2 occurred in the frontal and occipital regions.

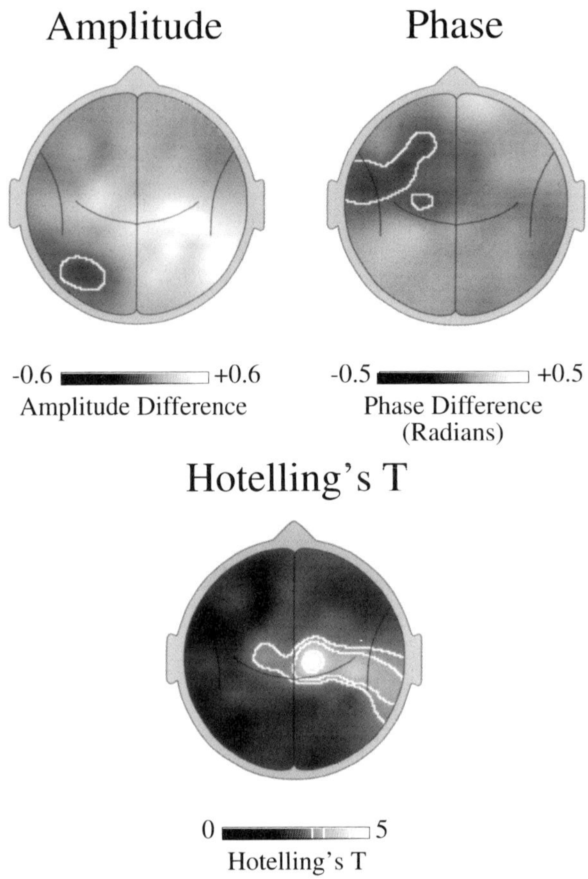

Figure 6-9. Topographic distribution of amplitude and phase differences and Hotelling's T 15 seconds into the circles of trials 2 and 3. The descriptions in the Figure 6-8 legend also apply to this figure. The main effect of increased vigilance at this time, while participants were waiting for the appearance of the "modified" circle, was a reduction in amplitude in the right parietotemporal region. This is highlighted by the Hotelling's T distribution.

effects suggest that variations in regional cortical activity are reflected in SSVEP amplitude changes, similar to the transient reductions in alpha activity associated with cognitive tasks or motor tasks (Pfurtscheller and Klimesch, 1990). The SSVEP amplitude changes are also consistent with the Probe-ERP paradigm, in which regional increases in cortical activity are associated with reductions in ERPs elicited by an irrelevant (or probe) stimulus (Papanicolaou and Johnstone, 1984).

Interpreting the SSVEP changes in terms of changes in cortical activity suggests a series of distinct changes associated with different phases of the vigilance task. The appearance of the circles elicited prefrontal and occipital changes, whereas the period when participants awaited the appearance of the modified circle was associated with right parietotemporal changes. The importance of these changes has been discussed previously (Silberstein et al, 1990). Briefly, these results suggest prefrontal activation when the participants were alerted to the possible appearance of the target circle. Such a finding is consistent with neuropsychological studies indicating prefrontal involvement in the mediation of attentional processes (Milner and Petrides, 1984; Roland, 1984). The pattern 15 seconds latter is dominated by changes in the right parietotemporal region, suggesting the involvement of different processes during this phase of the vigilance task. This right parietotemporal change may reflect the involvement of this region in the visual recognition memory aspect of the task (Milner, 1968). These changes could have been detected only with a technique possessing the required temporal resolution and continuity.

The visual vigilance task was examined with a temporal resolution of 10 seconds, appropriate for examining processes operating on a 10- to 180-second time scale. In contrast, the WCST requires participants to determine an operational strategy in 1 to 2 seconds. To examine the dynamics of the SSVEP topography in the WCST, a higher temporal resolution of 1 second is used.

SSPT and the WCST

The WCST is used widely as a neuropsychological test of frontal lobe function (Heaton, 1981; Milner, 1963). It consists of many cards (typically 128) containing geometrical objects that can vary in color, number, and shape. Participants are shown four key cards and requested to sort the cards presented under the key cards using some rule to guide them that must be guessed on the basis of trial and error. After each sort, participants are told whether they are correct or not correct. Having established the sorting criterion, the participant is allowed to sort successfully several consecutive cards (typically 10) before the sort criterion is changed by the test administrator. For each subject, this cycle is repeated several times. On average, healthy subjects encounter 7 to 10 criterion changes in a typical session lasting 10 minutes.

The need to dispense with the previous criterion and determine the new criterion places demands on the prefrontal cortex (Milner, 1963; Milner, 1964). Participants with frontal damage have difficulties in dispensing with the superseded sort criterion (perseveration errors) and in determining the new sort criterion (Milner, 1963; Drewe, 1974). Recent brain-imaging studies using regional cerebral blood flow and positron emission topography (PET) indicated prefrontal activation during the WCST (Weinberger et al, 1986; Berman et al, 1986; Goldberg et al, 1990). In a study reported by Weinberger and colleagues (1986), the increased prefrontal activation was observed only when healthy subjects performed the WCST, and not in a numbers-matching task designed to make comparable visuomotor demands. Although these results are consistent with neuropsychological evidence, an important limitation of the metabolic imaging methods is their poor temporal resolution and their very limited capacity for repeated measures in a single subject. The temporal resolution of the PET techniques, based on the short

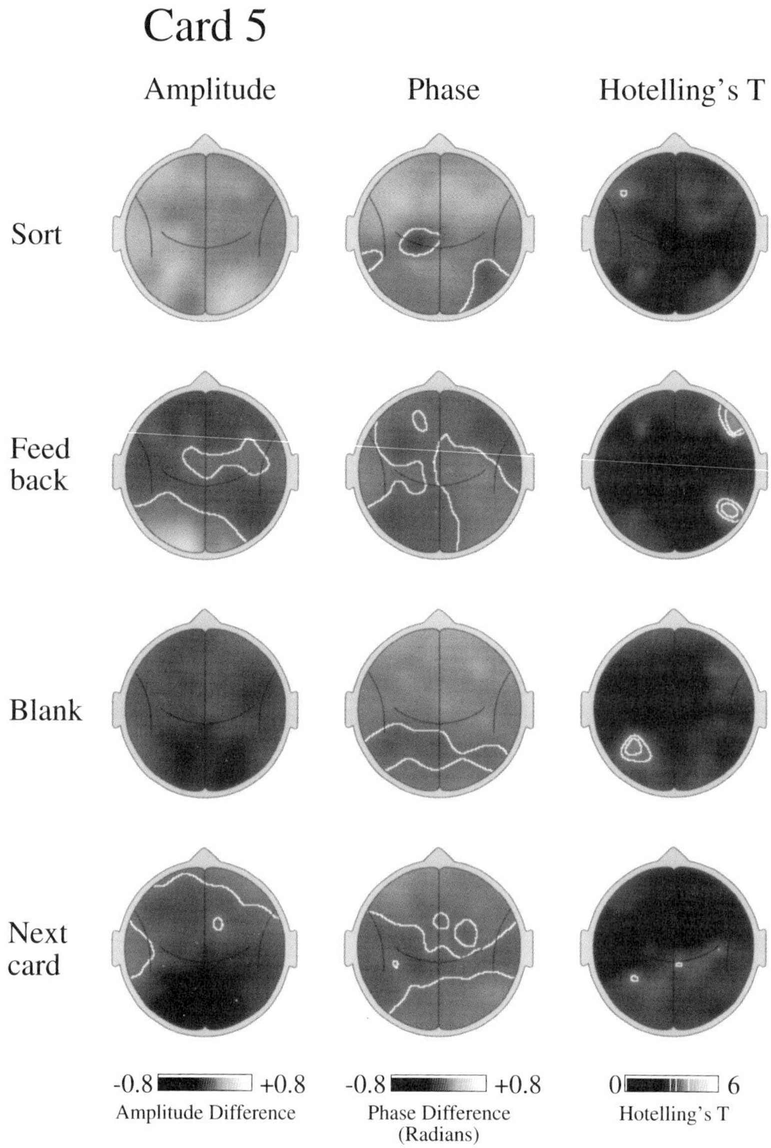

Figures 6-10 and 6-11. The differences in magnitude and phase between the SSVEP time series for cards 5 and 11 and the average of the SSVEP time series for cards 2 to 10. This illustrates the deviation about the mean response for the cards. The first row, labeled "sort," represents the deviations in magnitude and phase when the participants were sorting the given card in the sequence for a particular sort criterion. The grey scale conventions for the differences in magnitude and phase are the same as those in Figure 6-8, with the white contour line indicating those regions of zero difference in magnitude and phase. The third map illustrates the distribution of the corresponding Hotelling's T parameter. The iso-T contours delimit the T values of 4.10, 3.29, and 2.95, corresponding to P values of 0.1%, 0.5%, and 1.0%, respectively, for single comparisons. The second row, labeled

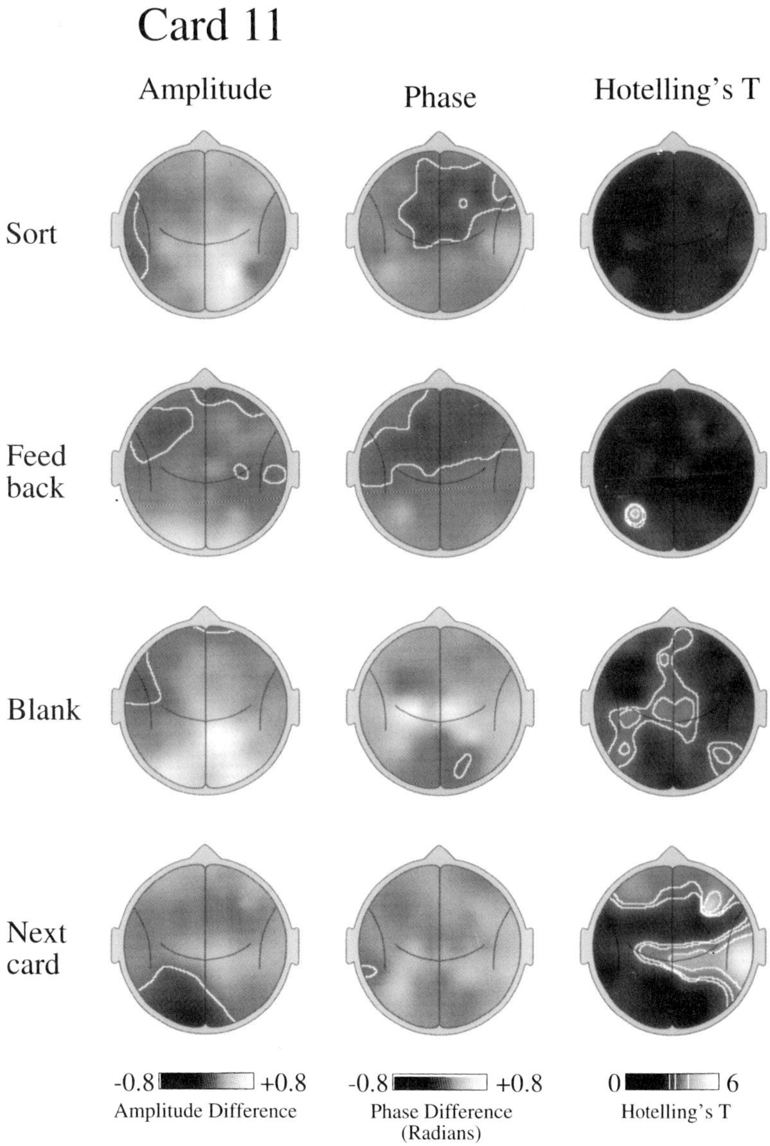

←

"feedback," illustrates the comparable topographies 1 second later when the subjects received feedback that their sort choice for card 5 was correct and card 11 was incorrect. The topography 0.75 seconds later, when the sort card was blanked in preparation for the next card, is illustrated in the third row, labeled "blank." The fourth row illustrates the situation 0.75 second later when the 6th and 12th cards appeared. Both cards 5 and 11 showed little deviation from the mean response during the "sort" and "feedback" times. During the "blank" and "next card" times, the card 5 sequence continued to show little deviation from the mean response, whereas the card 11 sequence showed pronounced changes. These changes were especially prominent in the prefrontal and right parietotemporal regions when card 12 (that is, next card) was presented.

half-life isotope O^{15}, is approximately 40 seconds (Petersen et al, 1988). During this interval, participants may have sorted as many as 12 cards and had experienced one to three criterion changes. These imaging methods are therefore inadequate to determine whether the prefrontal cortex is uniformly active during the WCST or preferentially active during the selection of the sort criterion. The association of perseverative errors with prefrontal damage (Milner, 1963, 1964) suggests increased demands on this region when the old criterion is being dismissed and the new one established.

Steady-state probe topography has been used to examine the changes in SSVEP topography associated with components of the WCST (Ciorciari et al, 1992; Silberstein, 1992; Silberstein, 1992, 1993). In this experiment, the timing of the WCST combined computer-paced and self-paced elements. After the appearance of a target card, subjects indicated their choice by pressing one of four buttons corresponding to the four key cards. When a button was pressed, the target card appeared under the key card. One second later, the word "right" or "wrong" appeared on the screen as feedback. The feedback remained on the screen for exactly 0.75 second. On the removal of the feedback word, the target card also was blanked in preparation for the appearance of the next target card. The duration of the "blank" target card was exactly 0.75 second. After this period elapsed, the next target card was presented and the cycle repeated. Except for the intervals between card presentation and subject choice, the duration of all components of the WCST were computer controlled.

To assess the changes in the SSVEP associated with sorting a specified card in a sequence of sorts performed correctly for a given sort criterion, the following procedure was used. The 4-second epochs of SSVEP centered on the feedback times were averaged for all occurrences of the specified card in the sequence for all criteria. This procedure was repeated for each card and electrode site, yielding 11 averages (one for each card) at each of the electrode sites. For purposes of brevity, the subsequent analysis is restricted to the sequences associated with cards 5 and 11. The topographic changes that occurred during card 5 were considered to be typical of changes that occur when participants were simply executing the sort criterion, whereas the changes that occurred during card 11 were considered to illustrate the changes associated with a criterion shift.

The topographic distribution of the deviations in amplitude and phase and their associated Hotelling's T for cards 5 and 11 about the mean formed from the average of cards 2 to 10 are illustrated in Figures 6-10 and 6-11. In each figure, four sets of three maps are shown. The first row shows the topography when the subject pressed one of four buttons to sort the card (labeled "sort"), the second row shows the topography 1 second later at the start of the feedback (labeled "feedback"), the third row illustrates the topography 0.75 second later when the card is blanked (labeled "blank"), and the final row shows the topography a further 0.75 second later when the next card is presented (labeled "next card"). For each point in time, the maps in the first columns illustrate the magnitude deviations, the second column illustrates the phase deviations, and the third column illustrates the Hotelling's T parameter associated with the deviations.

The similarities between the card 5 and 11 and the mean response SSVEP topographies stop after feedback. With the card 5 maps, the appearance of the blank card is associated with increased SSVEP amplitude in the occipitoparietal region. We interpret this as a transient reduction in occipitoparietal activity as participants having had their criterion choice confirmed, await the appearance of the next card. At the equivalent time for card 11, the SSVEP amplitude is attenuated in the occipitoparietal and prefrontal regions. The difference between card 5 and 11 topographies is most pronounced immediately after presentation of the "next card." With card 5, participants need only reapply the sort criterion that had proved successful the previous five times. With card 11, participants, having realized the sort criterion has changed, must test their choice of the new sort criterion. The card 5 topography is characterized by an occipitoparietal SSVEP amplitude increase. In contrast, the card 11 topography is characterized by widespread SSVEP amplitude attenuation, which is strongest in the prefrontal and right parietotemporal regions. This amplitude attenuation is also reflected in the Hotelling's T map, which highlights the importance of the features in the prefrontal and right parietotemporal region.

These card 11 SSVEP changes, interpreted as increases in regional activity, suggest a transient surge in activity when participants must determine the new sort criterion. The prefrontal focus of this increase is consistent with neurophysiologic and neuropsychological data pointing to a critical role for the prefrontal region at this point in the task. The transient nature of this increased prefrontal activity also indicates the involvement of this region at the time the old criterion must be dismissed and a new criterion determined. The consistent SSVEP changes observed in the right temporal region also suggest its involvement in this component of the WCST, perhaps mediating the visual recognition components of the task. Steady-state probe topography can thus quantify electrophysiologic changes occurring on a time scale consistent with the cognitive task being examined.

Some Constraints on the SSVEP as a Probe of Cortical Activity

Although SSPT appears to be a useful technique to measure changes in regional brain activity associated with cognitive processes, it is appropriate to consider the factors that may increase the technique's sensitivity and those that limit the range of applicability.

The sensitivity of the SSVEP to cognitive processes may be related to the sensitivity of the visual processes driven by the unstructured full-field visual stimulus used as an irrelevant probe. Such unstructured stimuli preferentially activate the M system, which is more sensitive than the P system to changes in states of arousal. Maffei and colleagues (1965) showed that lateral geniculate units (now identified as M cells) only responded to an unstructured visual stimulus when the EEG was desynchronized, suggesting an awake state. During periods of slow-wave synchronous EEG activity suggestive of sleep, these units were unresponsive to visual flicker. The precise mechanisms responsible for the variations in SSVEP amplitude and phase are unclear, although cortical and subcortical processes probably contribute. At the subcortical level, the pulvinar nucleus plays a role in processing visual information (LaBerge and Buchsbaum, 1990; Petersen et al, 1987; Robinson and Petersen, 1992). Use of an unstructured flicker as an "irrelevant" stimulus would be especially effective as an M system stimulus that could be modulated by the pulvinar nucleus. Similarly, the reticularis nucleus of the thalamus also may play a role in modulating the transmission of information through the pulvinar and lateral geniculate nuclei (Garey et al, 1984). Cortical mechanisms are less clear, although Papanicolaou and Johnstone (1984) have suggested a model to explain the changes observed with the Probe–ERP paradigm. They interpret reductions in the EP elicited by the irrelevant probe as a consequence of increased allocation of cortical resources to the principal task, thereby reducing the resources available to evoke an ERP by the probe stimulus.

One important issue, central to interpreting the changes in SSVEP amplitude, concerns the relation between the SSVEP amplitude and regional brain activity. Although several studies have suggested that increases in regional brain activity are associated with corresponding reductions in the SSVEP amplitude (Silberstein et al, 1990, 1993), this relation will probably not be true for the full range of states. Puce (1986) found that the 13-Hz SSVEP elicited by an unstructured visual flicker was reduced during general anaesthesia. Furthermore, we observed that drowsiness was associated with reduced SSVEP amplitude. This suggests that the relation between SSVEP amplitude and cortical activity is better described by an inverted U curve and that the negative correlation between cortical activity and SSVEP amplitude may only apply beyond a specific level of cortical activity or arousal.

Another issue warranting consideration is the extent of the cortical areas that can be probed using SSPT. Clearly the only areas that lend themselves to investigation with SSPT are those that respond directly or indirectly to the stimulus eliciting an SSVEP. Our previous studies indicate regional variations in the SSVEP that extend beyond the occipitoparietal region, the area considered to be the major visual processing zone. Changes in the SSVEP associated with cognitive processes have been identified in the temporal, central, frontal, and prefrontal regions.

At least two factors may contribute to the neuroanatomic extent of the changes observed. First, the spatially diffuse visual flicker is especially effective at stimulating the M system, which is directly and indirectly relayed through the lateral geniculate nucleus, pulvinar nucleus, and superior colliculus. As noted previously, different components of the pulvinar nucleus and superior colliculus project extensively to non-visual cortical regions. These regions include occipitoparietal regions, temporal cortex, primary sensory–motor cortex, and frontal and prefrontal cortices. Such wide-ranging projections could account for the widespread task-related changes in the SSVEP.

Wave propagation in the cortex could constitute another mechanism. The existence of such cortical waves suggest that many "nonvisual" cortical areas may be invaded by traveling waves elicited by the sinusoidal stimulus, thereby also accounting for widespread task-related changes in the SSVEP. These two factors are not mutually exclusive and both may be in operation, as discussed in Chapters 11 through 14.

In conclusion, driven activity offers a range of phenomena that shed light on neural processes underlying rhythmic activity and also a practical tool to investigate brain activity associated with higher cortical function.

References

Baker, C.L., Jr. and Hess, R.F. Linear and nonlinear components of the human electroretinogram. *J. Neurophysiol.* 51:952–957, 1984.

Bender, D.B. Electrophysiological and behavioral experiments on the primate pulvinar. In: *Progress in Brain Research.* (T.P. Hicks, and Benedek, G., Eds.) Vol. 75. New York: Elsevier Science Publishers, pp. 55–65, 1988.

Berman, K.F. Cortical "stress tests" in schizophrenia: Regional cerebral blood flow studies. *Biol. Psychiatry.* 22:1304–1326, 1987.

Bodis-Wollner, I., Brannan, J.R., Ghilardi, M.F., and Mylin, L.H. The importance of physiology to visual evoked potentials. In: *Visual Evoked Potentials.* (J.E. Desmedt, Ed.) pp. 1–24, 1990.

Burkitt, G., Silberstein, R.B., Cadusch, P.J., Nunez, P.L., and Wood, A.W. Steady state visually evoked potentials and travelling waves. In preparation (1994).

Burkitt, G., Silberstein, R.B., Cadusch, P.J., and Wood, A.W. Evidence of Travelling Waves on the Brain Surface from EEG and MEG Recordings. APSEM/BECON 92, Broadbeach, Queensland, Australia, p. 62, August 1992.

Cadusch, P.J., Breckon, W., and Silberstein, R.B. Spherical splines and the interpolation, deblurring and transformation of topographic EEG data. *Brain Topography.* 5:59, 1992.

Ciorciari, J., Silberstein, R.B., and Ma, S. Topography of the steady state visually evoked potential associated with the Wisconsin Card Sort Task. *Brain Topography.* 5:59–60, 1992.

Derrington, A.M. and Lennie, P. Spatial and temporal contrast sensitivities of neurons in lateral geniculate nucleus of macaque. *J. Physiol.* 357:219–240, 1984.

Drewe, E.A. The effect of type and area of brain lesion Wisconsin card sorting test performance. *Cortex.* 10:159–170, 1974.

Duffy, F.H., McAnulty, G.B., Jones, K., Als, H., and Albert, I. Brain electrical correlates of psychological measures: Strategies and problems. *Brain Topography.* 5:399–412, 1993.

Eskin, T.A. and Merigan, W.H. Selective acrylamide-induced degeneration of color opponent ganglion cells in macaques. *Brain Res.* 378:379–384, 1986.

Galambos, R. Tactile and auditory stimuli repeated in high rates (30–50 per sec) produce similar event related potentials. *Ann. NY Acad. Sci.* 388:722–727, 1982.

Galambos, R. and Makeig, S. Dynamic changes in steady-state responses. In: *Springer Series in Brain Dynamics.* (E. Basar, Ed.) Berlin: Springer-Verlag, pp. 103–122, 1988.

Garey, L.J., Dreher, B., and Robinson, S.R. The organization of the visual thalamus. In: *Development of Visual Pathways in Mammals.* (J. Stone, Dreher, B., and Rapaport, D.H., Eds.) New York: Alan R. Liss, pp. 176–234, 1984.

Gevins, A.S. and Cutillo, B.A. Signals of cognition. In: *Clinical Applications of Computer*

Analysis of EEG and Other Neurophysiological Signals. Handbook of Electroencephalography and Clinical Neurophysiology. (New Series). Vol. 2. (F.H. Lopes da Silva, Storm van Leeuwen, W., and Remond, A., Eds.) Amsterdam: Elsevier, pp. 335–384, 1986.

Goldberg, T.E., Berman, K.F., Mohr, E., and Weinberger, D.R. Regional cerebral blood-flow and cognitive function in Huntington's disease and schizophrenia. *Arch. Neurol.* 47:418–422, 1990.

Heaton, R.K. *A Manual for the Wisconsin Card Sorting Test.* Odessa, FL: Psychological Assessment Resources, 1981.

Hjorth, B. An on-line transformation of EEG scalp potentials onto orthogonal source derivations. *Electroencephalogr. Clin. Neurophysiol.* 39:526–530, 1975.

Hughes, J.R., Kuruvilla, A., and Fino, J.J. Topographic analysis of visually evoked potentials from flash and pattern reversal stimuli: Evidence for "travelling waves." *Brain Topography.* 4:215–228, 1992.

Karson, C.N., Coppola, R., Morihisa, J.M., and Weinberger, D.R. Computed electroencephalographic activity mapping in schizophrenia. The resting state reconsidered. *Arch. Gen. Psychiatry.* 44:514–517, 1987.

Kaufman, L. and Williamson, S.J. Responses to steady-state auditory stimulation. In: *Auditory Evoked Magnetic Fields and Electric Potentials.* (F. Grandori, Hoke, M., and Romani, M., Eds.) Basel: Karger, pp. 283–312, 1990.

LaBerge, D. and Buchsbaum, M.S. Positron emission tomographic measurements of pulvinar activity during an attention task. *J. Neurosci.* 10:613–619, 1990.

Le Grand, Y. Spectral luminosity. In: *Visual Psychophysics.* (D. Jameson and Hurvich, L.M., Eds.) Berlin: Springer-Verlag, pp. 413–433, 1972.

Linden, D.R., Picton, T.W., Hamel, G., and Campbell, K.B. Human auditory steady-state evoked potentials during selective attention. *Electroencephalogr. and Clin. Neurophysiol.* 66:145–159, 1987.

Lopes da Silva, F.H., Hoeks, A., Smits, A., and Zetterberg, L.H. The cortical alpha rhythm in dog: The depth and surface profile of phase. *Architectonics of the Cerebral Cortex.* (M.A.B. Brazier and Petche, H., Eds.) New York: Raven Press, pp. 319–333, 1978.

Lounasmaa, G.V., Williamson, S.J., Kaufman, L., and Tenenbaum, R. Visually evoked responses for non-occipital areas of the human cortex. In: *Biomagnetism, Applications and Theory.* (G. Weinberg, Stroink, G., and Katila, T., Eds.) New York: Pergamon, pp. 348–353, 1985.

Maffei, L., Moruzzi, G., and Rizzolatti, G. Influence of sleep and wakefulness on the response of lateral geniculate units to sinewave photic stimulation. *Arch. Ital. Biol.* 103:596–608, 1965.

Makeig, S. and Galambos, R. The CERP: Event-related pertubations in steady-state responses. In: *Springer Series in Brain Dynamics.* (E. Basar and Bullock, T.H., Eds.) Berlin: Springer-Verlag, 2:375–400, 1989.

Merigan, W.H. P and M Pathway specialization in the Macaque: In: *From Pigments to Perception.* (A. Valberg and Lee, B.B., Eds.) New York: Plenum Press, pp. 117–125, 1991.

Milner, B. Effects of different brain lesions on card sorting. *Arch. Neurol.* 9:90–100, 1963.

Milner, B. Some effects of frontal lobectomy in man. In: *The Frontal Granular Cortex and Behaviour.* (J.M. Warren and Akert, K., Eds.) New York: McGraw-Hill, pp. 313–334, 1964.

Milner, B. Visual recognition and recall after right temporal-lobe excision in man. *Neuropsychologia*. 6:191–209, 1968.

Milner, B. and Petrides, M. Behavioural effects of frontal-lobe lesions in man. *Trends in Neurosciences*. 7:403–407, 1984.

Nunez, P.L. *Electric Fields of the Brain: The Neurophysics of the EEG*. New York: Oxford University Press, 1981.

Nunez, P.L. Generation of human EEG by a combination of long and short range neocortical interactions. *Brain Topography*. 1:199–215, 1989.

Nunez, P.L. and Pilgreen, K.L. The spline-Laplacian in clinical neurophysiology: A method to improve EEG spatial resolution. *J. Clin. Neurophysiol*. 8:397–413, 1991.

Nunez, P.L., Silberstein, R.B., Cadusch, P.J., and Wijesinghe, R. Comparison of high resolution EEG methods having different theoretical bases. *Brain Topography*. 5:361–364, 1993.

Nunez, P.L., Silberstein, R.B., Cadusch, P.J., Wijesinghe, R., Westdorp, A.F., and Srinivasan, R. A theoretical and experimental study of high resolution EEG based on surface Laplacians and cortical imaging. *Electroencephalogr. Clin. Neurophysiol*. 90:40–57, 1994.

Papanicolaou, A.C. and Johnstone, J. Probe evoked potentials: Theory, method and applications. *Int. J. Neuroscience*. 24:107–131, 1984.

Petersen, S.E., Fox, P.T., Posner, M.I., Mintun, N., and Raichle, M.E. Positron emission tomographic studies of the cortical anatomy of single-word processing. *Nature*. 331:585–589, 1988.

Petersen, S.E., Robinson, D.L., and Morris, J.D. Contributions of the pulvinar to visual spatial attention. *Neuropsychologia*. 25:97–105, 1987.

Pfurtscheller, G. and Klimesch, W. Topographic display and interpretation of event-related desynchronization during a visual-verbal task. *Brain Topography*. 3:85–93, 1990.

Picton, T.W., Vajsar, J., Rodriguez, R., and Campbell, K.B. Reliability estimates for steady-state evoked potentials. *Electroencephalogr. Clin. Neurophysiol*. 68:119–131, 1987.

Puce, A. Evoked encephalographic changes during anaesthesia. Master of Applied Science Thesis. Swinburne Institute of Technology, Melbourne, 1986.

Regan, D. Some characteristics of average steady-state and transient responses evoked by modulated light. *Electroencephalogr. and Clin. Neurophysiol*. 20:238–248, 1966.

Regan, D. Evoked potentials and psychophysical correlates of changes in stimulus colour and intensity. *Vision Res*. 10:163–178, 1970.

Regan, D. *Evoked Potentials in Psychology, Sensory Physiology and Clinical Medicine*. London: Chapman & Hall, 1972.

Regan, D. *Human Brain Electrophysiology: Evoked Potentials and Evoked Magnetic Fields in Science and Medicine*. New York: Elsevier, 1989.

Robinson, D.L. How personality related to intelligence test performance: Implications for a theory of intelligence, ageing research and personality assessment. *Personality and Individual Differences*. 6:203–216, 1985.

Robinson, D.L. The neurophysiological bases of high IQ. *Int. J. Neuroscience*. 46:209–234, 1989.

Robinson, D.L. The neurophysiological bases of high IQ: A reply to Stowell. *Int. J. Neuroscience*. 54:135–138, 1990.

Robinson, D.L. and Petersen, S.E. The pulvinar and visual salience. *Trends in Neurosciences*. 15:127–132, 1992.

Rohbraugh, J.W., Varner, J.L., Paige, S.R., Eckardt, M.J., and Ellingson, R.J. Auditory and visual event-related perturbations in the 40 Hz auditory steady-state response. *Electroencephalogr. and Clin. Neurophysiol.* 76:148–164, 1990.

Rohrbaugh, J.W., Varner, J.L., Paige, S.R., Eckardt, M.J., and Ellingson, R.J. Event-related perturbations in an electrophysiological measure of auditory function: Measure of sensitivity during orientating? *Biol. Psychology.* 29:247–271, 1989.

Roland, P.E. Metabolic measurements of the working frontal cortex in man. *Trends in Neurosciences.* 7:430–435,. 1984.

Schier, M.A., Silberstein, R.B., and Cadusch, P.J. Steady state visually evoked potentials: A comparison of scalp and deconvolved data. Third International Brain Electromagnetic Topography Meeting, Amsterdam, The Netherlands, 1992.

Schiller, P.H. A model for the generation of visually guided saccadic eye movements. In: *Models of the Visual Cortex.* (D. Rose and Dobson, V.G., Eds.) New York: Wiley, pp. 62–70, 1985.

Silberstein, R.B. Topography and dynamics of the steady state visually evoked potential: A window into brain function? *Brain Topography.* 5:64–65, 1992.

Silberstein, R.B., Burkitt, G., and Nield, G. Spatio temporal characteristics of the steady state visually evoked potential. *Brain Topography.* 5:65, 1992a.

Silberstein, R.B., Burkitt, G., and Wood, S.R. Artifact sensitivity of Fourier based analysis of steady state visually evoked potential. Proceedings Second Annual Australasian Psychophysiology Conference, Nelson Bay, Australia, 1992.

Silberstein, R.B., Ciorciari, J., and Pipingas, A. Steady-state visually evoked potential topography during the wisconsin card sort. *Electroencephalogr. Clin. Neurophysiol.* In press, 1994.

Silberstein, R.B., Ciorciari, J., Pipingas, A., Schier, M.A., and Ma, S. Effects of the Wisconsin Card Sort test on the topography of the steady state visually evoked potential. Third ISBET Conference, Amsterdam, The Netherlands, 1992.

Silberstein, R.B., Pipingas, A., Ciorciari, J., and Schier, M.A. Steady state visually evoked scalp topography in a visual vigilance task: effects of eye movements. Second International Congress on Brain Electromagnetic Topography, Toronto, Canada, 1991.

Silberstein, R.B., Schier, M.A., Pipingas, A., Ciorciari, J., Wood, S.R., and Simpson, D.G. Steady-state visually evoked potential topography associated with a visual vigilance task. *Brain Topography.* 3:337–347, 1990.

Speckreijse, H., Estevez, O., and Reits, D. Visual evoked potentials and the physiological analysis of visual processes in man. In: *Visual Evoked Potentials in Man: New Developments.* (J.E. Desmedt, Ed.) Oxford: Clarendon Press, pp. 16–89, 1977.

Speckreijse, H. and Reits, D. Sequential analysis of the visual evoked potential system in man; nonlinear analysis of a sandwich system. *Ann. N.Y. Acad. Sci.* 388:72–97, 1982.

Stowell, H. IQ scores, brain waves, frequency response, and damping ratio: A weak mix. *Int. J. Neurosci.* 54:133–138, 1990.

Thatcher, R.W., Krause, P.J., and Hrybyk, M. Cortico-cortico associations and EEG coherence: A two-compartmental model. *Electroencephalogr. Clin. Neurophysiol.* 64:123–143, 1986.

Tyler, C.W., Apkarian, P., and Nakayama, K. Multiple spatial-frequency tuning of electrical responses from human visual cortex. *Exp. Brain Res.* 33:535–550, 1978.

Van Der Tweel, L.H. and Verduyn Lunel, H.F.E. Human visual responses to sinusoidally modulated light. *Electroencephalogr. and Clin. Neurophysiol.* 18:587–598, 1965.

Van Essen, D.C., Anderson, C.H., and Fellerman, D.J. Information processing in the primate visual system: An integrated systems perspective. *Science.* 255:419–423, 1992.

Wahba, G. Spline interpolation and smoothing on a sphere. *SIAM J. Sci. Stat. Comput.* 2:5–16, 1981.

Weinberger, D.R., Berman, K.F., and Zec, R.F. Physiologic dysfunction of dorsolateral prefrontal cortex in schizophrenia. *Arch. Gen. Psychiatry.* 43:114–124, 1986.

Williamson, S.J., Kaufman, L., and Brenner, D. Latency of the neuromagnetic response of the human visual cortex. *Vision Res.* 18:107–110, 1978.

Wilson, G.F. and O'Donnell, R.D. Steady state evoked responses: Correlations with human cognition. *Psychophysiology.* 23:57–61, 1986.

Wright, J.J. and Sergejew, A.A. Radial coherence, wave velocity and damping of electrocortical waves. *Electroencephalogr. Clin. Neurophysiol.* 79:403–412, 1991.

7

Neuroelectric Measures of Mind

ALAN S. GEVINS and BRIAN A. CUTILLO

Electroencephalography, Evoked Potentials, and Cognition

Scalp-recorded neural potentials have been used for more than 65 years to study brain activity associated with higher mental functions in humans, both as continuous electroencephalographic (EEG) and as event-registered evoked potentials (EP). Human cognitive neurophysiology is still in its infancy, however, awaiting more powerful tools to measure the minute signals of complex neurocognitive processes. Such tools will include recordings made with arrays of many channels of EEG (and magnetoencephalograms [MEG]), advanced signal processing, anatomic information from magnetic resonance images (MRI), and functional metabolic information from positron emission tomography, single photon emission computed tomography, and fMRI (functional MRI). With a combination of the most advanced techniques available, we can only observe some signs of the location, timing, and coordination of mass neural activity associated with cognition. The EEG's advantages of subsecond temporal resolution, ability to record in a natural situation, and its low cost are motivating the development of better recording and analytic techniques.

In 1929, Hans Berger reported that the alpha rhythm decreased in amplitude during mental arithmetic (Berger, 1929). Subsequently many EEG studies of cognition have been done, but their lack of precise time registration hinders resolution of the subsecond stages of cognitive processing. The solution has been use of EPs, which bring the temporal resolution into the millisecond range, and we will devote this chapter primarily to these studies.

Evoked potentials are a valuable tool to study the mass neural activity generated during cognitive processes. Usually they are studied by averaging several brief EEG segments time registered to the stimulus or response in a simple cognitive task (although methods exist to study EPs in a group of individual trials). Averaging enhances signals that are temporally consistent with respect to the event, and it suppresses unrelated background activity. An averaged EP waveform consists of a series of positive and negative "waves." (In evoked potential terminology, the word "wave" refers to the time series "waveform" or portion of waveform. No particular physical basis is implied.) A substantial change in latency, amplitude, or duration of an EP peak or wave between experimental conditions that differ in one specific cognitive factor is assumed to reflect the mass neural activity associated with that cognitive factor. Measuring changes in the amplitude and timings of peaks in the series of EP waves allows us to make inferences about the sequence and timing of task-associated processes, such as prestimulus preparation, encoding of stimulus features, operations such as matching or comparison of stimulus codes and memory codes, evaluation of the meaning of the stimulus, and response selection and execution.

The first reports of EP events related not only to external (exogenous) factors, such as stimulus properties or motor activity, but also to cognitive (endogenous) factors studied in the 1960s. In 1964, Grey Walter reported an EP event related to expectation (Walter et al, 1964). The "contingent negative variation" (CNV) is a low-frequency negative wave preceding an expected stimulus, often visible in the unaveraged EEG (Figure 7-1). The CNV varies during stages of conditioned learning, with motivation, attention, distraction, and other cognitive variables.

At almost the same time, Samuel Sutton, Victor Zubin, and E. Roy John discovered a positive wave peaking about 300 milliseconds after infrequent, task-relevant stimuli (Sutton et al, 1965; Figure 7-2). The P300 or P3 peak is considered endogenous because its scalp topography and behavior did not depend on physical stimulus properties per se, but rather on their meaning in the context of the task. P300 is evoked by many types of paradigms, but the strongest factors in its elicitation are stimulus frequency and task relevance. An especially cogent finding was the elicitation of P300 by the absence of a stimulus in a regularly timed sequence of stimuli. This missing stimulus EP, obtained by averaging brain potentials registered to the time the missing stimuli should have occurred, lacks early exogenous peaks, such as N100, but contains P300 and other endogenous waves.

Basic Aspects of the EP Method

The study of cognition using amplitude and timing measurements of EP waves and peaks is based on many of the same paradigms used in experimental psychology. In the most general terms, it is assumed that a cognitive behavior can be viewed as a combination of sequential (and in some cases parallel) subprocesses in which information from stimuli is encoded, compared with memory and previous experience, and acted on. The division into component subprocesses may be somewhat arbitrary and depends on the particular cognitive model used, but it is assumed that these subprocesses can be manipulated systematically and that the electric signals generated by these processes can be distinguished at the scalp. More extensive reviews of these issues can be found in Donchin et al, 1977; Thatcher and John, 1977; Gevins and Cutillo, 1986; and Meyer et al, 1990.

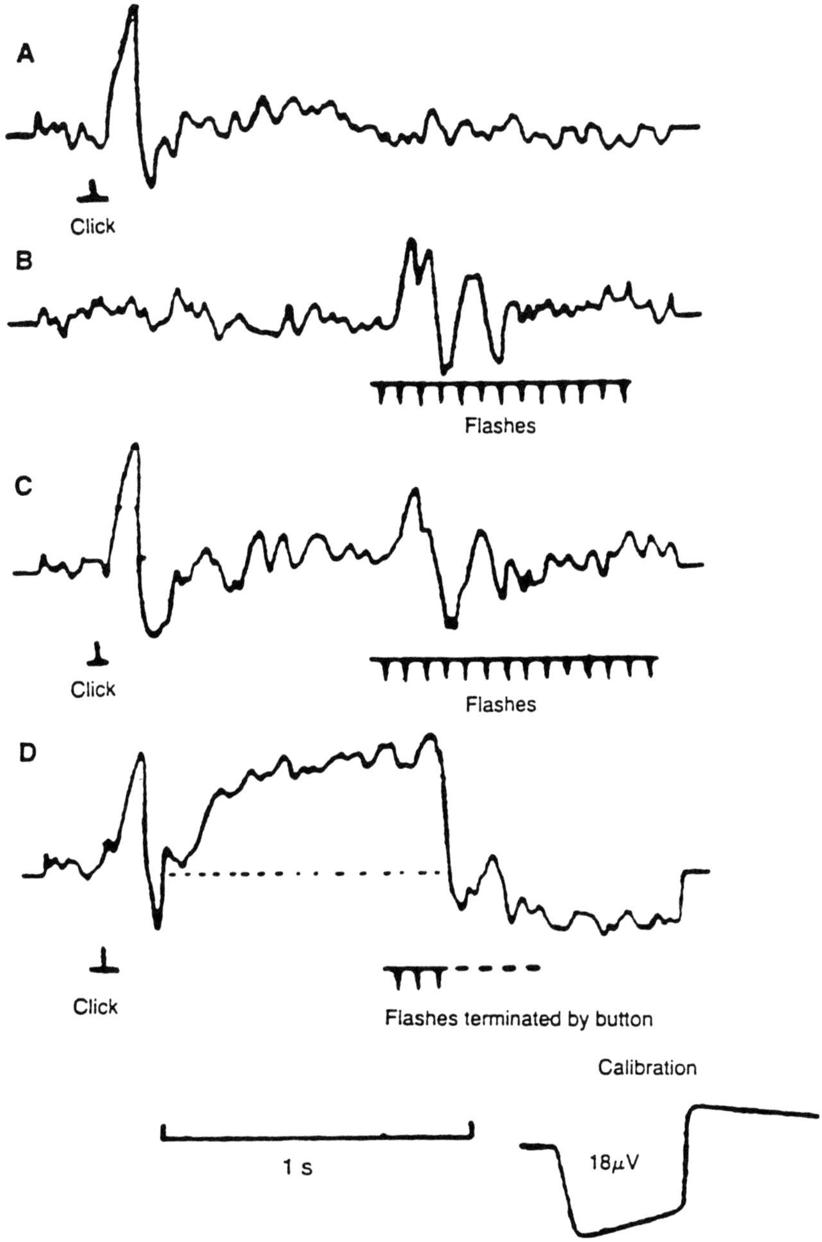

Figure 7-1. The contingent negative variation (CNV), reported to be related to expectation in the interval between warning and imperative stimuli, from the original report by Walter (Walter et al, 1964). Averaged waveforms (from vertex electrode referenced to mastoid) to unpaired click (**A**) and flash (**B**) stimuli, paired click and flash stimuli 1 second apart, with no task-relevant contingency (**C**), and CNV in the 1-second interval between the paired stimuli when they are made contingent by requiring a response (**D**).

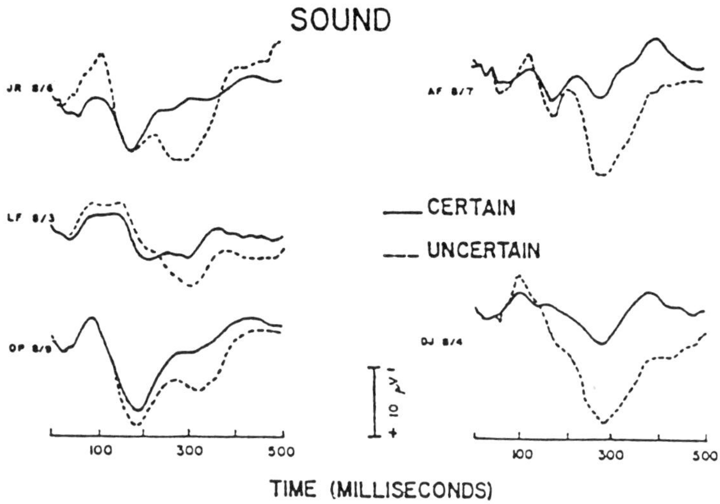

Figure 7-2. Illustration of P300 wave from the original report of Sutton and colleagues (Sutton et al, 1965). The P300 was observed as a large positive wave peaking about 300 milliseconds after the stimulus in these averaged waveforms from five persons elicited by infrequent unexpected (uncertain) and frequent expected (certain) auditory stimuli.

Cognitive Factors Can Be Systematically Manipulated

Mental events cannot be measured directly but can be inferred from measurements of the behavioral and neural activity associated with them. Psychological studies use behavioral measures such as reaction time and error to define component stages of cognitive processing and make inferences about their nature and timing. Thus the validity of a study depends on the ability to manipulate a specific cognitive factor while holding all other factors constant. This is also true for cognitive studies using measures of brain signals, in which the issue of holding irrelevant factors constant across conditions is somewhat more difficult because of the sensitivity of neuroelectric signals to factors such as the physical properties of stimuli and motor responses (see "Experimental Control," below).

The Timing of Neurocognitive Processes Is Consistent

As noted previously, the averaged EP method assumes that the component subprocesses comprising a cognitive behavior vary very little in timing among trials. This assumption should be made with the understanding that a certain amount of trial-to-trial variation may occur in the timing of neurocognitive processes that affect the latency and amplitude of EP components, because they are interdependent. Therefore, measures of the integrated amplitude (area) of an averaged wave are sometimes used, and "latency correction" of a particular peak before averaging can be done (Woody, 1967; McGillem and Aunon, 1987).

Overlapping Components Can Be Resolved

The average EP waveform is assumed to be a linear composite of spatially and temporally overlapping components generated in different neural systems. This overlap makes measurement of individual components in the composite waveform an important consideration. Sometimes relatively simple experimental or analytic methods may be effective in distinguishing components, as with the isolation of the N200 wave from the P200 by subtraction of the waveform to standard stimuli from the waveform to target stimuli. But often it is not possible to distinguish overlapping components by such simple methods. Principal components analysis (PCA) is often used as a more general solution to the problem of objective definition of components (Donchin and Heffly, 1978). The PCA method can be useful but is limited because physiologically independent neural generators may produce potential time series that are statistically correlated. Other practical problems have been described, such as the misallocation of variance among components and arbitrariness of the rotation used (Rosler and Manzey, 1981; Wood and McCarthy, 1984). Alternatives to PCA have been developed that may be more effective in extracting small signals in cases of low signal-to-noise ratio, including comparative factor analysis (Rogers, 1991).

Experimental Control Is Essential to Infer that a Signal Is Associated with a Particular Cognitive Factor

In any experiment, all factors not directly related to the intended experimental manipulation must be controlled. Special attention to experimental control is required in neurocognitive studies because brain signals are sensitive to many sensory, motor, and cognitive factors, and neurocognitive signals may be small in relation to other simultaneously occurring neural processes. The conditions should be controlled for irrelevant stimulus, physiologic-state and response-related factors by experimental design and also by a posteriori balancing of data sets. Such factors include physical stimulus properties, frequency and ordering of stimuli, task difficulty, automatization, and the timing, force, duration, hand, and nature of response movements (Gevins et al, 1979a, 1979b, 1979c; 1980, 1985; Gevins and Schaffer, 1980). Behavioral measures should be made for each trial to verify that the task was performed properly and to form balanced sets of trials differing only in the variable(s) being studied before hypothesis testing. In addition, brain signals vary with age, handedness, sex, level of automatic arousal, alertness and fatigue, habituation, and use of caffeine, nicotine, alcohol, and drugs. These factors should be taken into account when trying to measure physiological signs of mental activity in the brain.

EP Events Associated with Cognition: Two Major Lines of Research

Signals of Preparation: The Contingent Negative Variation

The CNV is a low-frequency (less than 1 Hz) "negative wave" (that is, negative potential waveform with respect to averaged ear potentials) that occurs between two stimuli that involve a contingency or association (Figure 7-1). It is best seen when the stimuli are separated by a regular interval with a response required after the second stimulus. About 200 milliseconds after the second stimulus, the CNV ends in a sharp positive-going (approximately 10 Hz) wave called the "CNV resolution." The CNV initially was considered a signal of expectancy (Walter, 1964), but subsequent studies showed that it is affected by many cognitive factors, including attention, distraction, preparation for cognitive tasks, anticipation of information, ambiguity, and task difficulty, and also by noncognitive factors such as stimulus intensity, modality and timing, reaction time, magnitude of movement, motivation, positive or negative reinforcement, noxious stimuli, arousal, age, fatigue, some drugs, and clinical disorders including learning disability, senility, neurosis, anhedonia, depression, and schizophrenia (reviewed in Tecce, 1972; Rockstroh et al, 1989; Rohrbaugh and Gaillard, 1983).

The idea that the CNV reflects preparatory processes assumes that the low-frequency wave (which appears as a negative potential shift when the time series is plotted conventionally) reflects an accumulation of cerebral potentiality that is released during the positive-going resolution after the second stimulus. The scalp distribution of the CNV (with linked ear or noncephalic reference) is widely distributed, usually largest at the midline central electrode, but also strong at precentral and frontal sites. The CNV reflects depolarization of apical dendrites in frontal and central cortex, but the theory that this facilitates neuronal action potentials has not been proved (Rebert, 1978; Rockstroh et al, 1989). The possible involvement of frontal cortex is of particular interest because this area is thought to mediate functions such as preparation and planning (Fuster, 1989; Goldman-Rakic, 1984). The theory that the CNV reflects task-specific cortical activation was questioned by repeated failure to localize amplitude with different types of tasks or with attention to different sensory modalities. More recently, however, evidence for localized, task-specific cortical activation during the CNV was found by recording from more scalp sites and using a spatial filter to reduce volume-conducted activity common to all electrodes (Gevins et al, 1987, 1989b; Gevins and Cutillo, 1993).

The extent to which the CNV reflects cognitive association of two stimuli is still unclear. Some researchers believe that the CNV is merely a composite of two separate negative waves and does not involve a contingent association between two stimuli (Rohrbaugh et al, 1980). But many others favor the view that the CNV reflects a cognitive association between stimuli (Donchin et al, 1974; Ritter et al, 1984). The CNV has been seen to develop when a contingency between two stimuli is learned and then decline when the contingency is removed. Contingent negative variation amplitude is reduced by distracting stimuli (Tecce, 1972), by instructions to change attentional focus (McCallum and Walter, 1968), and by equivocation of contingency through random omission of the second stimulus (Walter et al, 1964).

The issue of "cognitive association" now seems to be an academic point. The "contingent" negative variation can be viewed as just one type of low-frequency wave (or, in traditional terms, "slow potential shift" [SPS]). Positive and negative SPSs are seen frequently in EEG recordings, but they have been largely ignored. However, researchers are beginning to examine the functional significance of SPSs (Rockstroh et al, 1989; Harter et al, 1990; Rosler, 1991). Use of many recording sites and spatial enhancement techniques make possible the detection of the previously elusive variations in potential topography in response to task requirements, which will be discussed later.

Information and Expectation: The P300 and Slow Wave

Under appropriate conditions, task-relevant stimuli, or the omission of expected stimuli, elicit a sequence of overlapping positive waves in the 300 to 1,000 millisecond latency range. This is called the late positive complex and includes the P3a, P3b, and slow wave (SW). The P3b wave (P300, or simply 'P3') was first reported in 1965 (Sutton et al, 1965), and although it has been studied extensively, this robust, easily elicited wave has been resistant to a precise definition of its relation to cognition and behavior. Although P300 is complexly influenced by many factors, several well-established facts about its behavior are known (reviewed in Tueting, 1978; Donchin, 1979; Pritchard, 1981; Duncan-Johnson and Donchin, 1982). Task-relevant (attended) stimuli elicit substantial P300 waves with amplitudes that are larger for infrequent deviant stimuli, as in the popular "oddball" paradigm in which infrequent target stimuli must be distinguished from frequent nontargets. Its potential distribution is maximal at midline parietal or midline central sites (with linked ear or noncephalic references). The distribution is relatively unaffected by physical stimulus properties, such as modality or intensity, if they do not provide task-relevant information. The amplitude of P300 is inversely related to the probability of occurrence of stimuli that have different meanings in the context of the task.

The behavior of P300 is usually interpreted in terms of concepts from the field of cognitive psychology. However, its behavior may fit a particular theory in one study but not in another. No simple relation exists between P300 and cognitive factors, and thus a parsimonious model of P300 and cognition has not yet been developed. The difficulty of interpreting P300 in terms of psychological constructs was discussed by Chase and associates (1984) and by Verleger (1988). A few of the more popular models of P300 are described below.

P300 and Stimulus Evaluation

With one theory, P300 latency is related to the time required to evaluate stimuli. Increases in the latency of the onset and peak of the P300 have been produced by increasing the difficulty of stimulus discriminability (Squires et al, 1977) or stimulus complexity (Ritter et al, 1982). P300 latency is also lengthened by increasing categorization difficulty (Ritter et al, 1983b) or number of items in the target memory set (Ford et al, 1979). However, these factors also affect the N200 waves, which (unlike the P300) always precede response initiation and are more closely correlated with reaction time (Renault et al, 1982; Ritter et al, 1983a, 1983b), suggesting that they are associated more closely with actual stimulus evaluation.

P300 and Updating of an "Internal Model"

One explanation for the dissociation of P300 latency and reaction time and for its relation to stimulus evaluation is that P300 is associated with updating an internal schema or memory template after stimulus evaluation (Tueting, 1978; McCarthy and Donchin, 1983). This theory proposes that the internal schema cannot be updated until the importance of the stimulus has been fully evaluated, whereas a response can be initiated as soon as the information required to perform the current trial has been evaluated. Thus P300 latency would be correlated with reaction time only indirectly.

Two aspects of context updating are the amount of updating induced by the current stimulus and its effects on expectancy, which should be evident in the succeeding trial. The amount of updating aspect is supported by P300's larger amplitude for infrequent stimuli (global probability effect) and longer latency for "disconfirming" feedback (Squires et al, 1973), two instances in which more updating would be expected. Evidence for the expectancy aspect is the influence of local probability, which can modulate the effect of global probability on P300 amplitude (Squires et al, 1976). The order of preceding stimuli seems to create an expectancy set, resulting in larger amplitudes when an expectation is violated; the weakening of the effect of local probability at long interstimulus intervals suggests the decay of a memory trace. Context updating and memory also could account for the robust P300 for feedback stimuli and its tendency to be larger and longer in latency for disconfirming feedback.

P300, Controlled Processing, and Capacity

The psychological concepts of controlled processing and processing capacity have been applied to the behavior of P300. Controlled processing denotes a limited-capacity central process involving conscious effort and is distinguished from automatic processing, which does not make demands on processing capacity. Examples of automatic processes are initial encoding of sensory information and execution of well-practiced motor actions. Controlled processes include memory rehearsal and search, target detection, and several types of decision or judgment. Prominent P300 peaks are elicited when a task requires controlled processing, and P300 amplitude may be related to the amount of controlled processing required for some tasks (Rosler, 1983).

When two tasks that involve controlled processing are performed simultaneously, their interference is evident as a decline in performance measures such as reaction time and accuracy. If P300 is associated with controlled processing, it should reflect such interference. Studies using dual-task paradigms (Israel et al, 1980; Wickens et al, 1983) showed that P300 amplitude to infrequent targets in an oddball task is reduced when a second task is performed concurrently, and its amplitude to oddball targets varies inversely with the difficulty of the second task only if that task requires controlled processing. Increasing the difficulty of a well-learned, automatized, tracking task does not reduce the P300 amplitude in a concurrent oddball task, but increased difficulty of a monitoring task does. P300 amplitudes in the two tasks vary reciprocally as task difficulty is manipulated, suggesting that under those conditions it indexes the distribution of processing capacity between tasks. Even the instruction not to blink, which is usually given to experimental subjects, constitutes a secondary task that reduces the amplitude of the P300 of the primary task (Verleger, 1991).

The Slow Wave

Some tasks elicit a long-duration SW, which begins as early as 180 milliseconds and peaks at about 500 to 700 milliseconds. It has been distinguished from P300 by topography and behavior (Ruchkin and Sutton, 1983). Slow wave amplitude is larger for all task-relevant stimuli, regardless of whether they are targets, and thus can occur without a P300 (Squires et al, 1975). Its amplitude can even be larger for nontargets if they require more processing than targets (Friedman et al, 1981). Also SW amplitude increases with task difficulty, whereas P300 amplitude typically decreases (Ruchkin et al, 1980). The SW is associated with processes subsequent to stimulus evaluation, possibly the extraction of information necessary to maintain task performance over many trials (Stuss et al, 1980).

The SW is important because it is one of the first endogenous EP events whose scalp topography could be differentially manipulated by cognitive task factors. Its midline distribution for visual stimuli is typically negative at the front of the head and positive at the back. An experimental effect sometimes is seen only in the frontal negative or parietal positive portions of its topography, which suggests that the anterior and posterior portions may be generated by different neural processes (Picton and Stuss, 1980; Friedman et al, 1981).

The Variety of EP Events

Attention and Automaticity: Endogenous Negative Waves

Several phenomena in cognitive EP research have been researched more recently. In the past 15 years, the complexity of reported EP components has increased. We know that EP events first thought to be unitary phenomena consist of several waves, distinguishable by topography, experimental manipulations, and analytic methods. We will begin the discussion of this development by examining several negative waves that can occur in the first half second after a stimulus (reviewed in Näätänen and Michie, 1979).

Processing Negativity

The processing negativity (Näätänen et al, 1978) or "Nd" (Hansen and Hillyard, 1980), is a broad negative wave that is larger in amplitude for stimuli that must be selected on the basis of simple physical properties. It is a sign of early selective attention, sometimes called channel selection. Its onset and duration reflect the nature and difficulty of stimulus selection, and its topography reflects the modality and side of stimulation. Because it begins as early as 60 milliseconds and lasts for 500 milliseconds, it overlaps the N100 peak and causes an apparent increase in N100 amplitude, which is why researchers initially attributed the selective attention effect to N100 (Hillyard et al, 1973). It was distinguished from N100 by its behavior in response to experimental manipulations and by subtracting the averaged EPs for attended and unattended stimuli (Näätänen et al, 1978, 1981). The processing negativity may be composed of several components with different topographies and relations to task requirements (Hansen and Hillyard, 1983). The relation of these components to selective attention and sensory channels is important because it affects the issue of whether attentional selection occurs early or late in the course of stimulus processing. The behavior of the processing negativity tends to support early selection theories (Hansen and Woldorff, 1991).

The N200 Peaks

Infrequent stimuli that deviate from most stimuli elicit a negative wave at about 200 milliseconds (Roth, 1973). The stimuli need not be task relevant or attended (Snyder and Hillyard, 1976), and N200 amplitude is inversely related to the frequency of deviant stimuli (Squires et al, 1975). Because N200 closely overlaps the P200 peak, it is usually measured in the difference waveform by subtracting the EP to the frequent standard stimuli from the EP to deviant stimuli. The N200 wave consists of two separate peaks. The N2a, or "mismatch negativity," is elicited by infrequent deviant stimuli, regardless of whether it is task relevant. Its sensitivity to probability and magnitude of deviation led to the interpretation of N2a as a sign of neuronal mismatch in the orienting response to deviant stimuli, "an automatic, basic sensory process . . . irrespective of, perhaps even unmodified by, the task and subjective factors" (Näätänen, 1982). Its modality-specific topography suggests involvement of activity in and around sensory cortex, and its amplitude and timing are affected by physical factors such as stimulus discriminability, complexity, and nature and magnitude of deviation. The slightly later N2b peak is not sensitive to these factors but is affected by task-related factors such as attention and categorization difficulty (Ritter et al, 1979). N2b has a modality-independent frontocentral distribution similar to P3a, which appears always to follow it (Squires et al, 1975, 1977). A similar pair of peaks was observed in the missing stimulus negativity (Renault and Lesevre, 1979).

With certain tasks, N2b is preceded by a negative peak, called NA, that differs from the N2a because it is not affected by probability (Ritter et al, 1983a, 1983b). Because the N2a and the NA are affected by exogenous factors, whereas the behavior of N2b is more endogenous, and because an experimental manipulation that increases the latency of the earlier peak produces an identical increase in the timing of N2b (Ritter et al, 1979, 1983a; Renault, 1983), they are probably associated with successive, contingent stages of information processing (Figure 7-3). Several two-stage models have been proposed: pattern recognition and stimulus categorization (Ritter et al, 1982); two stages of the orienting response (Näätänen and Gaillard, 1983); automatic and controlled processing (Ritter et al, 1983b); and active perceptual processing (template matching) leading to evaluation of the importance of stimulus and response selection (Renault, 1983). All these models propose that the earlier wave is associated with automatic feature extraction processes that precede the endogenous processes associated with N2b, and that their

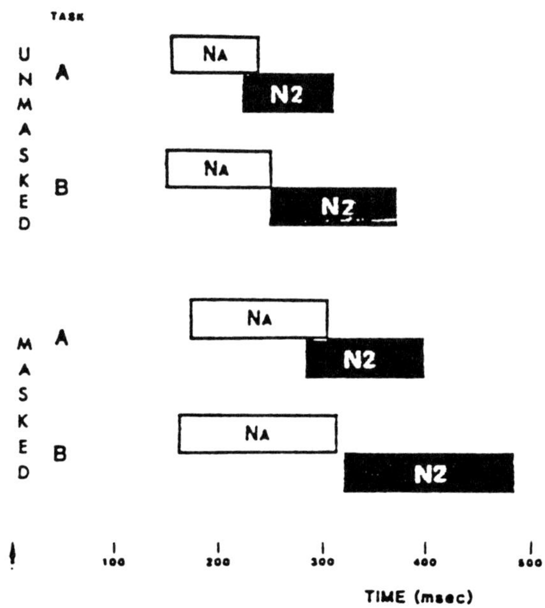

Figure 7-3. Differential manipulation of two overlapping peaks: the earlier NA and the later N2 (N2b). The bars span the onset and peak latencies of the waves. Increasing the difficulty of stimulus discrimination by stimulus masking increases the onset-to-peak time of NA and causes an identical increase in the onset time of N2. The increase in difficulty of stimulus categorization between task A and task B does not affect the timing of NA but increases the onset-to-peak time of N2. It was thus inferred that NA is related to feature extraction and N2 to the judgment of stimulus category. (Adapted with permission from Ritter et al, 1983.)

peak latency, onset, and duration reflect the timing of such processes. High correlations of peak latencies and reaction times have been reported (Renault et al, 1982; Näätänen and Gaillard, 1983), and differential manipulation of the amplitude and timing of the two waves by changes in physical (exogenous) and task-related (endogenous) factors, respectively, support this theory.

Neuroelectric Chronometrics

The term chronometrics refers to methods for inferring the sequence and timing of component stages of cognitive processes and to models of information processing, from behavioral or neuroelectric measures or both. This approach was pioneered by Donders in the mid-1800s, was brought back into popular use by Sternberg (1966), and was most elegantly applied in the work of Posner (1978). Detailed reviews are by Chase and associates (1984) and by Meyer and coworkers (1990). Chronometric analysis is well suited to EP studies, because the timing of onset, peak latency, and duration of the waves associated with cognitive factors can, in principle, be used to measure the temporal relations of processing stages directly. (Labeling of waves in the following discussion [such as N100] follows the convention of designating polarity ['P' or 'N'] and typical peak latency [such as 100].)

The short and medium latency peaks in the first 80 milliseconds after a visual stimulus are highly exogenous: Their latency and topography depend on the modality, intensity, and other physical properties of the stimulus. They reflect the arrival of the incoming sensory signals at subcortical and cortical structures. (The same is true of auditory and somatic stimuli, except that the initial processing is faster.) Next the P100 and the following N100 are usually considered exogenous. Their topography changes with modality and correlates with the assumption that they are generated primarily in sensory cortex. They reflect the encoding of basic features of stimuli. After the N100, a P200 peak occurs that has a frontocentral topography that is mainly independent of stimulus modality. If the task requires selection of stimuli on the basis of simple physical properties, the long-duration, low-amplitude processing negativity, thought to be a sign of early selective attention, also may occur in this latency range (Näätänen et al, 1978).

If the stimulus differs from most of the stimuli, the N2–P3a peak complex occurs at about 200 to 300 milliseconds (Squires et al, 1975). Task relevance is not required, and N2–P3a amplitudes vary inversely with probability. N2 consists of two successive peaks, as noted previously. The earlier peak (called N2a, mismatch negativity, or NA) and the succeeding N2b are differentially affected by task factors. Because N2b onset is delayed when NA peak latency is lengthened, and N2b peak latency is highly correlated with reaction time, N2a (or NA) and N2b reflect successive, contingent stages of task processing. If the stimulus is also task relevant, P3a will be followed by the P3b (P300) peak. The behavior of P3b is affected in a complex manner by many cognitive factors of an order higher than the preceding waves. P3b appears to be involved in almost all types of higher cognitive functions. Some tasks elicit later peaks, such as the long-duration SW, peaking between 500 and 700 milliseconds, which may reflect processes related to task performance over many trials.

A typical discrimination task might consist of identifying infrequent target stimuli in a sequence of standard stimuli and making a finger movement in response to the targets. An idealized averaged EP for the target stimuli might contain a sequence of peaks such as those in Figure 7-4: P90 (P1), N130 (N1), P190 (P2), N225 (N2a), N250 (N2b), P290 (P3a), P375 (P3b), a SW peaking at 575 milliseconds, and negative movement-related readiness potential and motor potential peaking at 500 milliseconds. The chronology of onset, peak latency, and duration of the component waves in this hypothetical waveform, as might be derived by PCA, subtraction, topographic, or other methods, is illustrated in the lower part of Figure 7-4. When the onset of a particular wave precedes the peak of the previous wave, the neural process indexed by the later wave appears to begin before the preceding stage culminates. If experimental manipulation indicates a contingency between two waves, the issue of discrete or continuous models of information transfer arises. If no direct contingency is evident, then the possibility of multiple parallel processing stages must be accounted for in the model (see Meyer et al, 1988).

Considering the hypothetical components of the EP waveform for target stimuli of our discrimination task in terms of information flow and processing stages, we can speculate that encoding of stimulus features begins with the mid-latency exogenous waves between 40 and 80 milliseconds and continues through P90, N130, and P190. The feature codes necessary for identification of target stimuli must be available by the N2a peak at 225 milliseconds because it is affected by the nature and degree of deviation from the standard stimuli. The N2b at 250 milliseconds is sensitive to endogenous factors that did not affect N2a, and the topographies of N2b and the P3a at 290 milliseconds are not affected by stimulus modality, suggesting that they are associated with processes involving a modality-independent common code. The increase in N2b latency caused by categorization difficulty and its high correlation with reaction time suggests that it is associated with evaluation of stimulus information required for response selection. The P3b (P300) at 375 milliseconds is elicited only by task-relevant stimuli. Its latency is sometimes (but not always) moderately correlated with N2b latency and reaction time. Its amplitude is larger for stimuli that match the memorized target but also becomes larger as the frequency of target stimuli is reduced. Considered along with its latency behavior, P3b is related to stimulus evaluation in the current trial and to the updating of an internal schema or expectancy set subsequent to stimulus evaluation in preparation for future trials. The slow wave also seems to be related to processes subsequent to stimulus evaluation and may also be involved in ongoing task performance, perhaps more than P3b, because it is often stronger for non-targets.

Recent Trends

In the last decade, EP research entered a phase characterized by two trends. First, many EP waves that were assumed to be simple, unitary phenomena were found to consist of several distinct components on the basis of their topography

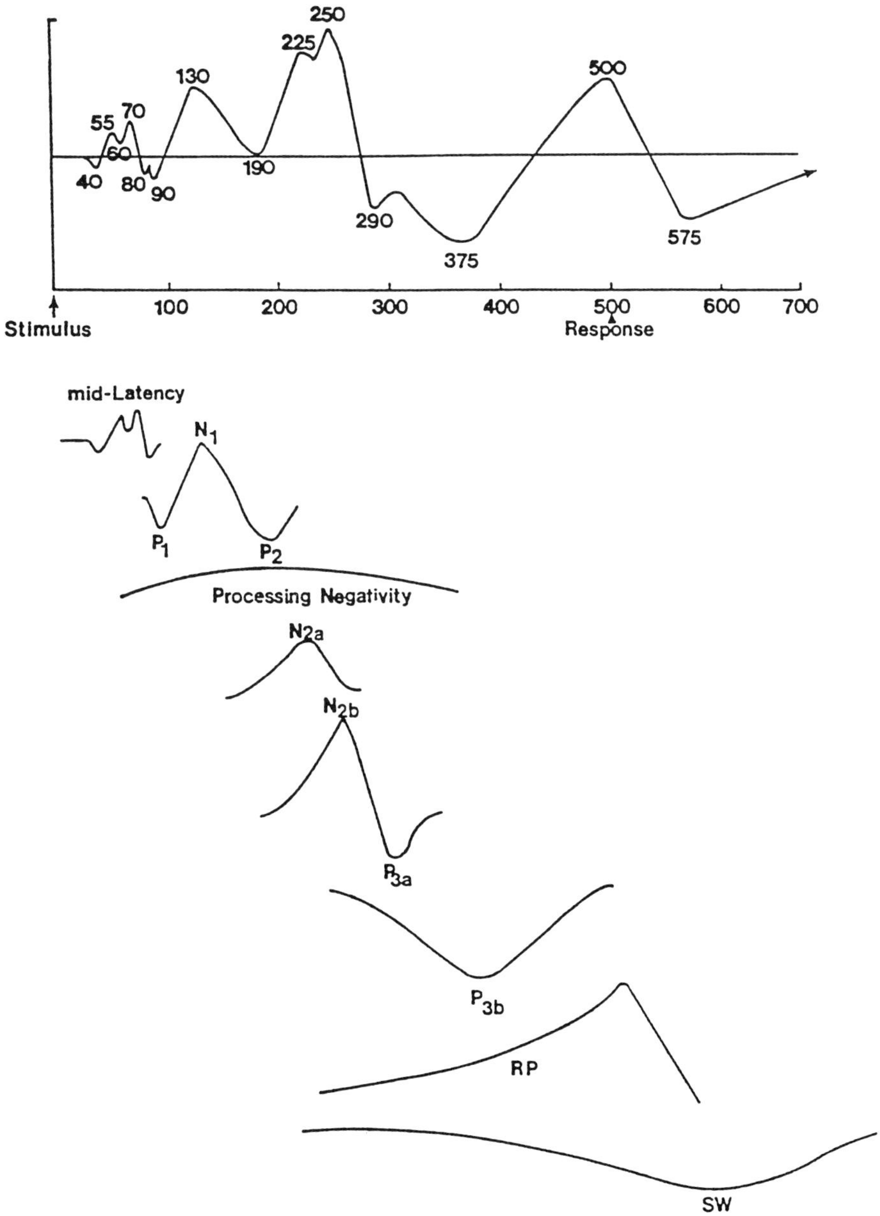

Figure 7-4. (*Upper*) Model averaged evoked potential waveform for infrequent target stimuli in a hypothetical visual discrimination task showing typical mid-latency and late peaks, the processing negativity, and the movement-related readiness potential. (*Lower*) Hypothetical components of the waveform, as might be inferred by subtraction, principal components analysis, and topographic methods, showing their onset times, peak latencies, and durations. Note the high degree of overlap of successive components. (Adapted with permission from Gevins and Cutillo, 1986.)

or their behavior in response to experimental manipulation. Second, the attempt to definitively describe the behavior of even the most well-studied EP waves in terms of simple psychological models has not been successful. The more closely an EP wave is studied, the more complex and resistant to simple description its behavior becomes. Even the auditory N100, long considered a simple exogenous event generated in primary sensory cortex, was found to consist of as many as six distinct waves (Näätänen and Picton, 1987). One of these, the "processing negativity," or Nd, elicited by sounds in attended stimulus channels, was, in turn, found to consist of three topographically distinct subcomponents with different behaviors (Giard et al, 1988), further complicating the complex issues in selective attention paradigms (Näätänen et al, 1978, 1981; Hillyard, 1984; Hansen and Woldorff, 1991).

The premiere example of these trends is the P300. When elicited by oddball or target-matching paradigms, the P300 typically has a maximum voltage at the midline parietal site, whereas the P300 elicited by "no-go" stimuli in a go/no-go task is more anterior in distribution (Simson et al, 1977), and the frontal or 'novelty' P300 elicited by unexpected stimuli is even more anterior (Courchesne et al, 1975). Furthermore, "multiple P3s" with differing topographies (Johnson and Donchin, 1985; Gevins et al, 1989b), and a "P4" with a slightly more posterior distribution for visual stimuli (see Roth, 1978) were reported. Changes in P300 topography with habituation (Courchesne, 1978) and stimulus modality (Snyder et al, 1980) were reported as well. The problem of trying to make psychologically based theories fit the behavior of the P3 wave is typified by Verleger's (1988) article on the P300 and by the comments by several other researchers. Few of them agree about what cognitive function P300 indexes; they do not even agree that the P300 results from excitatory or inhibitory neural activity. Investigators have begun to accept the complex nature of the P300 wave. For example, its behavior when the information content of stimuli is manipulated has been explained by proposing that the P300 is produced by multiple generators (Ruchkin et al, 1990). In a recent review, Picton (1992) treated the topics of the difficulty of specifying the cerebral generators of the P300 and its relation to psychological factors in much detail. However, in experiments conducted in the EEG Systems Laboratory using adequate spatial sampling and methods to reduce the blurring effects of volume conduction, the topography of the P300 varied systematically with task conditions (Gevins et al, 1987, 1989a, 1989b; Gevins and Cutillo, 1993), as we will show in the next section.

Many reported EP waves do not fit the behavior or distribution of the "canonical" peaks discussed so far. For example, a somatosensory "active search" positivity was found in the P300 latency range but is distinguished from P300 by its strong right-hemispheric lateralization for both left and right hands (Desmedt, 1977). Early attention-related shifts have been reported in addition to the "Nd effect" (Harter et al, 1990), and several distinct slow negative waves were observed to accompany such tasks as mental arithmetic, memory search, and mental rotation (Ruchkin et al, 1991; Wijers et al, 1989).

Similar situations can be cited in many lines of EP research. One way to resolve these issues may be to consider EP waves not just as epiphenomena that correlate with psychological constructs but rather as neurophysiologic processes underlying cognition. This approach requires consideration of the way in which the diverse cortical and subcortical systems of the brain might function in the task processing that creates EP signals. Some suggestions for this were provided by recent studies of the CNV, which has successfully survived a long controversy about its existence as a cognitive event (Rosler, 1991) and has given birth to an area of research into SPSs, of both positive and negative polarity, as signs of the regulation of cortical activity in specific cortical areas (Rockstroh et al, 1989; Harter et al, 1990).

Distributed Networks: A Metaphor for Neurocognitive Processing

The situation just outlined underscores the fact that EPs rarely reflect simple, unitary neural processes. This is not surprising, because neural processes are complex, as is their relation to psychological constructs. Although cognitive EP studies continue to produce interesting results, we have little reason to expect that simple peak amplitude and latency measurements from a few electrodes would adequately characterize processes that involve the integrated activity of many widely distributed neural areas. Because each cognitive task involves the organized processing of different types of sensory, motor, temporal, and mnemonic codes, a different sequence of coordinated neural subsystems must be invoked for each cognitive behavior. These metastable configurations or "processing stages" typically last about 100 to 200 milliseconds and represent the large-scale integration of distributed local processing. These large-scale integrations are evident in the brief stabilities in the topography of EP peaks and waves (Lehmann, 1981, 1987).

Exogenous EP components that accompany repetitive, meaningless sensory stimuli have scalp topographies that correspond to fairly compact neuronal generators in sensory cortex. In such cases, use of equivalent current dipole models may conveniently approximate the location of sources (Fender, 1987). However, the assumption that generators are simple or compact is particularly unrealistic with higher cognitive functions. Most cognitive EP components, such as P300, were thought to have a simple, broad spatial distribution at the scalp (such as parietal maximum; bilateral symmetry), which is supposed to be similar among paradigms. However, this view has arisen primarily from studies using only a few electrodes and a common reference such as linked ears. With those methods, EP events such as the P300 and CNV appear to be bilaterally distributed and similar in topography in different types of tasks. With a few exceptions, such as the SW, whose frontal negative and posterior positive components behave differently with just a few electrodes, most EP events reveal local between-condition differences in topography at the scalp only after recording from many sites and applying spatial enhancement signal processing methods (Gevins et al, 1989a, 1989b; Gevins and Cutillo, 1993). When this is done, many EP events show local variations in topography over cortical areas appropriate to the tasks used to envoke them. In support of this view, recent intracerebral recordings of N200, P300 and SW components directly from prefrontal, parietal, and temporal cortices indicate that the cortical generators of these events are widely distributed and vary in amplitude and (slightly) in timing between sites just a few centimeters apart (Smith et al, 1990). Also the mosaic-like structure of the cortical areas that appear to be involved in language processes and in the storage and retrieval of linguistic memory was shown by recordings and stimulation studies in humans during surgery (Ojemann, 1978).

A similar interpretation may be made of the results of an experiment on basic linguistic processes performed at the EEG Systems Laboratory (Gevins et al, 1993). The neuroelectric signals accompanying graphic, phonemic, semantic, and grammatic judgments had a high degree of commonality in topography and timing, suggesting that regulation of cued preparation, stimulus encoding, and decision and response selection evoked a dynamic sequence of distributed functional networks that were similar among conditions. However, within this framework of common activity, brief (about 100 to 300 milliseconds) intervals occurred in which particular task differences (such as language/nonlanguage, word/nonword, lexical/syntactic) evoked qualitatively or quantitatively different processing at one or more sites. This was reflected in brief, highly localized between-condition differences clearly observed in high-resolution Laplacian derivation EP waveforms and topographies.

The idea that EPs are manifestations of the integrated activity of widely distributed neural networks explains the tendency of EP components to become fractionated into an increasing number of subcomponents. An EP peak or wave is merely an indication that a group of neurons has been activated by a particular stimulus. There are not just a few types of fundamental EPs whose properties are fixed; in a sense, there are as many EPs as there are differing experiments. Given these facts, we can easily understand why explaining an EP component's behavior in terms of simple psychological theories has been so difficult. The "language" of brain processes is not the language of cognitive psychology. To observe the "language" of brain processes underlying cognition, we must use modern brain imaging technology with a sufficiently high temporal and spatial resolution.

Although no single brain imaging modality has both millisecond temporal information and millimeter spatial resolution, a combination of structural MRI, fMRI, and EEG (or MEG) seem to be the best techniques available. The high temporal and moderate spatial resolution possible with EEG permits detailed study of the subsecond relations between activity at different sites, whereas the high spatial and moderate temporal resolution of the fMRI allows us to determine exactly which neural areas are metabolically active during a 1- to 2-second interval. The combination of high-resolution EEG (Gevins et al, 1993) with fMRI is only beginning to be used successfully. In the meantime, we can discuss topographic variations in the CNV and P300 seen when EEGs are recorded from a sufficient number of scalp electrodes and when a method of spatial enhancement is applied to reduce blurring by volume conduction through the skull and scalp.

Measurement of Relations Between EPs at Different Sites

Studies of the inter-relation of event-related activity between different scalp locations try to find some indication of functional coordination or interdependency between neural areas. Such information can be useful for inferring the topology of task-related functional cortical networks. Relations between channels can be quantified by measures of similarity or interdependence of their activity, including spectral coherence (Walter, 1963); information–theoretic measures (Callaway and Harris, 1974; Saito and Harashima, 1981; Mars and Lopes da Silva, 1987); correlation (Livanov, 1977; Gevins, 1987); covariance (Gevins et al, 1989a, 1989b); multichannel time-varying autoregressive modeling (Gersch, 1987), and so on. Only a few of these methods can be applied to brief data segments, which is necessary for resolution of the subsecond stages of neurocognitive processing. For a measure of functional coordination to be anatomically and physiologically valid, it must be independent of reference location and should provide information about the temporal relation of interchannel signals, that is, whether the event-related signals of one channel lead to or mathematically predict those of another channel. Furthermore, scalp-recorded signals should be spatially enhanced, and confounded topographies due to tangentially oriented or distant generators must be resolved. (The latter problem has not been solved.)

We have been developing methods to measure relations between EPs at different sites during the sequential processing stages of cognitive tasks. Our method is called evoked potential covariance (EPC). Although the method does not solve the problem of confounded topographies, some interesting results have been obtained. The following represent some of our findings. In a bimanual visuomotor experiment (Gevins et al, 1987; 1989a, 1989b), seven participants performed a task that required graded finger-pressure responses with either the right or left hand proportional to visual numeric stimuli from 1 to 9. The hand to be used was cued 1 second before the stimulus. Feedback was presented 1 second after the response as a two-digit number indicating the exact response pressure made. Evoked potential covariances were computed on segments of the EP between the 120 pairwise combinations of 16 nonperipheral Laplacian derivation channels. The width of each segment was determined from the peaks and waves of the EP. Evoked potential covariances were tested for significance by reference to "noise" EPCs computed from randomly timed segments of the same data.

One EPC analysis interval spanned the late CNV to measure EP patterns that should differ according to the hand subjects expected to use. Evoked potential covariance patterns were computed in an interval from 500 to 875 milliseconds after subjects had been cued to prepare to make a graded pressure response with the index finger of either the right or left hand. Figure 7-5a shows the preparatory interval for the right hand for those trials for which the response was subsequently accurate or inaccurate. (Accurate trials were defined as those trials in which the response error was less than the mean error over the whole session that comprised several hundred trials.) Those trials with subsequently accurate responses are characterized by covariances of the left prefrontal electrode with electrodes over-

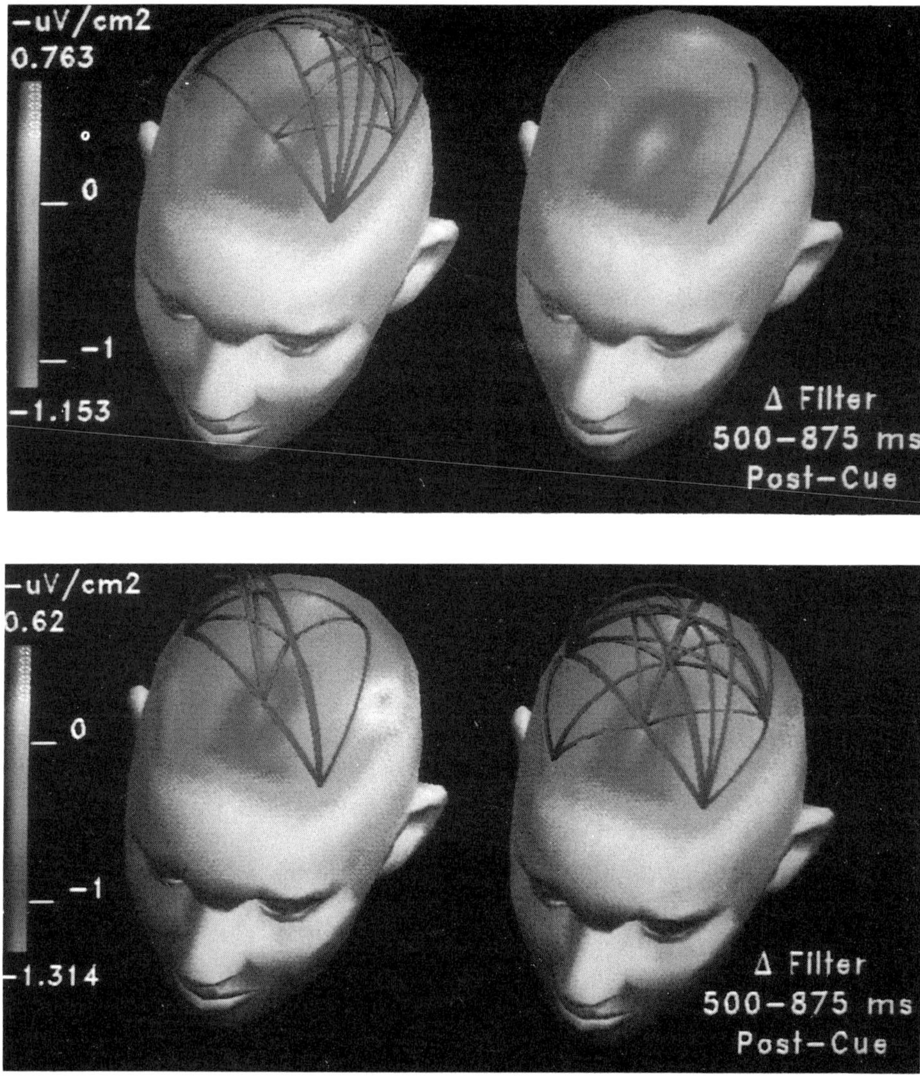

Figure 7-5. Evoked potential covariance (EPC) patterns related to preparation to respond to a visual stimulus number. **a.** right-hand cue. **b.** left-hand cue. The left side of each figure shows the preparatory pattern preceding accurate responses, whereas the right side shows the patterns preceding inaccurate responses. Data are averaged from seven right-handed subjects. Electrodes that appear to be involved in preparation for good performance overlie the left prefrontal cortex (a cognitive sequencing area), the supplementary motor area (mediator of voluntary movements), and the motor and parietal cortices contralateral to the cued hand. With right-hand (dominant) preparation, inaccurate performance is preceded by weak patterns, perhaps because of inattention. In contrast, inaccurate responses by the left hand (nondominant) are preceded by complex patterns, suggestive of a high level of attention but lack of formation of the necessary specific preparatory network. (Experimental data reproduced with permission from Gevins et al, 1989b.)

lying the same motor, somatosensory, and parietal areas that were involved in actual response execution. The accurate left-hand preparatory interval also had left frontal electrode EPCs with contralateral right-sided central and parietal EPCs (Figure 7-5b). The fact that the left frontal electrode was a focus of activity for both right and left hand preparation suggests that the same area of dorsolateral prefrontal cortex was involved in mediating the preparatory networks of both hands. (Because it is proximal to the recording electrode, because the geometry is such that predominantly radially oriented generators can be expected, and because a Laplacian operator was applied, we can reasonably infer that the left frontal electrode records activity of left dorsolateral prefrontal cortex in this instance.) The preparatory pattern preceding inaccurate responses differed markedly from that preceding accurate responses. Although the inaccurate right-hand pattern had fewer EPCs between the left frontal site and other electrodes (Figure 7-5a), inaccurate left-hand trials had a complex EPC pattern involving both right and left frontal, central, and parietal electrodes. Inaccurate performance of this task may be due, in part, to failure to produce a strong, well-focused neural network in which the left frontal cortex is coordinated with the cortical areas used subsequently to produce the response. This corroborates Walter's (1964) original theory that the CNV is a sign of facilitation of cortical processing regulated by areas of frontal cortex. The long controversy about the validity of this theory may have been caused largely by insufficient spatial resolution. If just a few channels of the data of this experiment are considered (without the Laplacian derivation), the CNV topography does not reveal the hand-specific and accuracy-related effects.

Another finding in the bimanual study was the existence of EPC patterns at the latency of the P300 in feedback-evoked EPs, which were different from the EPCs for the poststimulus P300 (Gevins et al, 1989b). Evoked potential covariance patterns associated with neural networks that might be involved in the adjustment of a sensory-motor system in response to feedback about the accuracy of the response pressure are shown in Figures 7-6a and 7-6b. The feedback-evoked EPC patterns for accurate trials of the left and right hands were very similar (bootstrap correlation = 0.91 +/− 0.01), involving midline anterocentral (overlying the supplementary motor area), central (motor), anteroparietal (possibly a locus of processing for reafferent somatosensory signals), parietal and antero-occipital sites; left anterocentral and anteroparietal sites; and right frontal, anterocentral, anteroparietal, and parietal sites. The patterns included many long-delay (32 to 79 milliseconds) EPCs, with the frontal and anterocentral sites lagging behind the more posterior sites. Evoked potential covariance patterns in the P300 interval in inaccurate trials were also very similar between hands (bootstrap correlation = 0.90 +/− 0.02) and involved most of the same sites as the accurate trials, with the notable inclusion of left and midline frontal sites. Because these EPC patterns were more alike between hands than between accurate and inaccurate trials, we infer that the adjustment of this motor system was not especially related to the responding hand. The inclusion of left frontal sites in the inaccurate patterns is consistent with the preparatory patterns reported previously, with the idea that left frontal cortical areas are involved in regulating motor memory, and with the

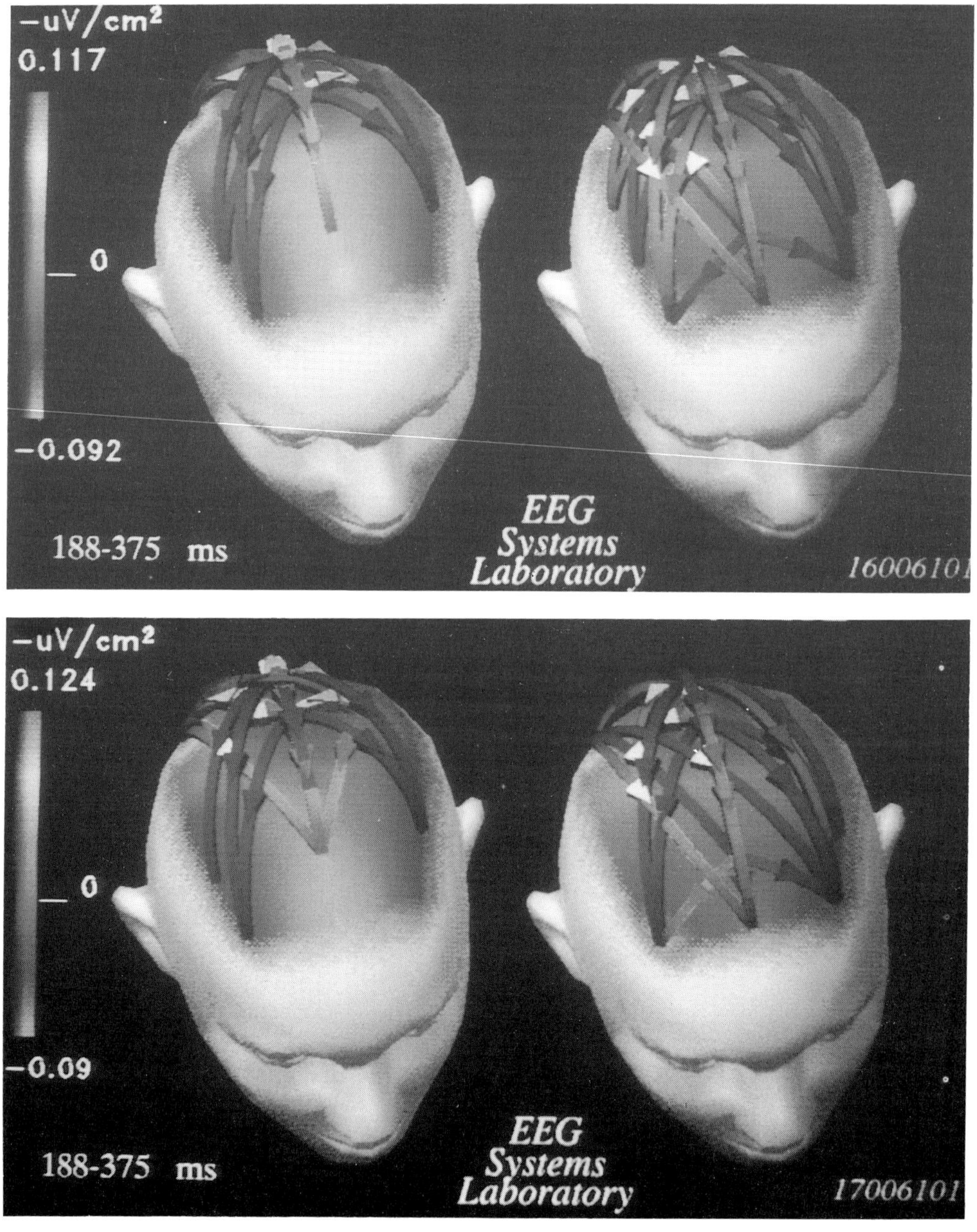

Figure 7-6. Feedback-evoked evoked potential covariances in an interval spanning the P300 wave elicited when participants were shown how accurately they responded. **a.** Right hand. **b.** Left hand. The most prominent features that differentiate feedback when subjects made accurate rather than inaccurate responses are covariances of the left and midline frontal sites for inaccurate responses, regardless of which hand was used. (Experimental data reproduced with permission from Gevins et al, 1989b.)

importance of the frontal lobes in the integration of sensory and motor activities (Fuster, 1989). As with the prestimulus CNV in this experiment, the feedback-evoked P300 would have appeared to be simply an ordinary P300 if it had been recorded with only the traditional few electrodes. However, the greater spatial resolution provided by the larger number of electrodes and the use of the Laplacian derivation provided more detailed topographic information.

Working memory was studied with a version of the same visuomotor finger pressure task that required subjects to remember two numbers and produce precise finger pressures according to the stimulus number seen two trials previously. Thus each stimulus number had to be maintained in working memory for about 12 seconds. On a random 20% of trials, the current stimulus number was the same as the number seen two trials earlier, and no response was to be made. The control condition was simply the graded pressure task described above, that is, pressures made with the right hand in response to the magnitude of the current stimulus number. In this control task, the no-response match trials were signaled by the stimulus number "0." Thus the control task required production of a graded pressure response based on perception of the current stimulus number; the working memory (WM) task required that participants remember two digits and their order and respond to the stimulus seen 12 seconds earlier.

Five U.S. Air Force test pilots practiced the memory task the day before the test recording, until performance measures such as reaction time and accuracy had reached asymptote. Twenty-seven channels of scalp-recorded EEG were used to determine 18 channels of nonperipheral Laplacian derivation EPs. Evoked potential covariance patterns were computed in brief intervals between all pairwise combinations of these 18 channels. The "awaiting stimulus" interval was an interval of 375-milliseconds spanning the late CNV, just before stimulus presentation, and the "memory match" interval was a 375-millisecond interval spanning the P300 peak in no-response match trials. Two other intervals, an early poststimulus ("stimulus processing") and a response-registered interval ("response execution") were analyzed, but their EPC patterns did not differ between conditions. Significant between-condition differences were found in the prestimulus and P300 intervals. In the prestimulus interval (Figure 7-7a), the control task had substantial covariances of midline central with bilateral anterocentral electrodes, and with right parietal and right anterior occipital electrodes. The pattern in the WM task was much stronger and more complex, having prominent covariances of the same midline central electrodes with bilateral anterocentral, parietal, and anterior occipital electrodes, and left anteroparietal to midline central and precentral electrodes. Also clearly evident were strong covariances involving frontal electrodes. In the memory match interval spanning the P300, the EPC patterns in the WM condition were also more left-sided than the control (Figure 7-7b), suggesting greater relative involvement of the left hemisphere. The greater posterior left-hemisphere EPCs in the memory task were consistent with the maintenance or processing of verbal/numeric codings. The greater prefrontal EPCs could be due to the activity of frontal cortex in the neural network subserving WM in this task, or perhaps in actual storage of mnemonic codes. Many inves-

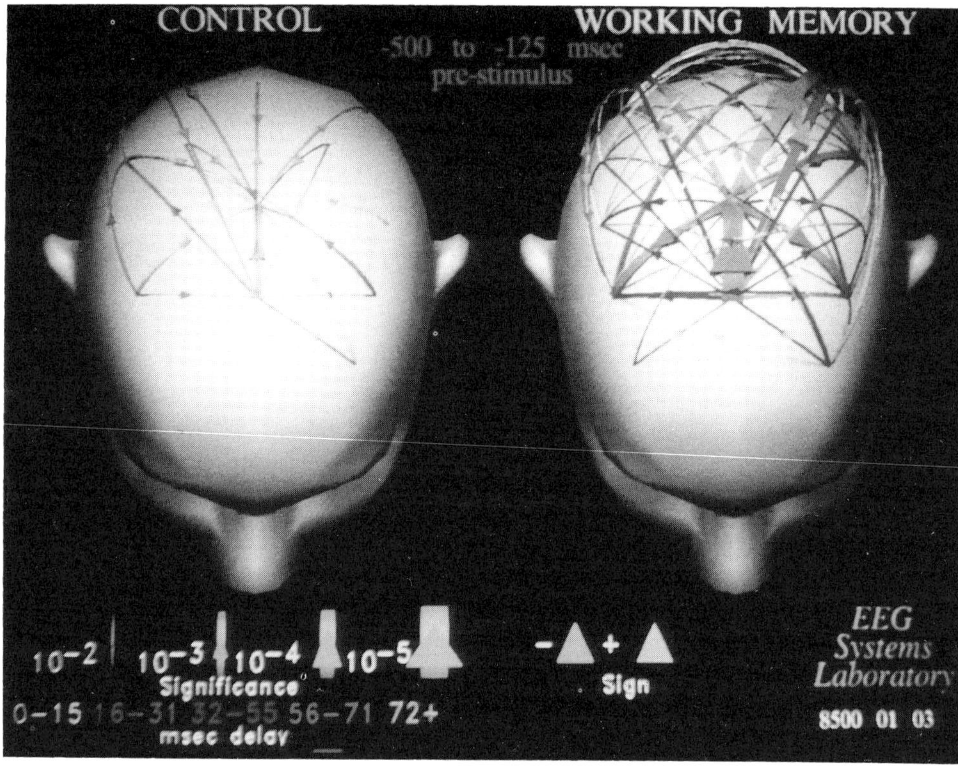
CONTROL
WORKING MEMORY
-500 to -125 msec
pre-stimulus
10−2 10−3 10−4 10−5
Significance
− +
Sign
0−15 16−31 32−55 56−71 72+
msec delay
EEG
Systems
Laboratory
8500 01 03

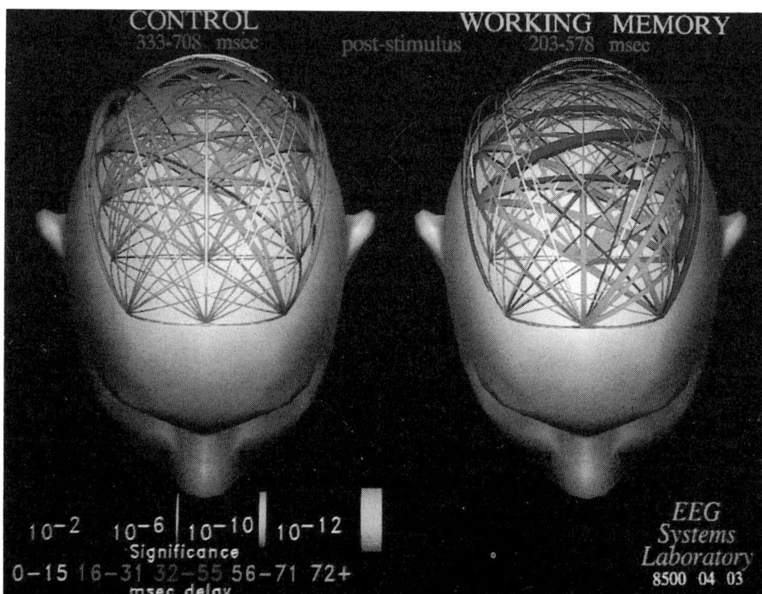
CONTROL
333-708 msec
post-stimulus
WORKING MEMORY
203-578 msec
10−2 10−6 10−10 10−12
Significance
0−15 16−31 32−55 56−71 72+
msec delay
EEG
Systems
Laboratory
8500 04 03

tigators thought the CNV and the P300 were related to some aspects of memory—the CNV to a learned association between two stimuli, and the P300 to a long-term storage. Based on these data, a broader view may be necessary. Just as some form of information storage and retrieval (memory) is involved in most cognitive behaviors, it's plausible that the CNV and P300, which are elicited by many EP paradigms, must be related to the many aspects of memory, expectation, and learned association.

The working memory task also was used in a study of leading indicator signs of mental fatigue due to extended sessions of task performance (Gevins et al, 1990). Changes in the EPCs with time on task occurred in the awaiting stimulus and memory match intervals during a recording session lasting from 10 to 14 hours (Figures 7-8a and 7-8b). The first substantial changes appeared after 7 or 8 hours of performance (labeled "middle" in Figure 7-8) but before behavioral signs of fatigue became important. Although the overall magnitude of the EPCs in both intervals was reduced with increasing time of the task, the topographic pattern was changed only in the prestimulus interval. The pattern changed from one strongly focused on midline central and precentral and left parietal sites, to one focused primarily on right-sided precentral and parietal sites. Extended task performance may have affected the neural strategy used for the complex processes involved in the preparatory interval of this task. These results provide evidence for another aspect of the behavior of these two familiar, easily elicited EP waves, which only becomes evident with increased spatial resolution.

Spatial Enhancement

Electric currents generated by sources in the brain are volume conducted through brain, cerebrospinal fluid, skull, and scalp to the recording electrodes. Therefore potentials due to a localized source are spread over a considerable area of scalp and, conversely, the potential measured at a scalp site represents the summation of signals from many sources over much of the brain. This is especially true when considering the signals of higher cognitive functions, such as the P300 and CNV, which occur in widely distributed neural networks. Thus signals corresponding to local variations in neurocognitive processes cannot be measured without suf-

←

Figure 7-7. Evoked potential covariance (EPC) patterns for the contingent negative variation (CNV) and P300 intervals of working memory (WM) and control tasks. Averaged data from five experimental subjects. **a.** Awaiting stimulus (CNV) interval. In the WM task (*right*), subjects had to remember the previous two stimulus numbers, whereas in the control task (*left*) they did not. The WM task has stronger evoked potential covariances (EPC) overall, with particularly stronger EPCs over the left hemisphere. **b.** Response inhibition (P300) interval. In the WM task, no response was required when the current stimulus number was the same as the number two trials back. With the control task, no response was required when "0" appeared. Note the relatively anterior, left-sided EPC patterns in the WM task compared with the more posterior distribution in the control task. (Adapted with permission from Gevins and Cutillo, 1993.)

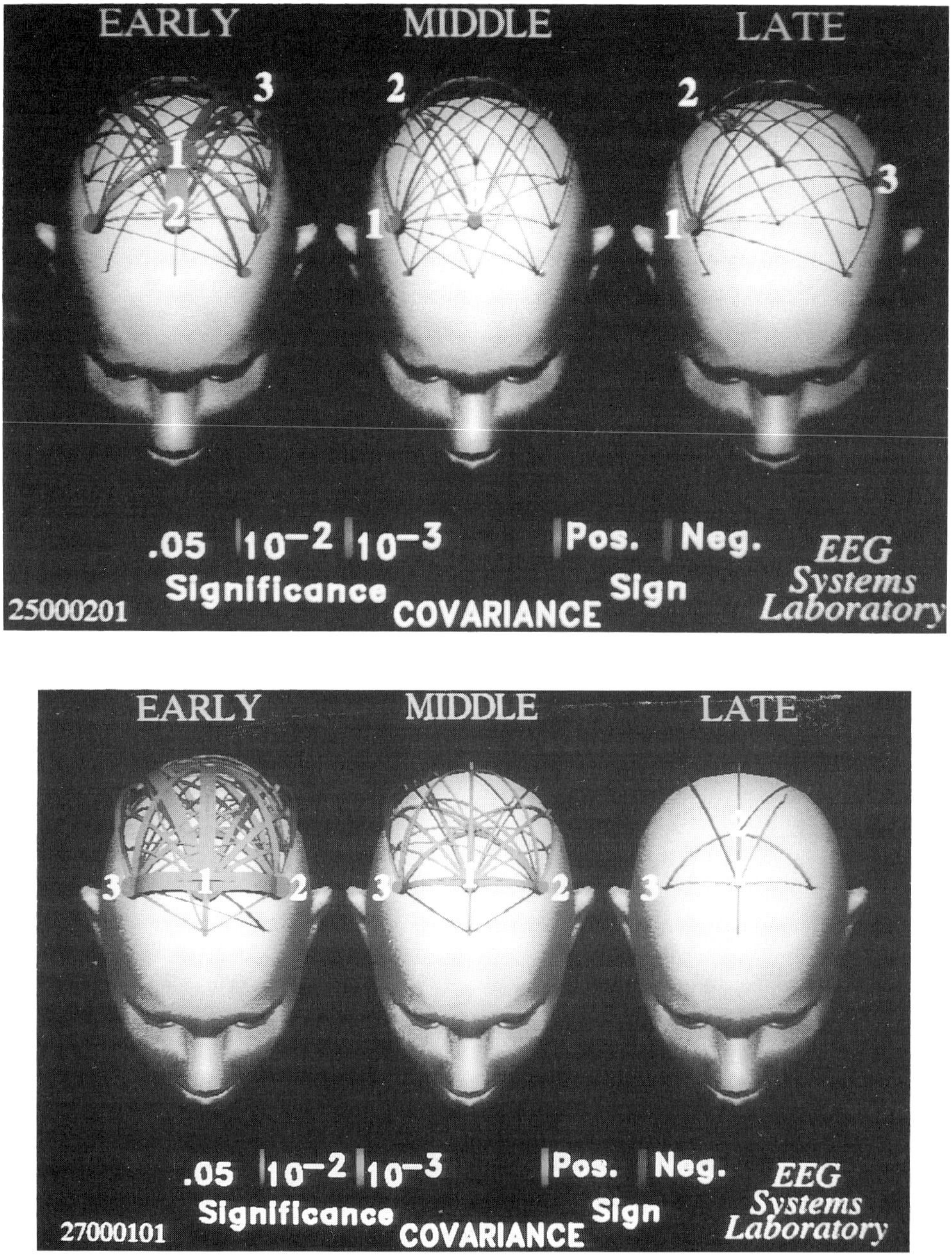

Figure 7-8. Evoked potential covariance (EPC) patterns for the contingent negative variation (CNV) and P300 intervals of the working memory (WM) task performed by five well-practiced participants during a 10- to 14-hour period. The task, intervals, and participants are the same as in Figure 7. "Early" signifies data recorded duing the first 6 hours of the session when the participants were fully alert. "Middle" corresponds to data during hours 6 to 8, just before overt signs of deteriorated performance. "Late" corresponds to data recorded after midnight, when performance accuracy had substantially declined. However,

ficiently fine spatial sampling and some technique for spatial sharpening. We used two spatial enhancement methods to correct for this blur distortion.

The more simple method computes an accurate estimate of the surface Laplacian derivation, which is proportional to local normal current at the scalp (Hjorth, 1975; Nunez, 1981). This has the advantage of eliminating the effect of the reference electrode used for recording and of eliminating much of the common activity due to the reference electrode or volume conduction from distant sources. Its disadvantages are that the Laplacian derivation may not produce accurate values at the outermost ring of electrodes and does not correct for local differences in skull thickness and conduction properties. Although computing the Laplacian derivation at first seems trivial, several subtle issues are involved (Nunez, 1989). The most accurate surface LD uses the actual measured electrode positions and estimates the Laplacian derivation over the actual shape of the head using a three-dimensional spline algorithm (Gevins et al, 1991), as discussed in Chapter 1. The ability of the Laplacian derivation to sharpen spatial detail and enhance weak signals has been well demonstrated (Thickbroom et al, 1984; Nunez, 1989; Nunez et al, 1991; Giard et al, 1988; Gevins et al, 1989a, 1989b). A dramatic increase in spatial detail is apparent with the Laplacian derivation compared with linked-ears–referenced potentials. Another improvement in spatial detail is obtained using a finite element model of the cortex, cerebrospinal fluid, skull, and scalp to estimate the potentials that would actually be recorded on the surface of the brain (Figure 7-9). We call our implementation of this cortical imaging method finite element deblurring (FED) (Gevins et al, 1991; Le and Gevins, 1993). The price of this improvement offered by FED is that MRIs must be recorded and processed and many more calculations must be performed. Unlike some other methods that estimate cortical potentials or currents, FEM is a true "downward continuation" method in that, without previous knowledge or assumptions about the generating sources, the cortical potential distribution is derived from the scalp potential distribution and a realistic model of the conducting volume between the scalp and cortical surfaces. Figure 7-10 shows the estimated cortical potentials of one subject in a recent language study. The time point sampled is 411 milliseconds after the presentation of closed-class (grammatic or syntactic) words. A focus of activity over the left frontal operculum, or Broca's language area, can be seen. In contrast, presentation of open-class (content) words pro-

to avoid confounding performance accuracy effects with those due to time on task, only accurately performed trials from the Early, Middle, and Late periods are shown. The numbers "1, 2, 3" signify the top three sites with the largest summed covariances with other sites. **a.** Prestimulus CNV interval. Preparatory EPC patterns decrease in overall strength and change in topographic pattern with a shift from left to right side. This change is evident by the Middle period, even before overt performance had substantially declined. **b.** Response inhibition P300. The P300 pattern also shows a decrease in signal strength with increasing time on task but not much change in pattern. (Adapted with permission from Gevins et al, 1990b.)

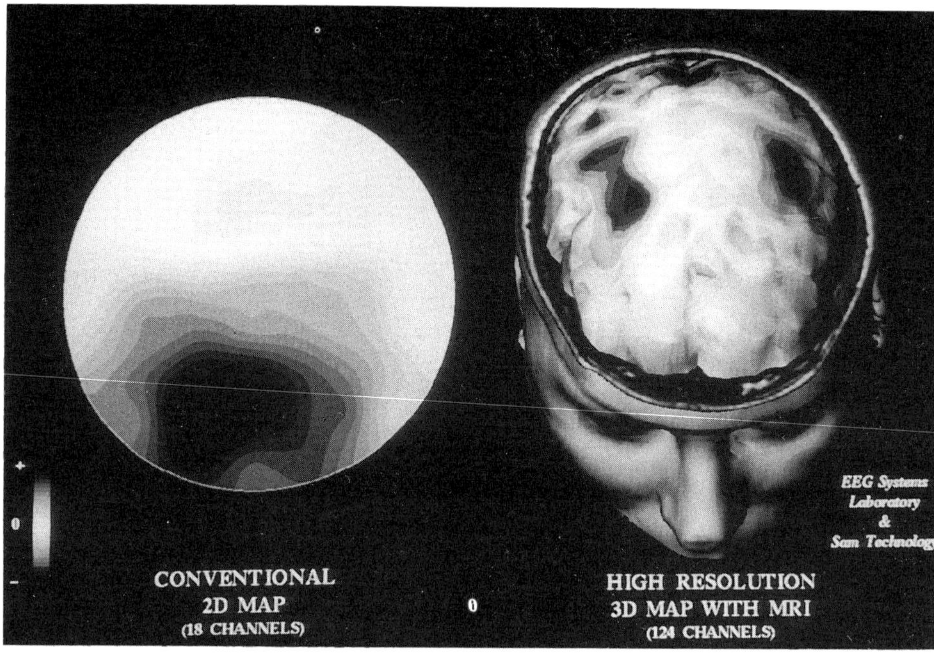

Figure 7-9. High-resolution somatosensory evoked potentials. A high-resolution, 124-channel, three-dimensional topographic map (*right*) of the steady-state potentials elicited by electric stimulation of the left-hand middle finger and right-hand index finger contains more useful localizing information than a more conventional two-dimensional topographic map of the same data sampled at 18 standard electrode locations from the 10-20 system (*left*). The high-resolution evoked potential maps are produced by recording from 124 channels and applying a spatial signal enhancement procedure that removes the blur distortion caused by conduction of potentials through the skull and scalp. With the high-resolution map, the left and right somatosensory cerebral cortices, corresponding to the right and left hands, were activated. (Adapted with permission from Gevins et al, 1994.)

duced a focus of activity in the posterior perisylvan area, corresponding approximately to the posterior language area.

Conclusion

Regardless of the specific findings we described, use of multielectrode arrays and suitable methods of spatial enhancement clearly constitutes a valuable new tool for EP researchers. Recent advances in recording and analysis technology will increase the sensitivity and specificity of measurements of the neurophysiologic basis of perception, cognition, and action. Information about distributed processing and its temporal relations may be provided by EPC or similar measures. The signs of rapidly shifting patterns of statistical interdependency between sites

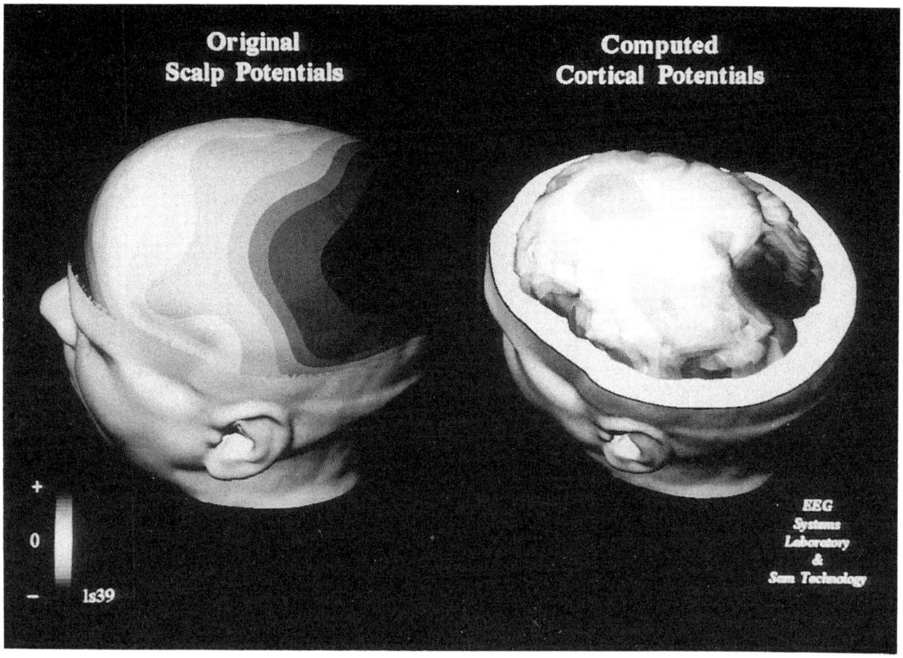

Figure 7-10. High-resolution evoked potentials of language processing. Data are shown from a participant doing the grammatic encoding task described in the text. The left side of the figure shows the 59-channel, linked-mastoid potential topography 422 milliseconds after the appearance of a single syllable closed-class (grammatic function) word. The topography is undifferentiated, as is typical of evoked potential data without spatial enhancement. The right side shows the same data after they have been deblurred and projected down to the cortical surface. The topography is well differentiated. Note particularly the activation over Broca's area of the left frontal hemisphere, an effect well known in neuropsychology but that has not previously been visualized so clearly with evoked potentials. (Adapted with permission from Gevins et al, 1994.)

that were reviewed here are particularly intriguing given their corroboration of historical and contemporary findings about localization and coordination of brain functions from clinical and experimental sources. Development of measurement technology is not complete. A crucial but difficult next step is removal of ambiguities in interpretating topographic maps in terms of cortical generators. With these developments, high-resolution EPs, by themselves and combined with other functional neuroimaging methods, will probably play an increasingly important role in cognitive neuroscience and clinical medicine.

The ability to characterize accurately the subsecond spatiotemporal dynamics of neurocognitive processes will probably promote the development of more realistic biological conceptions of mental functions. Preparatory processes that precede a stimulus and feedback processes that follow reception of information about performance accuracy are particularly interesting because they reveal aspects about the generation and updating of internal models of self and the environment. Although the frontal cortex plays a pivotal role in these high-level processes, it would be simplistic to consider the frontal lobes as only executive in nature. Rather many areas probably are involved in a constellation of rapidly changing functional networks that provide the delicate balance between stimulus-locked behavior and purely imaginary ideation. With further advances in brain imaging technology in the 1990s, we can expect to achieve increasingly detailed and direct measurements of the organization and inter-relations of the neural basis of basic and higher-level cognitive functions.

Acknowledgments

Sponsored by competitive grants and contracts from the following agencies of the United States government: The National Institute of Mental Health, The Air Force Office of Scientific Research, the National Institute of Neurological and Communicative Diseases and Strokes, The Office of Naval Research, The National Science Foundation, and The National Institute of Alcoholism and Alcohol Abuse.

References

Berger, H., Uber das Elektroenzephalogramm des Menschen. *Arch. Psychiatr. Nervenk.* 87:527–570, 1929.

Callaway, E. and Harris, P. Coupling between cortical potentials from different areas. *Science.* 183:873–875, 1974.

Chase, W., McCarthy, G., Squires, K., and Schvaneveldt, R. Mental chronometry. In: *Cognitive Psychophysiology: Event-Related Potentials and the Study of Cognition.* (E. Donchin, Ed.) Hillsdale, NJ: Erlbaum, pp. 249–301, 1984.

Courchesne, E. Changes in P3 waves with event repetition: Long-term effects on scalp distribution and amplitude. *Electroencephalogr. Clin. Neurophysiol.* 45:754–766, 1978.

Courchesne, E., Hillyard, S., and Galambos, R. Stimulus novelty, task relevance and the visual evoked potential in man. *Electroencephalogr. Clin. Neurophysiol.* 39:131–143, 1975.

Desmedt, J. Active touch exploration of extrapersonal space elicits specific electrogenesis in the right cerebral hemisphere of intact right-handed man. *Proc. Natl. Acad. Sci. USA.* 74:4037–4040, 1977.

Donchin, E. Event-related brain potentials: A tool in the study of human information processing. In: *Evoked Potentials and Behavior.* (H. Begleiter, Ed.) New York: Press, pp. 13–75, 1979.

Donchin, E. and Heffley, E.F. Multivariate analysis of event-related potential data: A tutorial review. In: *Multidisciplinary Perspectives in ERP Research.* (D. Otto, Ed.) *EPA-600/9-77-043.* Washington, DC: U.S. Government Printing Office, pp. 555–572, 1978.

Donchin, E., Kutas, M., and Johnson, R. The CNV does not behave like a 'motor potential.' *Electroencephalogr. Clin. Neurophysiol.* 37:484–496, 1974.

Donchin, E., Kutas, M., and McCarthy, G. Electrocortical indices of hemispheric utilization. In: *Lateralization in the Nervous System.* (S. Harnard, Ed.) New York: Academic Press, pp. 339–384, 1977.

Duncan-Johnson, C. and Donchin, E. The P300 component of the event-related potential as an index of information processing. *Biol. Psychol.* 14:1–52, 1982.

Fender, D. Source localization of brain electrical activity. In: *Handbook of Electroencephalography and Clinical Neurophysiology.* (Revised Series) Vol. 1. (A. Gevins, Remond, A., Eds.) Amsterdam: Elsevier, pp. 355–403, 1987.

Ford, J., Roth, W., Mohs, R., Hopkins, W., and Koppell, B. Event-related potentials recorded from young and old adults during a memory retrieval task. *Electroencephalogr. Clin. Neurophysiol.* 47:450–459, 1979.

Friedman, D., Vaughan, H.G. Jr., and Erlenmeyer-Kimling, L. Multiple late positive potentials in two visual discrimination tasks. *Psychol. Physiol.* 18:635–649, 1981.

Fuster, J. *Prefrontal Cortex: Anatomy, Physiology and Neuropsychology of the Frontal Lobe.* New York: Raven Press, 1989.

Gersch, W. Non-stationary multichannel time series analysis. In: *Handbook of Electroencephalography and Clinical Neurophysiology. Vol. 1. Methods of Analysis of Brain Electrical and Magnetic Signals.* (A. S. Gevins, Remond, A., Eds.) Amsterdam: Elsevier, pp. 171–193, 1987.

Gevins, A.S., Zeitlin, G.M., Doyle, J.C., Yingling, C.D., Schaffer, R.E., Callaway, E., and Yaeger, C.L. Electroencephalogram correlates of higher cortical functions. *Science* 203:665–668, 1979a.

Gevins, A.S., Zeitlin, G.M., Yingling, C.D., Doyle, J.C., Dedon, M.F., Schaffer, R.E., Roumasset, J.T., and Yeager, C.L. EEG patterns during "cognitive" tasks. I. Methodology and analysis of complex behaviors. *Electroencephalogr. Clin. Neurophysiol.* 47:693–703, 1979b.

Gevins, A.S., Zeitlin, G.M., Doyle, J.C., Schaffer, R.E., and Callaway, E. EEG patterns during "cognitive" tasks. II. Analysis of controlled tasks. *Electroencephalogr. Clin. Neurophysiol.* 47:704–710, 1979c.

Gevins, A.S., Doyle, J.C., Schaffer, R.E., Callaway, E., and Yeager, C. Lateralized cognitive processes and the electroencephalogram. *Science* 207:1005–1008, 1980.

Gevins, A. and Schaffer, R. A critical review of electroencephalographic correlates of higher cortical functions. In: *CRC Critical Reviews in Bioengineering.* Vol. 4. Boca Raton, FL: CRC Press, pp. 113–164, 1980.

Gevins, A.S., Doyle, J.C., Cutillo, B.A., Schaffer, R.E., Tannehill, R.S., and Bressler, S.L. Neurocognitive pattern analysis of a visuospatial task: Rapidly-shifting foci of evoked correlations between electrodes. *Psychophysiology.* 22:32–43, 1985.

Gevins, A.S. and Cutillo, B.A. Signals of cognition. In: *Handbook of Electroencephalography and Clinical Neurophysiology.* Vol. 2. (F. H. Lopes da Silva et al, Eds.) Amsterdam: Elsevier, pp. 335–381, 1986.

Gevins, A.S., Morgan, N.H., Bressler, S.L., Cutillo, B.A., White, R.M., Illes, J., Greer, D.S., Doyle, J.C., and Zeitlin, G.M. Human neuroelectric patterns predict performance accuracy. *Science* 235:580–585, 1987.

Gevins, A.S. Correlation analysis. In: *Handbook of Electroencephalography and Clinical Neurophysiology. Vol. 1. Methods of Analysis of Brain Electrical and Magnetic Signals.* (A.S. Gevins and Remond, A., Eds.) Amsterdam: Elsevier, pp. 171–193, 1987.

Gevins, S.A., Bressler, S.L., Morgan, N.H., Cutillo, B.A., White, R.M., Greer, D., and Illes, J. Event-related covariances during a bimanual visuomotor task. Part I: Methods and analysis of stimulus- and response-locked data. *Electroencephalogr. Clin. Neurophysiol.* 74:58–75, 1989a.

Gevins, A.S., Cutillo, B.A., Bressler, S.L., Morgan, N.H., White, R.M., Illes, J., and Greer, D. Event-related covariances during a bimanual visuomotor task. Part II: Preparation and feedback. *Electroencephalogr. Clin. Neurophysiol.* 74:147–160, 1989b.

Gevins, A.S., Bressler, S.L., Cutillo, B.A., Illes, J., Miller, J., Stern, J., and Jex, H. Effects of sustained mental work on functional brain topography. *Electroencephalogr. Clin. Neurophysiol.* 76:339–350, 1990.

Gevins, A.S., Le, J., Brickett, P., Reutter, B., and Desmond, J. Seeing through the skull: Advanced EEGs use MIRs to accurately measure cortical activity from the scalp. *Brain Topography.* 4:125–131, 1991.

Gevins, A.S. and Cutillo, B.C. Spatiotemporal dynamics of component processes in human working memory. *Electroencephalogr. Clin. Neurophysiol.* 87:128–143, 1993.

Gevins, A.S. High resolution evoked potentials of cognition. *Brain Topography.* (In press) 1994.

Gevins, A., Cutillo, B., and Smith, M. Regional modulation of evoked potentials during verbal and nonverbal matching tasks. *Electroencephalogr. Clin. Neurophysiol.* (Submitted, 1994).

Gevins, A.S., Le, J., Martin, N., Brickett, P., Desmond, J., Reutter, B. High resolution EEG: 124-channel recording, spatial enhancement, and MRI integration methods. *Electroencephalogr. Clin. Neurophysiol.* 90:337–358, 1994.

Giard, M., Perrin, F., Pernier, J., and Peronnet, F. Several attention-related waveforms in auditory areas: A topographic study. *Electroencephalogr. Clin. Neurophysiol.* 69:371–384, 1988.

Goldman-Rakic, P. The frontal lobes: Uncharted provinces of the brain. *Trends in Neuroscience.* 7:425–429, 1984.

Hansen, J.C. and Hillyard, S.A. Endogenous brain potentials associated with selective auditory attention. *Electroencephalogr. Clin. Neurophysiol.* 49:277–290, 1980.

Hansen, J. and Hillyard, S. Selective attention to multidimensional auditory stimuli. *J. Exp. Psychol. [Hum. Percept.]* 9:1–19, 1983.

Hansen, J. and Woldorff, M. Mechanisms of auditory selective attention as revealed by event-related potentials. In: *Event-Related Brain Research* (Electroencephologr. Clin. Neurophysiol. Suppl. 42). (C.H.M. Brunia, G. Mulder, and M. N. Verbaten, Eds.), Amsterdam: Elsevier, pp. 195–209, 1991.

Harter, M., Miller, S., Price, N., LaLonda, M., and Keyes, A. Neural processes involved in directing attention. *Journal of Cognitive Neurophysiology.* 1:223–237, 1990.

Hillyard, S. Event-related potentials and selective attention. In: *Cognitive Psychophysiology: Event-Related Potentials and the Study of Cognition.* Vol. 1. (E. Donchin, Ed.) Hillsdale, NJ: Erlbaum, pp. 51–72, 1984.

Hillyard, S., Hink, R., Schwent, V., and Piction, T. Electrical signs of selective attention in the human brain. *Science* 182:177–180, 1973.

Hjorth, B. On-line transformation of EEG scalp potentials into orthogonal source derivations. *Electroencephalogr. Clin. Neurophysiol.* 39:111–118, 1975.

Israel, J., Chesney, G., Wickens, C., and Donchin, E. P300 and tracking difficulty: Evidence for multiple resources in dual-task performance. *Psychophysiology* 17:259–273, 1980.

Johnson, R. and Donchin, E. Second thoughts: Multiple P300's elicited by a single stimulus. *Psychophysiology* 22:182–194, 1985.

Le, J. and Gevins, A.S. Method to reduce blur distortion from EEGs using a realistic head model. *IEEE Trans. Biomed. Eng.* 40:517–528, 1993.

Lehmann, D. Spatial analysis of evoked and spontaneous EEG potential fields. In: *Recent Advances in EEG and EMG Data Processing.* (N. Yamaguchi and Fujisawa, K., Eds.) Amsterdam: Elsevier, pp. 117–132, 1981.

Lehmann, D. Principles of spatial analysis. In: *Handbook of Electroencephalography and Clinical Neurophysiology. Vol. 1: Methods of Analysis of Brain Electrical and Magnetic Signals* (A.S. Gevins and Remond, A., Eds.) Amsterdam: Elsevier, pp. 309–354, 1987.

Livanov, M.N. *Spatial Organization of Cerebral Processes.* New York: Wiley, 1977.

Mars, N.J. and Lopes da Silva, F.H. EEG analysis methods based on information theory. In: *Handbook of Electroencephalography and Clinical Neurophysiology. Vol. 1: Methods of Analysis of Brain Electrical and Magnetic Signals.* Amsterdam: Elsevier, pp. 297–307, 1987.

McCarthy, G. and Donchin, E. Chronometric analysis of human information processing. In: *Tutorials in Event-Related Potential Research: Endogenous Components, Advances in Psychology.* Vol. 10. (A. Gaillard and Ritter, W., Eds.) Amsterdam: Elsevier: pp. 251–268, 1983.

McGillem, C.D. and Aunon, J.I. Analysis of event-related potentials. In: *Handbook of Electroencephalography and Clinical Neurophysiology. Vol. 1: Methods of Analysis of Brain Electrical and Magnetic Signals.* (A.S. Gevins and Remond, A., Eds.) Amsterdam: Elsevier, pp. 131–169, 1987.

Meyer, D., Osman, A., Irwin, D., and Yantis, S. Modern mental chronometry. *Biol. Psychol.* 26:3–67, 1990.

Näätänen, R. The N2 component of the evoked potential: A scalp reflection of neuronal mismatch of orienting theory? In: *Biological Foundations of Personality and Behavior.* (J. Strelau, Farley, F., and Gale, A., Eds.) Washington, DC: Hemisphere Press, pp. 116–127, 1985.

Näätänen, R. and Gaillard, A. The orienting reflex and the N2 detection of the ERP. In: *Tutorials in Event-Related Potential Research: Endogenous Components Advances in Psychology.* Vol. 10. (A. Gaillard and Ritter, W., Eds.) Amsterdam: Elsevier, pp. 119–142, 1983.

Näätänen, R. and Michie, P.T. Different variants of endogenous negative brain potentials in performance situations: Review and classification. In: *Human Evoked Potentials, Applications and Problems: NATO Conf. Ser., Ser. III: Human Factors.* Vol. 9. (D. Lehmann and Callaway, E., Eds.) New York: Plenum, pp. 251–268, 1979.

Näätänen, R. and Picton, T. The N1 wave of the human electric and magnetic response to sound: A review and analysis of the component structure. *Psychophysiology.* 24:375–425, 1987.

Näätänen, R., Gaillard, A., and Montysalo, S. The N1 effect of selective attention reinterpreted. *Acta Psychol. (Amst.).* 42:173–187, 1978.

Näätänen, R., Gaillard, A., and Varey, C. Attention effects on auditory EPs as a function of inter-stimulus interval. *Biol. Psychol.* 13:173–187, 1981.

Nunez, P.L. *Electric Fields in the Brain: The Neurophysics of EEG.* New York: Oxford University Press, 1991.

Nunez, P. Estimation of large-scale neocortical source activity with EEG surface Laplacians. *Brain Topography.* 2:141–154, 1989.

Nunez, P., Pilgreen, K., Westdorp, A., Law, S., and Nelson, A. A visual study of surface potentials and Laplacians due to distributed neocortical sources: Computer simulations and evoked potentials. *Brain Topography* 4:151–168, 1991.

Ojemann, G. Organization of short-term verbal memory in language areas of human cortex evidence from electrical stimulation. *Brain Lang.* 5:331–340, 1978.

Picton, T.W. and Stuss, D.T. The component structure of the human event-related potentials. In: *Motivation, Motor and Sensory Processes of the Brain: Electrical Potentials, Behavior and Clinical Use. Progress in Brain Research.* Vol. 54. (H. Kornhuber and Deecke, L., Eds.) Amsterdam: Elsevier, pp. 17–49, 1980.

Picton, T. The P300 wave of the human event-related potential. *J. Clin. Neurophysiol.* 9:456–479, 1992.

Posner, M. Chronometric explorations of mind. Hillsdale, NJ: Erlbaum, 1978.

Pritchard, W. Psychophysiology of the P300. *Psychol. Bull.* 90:506–540, 1981.

Rebert, C. Electrogenesis of slow potential changes in the central nervous system: A summary of issues. In: *Multidisciplinary Perspectives in Event-Related Brain Potential Research.* (D. Otto, Ed.) EPA-600/9-77-043, Washington, DC: U.S. Government Printing Office, pp. 3–11, 1978.

Renault, B. The visual emitted potentials: Clues for information processing. In: *Tutorials in Event-Related Potential Research: Endogenous Components. Advances in Psychology.* Vol. 10. (A. Gaillard and Ritter, W., Eds.) Amsterdam: Elsevier, pp. 159–176, 1983.

Renault, B. and Lesevre, N. A trial-by-trial study of the visual omission response in reaction time situation. In: *Human Evoked Potentials.* (D. Lehman and Callaway, E., Eds.) New York: Plenum Press, pp. 317–329, 1979.

Renault, B., Ragot, R., Lesevre, N., and Remond, A. Onset and offset of brain events as indices of mental chronometry. *Science*, 215:1413–1415, 1982.

Ritter, W., Simson, R., Vaughan, H., and Friedman, D. A brain event related to the making of a sensory discrimination. *Science* 203:1358–1361, 1979.

Ritter, W., Simson, R., Vaughan, H., and Macht, M. Manipulation of event-related potential manifestations of information processing stages. *Science* 218:909–911, 1982.

Ritter, W., Vaughan, H., and Simson, R. On relating event-related potential components and stages of information processing. In: *Tutorials in Event-Related Potential Research: Endogenous Components. Advances in Psychology.* Vol. 10. (A. Gaillard and Ritter, W., Eds.) Amsterdam: Elsevier, pp. 143–158, 1983a.

Ritter, W., Simson, R., and Vaughan, H. Event-related correlates of two stages of information processing in physical and semantic discrimination tasks. *Psychophysiology* 20:168–179, 1983b.

Ritter, W., Kelso, S., Kutas, M., and Shiffrin, R. Preparatory processes. *Cognitive Psychophysiology: Event-Related Potentials and the Study of Cognition.* (E. Donchin, Ed.) Hillsdale, NJ: Erlbaum, pp. 179–219, 1984.

Rockstroh, B., Elbert, T., Canavan, A., Lutzenberger, W., and Birbaumer, N. *Slow Cortical Potentials and Behavior.* Baltimore: Urban and Schwartzberger, 1989.

Rogers, L. Determination of the number and waveshapes of event related potential components using comparative factor analysis. *Int. J. Neuroscience* 56:219–246, 1991.

Rohrbaugh, J. and Gaillard, A. Sensory and motor aspects of the contingent negative variation. In: *Tutorials in Event-Related Potential Research: Endogenous Components. Advances in Psychology.* Vol. 10. (A. Gaillard and Ritter, W., Eds.) Amsterdam: Elsevier, pp. 269–310, 1983.

Rohrbaugh, J., Syndulko, K., Sanquist, T., and Lindsley, D. Synthesis of the contingent variation brain potential from noncontingent stimulus and motor elements. *Science* 208:1165–1168, 1980.

Rosler, F. Endogenous ERPs and cognition: Probes, prospects and pitfalls in matching pieces of the mind-body puzzle. In: *Tutorials in Event-Related Potential Research: Endogenous Components. Advances in Psychology.* Vol. 10. (A. Gaillard and Ritter, W., Eds.) Amsterdam: Elsevier, pp. 9–36, 1983.

Rosler, F. and Manzey, D. Principal components and Varimax-rotated components in event-related potential research: Some remarks on their interpretation. *Biol. Psychol.* 13:3–26, 1981.

Rosler, F. Perception or action: Some comments on preparatory negative potentials. In: *Electroencephalogr. Clin. Neurophysiol.* 42(Suppl.):116–129, 1991.

Roth, W. Auditory evoked responses to unpredictable stimuli. *Psychol. Physiol.* 10:125–137, 1973.

Roth, W.T. How many late positive waves are there? In: *Multidisciplinary Perspectives in Event-Related Brain Potential Research.* (D. Otto, Ed.) EPA-600/9-77-043, Washington, DC: U.S. Government Printing Office, pp. 170–172, 1978.

Ruchkin, D. and Sutton, S. Positive slow wave and P300: association and disassociation. In: *Tutorials in Event-Related Potential Research: Endogenous Components. Advances in Psychology.* Vol. 10. (A. Gaillard and Ritter, W., Eds.) Amsterdam: Elsevier, pp. 233–250, 1983.

Ruchkin, D., Sutton, S., Kietzman, M., and Silver, K. Slow wave and P300 potentials and variation in stimulus probability. *Psychophysiology* 12:233–250, 1980.

Ruchkin, D., Johnson, R., Canoune, H., Ritter, W., and Hammer, M. Multiple sources of P3b associated with different types of information. *Electroencephalogr. Clin. Neurophysiol.* 27:157–176, 1990.

Ruchkin, D., Johnson, R., Canoune, H., and Ritter, W. Event-related potentials during arithmetic and mental rotation. *Electroencephalogr. Clin. Neurophysiol.* 79:473–487, 1991.

Saito, Y. and Harashima, H. Tracking of informations within multichannel EEG record—Causal analysis in EEG. In: *Recent Advances in EEG and EMG Data Processing* (N. Yamaguchi and Fujisawa, K., Eds.) Amsterdam: Elsevier, pp. 133–177, 1981.

Simson, R., Vaughan, H.G., and Ritter, W. The scalp topography of potentials in auditory and visual go/no-go tasks. *Electroencephalogr. Clin. Neurophysiol.* 43:864–875, 1977.

Smith, M., Halgren, E., Sokolik, M., Baudena, P., Musolino, A., Liegeois-Chauvel, C., and Chauvel, P. Intracranial topography of the P3 event-related potential during auditory oddball. *Electroencephalogr. Clin. Neurophysiol.* 76:235–248, 1990.

Snyder, E. and Hillyard, S.A. Long-latency evoked potentials to irrelevant, deviant stimuli. *Behav. Biol.* 16:319–331, 1976.

Snyder, E., Hillyard, S., and Galambos, R. Similarities and differences among the P3 waves to detected signals in three modalities. *Psychol. Physiol.* 17:112–122, 1980.

Squires, K., Hillyard, S., and Lindsay, P. Cortical potentials evoked by feedback confirming and disconfirming an auditory decision. *Percept. Psychophysiol.* 13:25–31, 1973.

Squires, N., Squires, K., and Hillyard, S. Two varieties of long latency positive waves evoked by unpredictable auditory stimuli in man. *Electroencephalogr. Clin. Neurophysiol.* 38:387–401, 1977.

Squires, K., Wickens, C., Squires, N., and Donchin, E. The effect of stimulus sequence on the waveform of the cortical event-related potential. *Science* 193:1142–1146, 1976.

Squires, N., Donchin, E., Squires, K., and Grossberg, S. Bisensory stimulation: Inferring decision-related processes from the P300 components. *J. Exp. Psychol. [Hum. Percept.]* 3:299–315, 1975.

Sternberg, S. High speed scanning in human memory. *Science* 153:652–654, 1966.

Stuss, D.T., Toga, A., Hutchinson, J., and Picton, T.W. Feedback evoked potentials during an auditory concept formation task. In: *Motivation, Motor and Sensory Processes of the Brain: Electrical Potentials, Behavioral and Clinical Use. Progress in Brain Research*. Vol. 54. Amsterdam: Elsevier, pp. 403–409, 1980.

Sutton, S., Braren, M., Zubin, J., and John, E. Evoked potential correlates of stimulus uncertainty. *Science* 150:1187–1188, 1965.

Tecce, J. Contingent negative variation (CNV) and psychological processes in man. *Psychol. Bull.* 77:73–108, 1972.

Thatcher, R. and John, E. *Functional Neuroscience. Vol. 1. Foundations of Cognitive Processes*. Hillsdale, NJ: Erlbaum, 1977.

Thickbroom, G., Mastaglia, F., Carroll, W., and Davies, H. Source derivation: application to topographic mapping of visual evoked potentials. *Electroencephalogr. Clin. Neurophysiol.* 59:279–285, 1984.

Tueting, P. Event related potentials, cognitive events and information processing: A summary of issues and discussion. *Multidisciplinary Perspectives in Event-Related Brain Potential Research*. (D. Otto, Ed.) EPA-60019-77-043. Washington, DC: U.S. Government Printing Office, pp. 159–169, 1978.

Verleger, R. Event-related potentials and cognition: A critique of the context updating hypothesis and an alternative interpretation of P3. *Behavioral and Brain Sciences* 11:343–427, 1988.

Verleger, R. The instruction to refrain from blinking affects auditory P3 and N1 amplitudes. *Electroencephalogr. Clin. Neurophysiol.* 78:240–251, 1991.

Walter, D.O. Spectral analysis for electroencephalograms: Mathematical determination of neurophysiological relationships from records of limited duration. *Exp. Neurol.* 8:155–181, 1963.

Walter, W.G. The contingent negative variation: An electrocortical sign of significant association in the human brain. *Science* 146:434, 1964.

Walter, W.G., Cooper, R., Aldridge, V., McCallum, W., and Winter, A. Contingent negative variation: An electrical sign of sensorimotor association and expectancy in the human brain. *Nature* (London). 203:380–384, 1964.

Wickens, C., Kramer, A., Vanasse, L., and Donchin, E. Performance of concurrent tasks: Physiological analysis of reciprocity of information-processing resources. *Science* 221:1080–1082, 1983.

Wijers, A., Otten, L., Feenstra, S., Mulder, G., and Mulder, L. Brain potentials during mental rotation. *Psychophysiology*. 26:452–467, 1989.

Wood, C. and McCarthy, G. Principal components analysis of event-related potentials: Simulation studies demonstrate misallocation of variance across components. *Electroencephalogr. Clin. Neurophysiol.* 59:249–260, 1984.

Woody, C.D. Characterization of an adaptive filter for the analyses of variable latency neuroelectric signals. *Med. Biol. Engrg.* 5:539–553, 1967.

8

Discrete Linear Systems of Physics and Brain

PAUL L. NUNEZ

The history of physical science and engineering is concerned primarily with the study of linear systems. This emphasis on linear rather than nonlinear systems is not due to any illusion that the most interesting natural phenomena are perfectly linear. Rather many systems behave in an approximately linear manner under conditions that are of practical interest. Linear systems typically are easier to study theoretically and experimentally. Furthermore, results from one field of study often can be extrapolated to other fields. Therefore, the study of many new phenomena often begins as a linear systems analysis. Of course, nearly all physical systems display nonlinear characteristics under sufficiently extreme input conditions. For example, a capacitor passes current proportional to an increasing voltage time derivative only to some magnitude at which arcing occurs across the capacitor plates. A mechanical spring is extended proportional to applied force only over a relatively narrow range of force. In the classic example of electrophysiology, transmembrane current is proportional to transmembrane voltages that are well below the threshold level. As threshold is approached, the voltage–current relation (Ohm's Law) becomes more and more nonlinear. When threshold is achieved, an entirely new phenomena occurs that cannot be predicted by any linear theory: the propagation of the action potential.

Underlying the concise definition of linear systems are more subtle issues. For example, membrane biophysics (and all of chemistry) is governed by the Schrodinger equation of quantum mechanics combined with the microscopic version of Maxwell's equations of electrodynamics which are all linear equations. Yet, when many molecular fields interact within the membrane, the action potential, a highly nonlinear phenomenon, can occur. Ohm's Law may be violated in all membranes in a mass of neural tissue, while at the same time a macroscopic mass of tissue satisfies Ohm's Law (because most current flows through the extracellular fluid). Thus, in this example, the three hierarchical levels, molecular, membrane, and neural mass, simultaneously exhibit linear, nonlinear, and linear characteristics, respectfully.

Many similar examples from the physical sciences show that linearity depends on spatial and temporal scale. For instance, materials may be linear over some frequency ranges and nonlinear over others. In this context, "linear" means that the usual constitutive relations required to supplement the macroscopic version of Maxwell's equations are linear. That is, the conductive, dielectric, or magnetic properties are linear. Of course, a material may be linear in one sense and nonlinear in another. For example, a linear dielectric can also be a nonlinear conductor, as with the active neural membrane. In future experimental and theoretical studies of neocortex, the issues of spatial and temporal scale will probably reoccur continually, especially in the context of linear versus nonlinear approaches to quantitative description.

Although the label "linear systems analysis" may evoke thoughts of simple electric circuits, mechanical oscillators, or perhaps ordinary differential equations, systems can be very complicated but still linear. A linear system may have many components (with associated degrees of freedom.) In this case, the mathematical description may consist of a large set of coupled ordinary differential equations with dependent variables X_1, X_2, X_3, . . . X_N, representing perhaps the voltage at N nodes in a circuit, to be expressed as a function of the single independent variable t. When N is very large, the medium can often be viewed as a continuum so that the dependent variables $X_i(t)$ are replaced by a single dependent variable $\Psi(\mathbf{r}, t)$, which is then a function of the four scalar independent variables $(\mathbf{r}, t)$. Typically $\Psi(\mathbf{r}, t)$ satisfies a partial differential equation, as shown in many of the examples in Chapter 9. But differential equations can only describe local interactions so that, for example, the potential at one location can affect the potential at a distant location only by action through the intervening medium. Local interactions in the time domain are called Markovian. In a Markovian system, the state of the system at a designated time (perhaps the potential everywhere in a volume conductor) is determined completely by the state of the system just before that time. Systems with nonlocal interactions in either space or time do not satisfy differential equations: rather they are often described by integral equations.

Simple Linear Systems

Often a system is represented by a black box with some input v(t) and resulting output X(t), as indicated in Figure 8-1a. The problem of identifying the quantitative relation between input and output is called system characterization. The classic example from mechanical engineering is the mass attached to a spring in Figure 8-1b, in which the instantaneous position of the oscillating mass is the output X(t), and the external force v(t) is the input. An electrical analog is the parallel RLC circuit Figure 8-1c in which the input current v(t) causes an output voltage X(t). Whereas the relation between input and output for these and many other systems is governed by linear differential equations, the general concept of a linear system is not so limited. That is, the system shown in Figure 8-1a is identified as linear or nonlinear by the following experiment: A certain input $v_1(t)$ is applied to the

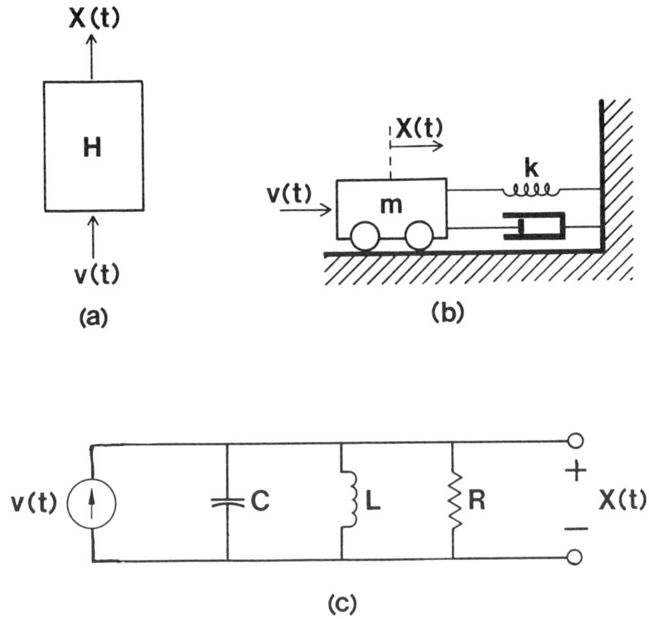

Figure 8-1. **a.** General input–output in a linear system with transfer function $H(\omega)$. **b.** Linear mass–spring system with external force $v(t)$ and displacement $X(t)$. Damping force is proportional to velocity. **c.** Linear, parallel RLC circuit with input current source $v(t)$ and output voltage $X(t)$. The passive elements are a resistor (R), indictor (L), and capacitor (C). The outputs in examples b and c satisfy the differential equation (8.1), except that $v(t)$ is either proportional to force (b) or the time derivative of the current source (c).

system with resulting output $X_1(t)$. Another input $v_2(t)$ elicits the output $X_2(t)$, and so on to N inputs. The system is linear if the combined input $v_1(t) + v_2(t) + \cdots + v_N(t)$ results in the combined output $X_1(t) + X_2(t) + \cdots + X_N(t)$. Any other result indicates that the system is nonlinear. Therefore, nearly all macroscopic physical and biological systems are nonlinear. However, use of linear systems analysis has proved invaluable because many systems are approximately linear over interesting ranges of input $v(t)$ and the system parameters. Furthermore, linear systems analysis for limiting cases often provides the first step in the analysis of nonlinear systems.

The relations between input and output for many systems similar to those shown in Figures 8-1b and c are described by the ordinary differential equation

$$\frac{d^2X}{dt^2} + 2\alpha \frac{dX}{dt} + \omega_0^2 X = v(t) \tag{8.1}$$

where the damping constant α and the undamped natural frequency ω_0 are determined by the appropriate mechanical or electrical parameters. With electrical systems, the dissipative term involving the first time derivative in (8.1) is often an excellent representation of the actual system. However, mechanical systems with damping often have frictional forces that are not proportional to velocity, so (8.1) is not strictly valid. Nevertheless, the engineer is likely to use (8.1), or its equivalent version in more complicated systems, because it may provide a fairly good semiquantitative representation of system behavior, which then may be used in a more exact, perhaps nonlinear, analysis. We suggest that an analogous approach may be valuable to study physiologic systems that are likely to be nonlinear.

When $v(t) = 0$, system oscillations must be started by initial conditions at $t = 0$, such as pushing the mass or closing a switch. The resulting motion or voltage results in underdamped free oscillations for the parameter range $\alpha < \omega_0$, with exact functional form $X(t)$ dependent on the initial conditions. For example, voltage oscillations in a circuit may be initiated by rapid motion of a magnet near the circuit. If, however, the input $v(t)$ is applied for $t > 0$, the resulting motion or voltage is called a forced oscillation. In general, the solution to (8.1) or other linear differential equation may be expressed as the sum of two parts, that is

$$X(t) = \text{transient solution} + \text{steady state solution} \tag{8.2}$$

where only the transient solution depends on initial conditions and the steady-state solution is zero when the input function $v(t) = 0$. In practice, this separation of the solution into two parts is very convenient. In electric circuits, for example, the transient solution typically dies out exponentially in times of the order of milliseconds, thereby leaving only the steady-state solution. In circuit design, one study is typically concerned with ensuring that no circuit elements will be damaged by high-voltage transients, whereas a separate study is concerned with the steady-state output produced by the input $v(t)$. This separation of output $X(t)$ into two parts is fundamental to linear systems but is generally not possible is nonlinear systems, an issue considered further in Chapter 10.

Input/Output Relations

When studying the characteristics of a system with inner workings that are largely unknown, it is often valuable to consider the Fourier transform of the output defined by

$$X(\omega) = \int_{-\infty}^{+\infty} X(t)e^{-j\omega t}\, dt \tag{8.3}$$

The Fourier transform of the input $v(\omega)$ is defined similarly, and the angular frequency is $\omega(\text{sec}^{-1}) = 2\pi f$ (cycles/second or Hertz). With a constant-parameter linear system (for example, one described by (8.1) with α and ω_0 independent of either t or X), input and output are related by

$$X(t) = \int_{-\infty}^{+\infty} h(\tau)v(t - \tau)\, d\tau \tag{8.4}$$

where $h(\tau)$ is the weighting function of the system and the lower limit on the integral may be replaced by zero because the requirement of causality for any real system ensures that $h(\tau) = 0$ for $t < 0$. Equation (8.4) merely expresses mathematically the general idea that the output v(t) at one time depends on the input at all earlier times, but with some unequal weighting function of the time delay τ, given by $h(\tau)$. Thus, (8.4) defines the function $h(\tau)$, but such simple definition is possible only for constant parameter, linear systems. Extension of this concept to nonlinear systems is accomplished with nonlinear transfer functions or kernels.

The Fourier transform of the weighting function

$$H(\omega) = \int_{-\infty}^{+\infty} h(t)e^{-j\omega t}\,dt \tag{8.5}$$

is called the frequency response function for the system. The transfer function for the system refers to the Laplace transform of the weighting function

$$H(s) = \int_{0}^{+\infty} h(t)e^{-st}\,dt \tag{8.6}$$

Equations (8.5) and (8.6) are consistent because $h(t) = 0$ for $t < 0$ and ω and s are generally complex.* Laplace transform methods typically are used in problems for which transient solutions are required, whereas Fourier transform methods are better suited to studies of steady-state solutions, as emphasized in later chapters. The definitions (8.5) and (8.6) are sufficiently similar so that the label transfer function often is also applied to (8.5).

The standard relations between input and output for a constant-parameter, linear system in terms of the frequency response function is obtained by calculating the Fourier transform of both sides of (8.4), a procedure that yields

$$X(\omega) = H(\omega)v(\omega) \tag{8.7}$$

That is, the Fourier transform of the output is simply the frequency response function multiplied by the Fourier transform of the input. The same relation is, of course, valid for Laplace transforms and transfer functions with the transformation $\omega = -js$. Examples are the mechanical or electrical systems of Figures 8-1b and 8-1c, which have the frequency response function

$$H(\omega) = [\omega_0^2 - \omega^2 + 2j\alpha\omega]^{-1} \tag{8.8}$$

Thus, when the damping constant α is relatively small, any input function v(t) that contains frequency components ω_0 tends to produce large (resonant) output X(t) in the range of frequencies near ω_0. Another important implication of (8.7) is that only the frequency components (or frequency ranges) in the input function v(t) can appear in the output X(t), regardless of the nature of the constant-parameter, linear system described by $H(\omega)$. This is in marked contrast to nonlinear systems in which the frequency response function depends on the input, and the

*Some texts use the notation $H(j\omega)$ for the frequency response function, where H(s) is the transfer function. To keep the notation simple, we use $H(\omega)$ with the implicit understanding that frequency response functions are obtained from transfer functions by substituting $s = j\omega$.

output may contain an abundance of frequency components not present in the input.

Experimental Measures of Linear Systems

The output of a physical or biological system that produces sustained oscillations is conveniently characterized by its spectral density function (or "power spectrum") $G(\omega)$, defined in terms of the output Fourier transform

$$G(\omega) = |X(\omega)|^2 \tag{8.9}$$

with a similar definition for the spectral density function of the input. Unlike the Fourier transform, the spectral density function is a real function of ω. The spectral density function has the following physical interpretation: The power dissipated in a 1-ohm resistor with voltage $X(t)$ is expressed by $X^2(t)$ watts. The total energy dissipated (that is, converted to thermal energy) over the time interval $(-T, T)$ is then

$$E = \int_{-T}^{T} X^2(t)\, dt \quad \text{joules} \tag{8.10}$$

If an estimate of the Fourier transform of $X(t)$ is made for this signal on the same interval $(-T, T)$, Parseval's theorem of Fourier transforms shows that if T is large (in practice, many cycles of $v(t)$ in the frequency range studied occur on the interval $2T$), then

$$E \cong \frac{1}{2\pi} \int_{-\infty}^{+\infty} G(\omega)\, d\omega \quad \text{joules} \tag{8.11}$$

where the approximation becomes exact as $T \to \infty$. A comparison of (8.10) and (8.11) shows that the total energy in the voltage signal is distributed over frequency. For example, we might say that 50% of the energy or power in some signal occurs over the frequency range $f = \omega/2\pi = 0$ to 10 Hz. Many experiments involve transducers that convert physical quantities (displacement, pressure, and so on) into voltage records. Thus the term "power spectrum" is applied to $G(\omega)$, even when the experimental or other record $X(t)$ is not voltage.

The spectral density function lacks phase information. But the phase of the output function (relative to the input function, for example) at each frequency is given by (8.7). The output may be characterized by its spectral density function and its phase spectrum. When the system has multiple output $X_1(t)$, $X_2(t) \cdots X_N(t)$, as in a multichannel electroencephalographic (EEG) record, particularly useful quantities are the coherence functions that measure the phase consistency of pairs of outputs, typically over many epochs of Fourier transformed data. For example, the coherence function (or "squared coherency") between channels 1 and 2 of data is (Bendat and Piersol, 1986)

$$\gamma_{12}^2(\omega) = \frac{|G_{12}(\omega)|^2}{G_1(\omega)G_2(\omega)} \tag{8.12}$$

Here $G_1(\omega)$ and $G_2(\omega)$ are the spectral density functions for data channels 1 and 2, respectively, and $G_{12}(\omega)$ is a complex quantity called the cross-spectral density function expressed by

$$G_{12}(\omega) = X_1(\omega)X_2^*(\omega) \tag{8.13}$$

where $X_2^*(\omega)$ denotes the complex conjugate. The coherency is a correlation coefficient defined as a function of frequency so that

$$0 \leq \gamma_{12}^2(\omega) \leq 1 \tag{8.14}$$

Two random variables whose correlation coefficient is zero are said to be uncorrelated. It may be shown that statistically independent random variables are necessarily uncorrelated. The reverse is not always true; however, for physically important situations involving two or more normally distributed random variables, "mutually uncorrelated" implies statistical independence (Bendat and Piersol, 1986.)

If the two data channels contain common frequency components but different phases, the coherency function is a measure of whether the phase difference changes with sample epoch. Thus, if the phase difference between channels is always the same at ω_1, the coherence function equals one at $\omega = \omega_1$. If v(t) and X(t) are completely unrelated (uncorrelated) at frequency ω_1, the coherence function will be zero at $\omega = \omega_1$. Of course, the coherency function will have different values at different frequencies. The coherency function relating input v(t) to output X(t) for any constant-parameter, linear system is equal to 1 at all frequencies. If the coherence function is greater than zero but less than 1 at any frequency, one or more of the following must be true (Bendat and Piersol, 1986):

1. Extraneous noise occurs in the measurements.
2. The system relating v(t) and X(t) is nonlinear or has time-varying parameters.
3. The output X(t) is due not only to v(t) but also to other inputs.

These statements refer to actual coherence functions. When working with experimental data, we can only estimate coherence functions. Confidence intervals for estimated coherence functions, based on number of data epochs averaged, are given in Chapter 3. Because noise is unwanted input, case 1 above may be a special instance of case 3.

With the application of systems analysis methods (linear or nonlinear) to physiology, considerable problems may occur because we cannot control system inputs. For example, we can control the physical parameters of a visual stimulus to the retina, but many additional inputs (and feedback) may occur along the pathway leading to the visual cortex. Where do we draw our system boundaries? Large neural systems may appear hopelessly complex, whereas small systems probably receive many inputs from other parts of the brain. Several examples of ordinary coherence functions when multiple inputs and outputs occur and examples of partial coherence functions are presented in the literature (such as Bendat and

Piersol, 1986). The partial coherence functions can be used in neurophysiologic studies of the following general nature. Suppose a high ordinary coherence between EEG activity recorded between two neural systems (say A and B) is observed. This may sugest functional connections between A and B. However, another explanation is that A and B are not substantially interconnected but rather both are connected to a third system C. The partial coherence function between A and B is a measure of the coherence between A and B when the influences of C on A and B have been removed. Partial coherence functions have been estimated for canine EEG to determine whether the large coherence between alpha rhythms recorded from different cortical sites (A and B) might be accounted for by a common thalamic site (C) (Lopes da Silva et al, 1980). These studies generally suggest a small to moderate influence from the thalamus on corticocortical coherence in the dog.

Resonance

If a simple mechanical or electrical system similar to the examples of Figure 8-1 is driven by an external forcing function $v(t) = B \cos \Omega t$, representing force, voltage, or current, the output $X(t)$ is governed by (8.1) which has an underdamped solution

$$X(t) = e^{-\alpha t}(A_1 \cos \omega t + A_2 \sin \omega t) + \frac{B \cos(\Omega t - \Theta)}{\sqrt{(\omega_0^2 - \Omega^2)^2 + 4\alpha^2\Omega^2}} \qquad (8.15)$$

which is a special case of (8.2). Here the arbitrary constants A_1 and A_2 are determined by the initial conditions. The underdamped solution occurs when damping is sufficiently small ($\alpha < \omega_0$), in which case the frequency of the free oscillation is

$$\omega = \sqrt{\omega_0^2 - \alpha^2} \qquad (8.16)$$

After times t of a few $1/\alpha$, the exponential factor in (8.15) causes the free oscillation (transient solution) to be negligible with respect to the forced oscillation (steady-state solution), which occurs at the forcing frequency Ω. Resonance occurs when the forcing frequency Ω is close to the undamped natural frequency ω_0. In this case, the amplitude of the forced oscillation is large because the quantity under the square root sign is small for small damping factor α. The response curve that shows the normalized amplitude of $X(t)$ or the "magnification factor" as a function of forcing frequency is shown in Figure 8-2. The bandwidth β, defined as the range of frequencies in which the amplitude of the output is greater than its maximum value divided by the square root of two, is 2α ($1/RC$ for the parallel electrical circuit of Figure 8-1c). For a circuit intended to be frequency selective, the sharpness of the response is a measure of the quality of the circuit. The quality factor Q is a nondimensional quantity defined as the ratio of the resonant frequency ω_0 to bandwidth β (Nilsson, 1986). In a physiologic example, an EEG from a person with a "good" alpha rhythm may show a 10-Hz rhythm with an apparent

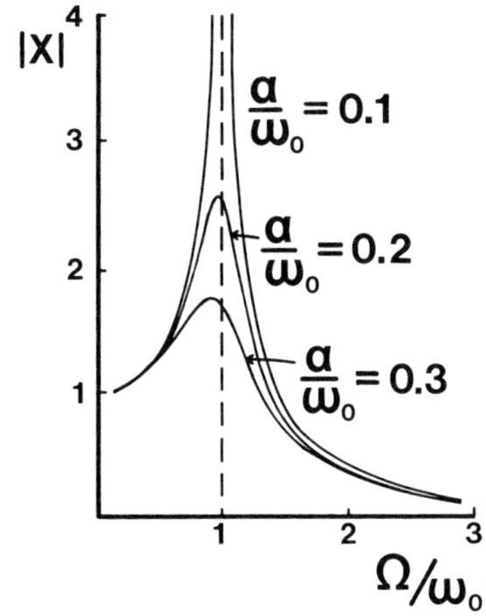

Figure 8-2. Amplitude of the response (that is, the magnitude of the output X(t)) of linear systems as a function of the frequency Ω of the input v(t). The width or "sharpness" of this curve is measured by the bandwidth or quality factor, which depends on the relative damping constant α/ω_0. These particular curves are obtained from the right-most term of (8-15).

bandwidth of 1 Hz, or an apparent Q of 10. However, the actual Q of the underlying neural system might be much larger because some of the observed spread of 1 Hz in the average EEG spectrum is typically due to the nonstationary behavior of the EEG signal. For example, in one study of steady-state visual evoked potentials, many participants showed Q values greater than 50 or 100 (Robinson, 1983). If the external forcing function contains N frequency components Ω_n, that is

$$v(t) = \sum_{n=1}^{N} B_n \cos(\Omega_n t - \phi_n) \tag{8.17}$$

linearity of the system requires that the output X(t) be expressed by

$$X(t) = e^{-\alpha t}(A_1 \cos \omega t + A_2 \sin \omega t) + \sum_{n=1}^{N} \frac{B_n \cos(\Omega_n t - \Theta_n)}{\sqrt{(\omega_0^2 - \Omega_n^2)^2 + 4\alpha^2\Omega_n^2}} \tag{8.18}$$

where the Θ_n represent the output phases. Thus the forced oscillation contains the same frequency components as the forcing function, but with varying magnitudes depending on the coefficients B_n and the closeness of each forcing frequency Ω_n to the undamped natural frequency ω_0. Because nearly any forcing function v(t) can be decomposed into a series of cosine functions with phase ϕ_n by the methods of Fourier series, (8.18) can be regarded as the general solution to (8.1) for any input v(t). This result for linear systems is in marked contrast to that of nonlinear systems in which higher harmonics and subharmonics of the forcing frequency and combination frequencies $(\omega_0 \pm \Omega_n)$ may occur in the output X(t). In highly nonlinear systems, chaotic "motion" may occur in which a broad spectrum of frequencies is observed as the result of even a single forcing frequency Ω. This topic is discussed in Chapter 10.

The effect of varying the frequency Ω of a sinusoidal input v(t) on the output X(t) in an electric circuit is the frequency response of the circuit. In engineering applications, this is valuable for at least two reasons. First, circuits that transmit some frequencies noticeably better than others allow us to filter signals in unwanted frequency ranges. The design of such circuits makes radio, telephone, and television receivers possible and allows us to use analog filters in EEG machines. Second, if the frequency response of a linear circuit is known, the response (or output X(t)) due to a nonsinusoidal input v(t) may be predicted using Fourier analysis methods. A circuit containing an operational amplifier and its frequency response curve are shown in Figure 8-3 (Schwarz and Oldham, 1984). A different choice of resistances and capacities in the circuit results in a broader or narrower frequency response band. A narrow response, that is, a larger Q, is associated with resonance phenomena. This circuit also illustrates the concept of feedback from the output to the input of the amplifier.

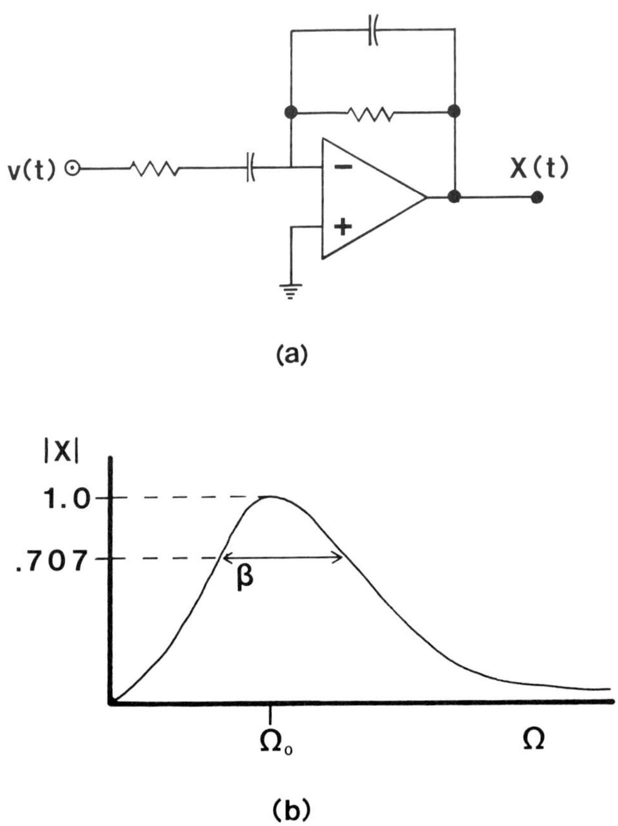

Figure 8-3. **a.** Operational amplifier circuit with input v(t) and output X(t), which is fed back into input. **b.** Typical frequency response curve of operational amplifier showing bandwidth β.

Coupled Oscillators

In contrast to the simple mechanical and electrical system of Figure 8-1, many physical and especially physiologic systems normally have multiple inputs and outputs, as indicated in Figure 8-4. In this case, there are N outputs $X_1(t)$, $X_2(t)$ $\cdots$ $X_N(t)$. If the system is governed by ordinary differential equations, typically there are N second-order differential equations for the N dependent variables or outputs that result from the N inputs $v_1(t)$, $v_2(t)$ $\cdots$ $v_N(t)$. For this to be considered a single system, rather than N independent systems, interactions should occur between the subsystems represented by the individual boxes. Both nearest-neighbor and more distant interactions are shown. We can imagine each subsystem n, characterized by its frequency response function $H_n(\omega)$, to represent a mechanical or electrical oscillator. Or perhaps each box, distributed over two spatial dimensions, represents a neocortical column with synaptic input $v_n(t)$ from the midbrain, and output $X_n(t)$ representing some measured quantity. For example, $X_n(t)$ might be the number of action potentials fired between times t and $t + \Delta t$ from within the column. Alternately, $X_n(t)$ might represent the extracellular potential, averaged over the volume of the column. The question of the surface area of cortex represented by each box is critical in this example and is closely related to electrode size in imagined experiments and to the nature of intracortical connections. The neocortical system also provides an example with short-range interactions through the intracortical connections and with long-range interactions through cortico-cortical fibers. The latter are fundamentally different than the intracortical fibers because their range is about two orders of magnitude longer, and because they provide a means for distant columns to interact directly without acting through the intervening tissue (the case of non-Markovian spatial variables).

A simple mechanical system of coupled oscillators composed of two identical

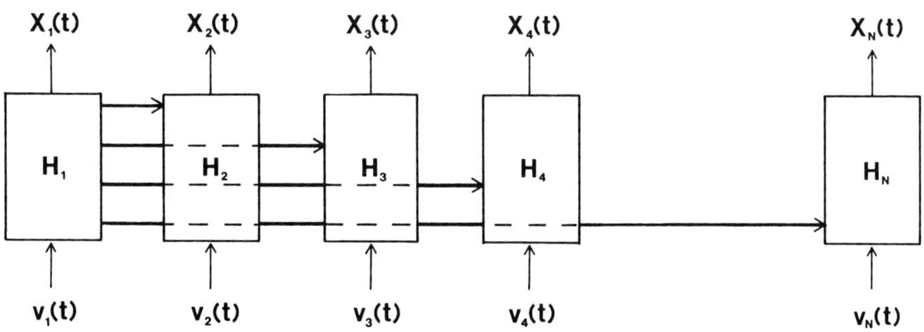

Figure 8-4. Large system composed of subsystems with multiple inputs $v_n(t)$ and outputs $X_n(t)$. If interactions between subsystems are sufficiently strong, it may be appropriate to treat the entire system as having a single spatially dependent input $v(\mathbf{r}, t)$ and single spatially dependent output $X(\mathbf{r}, t)$. The subsystems might, for example, represent single cortical macrocolumns, the large system then representing the entire neocortex. When sufficiently strong interactions occur between subsystems, the subsystems may lose their separate identities.

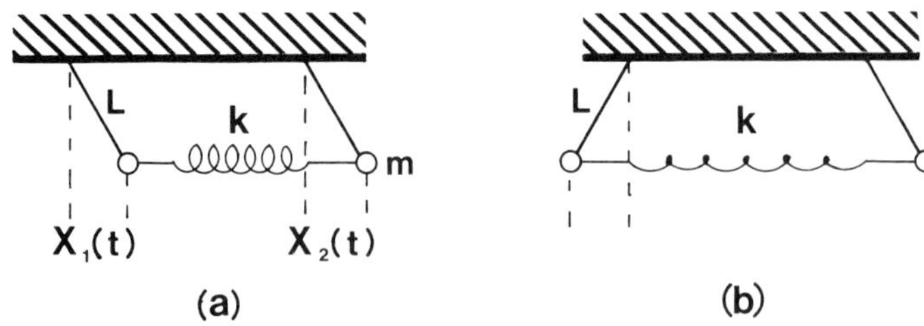

Figure 8-5. Two pendulums connected by a spring (k) with displacements from equilibrium expressed by $X_1(t)$ and $X_2(t)$. **a.** Masses move together and frequency is that of a simple pendulum. **b.** Masses move in opposite directions at a higher frequency.

pendulums of length L supporting masses m coupled by a weightless spring of stiffness k is shown in Figure 8-5. Application of Newton's law of motion yields two ordinary differential equations for the displacements $X_1(t)$ and $X_2(t)$ of the two masses from their equilibrium positions. It is then convenient to transform these dependent variables to a new set (x, y, called "normal coordinates")

$$\begin{aligned} x &= X_2 + X_1 \\ y &= X_2 - X_1 \end{aligned} \tag{8.19}$$

so that the differential equations assume the simple forms (Pain, 1968)

$$\frac{d^2x}{dt^2} + \omega_1^2 x = 0 \tag{8.20}$$

$$\frac{d^2y}{dt^2} + (2\omega_0^2 + \omega_1^2)y = 0 \tag{8.21}$$

The form of (8.20) and (8.21) show that both new dependent variables undergo simple harmonic motion. Two familiar frequency parameters are involved; the oscillation frequency for a mass attached to a spring (with no friction), as in Figure 8-1b and (8.1)

$$\omega_0 = \sqrt{\frac{k}{m}} \tag{8.22}$$

and the oscillation frequency of a simple pendulum of length L

$$\omega_1 = \sqrt{\frac{g}{L}} \tag{8.23}$$

where g is the acceleration of gravity. If the masses are set in motion, perhaps by pulling both an equal distance to the right, $X_1 = X_2$ and $y = 0$ at all times. In this case, the spring remains at its equilibrium length so the motion is completely described by (8.20); the motion is that of a single simple pendulum. Alternately, if the masses are pulled equally in opposite directions from their equilibrium positions, $X_1 = -X_2$ and $x = 0$ at all times so the motion is completely described by (8.21). The motion occurs with the higher frequency $(2\omega_0^2 + \omega_1^2)^{1/2}$ because of the effective coupling of the individual oscillators. If the coupling between oscillators becomes weak (that is, the spring constant k becomes small), $\omega_0 \rightarrow 0$ and the pendulums both oscillate at the frequency ω_1. Oscillations at the frequencies ω_1 and $(2\omega_0^2 + \omega_1^2)^{1/2}$ are called normal modes of vibration because each can be described by one normal coordinate x or y. Of course, the motion of the system can be started in many ways, and each such initial condition will cause a different motion.

This example of a simple mechanical oscillator can be extended to other fields. For example, atoms in polyatomic molecules are held together by chemical bonds that provide restoring forces analogous to masses on springs. The normal modes of vibration of the water molecule are 4.78×10^{13}, 11.0×10^{13}, and 11.27×10^{13} second^{-1}. Resonance effects can be expected due to external forces applied at these frequencies. Thus electromagnetic fields transmitted through the atmosphere are more strongly absorbed by water vapor in these frequency ranges. The same principle has been applied to the detection of toxic gases (such as on a battlefield or near a chemical plant). A laser beam with frequency tuned to one of the resonant frequencies of the suspected gases is passed through the region in question. Because its characteristic resonant frequencies provide an excellent signature for each molecule, measurement of laser energy absorbed at a specific frequency determines if the suspected gas is present.

Another mechanical example (which helps provide the transition from the study of discrete to continuous systems, discussed in Chapter 9) is the coupled oscillations of a loaded string. In Figure 8-6, a light string supports N equal masses m, spaced at equal distances a along its length. The string is fixed at both ends, has a length (N + 1)a, and a constant tension T, which pulls displaced masses toward their equilibrium positions (Pain, 1986). The equation of motion of the ith

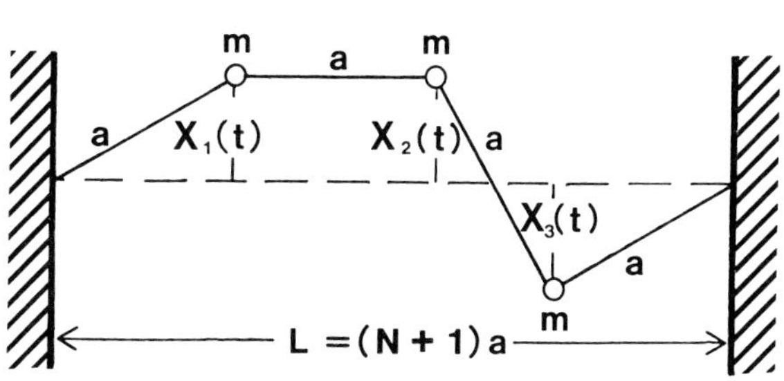

Figure 8-6. A stretched string of negligible mass and constant tension T, loaded with N equally spaced masses. Small displacements are greatly exaggerated in the figure. Each mass oscillates with a linear combination of the N normal mode frequencies given by (8-25). This system has only nearest-neighbor interactions, that is, each mass is connected only to one or two adjacent masses. A more complicated example is given in Chapter 10, in which each mass has multiple strings to allow more distant (non-local) interactions.

mass is

$$\frac{d^2X_i}{dt^2} = \frac{T}{ma}(X_{i-1} - 2X_i + X_{i+1}) \quad i = 1, N \tag{8.24}$$

Thus there are N equations for the N displacements of the individual masses. There are N normal modes, and the oscillation of any mass will be a combination of these modes. The frequency of each normal mode is given by

$$\omega_n^2 = \frac{2T}{ma}\left(1 - \cos\frac{n\pi}{N+1}\right) \quad n = 1, N \tag{8.25}$$

To provide an example, let $N = 10$ and normalize frequencies such that the fundamental frequency is $\omega_1 = 1$. The 10 normal mode frequencies obtained from (8.25) are 1.00, 1.98, 2.92, 3.81, 4.61, 5.32, 5.92, 6.40, 6.75, and 6.97. For comparison, if the total mass of Nm were continuously distributed over the length of the string L, the fundamental frequency and overtones are given by

$$\omega_n = \frac{n\pi}{L}\sqrt{\frac{T}{\text{mass/unit length}}} \quad n = 1, 2, 3, \ldots \tag{8.26}$$

Equation (8.26) may be obtained directly from (8.25) by letting $N >> n$ or derived separately in Chapter 9. By using the same values for parameters as in the case of discrete masses, (8.26) yields frequencies of 1.05, 2.11, 3.16, 4.21, 5.27, 6.32, 7.38, 8.43, 9.48, 10.54, and so on. Thus the lower normal modes for the discrete mass system are close to the lower normal modes for the continuous string, but the relative error is much larger for higher modes. This occurs because the eigenfunctions (spatial shapes of string displacement corresponding to each normal mode frequency) for the discrete and continuous systems are more similar for the lower modes. Only a finite number of modes exist for the discrete system, but there are an infinite number for the continuous system. Of course, if we included either the mass of the string or the finite size of the masses in the discrete system, an infinite number of normal modes would also result.

The number of dependent variables (mass displacements, voltages, and so on) required to specify the state of a system is the number of degrees of freedom of the system. For example, both mechanical systems shown in Figure 8-7 have four degrees of freedom. Figure 8-7a shows two masses, each of which can move in both the horizontal and vertical directions. Figure 8-7b has four masses, but each can move only vertically. Figure 8-7b also provides an example of a system with non–nearest-neighbor interactions. When the springs k_1 and k_2 are absent, the four normal mode frequencies of the system (normalized so that the fundamental frequency is $\omega_1 = 1$) are $\omega = 1$, 2.70, 4.83, and 9.43 (Seto, 1964). Additional coupling provided by the springs k_1 and k_2 causes the normal mode frequencies to move closer together. In the limit of very stiff springs, that is, large k_1 and k_2, the system approaches a two-degree of freedom system consisting of the relative motion of mass 2m and that of the combined masses m, 3m, and 4m. In this case,

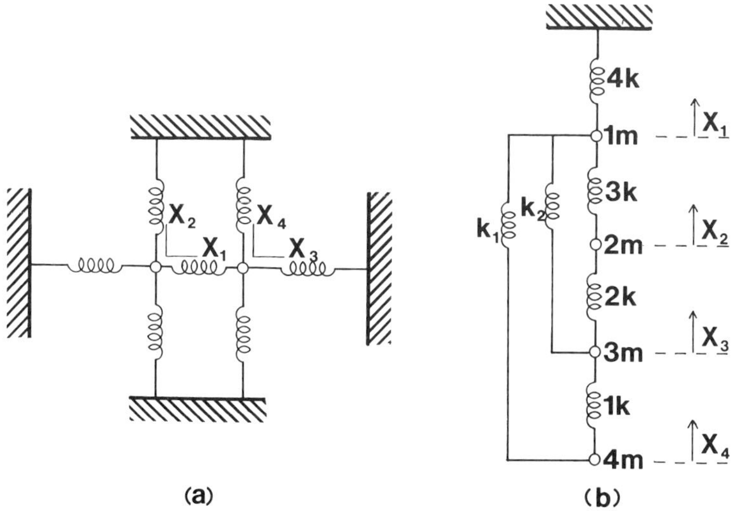

Figure 8-7. Systems with four degrees of freedom. **a.** Two masses move in a plane. **b.** Four masses move in one dimension. The springs k_1 and k_2 provide for longer ranges of interaction than simple nearest-neighbor coupling. If these springs are sufficiently stiff, the effective number of degrees of freedom is reduced to a value near two as a result of the non-local interactions produced by the k_1 and k_2 springs.

three of the four normal mode frequencies are close together, and the motion is generally simplified. Essentially the number of effective degrees of freedom is less than the actual number of degrees of freedom. We will return to this important idea in Chapter 10.

To provide another example, note that a room full of N air molecules has 6N external degrees of freedom, three for translational motion and three for rotation of each molecule. In addition, a molecule consisting of several atoms has internal (vibrational) degrees of freedom. To list some fairly general characteristics of linear oscillators, consider a system of N degrees of freedom, held together by linear forces that tend to bring each of the N displacements back to equilibrium. Of course, displacement of one coordinate toward equilibrium may make another coordinate move away from equilibrium, as is characteristic of coupled systems. The N coordinate values at any time specify the state of the system and satisfy the coupled set of differential equations (Morse and Ingard, 1968)

$$\frac{d^2X_i}{dt^2} + 2\alpha_i \frac{dX_i}{dt} + \sum_{n=1}^{N} B_{in}X_n = v_i(t) \quad i = 1, N \tag{8.27}$$

where the coefficients B_{in} determine the coupling of the system elements (such as masses) and the $v_i(t)$ are external forces applied to the ith element. If all the applied forces are simple harmonic so that $v_i(t) = |F_i e^{-j\Omega t}|$ for $i = 1, N$, the steady-state motion of the system is given by the real part of

$$X_i(t) = \sum_{n=1}^{N} \frac{A_{in}(\Omega)e^{-j\Omega t}}{[\omega_{R1}^2 - (\Omega + j\gamma_1)^2] \cdots [\omega_{RN}^2 - (\Omega + j\gamma_N)^2]} \quad i = 1, N \tag{8.28}$$

Here the A_{in} are coefficients determined by the parameters in (8.27). The N normal mode frequencies have both real and imaginary parts; that is,

$$\omega_n = \omega_{Rn} - j\gamma_n \tag{8.29}$$

where the imaginary parts γ_n result from the damping constants α_i in (8.27), due to friction in mechanical systems or resistive losses in electrical systems. If all the damping coefficients α_i are small, the γ_n will generally be small, and the system will exhibit resonance whenever the external forcing frequency Ω is close to any of the real parts of the normal mode frequencies ω_{Rn}. When a single oscillator becomes uncoupled from the other oscillators (N = 1), the imaginary part of the frequency is given by $\gamma_1 = \alpha$, but for coupled oscillators each of the γ_n depend on all the α_i in (8.27).

Linear Models for Neurons

Discussions of electrical and mechanical systems as given here and in most textbooks sometimes assume a rather cavalier attitude about the distinction between real systems and models of systems. There are, of course, valid pedagogic motivations for this. Ideally physical scientists first fully understand the behavior of the model system before considering what happens when the real system does not conform to the model. In this manner, a scientist or engineer can obtain a far deeper understanding of the system than could have been obtained without the model, even though the model is imperfect. With mechanical, and especially electrical systems, our models are often excellent representations of real systems. After all, the fundamental laws are known and an inadequate model usually can be replaced by a better model, given enough brain and computer power. Exceptions to this rule occur mainly with systems with many degrees of freedom, the behavior of a turbulent fluid being a prime example. Also we now appreciate that nonlinear systems with even a few degrees of freedom can undergo chaotic behavior, which is characterized by exquisite sensitivity to initial conditions, system parameters, or both, so that precise predictions of the model may be difficult or impossible to verify experimentally which is an issue considered further in Chapter 10.

Neural models must generally lie on less solid foundations than those of physical systems. We can, for example, purposely design electric circuits with linear elements or with nonlinear elements with known input/output relations; but practical alterations of neural systems are far more limited. Also even a very simple neural system, such as a patch of membrane, is a system with many degrees of freedom (if only we consider the system in sufficient detail). Nevertheless, membrane models, models of single neurons, and, to some extent, models of neural networks or mases have provided not only a framework for discussion but also quantitative predictions of experimental results. The remaining discussions of this chapter rely heavily on the published works of one of the principal architects of neurophysiologic systems analysis (Freeman, 1975, 1987), with some modifications to fit our discussion of neocortex.

Because about 85% of the neurons of mammalian neocortex are pyramidal cells, it is appropriate to consider a large pyramidal cell with its major parts: dendrites, cell body, and axon, as shown in Figure 8-8. The input consists of synaptic activity from the axons of other neurons on the dendrites and cell body of the output neuron. The number of synapses on cortical pyramidal cells is about 10^4 to 10^5. These inputs come from cortical interneurons, other pyramidal cells through the recurrent collaterals (branches of the axon that remain within the local cortex), corticocortical axons from more distant regions of cortex, and commissural axons from the opposite cortical hemisphere. Input from interneurons is partly inhibitory; the other inputs are exclusively excitatory. The inputs $v_n(t)$ are determined by the presence or absence of an action potential on the nth input axon at time t. The axon terminals release neural transmitters contained in the synaptic vesicles at rates that depend on the occurrence of action potentials. The transmitter substances change the local transmembrane potential $X_m(t)$ either toward (depolarization, excitatory) or away (hyperpolarization, inhibitory) from values tending to cause the output (postsynaptic) neuron to fire its own action potential. A diffusion process due to the capacitive—resistive (cable) properties of the membrane causes the dendritic input to be felt at the trigger zone for action potentials (usually the initial segment of the axon, just below the cell body in Figure 8-8). This diffusion process is described quantitatively in Chapter 9, but for purposes of this discussion, the soma or initial segment transmembrane potential is considered spatially independent and denoted by $X_s(t)$. If $X_s(t)$ exceeds the threshold value, an action potential X(t) propagates along the axon and provides input to many other neurons. This input occurs locally and at distant cortical locations, with perhaps substantial time delay due to finite velocity of the action potential. Thus the inputs $v_n(t)$ are related to the output X(t) of the single neuron through several serial stages.

In experimental studies of the neuron, the input may be due to a pair of transmembrane-stimulating electrodes providing an initial condition $X_m(0)$ or to extracellular single-shock stimulation of carefully defined central tracts or peripheral nerves providing the input $v_n(t)$. Sensory stimuli are not useful in this application because the transformation to action potentials is too complex to provide known input functions $v_n(t)$. In general, the relation between the amplitude of the stimulus (magnitude of the current injected into the extracellular fluid near the nerve) and the functions $v_n(t)$ is nonlinear; however for a limited range over relatively small stimulus values, the crest amplitude of the postsynaptic potential (PSP or $X_s(t)$) changes in proportion to the stimulus amplitude. No action potential is fired by the postsynaptic neuron over this range of stimulus. For this linear range, experiments indicate that the soma PSP may be approximated by

$$X_s(t) = C[e^{-a(t-T_c)} - e^{-b(t-T_c)}], \qquad t \geq T_c \tag{8.30}$$

as shown in Figure 8-9b. Here C is an arbitrary constant. The parameter a is interpreted as the reciprocal of the passive membrane time constant. The parameters b and T_c are combined representations of serial distributed delays (including

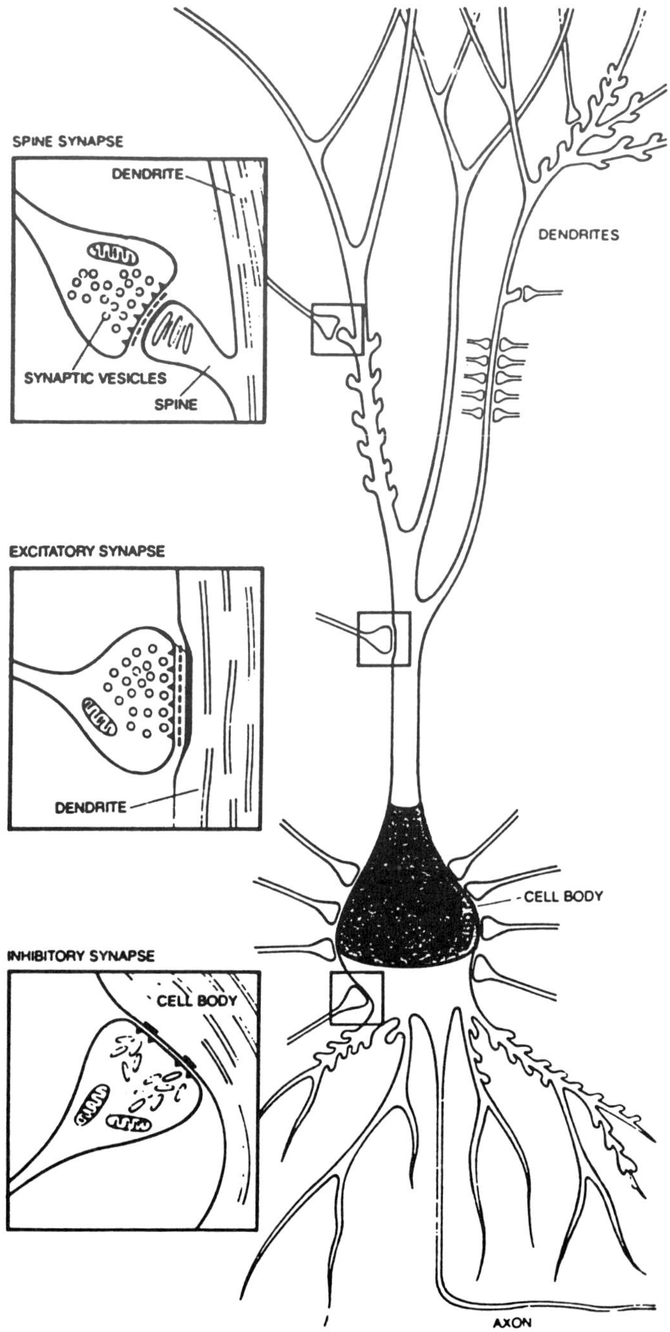

Figure 8-8. Pyramidal cell and several synapses. Synaptic vesicles carry chemical transmitters that determine whether the synapse on the postsynaptic neuron is excitatory or inhibitory. A large cortical pyramidal cell can receive 10^4 or more synapses. (Reproduced with permission from Iversen, 1979).

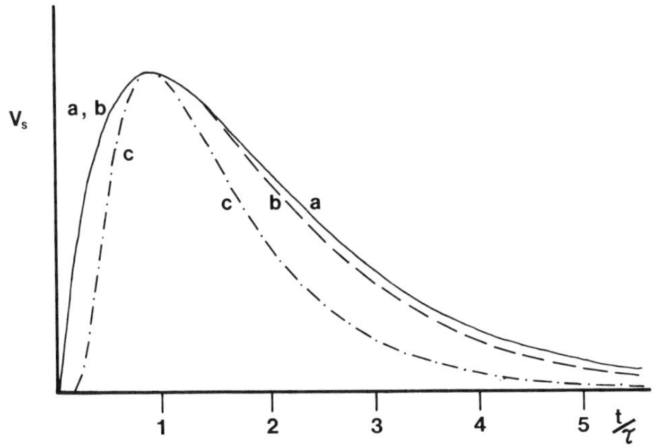

Figure 8-9. Three functions X(t) representing transmembrane potential at fixed location due to a synaptic input at some other location on the neuron. **a.** te^{-t}; **b.** $e^{-at} - e^{-bt}$; **c.** $t^{-1/2}e^{-(A/t+t)}$. The parameters a, b, and A were chosen so that all three functions peak at a normalized time, $t/\tau = 1$. X(t) was also normalized so that all three peaks would have unit magnitude. Functions (**a**) and (**b**) were chosen only as fits to experimental data. Function (**c**) was derived theoretically from the core-conductor neuron model and accounts for the spatial separation of synapse and field point (see Chapter 9).

temporal dispersion of action potentials in the afferent tract), synaptic diffusion, and capacitive–resistive delay in the dendrites. The latter delay depends on the manner in which synapses are distributed over the dendrites and soma and is examined further in Chapter 9. Another possible delay is due to the effects of residual transmitter substance on or in the postsynaptic membrane. The delays are combined because the PSP rise time is brief, typically about 1 to 4 milliseconds, and the processes are so similar that they cannot be readily distinguished (Freeman, 1975). To apply local EEG theories, a simpler version of (8.30) involving only one parameter has been suggested (van Rotterdam et al, 1982)

$$X_s(t) = C\ at\ e^{-at}, \qquad t \geq 0 \tag{8.31}$$

which, for EEG theory, may be close enough to (8.30) because the delay T_c is normally short compared with EEG cycle times (see Figure 8-9a). The parameter a may be longer than the membrane time constant and may depend on whether the input is excitatory or inhibitory. See Chapter 5 for application of PSP rise times to a local circuit theory of EEG.

Linear Models of Neural Masses

Models of neural masses are based on the idea, discussed in Chapters 1, 2, 3, 5, 11, 13, and 14, that the existence of many neurons with locally dense synaptic (and perhaps other chemical or direct electric field) interaction can result in the emergence of this more macroscopic entity. The resultant coupling of neurons within the mass is sufficiently strong so that new macroscopic properties emerge that define the instantaneous state of the mass. These neural mass "mesostates" are characterized by highly cooperative activity of the neurons. Neither the mesoscopic properties nor the cooperative activity can be explained at the level of a single neuron, any more than the temperature or viscosity of a gas can be explained at the level of a single molecule (Freeman, 1975). In neocortical EEG applications at the higher hierarchical levels associated with scalp potentials, the relevant neural mass is the cortical column with a diameter of perhaps 1 mm (such as a macrocolumn containing about 10^5 neurons), and a relevant mesoscopic property is the (columnar) dipole moment per unit volume **P**. A collection of about 10^5 of these columns forms a neocortical hemisphere with a state partly defined by the probability density function $f(\mathbf{r}, \mathbf{P}, t)$, defined such that $f(\mathbf{r}, \mathbf{P}, t)\, d^2\mathbf{r}\, d^3\mathbf{P}$ is the number of cortical columns at surface locations between **r** and $\mathbf{r} + d\mathbf{r}$ having dipole moments per unit volume between **P** and $\mathbf{P} + d\mathbf{P}$ at time t, as described in Chapter 1.

Electrophysiologic studies involving extracellular "micro-EEG" electrodes with a tip diameter of approximately 10^{-2} to 10^{-3} cm or intracellular "microelectrodes" with a tip diameter of about 10^{-4} cm must, of course, be concerned with lower hierarchical levels than those usually associated with human EEG (recorded from the scalp). The hierarchy of neural masses has been characterized in terms of "K sets" (Freeman, 1975). A KO set is a collection of perhaps 10^3 to 10^8 neurons that have common input (for example, a set of sensory receptors of the first-stage neurons to which they project) and a common sign of output (excitatory or inhibitory) and having no functional interconnections. One example is the monosynaptic reflex pathway of the gastrochemius nerve in feline spinal cord (Rall, 1955a). As shown in Figure 8-10a, a single shock stimulus to the nerve fiber produces an approximately synchronous input v(t) of action potentials in a certain fraction of the several hundred afferent axons stimulated. Some of these afferent fibers distribute many presynaptic terminations directly to motoneurons of the pathway (A).

The total transmembrane potential change from equilibrium at each motoneuron resulting from these synaptic inputs depends on the number and arrangement of the active terminals received by it. Spatial summation of the excitation produced by the active terminals is thus an essential feature of this process. The output of the system X(t) is the magnitude of the compound action potential of the nerve, which is determined by the number of motoneurons receiving at least a threshold intensity of spatially summed synaptic excitation. The experimental input–output relation is shown in Figure 8-10b. The reflex excitability of the pathway was changed by adjusting depth of anesthesia and by tetanic conditioning (50 volleys of input stimulation ending 150 milliseconds before the test volley was evoked). By this means, four sets of input–output results were obtained from a single animal. The magnitude of the output action potential was linearly related to the magnitude of the input potential over the input range of about 20% to 60% of its maximum.

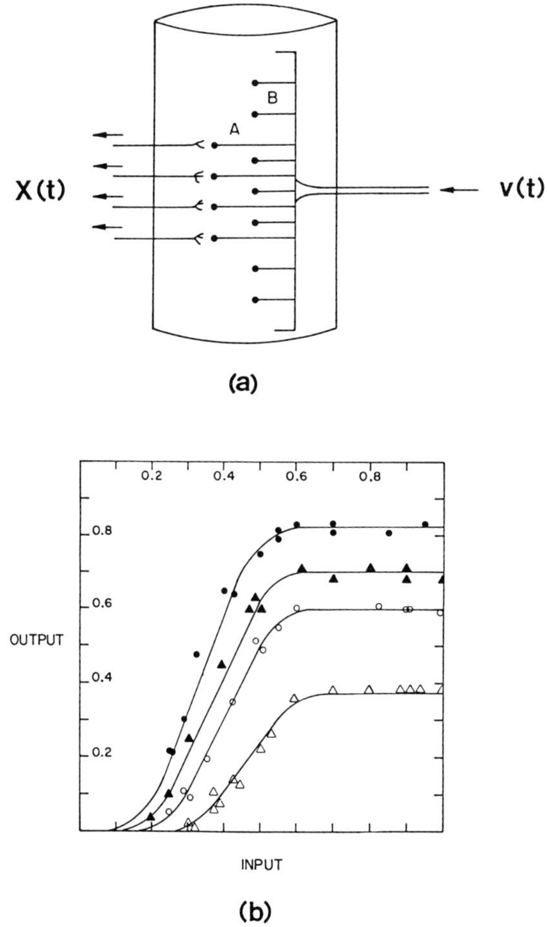

Figure 8-10. **a.** Shock stimulus v(t) is input to the spinal cord. Synaptic transmission is of two types: the monosynaptic reflex (A), in which synaptic input directly stimulates the motoneurons of the pathway, and the diffuse reflex mechanism (B), in which synpatic input stimulates an interneuron, which, in turn, acts on the motoneurons (latter not shown). **b.** Experimental relation between input and output in the reflex pathway of the spinal cord shown in (a). The input is approximately proportional to number of input fibers stimulated, and the output is roughly proportional to number of output fibers activated. (Reproduced with permission from Rall, 1955a.)

The magnitudes of the input and output compound action potentials are each approximately proportional to the corresponding number of active fibers. Thus Figure 8-10b implies a linear relation between number of input fibers stimulated and number of output fibers activated within the neural mass. Furthermore, the asymptotic approach to output maximum for each of the four curves of Figure 8-10b was not due to approaching saturation of pool discharge. Rather the afferent impulses in the higher threshold fibers, which contribute to the last 30% of a maximum input record, do not contribute to excitation of the monosynaptic reflex (A) but rather stimulate the interneurons at (B). Thus we can consider the effective monosynaptic input, which is due only to stimulation of 70% of input fibers having the lowest thresholds. The implication is that the relation of output to effective input is linear over most of the range of this effective input. The experimental results are explained largely by a statistical input–output theory based on random distributions of thresholds and locations of synaptic knobs in the motoneuron pool (Rall, 1955b).

Spontaneous and Evoked Potentials in Olfactory Cortex

A schematic of principal neurons, pathways, and synaptic connections in the feline olfactory mucosa, bulb, and olfactory cortex is shown in Figure 8-11 (Freeman, 1975). The approximately 10^8 olfactory receptors (R) lie in the mucosa that lines the nasal cavity. Sensory information is carried along the axons (one for each receptor) of the primary olfactory nerve to the bulb, a relatively isolated neural structure with the size and shape of a lima bean (in cats) and containing approximately 10^5 neurons of several types oriented radially within the bulb. After processing its input, the olfactory bulb sends its output along the lateral olfactory nerve tract to the olfactory (that is, prepyriform) cortex, which extends over 1 cm anteriorly from the anterior edge of the bulb. There is no obvious topographic projection, that is, axons from each part of the bulb end in all parts of the olfactory cortex.

Both bulb and cortex produce bursts of "spontaneous" (or background) sinusoidal activity of about 40 Hz (with a typical apparent Q of perhaps 5 to 10). The bursts may be abolished by holding the nostrils closed to prevent activation of the olfactory receptors. There is a consistent relation between the size of the olfactory bulb and EEG frequency, for example, about 90 Hz in the mouse, 60 Hz in the rabbit, and 30 Hz in the pig (Freeman, 1991), as discussed in Chapter 2. This background EEG tends to be spatially coherent over the olfactory cortex. A comparison of the amplitude spectrum (square root of spectral density function) for background EEG and average potentials evoked by a sequence of electric shocks to the lateral olfactory tracts is shown in Figure 8-12 (Freeman, 1987). The characteristic effect of increasing the stimulus intensity from 1.0 (arbitrary units) to 76.4 is to shift the output spectrum toward lower frequencies. The asterisk shows the magnitude of stimulus threshold at which behavioral responses are observed and single evoked potentials are close in amplitude to that of the background EEG. Increased stimulus intensity causes an increase in active input axons, which presumably accounts for the altered spectra. Because of the temporal dispersion of action potentials with different velocities in the lateral olfactory tract, it is not clear whether these curves illustrate linear or nonlinear behavior of the olfactory cortex.

Average evoked potentials recorded in olfactory cortex (and in olfactory bulb)

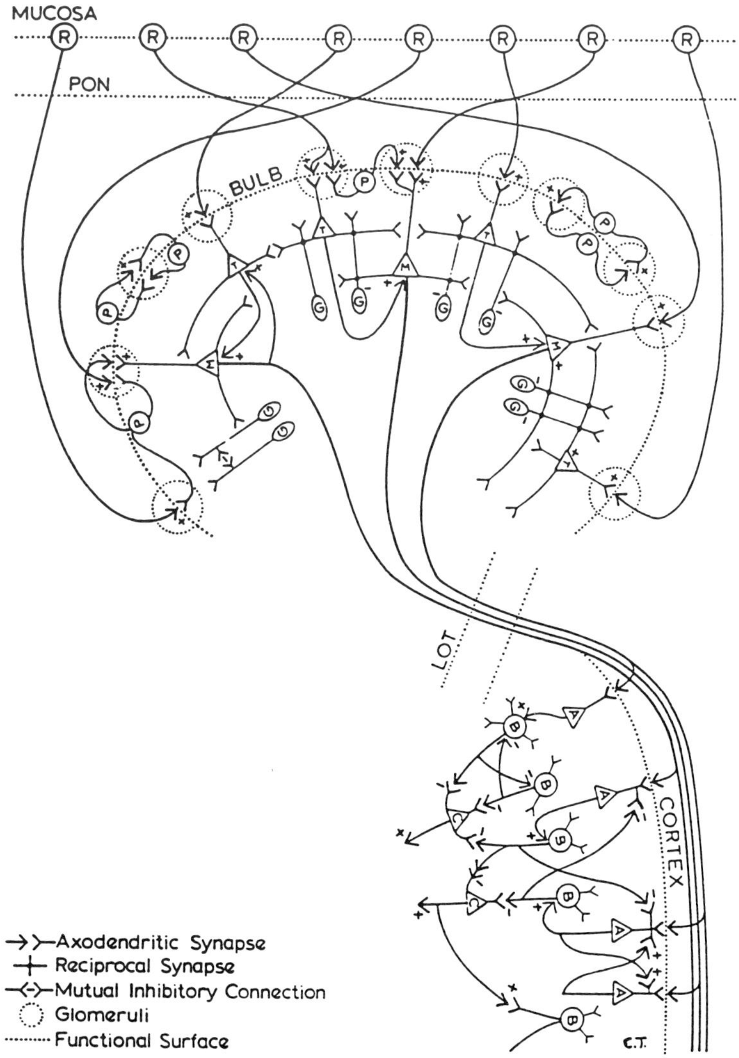

Figure 8-11. Principal types of neurons, pathways, and synpatic connections in the olfactory mucosa, bulb, and cortex. PON is primary olfactory curve. LOT is lateral olfactory tract connecting the olfactory bulb to olfactory cortex. (Reproduced with permission from Freeman, 1975.)

qualitatively resemble the transient responses of classical linear systems, as discussed previously (Freeman, 1964a, 1964b, 1975, 1987). Cortical excitatory neurons receiving afferent input excite inhibitory interneurons, which provide negative feedback to the excitatory neurons. Although the details of the operation of neural circuits are poorly understood, this general type of feedback circuit has been studied widely in electrical engineering applications. It typically results in

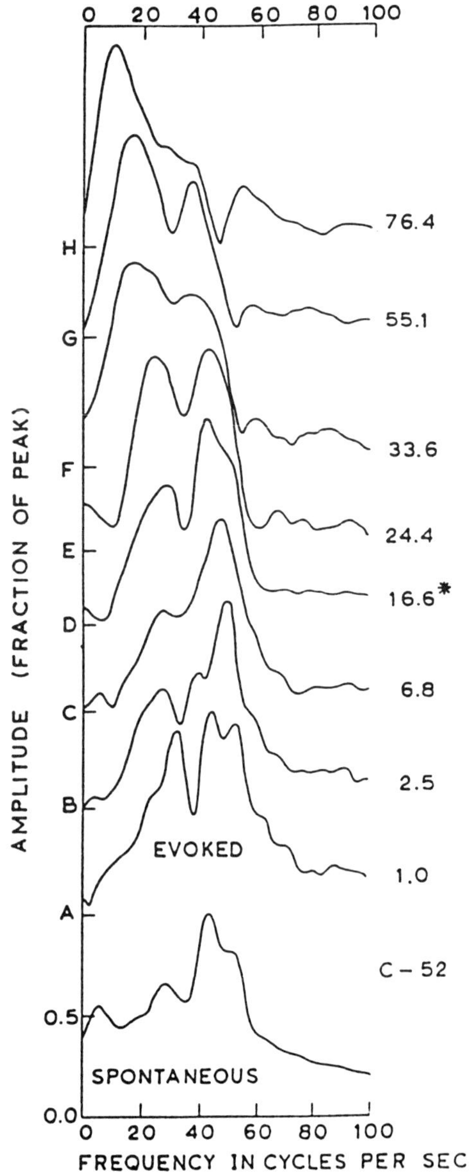

Figure 8-12. The characteristic effect on event-related potentials (ERP) of increasing the stimulus intensity is a spectral shift to the left. The lowest curve is the amplitude spectrum of the spontaneous EEG recorded from olfactory cortex in a cat. The remaining curves in ascending order are the amplitude spectra of the Fourier transforms of ERPs (normalized to equal maximal amplitude) over a range of increasing stimulus intensity. The asterisk shows the level of the threshold for behavioral responses to the electrical stimulation, at which the single evoked potentials are close in amplitude to the background EEG. At this level ERP spectrum most closely conforms to the EEG spectrum. (Reproduced with permission from Freeman, 1975.)

underdamped or overdamped responses to input pulses as illustrated by the first two terms on the right side of (8.15), except that systems with many degrees of freedom generally are composed of a superposition of many such responses, as in (8.28).

Given this background, evoked potentials in cat cortex are appropriately fit to the complex exponential waveforms

$$X(t) = \sum_{n=1}^{N} C_n e^{-j\omega_n t} \tag{8.32}$$

by nonlinear regression techniques. The coefficients C_n and corresponding frequencies ω_n are, in general, complex so that 4N parameters are required to describe an Nth order system. Olfactory potentials are typically well fit by second- or third-order systems, although detailed analysis of cortical circuits might predict systems of much higher order because of the apparent complexity of cortical interactions. The relative simplicity of observed waveforms appears to support the neural mass concept, which depends on dense collective interaction between neurons, thereby reducing the effective number of degrees of freedom.

When very deep anesthesia is used to suppress the background EEG of olfactory cortex, the average evoked potential is rendered nonoscillatory because the inhibitory postsynaptic potentials no longer occur; that is, negative feedback is eliminated. (This may be called the open loop state because the feedback loop is removed.) As with apparently similar physical systems, the open loop frequencies in (8.32) are nearly pure imaginary, that is, $\omega_n = \omega_{Rn} - j\gamma_n$ with $\omega_{Rn} \cong 0$ for n = 1, 2, and the result is overdamped output similar to the output of a single neuron (soma PSP), expressed by (8.30) with $T_c = 0$, and damping factors $\gamma_1 =$ a, and $\gamma_2 =$ b. In one reported experiment, $\gamma_1 \sim 200$ and, $\gamma_2 \sim 700$ sec^{-1}, which yields a rise time of roughly 5 milliseconds (Freeman, 1975). In the awake state, damped oscillations in (8.32) occur with real frequencies ω_{R1}, ω_{R2} typically of about 200 to 400 second^{-1}, reflecting the natural background EEG frequency of approximately $f = 40$ Hz or $\omega = 2\pi f = 251$ second^{-1}, and damping factors γ_1, γ_2 typically about 30 to 80 second^{-1} (Freeman, 1964a). Because (8.32) is the output X(t) due to an impulse or delta function input $v(t) = \delta(t)$, the Fourier or Laplace transforms of (8.32) yield an estimate of frequency response $H(\omega)$ or transfer function H(s) for the olfactory cortex.

Circuits with Negative Feedback

An important feature of neocortical dynamics in negative feedback from interneurons acting back on excitatory pyramidal cells. Thus we can consider apparently analogous effects that occur in electric circuits. In the analyses of the feedback circuit of Figure 8-13a, we use transfer functions relating input to output. Of course, the following could have been calculated using frequency response functions (8.7) with the replacement of s by $j\omega$. The input v(s) is fed into a circuit component (typically an operational amplifier) that subtracts some multiplier (gain) A of the feedback $X_2(s)$ from the output. The resulting difference is input to a linear subsystem with transfer function $H_1(s)$. The output from $H_1(s)$ is multiplied

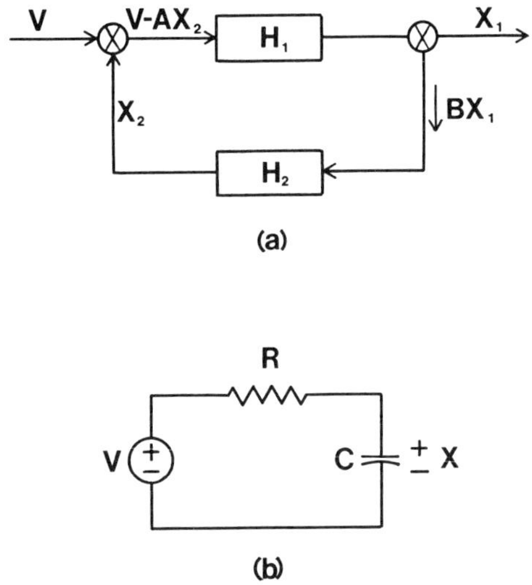

Figure 8-13. a. General feedback circuit. In one model of EEG, H_1 and H_2 represent pools of excitatory and inhibitory neurons, respectively. The gain A is proportional to the number of inhibitory synapses (fed back) on excitatory neurons. b. Simple, linear RC circuit with input and output voltages v(t) and X(t), respectively. Two such circuits (with different resistors and capacitors) might be used as subsystems H_1 and H_2. External control of the system may be obtained by changing the R and C (control) parameters.

by the gain B and then fed back through another linear subsystem with transfer function $H_2(s)$. The system equations follow directly from (8.7)

$$\begin{aligned} X_1(s) &= H_1(s)[v(s) - AX_2(s)] \\ X_2(s) &= BH_2(s)X_1(s) \end{aligned} \tag{8.33}$$

which yields

$$X_1(s) = H(s)v(s) \tag{8.34}$$

where H(s), the effective transfer function for the entire system, is given by

$$H(s) = \frac{H_1(s)}{1 + ABH_1(s)H_2(s)} \tag{8.35}$$

For an example of a feedback circuit, let both subsystems be simple RC circuits, as shown in Figure 8-13b with input voltage (for subsystem 2) $X_1(t)$ and output $X_2(t)$ across the capacitor. The individual transfer functions are expressed by

$$H_1(s) = \frac{a}{s + a} \quad \text{and} \quad H_2(s) = \frac{b}{s + b} \tag{8.36}$$

where the inverse time constants of the two subsystems are $a = (R_1C_1)^{-1}$ and $b = (R_2C_2)^{-1}$. Substitution of (8.36) into (8.35) yields the total system transfer function

$$H(s) = \frac{a(s + b)}{(s + a)(s + b) + ABab} \tag{8.37}$$

The system output $X_1(t)$ as a result of a delta function input $v(t) = \delta(t)$ is the weighting function h(t), which for general forms of H(s) may be obtained by inverting the Laplace transform of (8.6), that is

$$h(t) = \frac{1}{2\pi j}\int_{-\infty+j\sigma}^{+\infty+j\sigma} H(s)e^{st}\, ds \tag{8.38}$$

Here the integral is carried out in the complex s plane along the line $\sigma + js_y$ with $-\infty < s_y < +\infty$, and σ is sufficiently large so that the contour lies to the right of all singularities of H(s). However, when H(s) is a rational fraction of s (that is, one expressed as the ratio of two polynomials, as in the example of (8.37)), the sometimes difficult contour integral can be avoided, and standard cookbook techniques of electrical engineering can be used to invert the transform (as described in nearly any text on electric circuits). When H(s) is a rational fraction, the inverse transform of (8.37) is of the form

$$h(t) = Ce^{-\gamma t}\cos(\omega_R t + \theta) \tag{8.39}$$

where the constants C and θ depend on circuit parameters and initial conditions. The main point is that h(t) is a damped sinusoidal oscillation with a damping decrement γ and frequency ω_R given by

$$\gamma = -1/2(a + b) \tag{8.40}$$

$$\omega_R^2 = ab(1 + AB) - \gamma^2 \tag{8.41}$$

The damping of the feedback system is simply the average damping of the uncoupled subsystems, but unlike the uncoupled systems, the feedback system produces oscillations that are weakly damped if $|\gamma/\omega_R| << 1$. Linear systems analysis often is not concerned with the exact functional form of the output h(t) (which is only valid for a delta function input in any case) but rather only with the frequencies and damping decrements of the output, which are independent of the initial conditions. When H(s) is equal to a rational fraction of s, frequencies and damping decrements are determined by the poles of H(s), that is by location in the complex s plane where the denominator of (8.35) is zero. There are, in general, N poles $s_1, s_2, \ldots s_N$, each having a real and imaginary part, that is,

$$s_n = \gamma_n + j\omega_{Rn} \quad n = 1, N \tag{8.42}$$

If the transformation $s_n = j\omega_n$ is applied to (8.42), (8.29) is recovered. Complex poles appear in pairs with positive and negative real frequencies ω_R. An Nth order system (highest power of s in the denominator of H(s)) can produce as many as N poles. The number of natural frequencies observed in the output then can be anything from 0 to N/2, depending on the number of overdamped poles, which correspond to exponential damping rather that oscillations. The locations of the poles (or other singularities such as branch points in more complicated systems) then yield the general character of the system. If the only singularities are poles, the following principles apply: (1) The system is stable only if all the poles have negative or zero real parts, that is, $\gamma_n \leq 0$ for all $n = 1, N$. Otherwise a random fluctuation producing a transient solution will increase exponentially in time rather than damp out. In real systems, these instabilities typically grow until they are limited by nonlinear effects. We can speculate that epileptic phenomena are essentially brain instabilities that rapidly grow beyond quasi-linear states. (2) Oscillations at frequency ω_{Rn} may be observed in the output of the system only if $|\gamma_n/\omega_{Rn}|$ is typically less than approximately 0.1 to 0.5, depending on system noise level. Some poles have only real parts ($\omega_R = 0$) corresponding to exponentially damped parts of the output. Linear electric circuits with 50 or 100 poles are not uncommon in industrial applications; the output waveforms (linear) can be complicated.

Negative Feedback in Neocortical Models

The system pictured in Figure 8-13 is of interest in neurophysiology partly because the predicted oscillations occur in a simple system with only linear resistive and capacitive properties, as with the passive membrane. If the system $H_1(s)$ represents many excitatory neurons that receive subcortical input v(s) and excite an interneuron pool $H_2(s)$ to provide negative feedback to the excitatory pool, the gain A is proportional to the number of inhibitory synapses from system $H_2(s)$ on the excitatory neurons of system $H_1(s)$. The gain B is proportional to the number of excitatory synapses from system $H_1(s)$ that feed back to the inhibitory neurons of system $H_2(s)$. If $a = b$ in (8.40), weakly damped oscillations ($|\gamma/\omega_R| \leq 0.2$) are possible only for the relatively large gains $A \cdot B \sim 25$. Membrane time constants for cortical pyramidal cells are about 8 milliseconds (Lux and Pollen, 1966). Thus, if we choose $a = b = 1/8$ millisecond^{-1} = 125 second^{-1}, weakly damped oscillations are possible only for $\omega_R \sim 600$ second^{-1} or more, that is, $f_R > 100$ Hz. The only way to obtain weakly damped oscillations at lower frequencies from this model system is to imagine much longer decay times, that is smaller a's and b's than appear justified by neocortical time constants.

The simple RC circuits of Figure 8-13b do not, of course, match the qualitative features of input–output from a KO neural mass (that is, the open loop case), as described by (8.30) or (8.31) because the rise period is missing. Both rise and decay times may be included without additional parameters by using the approximation (8.31) as the response of KO neural mass. By taking the Laplace transform of this relation (neglecting multiplying constants), we obtain transfer functions for the two subsystems of Figure 8-13a, which appears to be the most simple plausible representation of a KO neural population. That is

$$H_1(s) = \frac{a}{(s+a)^2} \qquad (8.43)$$

$$H_2(s) = \frac{b}{(s+b)^2}$$

Here a and b are reciprocal rise times of the excitatory and inhibitory neurons, respectively; the total system transfer function is then

$$H(s) = \frac{a(s + b)^2}{(s + a)^2(s + b)^2 + abAB} \tag{8.44}$$

Equation (8.44) is one of the transfer functions proposed as a model for local neocortical interaction, as discussed in Chapter 5 (van Rotterdam et al., 1982).

Dispersion functions D(k, ω) (see Chapter 9) describe systems with spatial extent for which descriptions in terms of both spatial (k) and temporal (ω) frequencies are needed. With minimal spatial variation (that is, low spatial frequencies), we can set $k = 0$ in dispersion functions. In this limiting case, dispersion functions are simply the inverse of the simple transfer functions of this chapter, that is

$$H(s) = D^{-1}(0, s) \tag{8.45}$$

The transfer function (8.44) is identical to the dispersion function (5.1) suggested by Lopes da Silva's limiting linear model for local neural circuits, with the additional approximation $k = 0$ and the substitution $j\omega = s$ in (5.1).

Several more complicated transfer functions also have been proposed. For example, the next obvious complication is to use the KO input–output relation (8.30) rather than (8.31) to include rise and decay times as separate parameters (Lopes da Silva et al, 1974; Freeman, 1975). The subsystem transfer functions are then simply those of the overdamped RLC circuit whose transient response is expressed by (8.30). That is, when $T_c = 0$

$$\begin{aligned} H_1(s) &= \frac{(a_1 - a_2)s}{(s + a_1)(s + a_2)} \\ H_2(s) &= \frac{(b_1 - b_2)s}{(s + b_1)(s + b_2)} \end{aligned} \tag{8.46}$$

which when applied to the system shown in Figure 8-13a yields the total system transfer function

$$H(s) = \frac{(a_1 - a_2)s(s + b_1)(s + b_2)}{(s + a_1)(s + a_2)(s + b_1)(s + b_2) + AB(a_1 - a_2)(b_1 - b_2)s^2} \tag{8.47}$$

More complicated transfer functions involving multiple feedback loops in KI and KII neural masses also have been proposed (Freeman, 1975) that appear to provide good fits to feline cortical evoked potentials. It is not clear, however, that a realistic choice of physiologic parameters at the local level can result in the prediction of the low natural frequencies $f \sim 1$ to 15 Hz characteristic of human EEG, an issue considered in multiple contexts in Chapters 9 through 14.

References

Bendat, J.S. and Piersol, A.G. *Random Data: Analysis and Measurement Procedures. 2nd Ed.* New York: Wiley, 1986.

Freeman, W.J. Use of digital adaptive filters for measuring prepyriform evoked potentials from cats. *Exp. Neurol.* 10:475–492, 1964a.

Freeman, W.J. A linear distributed feedback model for prepyriform cortex. *Exp. Neurol.* 10:525–547, 1964b.

Freeman, W.J. *Mass Action in the Nervous System.* New York: Academic Press, 1975.

Freeman, W.J. Analytic techniques used in the search for the physiological basis for EEG. In: *Handbook of Electroencephalography and Clinical Neurophysiology.* (Revised series) Vol. 1. *Methods of Analysis of Brain Electrical and Magnetic Signals.* (A.S. Gevins and Remond, A., Eds.) New York: Elsevier, pp. 583–664, 1987.

Freeman, W.J. The physiology of perception. *Sci. Am.* 264:34–41, 1991.

Iversen, L.L. The chemistry of the brain. *Sci. Am.* 241(Sept):118–129, 1979.

Lopes da Silva, F.H., Hoeks, H., Smith, H., and Zetterberg, H. Model of brain rhythmic activity. *Kybernetik.* 15:27–37, 1974.

Lopes da Silva, F.H., Vos, J.E., Mooibroek, J., and van Rotterdam, A. Partial coherence analysis of thalamic and cortical alpha rhythms in dog—A contribution towards a general model of the cortical organization of rhythmic activity. In: *Rhythmic EEG Activities and Cortical Functioning.* (G. Pfurtscheller, Busar, P., Lopes da Silva, F.H., and Petsche, H., Eds.) Amsterdam: Elsevier, pp. 33–59, 1980.

Lux, H.D. and Pollen, D.A. Electrical constants of neurons in the motor cortex of the cat. *J. Neurophysiol.* 29:207–220, 1966.

Morse, P.M. and Ingard, K.U. *Theoretical Acoustics.* New York: McGraw-Hill, pp. 70–80, 1968.

Nilsson, J.W. *Electric Circuits.* Reading, MA: Addison-Wesley, pp. 457–488, 1986.

Pain, H.J. *The Physics of Vibrations and Waves.* London: Wiley, pp. 56–68, 1968.

Rall, W.A. A statistical theory of monosynaptic input-output relations. *J. Cell. Comp. Physiol.* 46:373–411, 1955a.

Rall, W.A. Experimental monosynaptic input–output relations in mammalian spinal cord. *J. Cell. Comp. Physiol.*, 46:413–437, 1955b.

Robinson, D.L. An analysis of human EEG responses in the alpha range of frequencies. *Int. J. Neurosci.* 22:81–98, 1983.

Schwarz, S.E., and Oldham, W.G. *Electrical Engineering: An Introduction.* New York: Holt, Rinehart, and Winston, 1984.

Seto, W.W. *Theory and Problems of Mechanical Vibrations.* New York: Schaum, pp. 103–104, 1964.

van Rotterdam, A., Lopes da Silva, F.H., van der Ende, J., Viergever, M.A., and Hermans, A.J. A model of the spatial-temporal characteristics of the alpha rhythm. *Bull. Math. Biol.* 44:283–305, 1982.

9

Continuous Linear Systems of Physics and Brain

PAUL L. NUNEZ

Transition from Discrete to Continuous Systems

Another method to depict a linear system with multiple inputs and outputs is to express input and output in terms of continuous spatial variables. For example, in the core conductor network model of the cylindrical axon, each box in Figure 8-4 might represent a short segment Δx of membrane and intracellular and extracellular fluid with appropriate capacitive-resistive properties. In this case, the inputs $v_n(t)$ are local current sources produced by synapses or electrodes. The outputs $X_n(t)$ are local transmembrane potential at discrete locations, $n = 1, N$. When making the transition from a discrete to a continuous system, the N inputs $v_n(t)$ and outputs $X_n(t)$ are replaced by the single input–output pair $v(x, t)$, $\Psi(x, t)$, where x is the coordinate along the axon. Similarly, the subsystem frequency response functions $H_n(\omega)$, or corresponding transfer functions $H_n(s)$, are replaced by the single frequency response function $H(k, \omega)$, where k is the wavenumber (or spatial frequency). Mathematically, a decrease in the number of dependent variables (or "unknowns") $X_n(t)$ from N to one occurs at the expense of increasing the independent variables from one (t) to two (x and t). The N ordinary differential equations for $X_n(t)$ are then typically replaced by a single partial differential equation for $\Psi(x, t)$. In more complex systems (such as the stochastic systems described in Chapter 14), a "field" $\Phi[\Psi(x, t)]$ may be defined. The function $\Psi(x, t)$ may then satisfy a partial differential equation only in certain limiting approximations. In less limiting approximations, a partial differential equation may describe $\Phi[\Psi(x, t)]$.

Of course, many systems require more than one spatial variable for description so that, in general, we are concerned with output $\Psi(\mathbf{r}, t)$ due to input $v(\mathbf{r}, t)$ with frequency response function $H(\mathbf{k}, \omega)$, where the vector $\mathbf{k}$ denotes wavenumbers in three spatial directions. For example, each box in Figure 8-4 might represent a neocortical column (at some arbitrary scale), and some macroscopic property

$\Psi(\mathbf{r}, t)$ may be associated with each two-dimensional location $\mathbf{r}$ of a column on the cortical surface. (Limitations of this approach, involving the spatial resolution of the sensor system used to measure $\Psi(\mathbf{r}, t)$, are discussed in Chapters 1, 2, and 3.) In the neocortical example in which the ouput $\Psi(\mathbf{r}, t)$ is macroscopic EEG or some quantity directly related to it, two spatial dimensions are appropriate for the description so we are concerned with the cortical frequency response function $H(k_x, k_y, \omega)$. Alternately, micro-EEG studies in the cortical depths might require a description in all three spatial dimensions $H(k_x, k_y, k_z, \omega)$.

All but the sections Collective Effects in Neocortical and Physical Systems and Hot Plasma and Neocortex of this chapter address systems with output $\Psi(\mathbf{r}, t)$ due to some input $v(\mathbf{r}, t)$ described by the linear, partial differential equation

$$\frac{\partial^2 \Psi}{\partial t^2} + 2\alpha \frac{\partial \Psi}{\partial t} - \nabla \cdot c^2 \nabla \Psi + \omega_0^2 \Psi = v(\mathbf{r}, t) \tag{9.1}$$

where α, c, and ω_0 may be constant parameters or, in inhomogeneous systems, spatially dependent. However, even in homogeneous systems, the damping parameter α is typically frequency dependent. The usual Laplacian operator is expressed by

$$\nabla^2 \equiv \frac{\partial^2}{\partial x^2} + \frac{\partial^2}{\partial y^2} + \frac{\partial^2}{\partial z^2} \tag{9.2}$$

in rectangular coordinates. Other coordinate systems may be required for particular geometric shapes of the medium (the surfaces of a sphere or neocortex, for example), so the general Laplacian operator is introduced to address this possibility. Equation (9.1) has an infinite number of solutions; however, the relevant unique physical or physiologic solution is the one that satisfies known initial and boundary conditions, consistent with the specification of typically either $\Psi(\mathbf{r}_s, t)$ or its normal derivative at the surface ($\mathbf{r} = \mathbf{r}_s$) of the system being studied. For example, a special case of (9.1) is Poisson's equation

$$\nabla \cdot c^2 \nabla \Psi = -v(\mathbf{r}, t) \tag{9.3}$$

which describes the manner in which the macroscopic potential $\Psi(\mathbf{r}, t)$ is distributed in a generally inhomogeneous volume conductor due to a known volume current source distribution $v(\mathbf{r}, t)$ (Rush and Driscoll, 1969; Nunez, 1981). In this case, $c^2 = \sigma$ is the electric conductivity of the medium. For a conductor surrounded by an insulator (perhaps the head surrounded by air), the appropriate boundary condition requires that current flow normal to the bounding surface be zero, a condition expressed by

$$\left(\frac{\partial \Psi}{\partial n}\right)_{\mathbf{r}=\mathbf{r}_s} = 0 \tag{9.4}$$

where $\mathbf{r}_s$ defines the surface of the conductor and n is a coordinate everywhere normal to this surface. Equation (9.3) when combined with (9.4) then has a unique solution for every source distribution $v(\mathbf{r}, t)$ and conductor shape. Equation (9.1)

was chosen to provide most of the physical examples in this chapter because it is sufficiently general to account for various diffusion processes, simple wave phenomena, and volume conduction phenomena that occur in neocortex.

Types of Equations and Boundary Conditions

Much of linear systems analysis in the physical sciences concerns three types of second-order partial differential equations (examples are in parentheses): hyperbolic (wave equations), parabolic (diffusion equations), and elliptic (Poisson's equation). Equation (9.1) encompasses all three types, with particular type determined by the relative values of the coefficients $\alpha(\mathbf{r}, t)$, $c(\mathbf{r}, t)$, and $\omega_0(\mathbf{r}, t)$, which may vary with location $\mathbf{r}$ in an inhomogeneous medium and with time t in a nonstationary medium. The importance of these labels for partial differential equations is due to two considerations: the different kinds of boundary and initial conditions required to ensure the existence of unique solutions to (9.1) and the different character of the resulting solutions. For example, small values of the damping parameter $\alpha(\mathbf{r}, t)$ causes (9.1) to behave like a wave equation and large values make it behave like a diffusion equation. The analogous consideration of α in discrete systems, described by (8.1), determines the distinction between underdamped and overdamped solutions. The fundamental difference between wave and diffusion processes is illustrated in Figure 9-1. Because the coefficients may vary spatially, a solution may be more wave-like in one part of the medium and more diffusion-like in another. An example is the transmission of light through fog in which a sufficiently dense region of fog causes the electromagnetic field to attenuate exponentially with distance rather than oscillate spatially in the usual manner of a wave (Morse and Feshbach, 1953).

If (9.1) is to be solved in some bounded spatial region, the existence of a unique solution is guaranteed if either Ψ or its normal derivative $\partial\Psi/\partial n$ is specified on all parts of the bounding surface, as in the example of (9.4). A unique solution also may be obtained if Ψ is specified on one part of the boundary and $\partial\Psi/\partial n$ on another part. In a volume-conduction example, suppose Ψ were known everywhere on some inner surface of a three-dimensional body (perhaps the surface of the cortex). The normal derivative of Ψ (proportional to the normal current density) is zero on the outer surface because of electrical isolation at the surface of the scalp. If, in addition, no sources occur between the two closed surfaces, the potential is uniquely specified everywhere between the two surfaces and can, in principle, be calculated.

In electroencephalographic (EEG) applications, cortical imagining algorithms (see Chapters 1, 6, and 7) make use of our knowledge of Ψ (measured scalp potential) and its normal derivative (equal to zero on the outer surface) to estimate Ψ on an inner surface (such as cortical potential). There are, however, several engineering limitations of cortical imaging due primarily to limited spatial sampling over the scalp and incomplete knowledge of the head volume conductor, especially

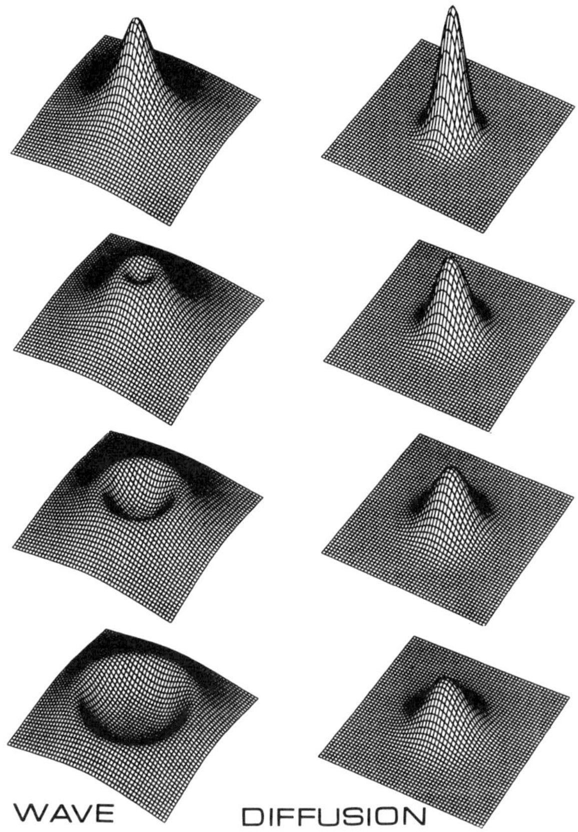

Figure 9-1 At t = 0, some initial disturbance is created in a medium. Depending on the nature of the medium, the disturbance may diffuse away from its origin or propagate as a traveling wave. Either case can be described by (9.1) depending on the relative magnitudes of the parameters α and c^2.

local tissue resistivities. In contrast to geometric information about the head, electrical properties cannot be obtained directly from computed tomographic or magnetic resonance imaging scans. Methods to obtain such electrical images are being studied.

Another type of boundary condition is the periodic boundary condition. For example, with either wave or diffusion processes on the surface of a three-dimensional body of arbitrary shape, the solution must be a single valued function of tangent (or angular) coordinates as we move all around the surface in any direction to obtain a mathematical solution that is physically possible. Examples are waves on the surface of a sphere or prolate spheroid, considered later. The question of required initial conditions is easier to describe than that of boundary conditions. Hyperbolic systems (such as wave equations) require that both Ψ and $\partial\Psi/\partial t$ be specified at $t = 0$, whereas parabolic equations (such as diffusion equations) have a unique solution if either Ψ or $\partial\Psi/\partial t$ is specified at $t = 0$. Discussion of boundary and initial conditions occurs throughout the physical science literature (for example, see Morse and Feshbach, 1953).

Because attempts to make mathematical descriptions of neural interaction probably involve much more complicated issues than those found in simple systems, we should first consider some complications in physical systems. Several distinct ways exist in which the relatively simple problems, such as those of the vibrating string, transmission line, and membrane potential, can be made more complicated. The following examples are discussed in various parts of this book:

1. The fundamental equations relating input to output in the medium may be nonlinear. This is the most serious complication to address (and perhaps the most interesting). Nonlinear systems are discussed in Chapters 10 and 14.
2. The medium may be anisotropic, inhomogeneous, or nonstationary. In the latter two examples, at least one of the coefficients in (9.1) will be a function of r or t. Solutions of volume conduction problems, such as Poisson's equation (9.3) in the inhomogeneous head, are discussed in Nunez (1981). Wave phenomena in inhomogeneous media are considered in Morse and Ingard (1968) and later in this chapter.
3. The boundary conditions may be complicated. Standing waves on the surface of hollow shells are considered in this chapter to introduce concepts related to the standing neocortical waves, proposed in Chapter 11. Periodic boundary conditions are required in this example.
4. Interactions may be nonlocal. In this case, the fundamental rules relating input to output cannot be expressed by a differential equation. However, an integral equation formulation may be appropriate. An example from the physical sciences, which also introduces the idea of statistical approaches to complex systems such as plasmas or neocortex, is provided in this chapter. Neocortical interactions are also partly nonlocal, as shown in Chapters 2 and 11 because of the corticocortical fibers. Furthermore, nonlocal stochastic interactions among columns within a region and among regions are described in Chapter 14. The probability distribution of neuronal firing fields may satisfy an integral equation in this case.

Free Vibrations of Stretched Strings and Membranes

The stretched string shown in Figure 9-2 provides an effective example of the transition from discrete to continuous systems and a prototype to study more advanced wave phenomena. The discrete masses in Figure 8-6 are here imagined to be distributed uniformally over the string. The tension in the string provides the restoring force that tends to return a displaced portion of the string $\Psi(x, t)$ to its equilibrium position. Application of Newton's Law then yields (9.1) as the equation of motion for the string. In the limiting case of a simple, undriven and undamped string, the parameters α and ω_0 and the forcing function $v(x, t)$ are zero. Viscous damping (due to surrounding air, for example) may be described approximately by the term involving α, and additional stiffness forces provided

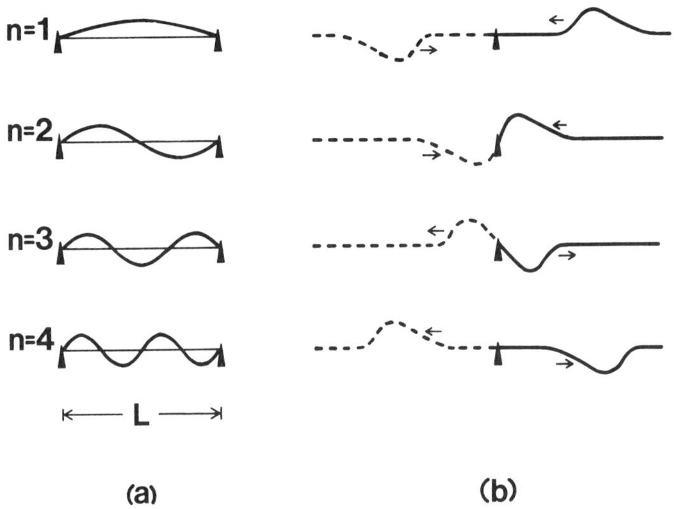

Figure 9-2. The stretched string. **a.** The first four eigenfunctions of the string, $\sin(k_n x)$, with wave numbers k_n given by (9.7). Corresponding oscillation frequencies are determined by (9.9). **b.** A traveling wave in the string reflects from a fixed support. The solid line indicates shape of string at successive times. Dotted lines show imaginary extension of the wave beyond the end of the string. A combination of traveling waves produces standing waves, as in (a), by constructive and destructive interference (Reproduced with permission from Morse and Ingard, 1968.)

by the medium surrounding the string are described by the term involving ω_0^2 (string embedded in a sheet of rubber or a series of closely spaced equal springs attached to the string, as in Figure 9-3 for example). The particular symbols for the parameters α and ω_0 are chosen to make their physical units clear (second^{-1}) and to retain consistency with the classical, discrete linear system described by (8.1). For example, the propagation velocity for waves in the string is

$$c = (\text{tension/mass per unit length})^{1/2} \tag{9.5}$$

In the limit of very small propagation velocities ($c \to 0$), that is, a string with no tension or infinite mass, the third term on the left of (9.1) vanishes and the

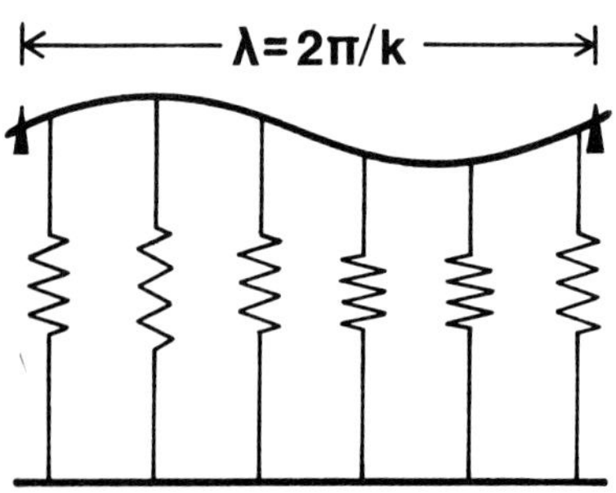

Figure 9-3. A stretched string with attached springs. The dispersion relation for the oscillating system is given by (9.8), where ω_0 is the resonant frequency associated with a single spring. This system is the mechanical analog of the transmission line, Figures 2-3 and 9-7.

simple equation for a mass on a spring (8.1) is again obtained. With a string with attached springs (Figure 9-3), each portion of the string is attached to its own spring and oscillates independently if $c \to 0$, because the coupling between different portions of the string has been removed in a string with no tension.

The shape of the string $\Psi(x, t)$ at any instant is described by (9.1) if the string undergoes only small displacements from equilibrium. The solution depends on both boundary and initial conditions. The usual boundary conditions require the ends of the string to be fixed, that is, $\Psi(0, t) = \Psi(L, t) = 0$ at all times $t > 0$, although strings with flexible supports also have been studied (Morse and Ingard, 1968). The unforced solution ($v(x, t) = 0$, or transient solution) is expressed by an equation similar to the first two terms on the right side of (8.15) describing the motion of the discrete oscillator. That is, instantaneous string shape due to an initial disturbance at $t = 0$ is expressed by

$$\Psi(x, t) = \sum_{n=1}^{\infty} e^{-\alpha_n t}(A_n \cos \omega_n t + B_n \sin \omega_n t)\sin k_n x \tag{9.6}$$

where the damping parameters α_n are mode (that is, frequency) dependent and represent a simple generalization of the parameter α in (9.1). Here the choice of the eigenfunctions $\sin k_n x$ (spatial shapes of string corresponding to each of the normal mode frequencies) with discrete wave numbers

$$k_n = n\pi/L \qquad n = 1, 2, 3 \ldots \tag{9.7}$$

forces the solution (9.6) to be zero at the ends of the string. In other words, only the specific wavelengths $\Lambda_n = 2\pi/k_n = 2L/n$ are allowed over the span of the string. Other boundary conditions will, of course, require other eigenfunctions in the solution. For (9.6) to satisfy the partial differential equation (9.1), the normal mode frequencies ω_n must satisfy the dispersion relation relating temporal to spatial frequencies (or wave numbers), that is

$$\omega_n^2 = \omega_0^2 + c^2k_n^2 - \alpha_n^2 \qquad n = 1, 2, 3 \ldots \tag{9.8}$$

which agrees with (8.16) in the limit of infinite spatial wavelengths ($k_n \to 0$). If the damping constants α_n and the stiffness parameter ω_0 are zero, the usual dispersion relation for electromagnetic waves in a vacuum, sound waves in a neutral gas, and many other physical phenomena is obtained, that is, frequency is proportional to wave number or inverse wavelength

$$\omega_n = ck_n \qquad n = 1, 2, 3 \ldots \tag{9.9}$$

Generally wave phenomena are normally defined by the existence of a dispersion relation $\omega = \omega(k)$ for which the imaginary part of ω is small compared with the real part (so waves are not overdamped), and in which ω is an increasing function of k (so the group velocity of a pulse is positive) over most of the wave number range. In complex media, there may be narrow wave number ranges of anomalous dispersion, such as regions in which ω changes so rapidly with wave number that group velocity is greater than the speed of light or in which group velocity is negative. In these cases, group velocity has no simple physical interpretation (Montgomery and Tidman, 1964; Jackson, 1975).

Waves in an infinite medium ($L \rightarrow \infty$) are not restricted to discrete wave numbers so that (9.9) also allows for a continuum of frequencies. For example, visible light (like string motion consisting of transverse waves) occurs with spatial wavelengths $\Lambda = 2\pi/k$ just below 1 μm. From (9.9) with c equal to the velocity of light in a vacuum, this wavelength corresponds to a frequency

$$f = \frac{\omega}{2\pi} = \frac{c}{\Lambda} = \frac{3 \times 10^{10}\ \text{cm/second}}{10^{-4}\ \text{cm}} = 3 \times 10^{14}\ \text{Hz} \tag{9.10}$$

The exquisite sensitivity of the rods and cones of the retina, which covers the narrow frequency band 4.3 to 7.0×10^{14} Hz (compared with the typical frequency range of 10^4 to 10^{22} Hz between radio waves and gamma rays), is apparently due to electronic resonance phenomena in specific chemicals in the retina.

Unlike light, which is composed of transverse waves and may occur in a vacuum, sound waves are created by the longitudinal motion of some wave medium. If the velocity of light is replaced by the velocity of sound in air at zero °C ($c = 3.31 \times 10^4$ cm/second) in (9.10), audible frequencies of 20 to 2×10^4 Hz correspond to spatial wavelengths ranging from about $\Lambda = 1.7$ cm to 17 m. We can, however, produce ultrasonic frequencies as high as 6×10^8 Hz by applying an alternating electric field at the resonant frequency of a quartz crystal that produces elastic vibrations (piezoelectric effect) and corresponding sound waves in air with wavelengths of about 5×10^{-5} cm, approximately the same wavelength as that of visible light.

Dispersion relations, as expressed by (9.8), (9.9), or (9.10), depend only on the wave medium, that is, the equation that describes the medium's properties. They are independent of standard boundary or initial conditions. Thus the vibrating string can undergo an infinite variety of motion (with corresponding sounds in stringed musical instruments), but the dispersion relation does not change. Waves with the simple linear dispersion relation (9.9) or (9.10) are called nondispersive. Most waves in nature are, however, dispersive. Unlike nondispersive waves, they distort as they propagate. General examples are described by (9.8), including electromagnetic propagation along transmission lines and high-frequency plasma waves. Water waves, electromagnetic radiation through a material medium, the compound action potential (with dispersion due to multiple axons with different action potential velocities), and, as suggested in Chapter 11, neocortical waves generally have more complicated dispersion relations than those shown in this section.

The general motion of even the simple vibrating string is very complicated, because it is composed of many modes of unequal intensity. The manner in which the total intensity is distributed among the modes (that is, the A_n and B_n's in (9.6)) depends on how and where the string is struck or plucked. An initial disturbance $\Psi(x, 0)$ near the center of the string will travel with velocity c toward the supports at the ends, as indicated in Figure 9-2b. This traveling wave is reflected at the end and propagates toward the center, where it meets another wave that has been reflected from the opposite end. The traveling waves combine to form standing waves whose half wavelengths must be integral multiples of the length of the string to satisfy the boundary conditions, as indicated by (9.7). The lowest frequency ω_1, with its corresponding wave number k_1, is called the fundamental mode of vibration; higher frequencies are called the overtones, ω_2 being the first overtone and so on. In the special case of a string with no stiffness or damping (9.9), the overtones are integral multiples of the fundamental. Overtones bearing this simple relation to the fundamental are called harmonics. Very few vibrating systems have harmonic overtones, but these few are the basis for nearly all musical instruments because humans find harmonic overtones more pleasing. These ideas concerning wave motion in a string extend naturally to more complex systems. (This is, of course, why most texts on wave phenomena begin with a discussion of the stretched string). An obvious extension is from one to two spatial dimensions; that is, the string is replaced by a vibrating membrane, such as a drum. The first

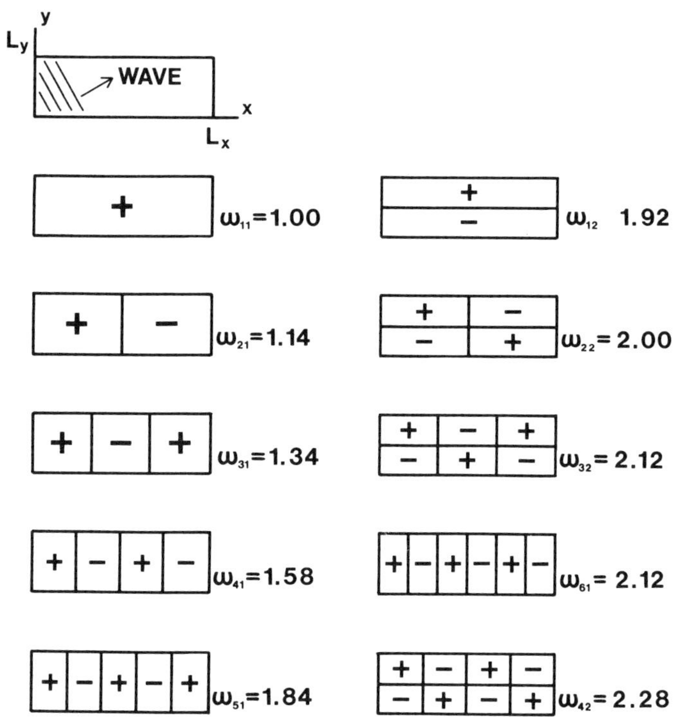

Figure 9-4. Ten eigenfunctions, $\sin(k_{xn}x)\sin(k_{ym}y)$, and corresponding normal mode frequencies for a rectangular membrane (such as a drum) with dimensions $L_x = 3L_y$. Plus and minus signs indicate membrane deflections in and out of the plane of paper. Normal mode frequencies ω_{nm} are normalized so that $\omega_{11} = 1.00$. Higher modes are proportional to $[n^2 + (L_x/L_y)^2m^2]^{1/2}$, where n and m are eigenvalues (similar to quantum numbers) for standing waves in the x and y directions, respectively. Some of the degenerate modes are $\omega_{32} = \omega_{61} = 2.12$ and $\omega_{91} = \omega_{33} = 3.00$ (not shown).

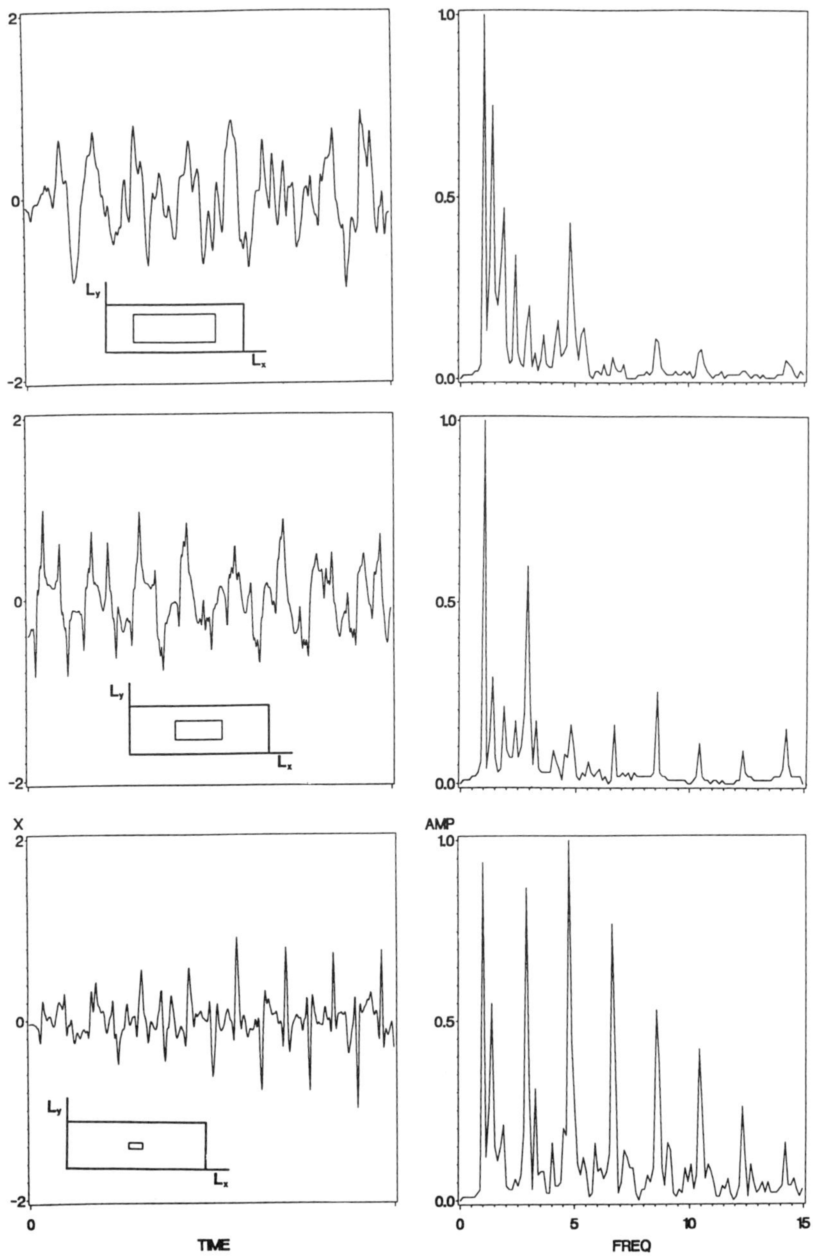

Figure 9-5. (*Left*) A few typical waveforms composed of the normal mode frequencies at fixed location on the membrane, that is, $\Psi = \Psi(x_1, y_1, t)$. Generally the amplitude associated with each normal mode frequency is determined by the spatial properties of the input, that is, either the initial deflection of the membrane (with transient oscillations) or spatial distribution of the forcing function (with steady-state oscillations). All oscillations shown here are due to the initial rectangular displacements of different sizes, as shown in the insets. (*Right*) Smaller initial deflections excite higher frequencies, as shown explicitly by the amplitude spectra to the right of each corresponding waveform.

few eigenfunctions (corresponding to the 10 lowest normal mode frequencies) for standing waves in a rectangular membrane of length (L_x) three times its width (L_y) are shown in Figure 9-4. Generally the overtones are not harmonics of the fundamental frequency or multiples of any number. The appearance of harmonics in most systems suggests the occurrence of nonlinear effects, as discussed in Chapter 10.

The actual waveform at some fixed location $\Psi(x_1, y_1, t)$ is composed of a linear combination of eigenfunctions, as in (9.6). However, the manner in which the various modes contribute to this waveform depends on the initial conditions, that is, the manner in which the membrane is set in motion. For example, if the initial membrane deflection $\Psi(x, y, 0)$ is over a small surface area, high frequencies tend to occur more in the signal than if the initial deflection is over a large surface. This effect is illustrated in Figure 9-5, in which waveforms due to three initial deflections are indicated by the rectangular inserts shown on the membrane. A wide variety of waveforms can be generated from this simple linear system. In technical terms, these waveforms are called quasi-periodic to distinguish them from chaotic motion (discussed in Chapter 10). However, because of the many modes that contribute to the motion, the waveforms may not even be close to periodic and may be difficult to distinguish from chaotic signals, especially when noise is present and data records are not large.

Forced Vibrations of a Stretched String

One of the most interesting kinds of experiment in EEG research involves driving EEG with modulated light whose amplitude varies as a sinusoidal function of time, as discussed in Chapter 6. Past interpretations of these results usually were based only on oscillator models that had no spatial dependence, as described in Chapter 8. However, we must understand how forced oscillations behave in the spatial–temporal domain to follow arguments on resonant effects in EEG. The motion of a string due to an external driving force exhibits some of the properties of a simple oscillator; it also displays new properties arising from the system's spatial extension. The relative intensities of the various modes driven by the external force depend on the temporal and spatial properties of the force. For example, if an isolated point force (delta function in x) is applied, the modes having nodes at the point of application will be absent from the motion. Thus, if the string is driven by a sinusoidal oscillation of frequency equal to one of the normal mode frequencies of the string, a resonance phenomenon occurs only if the point of application of the force does not coincide with one of the nodes of this normal mode. This effect is similar to that which occurs for transient oscillations, as in the prolate spheroidal waves illustrated in Figure 2-12. Of course, in the general case, both the location of application of the driving force and its spatial extent are arbitrary. These variables (together with the damping constant of the system) determine the "amount" of resonance observed, that is, the amplitude of the oscillation in response to an external force having a frequency equal to one of the normal modes of the string.

For example, if a point input is close to a nodal line, but not directly on it, only a small resonance response will occur at the driving frequency equal to the corresponding normal mode.

Consider the effect of driving forces of frequency Ω, as depicted in Figure 9-6. In one instance (a), a distributed force is applied along the whole string so only the fundamental mode is excited. In the following cases (b–e), two point forces of opposite sign are applied at two locations x_1 and x_2 along the string. The forcing function for cases (b–e) is given by

$$v(x, t) \sim [\delta(x - x_1) - \delta(x - x_2)]\cos(\Omega t) \tag{9.11}$$

If the damping is small, the resonant frequencies of the string with damping are only slightly altered from the undamped case, expressed by the combination of (9.7) and (9.9) with the dispersive term due to stiffness (ω_0) here assumed negligible, that is

$$\omega_n = n\pi c/L \qquad n = 1, 2, 3 \ldots \tag{9.12}$$

Thus we can expect resonance effects when the driving frequency Ω is near the frequency of one of the normal modes ω_n. After the initial disturbance has died down ($t >> \alpha_n^{-1}$), the amplitude of the string motion is expressed by a sum of contributions from each spatial mode, $k_n = n\pi/L$, that is

$$\Psi(x, t) \cong \sum_{n=1}^{\infty} A_n \sin(k_n x)\cos(\Omega t - \Theta_n) \tag{9.13}$$

where the coefficient of each (nth) mode is expressed by

$$A_n \sim \frac{\left(\sin\dfrac{n\pi x_1}{L} - \sin\dfrac{n\pi x_2}{L}\right)}{\sqrt{\left(n^2 - \dfrac{\Omega^2}{\omega_1^2}\right)^2 + \dfrac{4\alpha_n^2\Omega^2}{\omega_1^4}}} \tag{9.14}$$

and ω_1 is the fundamental mode of the string. The phase (with respect to the forcing function) of each mode is given by

$$\cos\Theta_n = \frac{\omega_n^2 - \Omega^2}{\sqrt{(\omega_n^2 - \Omega^2)^2 + 4\alpha_n^2\Omega^2}} \tag{9.15}$$

In Figure 9-6 (a–f), the responses of the string (amplitude of the motion at any fixed location) are shown as a function of the normalized driving frequency. All curves are drawn for the special case of damping constants, $\alpha_n/\omega_1 = 0.2$. In case (a), the force is applied to excite only the fundamental mode. The response is identical to that of the simple oscillator, described by the far right term of (8.15) and shown in Figure 8-2. In cases (b–e), two point forces of opposite sign are applied at the locations shown. Different modes of the string tend to be excited at resonance, depending on the location of the forces. For example, in case (e),

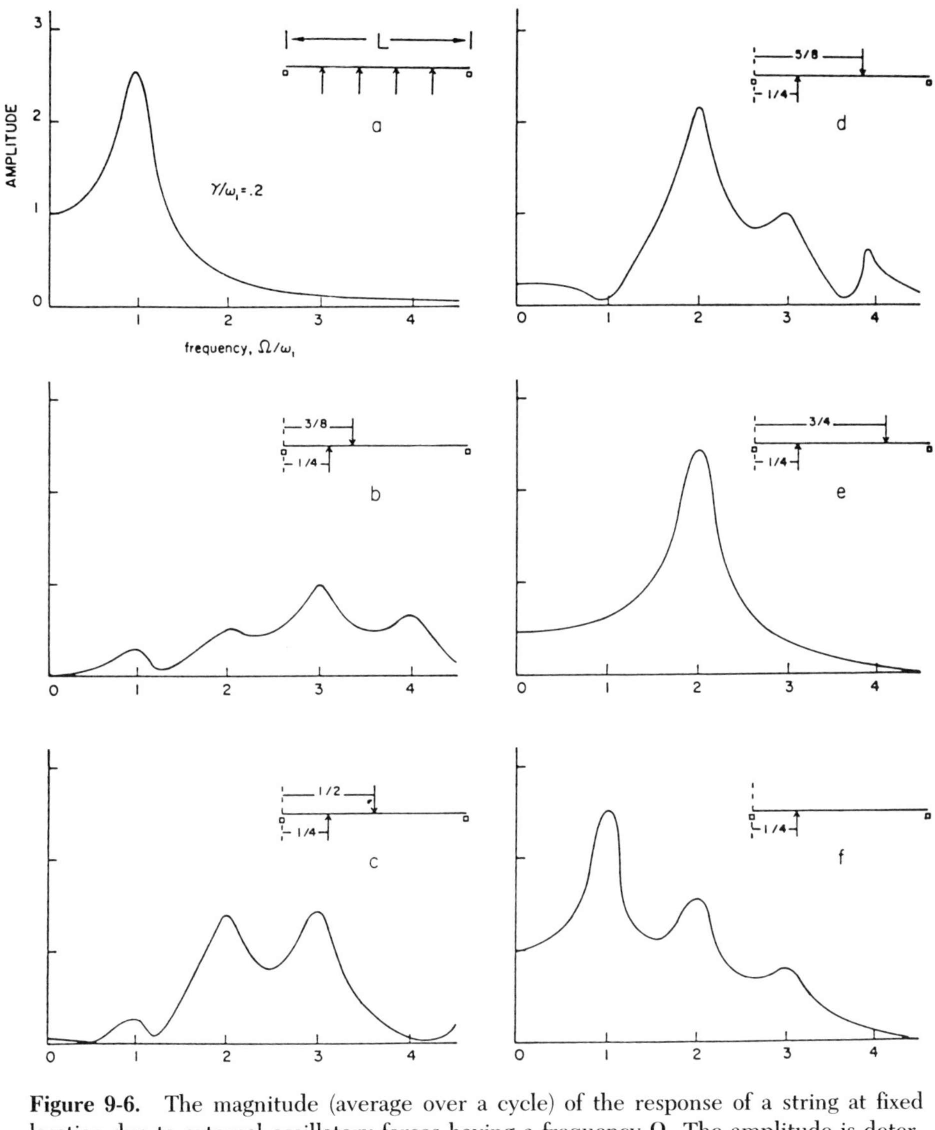

Figure 9-6. The magnitude (average over a cycle) of the response of a string at fixed location due to external oscillatory forces having a frequency Ω. The amplitude is determined by (9.13) and (9.14); the fundamental frequency of the string (n = 1) is given by (9.12). All curves are drawn for the special case of string damping $\alpha_n/\omega_1 = 0.2$. **a.** The driving force is distributed along the string to produce the sinusoidal-shaped deflection of the first eigenfunction (n = 1). **b–e.** The driving consists of two forces of equal magnitude and opposite sign (9.11), applied to the string at the locations shown. **f.** A single force is applied at the location shown. (Reproduced with permission from Nunez, 1981.)

only the second harmonic exhibits a resonance phenomenon. In case (f), a single point force is applied, and the higher harmonics show progressively weaker responses at the higher resonant frequencies of the string.

This description applies to the amplitude of the motion of the string of any fixed location x. Furthermore, the location of maximum amplitude in each instance does not necessarily coincide with one of the points of application of the forces. When two forces of opposite sign are applied to close locations, the maximum amplitude lies at some distance away from the locations of the forces. On the other hand, if point forces of the same sign are applied to close locations of the string, the amplitude of the motion is maximum in this region. We should remember this result when considering the variation, with location on the scalp, of the magnitude of evoked potentials, which may consist of excitatory cortical input with an inhibitory surround, as discussed in Chapter 6.

The Transmission Line

Transmission lines are used to transmit electric power and information (such as telephone, television, computer lines). The transmission line consists of two conductors separated by a dielectric (insulating) medium and may have any of several geometric cross-sections (see Figure 2-3). The line carries transverse electromagnetic waves; that is, the electric and magnetic fields are both perpendicular to the direction of propagation and perpendicular to each other. The equivalent circuit for an incremental length of transmission line is shown in Figure 9-7. With the coaxial line, outer and inner conductors are represented by a series resistance R and inductance L_I per unit length. The dielectric is represented by a capacitance C and conductance G per unit length (conductance is inverse resistance), the latter included to account for current leakage across the dielectric. An applied voltage $\Psi(0, t)$ across one end of the transmission line then propagates along the line, with potential difference between the two conductors $\Psi(x, t)$

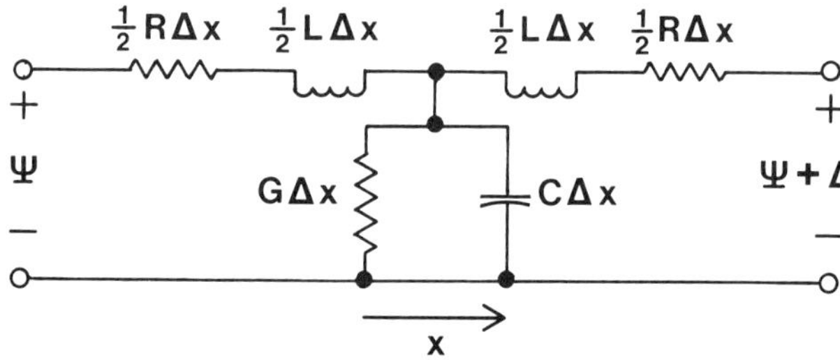

Figure 9-7. Equivalent circuit for the transmission line shown in Figure 2-3. The same circuit (with the inductance $L_I = 0$) applies to the subthreshold membrane with intracellular and extracellular fluid analogous to the outer and inner conductors and membrane analogous to the dielectric (see Figure 9-10). Transmission line forming a closed loop illustrates periodic boundary conditions for standing electromagnetic waves.

governed by the same equation used to describe the vibrating, stiffened string (9.1). In this example, however, the propagation velocity c is determined by the inductive–capacitive properties of the line, that is

$$c = (L_I C)^{-1/2} = (\mu\varepsilon)^{-1/2} \tag{9.16}$$

where μ and ε are the conductor permeability and dielectric permittivity, respectively. When μ_0 and ε_0, the values of these parameters in empty space, are used in (9.16), c is just the velocity of light in vacuum, but propagation in a transmission line is somewhat slower. The damping constant, due to resistive losses (conversion of wave energy to thermal energy) in both conductor and dielectric is expressed by

$$\alpha = \frac{RC + L_I G}{2L_I C} \tag{9.17}$$

and the "stiffness" parameter associated with wave dispersion is

$$\omega_0^2 = RG/L_I C \tag{9.18}$$

Transmission lines are normally designed to avoid reflection at the ends of the line, which disrupts its communication function. However, if the right boundary conditions are applied to the line (such as shorting both ends), creation of a disturbance somewhere in the middle results in standing waves of electric potential analogous to waves in a stretched string. That is, wave numbers of the standing waves are restricted to those given by (9.7) and corresponding normal mode frequencies are given by (9.8). On the other hand, if the line forms a closed loop so that waves may propagate without reflection, as shown in Figure 2-3, only the even modes ($n = 2, 4, 6 \ldots$) can persist, but with normal mode (that is, resonant) frequencies still expressed by (9.8).

Frequency Response and Spectral Density Functions for Continuous Systems

The concepts of Fourier transform, frequency response function (or transfer function), and spectral density function, so important when analyzing discrete linear systems, are easily extended to continuous systems of infinite spatial extent. In practice, an "infinite medium" is simply one whose spatial extent is large compared with some relevant wavelength range. The Fourier transform of a two-dimensional system output $\Psi(x, y, t)$ is given by

$$\Psi(k_x, k_y, \omega) = \int_{-\infty}^{+\infty} dt \int_{-\infty}^{+\infty} dx \int_{-\infty}^{+\infty} dy\, \Psi(x, y, t) e^{-j(\omega t + k_x x + k_y y)} \tag{9.19}$$

Here $\Psi(k_x, k_y, \omega)$ is a function of two wave numbers k_x and k_y and the temporal frequency ω. For one-dimensional problems, the integral over y is omitted, the subscript on k_x is no longer required, and $\Psi(k_x, k_y, \omega)$ is replaced by $\Psi(k, \omega)$. As in discrete linear systems, an input $v(x, y, t)$ results in some output $\Psi(x, y, t)$. Also the frequency response function $H(k_x, k_y, \omega)$ relates input and output in a manner analogous to (8.7), that is

$$\Psi(k_x, k_y, \omega) = H(k_x, k_y, \omega)v(k_x, k_y, \omega) \tag{9.20}$$

The frequency response function $H(k_x, k_y, \omega)$ reflects the fact that system response generally depends as much on the spatial properties of the input $v(x, y, t)$ as its temporal properties, as illustrated by the examples of forced oscillation of a stretched string, transmission line, or membrane depicted in Figures 9-4 and 9-5. If the effects of system boundary conditions are included in $H(k_x, k_y, \omega)$, the Fourier transform (9.19) must be replaced by the finite Fourier transform. In practice, however, it is often more convenient and illuminating first to treat complicated systems as if infinite, and consider the effects of boundary conditions separately. For example, if the input $v(\mathbf{r}, t)$ in (9.1) is taken as the delta function in two spatial and the time dimensions, $v(x, y, t) = \delta(x)\,\delta(y)\,\delta(t)$, the frequency response function is obtained using the Fourier transform (9.19), that is

$$H(k_x, k_y, \omega) = [\omega_0^2 - \omega^2 + j2\alpha\omega + c^2(k_x^2 + k_y^2)]^{-1} \tag{9.21}$$

which can be compared with the frequency response function for the analogous discrete system given by (8.8). Setting the denominator of (9.21) to zero (that is, finding the poles of the frequency response function) yields the dispersion relation (9.8), except that the waves occur in two spatial dimensions so that k is replaced by $(k_x^2 + k_y^2)^{1/2}$. Closely related to the weighting function $h(\tau)$ for discrete systems is the Green's function for continuous systems, which is a solution $\Psi_G(x, y; x_1, y_1)$ to (9.1) that satisfies the boundary conditions when the input $v(x, y, t)$ is of the form $\delta(x - x_1)\,\delta(y - y_1)f(t)$. The solution $\Psi(x, y, t)$ for arbitrary input $v(x, y, t)$ may then be constructed from the Green's function $\Psi_G(x, y; x_1, y_1)$ by integrating the product $v(x_1, y_1, t)\Psi_G(x, y; x_1, y_1)$ over the surface (or volume in the three-dimensional case) of the system (Morse and Feshbach, 1953).

The spectral density function expresses power in a multichannel signal in terms of its frequency and wave number by analogy to its equivalent for discrete systems given by (8.9), that is

$$G(k_x, k_y, \omega) = |\Psi(k_x, k_y, \omega)|^2 \tag{9.22}$$

This quantity is particularly applicable in electrophysiology partly because various experimental approaches (such as electrode size and spacing, cortical versus scalp recordings, and reference electrode) effectively filter multichannel EEG records in the spatial domain. Thus any particular experimental approach will suppress some parts of the spectral density function $G(k_x, k_y, \omega)$ and emphasize others.

One important type of spatial filtering of EEG occurs because scalp electrodes are separated from sources and because of the poorly conducting skull, both of which smear potentials. This effect can be simulated using a three concentric sphere model of the head (Rush and Driscoll, 1969; Nunez, 1981, 1988). The resulting theoretical spectral density function expected at the scalp surface due to white noise sources in neocortex, that is, $G(k_x, k_y, \omega)$ = constant, is shown in

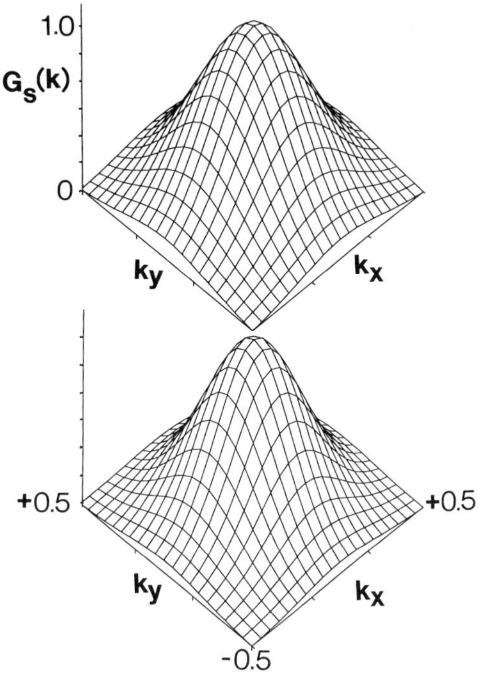

Figure 9-8. Theoretical estimates of scalp spectral density function when cortical power is white noise, that is, $G_c(k_x, k_y, \omega)$ = constant. Based on a three concentric sphere model of radii (8.0, 8.6, 9.2 cm) and ratio of brain to skull conductivity of 40 in the upper plot and 80 in the lower plot. These spectra may be compared with experimental EEG spectra shown in Figure 1-21. (Reproduced with permission from Nunez, 1988.)

Figure 9-8. With a brain–skull conductivity ratio of 80 (Rush and Driscoll, 1968), the theoretical scalp spectral density function is attenuated by 99% (potential down by 90%) at $k = 1.6 \text{ cm}^{-1}$ (that is, 0.26 cycles/cm or wavelength = 3.8 cm). Thus scalp recordings emphasize only the part of $G(k_x, k_y, \omega)$ corresponding to small k_x and k_y, that is, long wavelengths. The behavior of the resulting signal can be quite different at the short wavelengths typically emphasized with intracranial recordings.

An example of a portion of the estimated spectral density function (at two discrete frequencies $f = \omega/2\pi = 8.0$ and 9.5 Hz) for an awake person with eyes closed is shown in Figure 1-21. Here y is the midline scalp coordinate and x is the transverse coordinate. In contrast to the theoretical spectra, these experimental spectra have low power near the origin ($k_x = k_y = 0$) due to the use of average reference data, which essentially filters out power in small wave numbers. The alpha (9.5 Hz) part of the spectral density function shows nearly equal peaks for positive and negative k_y, consistent with standing wave phenomena. The "mu" (8.0 Hz) part of the spectrum shows a larger peak in the positive k_y region, more consistent with posterior-to-anterior traveling waves. Technical problems of estimating the spectra with arrays of finite size severely limit spatial resolution in these examples.

If cortical EEG activity is actually composed of waves (in the sense that this term is used in the physical sciences), we can expect a relation (the dispersion relation) between the temporal and spatial frequency spectra. For most waves, low pass spatial filtering implies low pass temporal filtering as observed in the EEG data discussed in Chapter 2, although multiple branches of dispersion re-

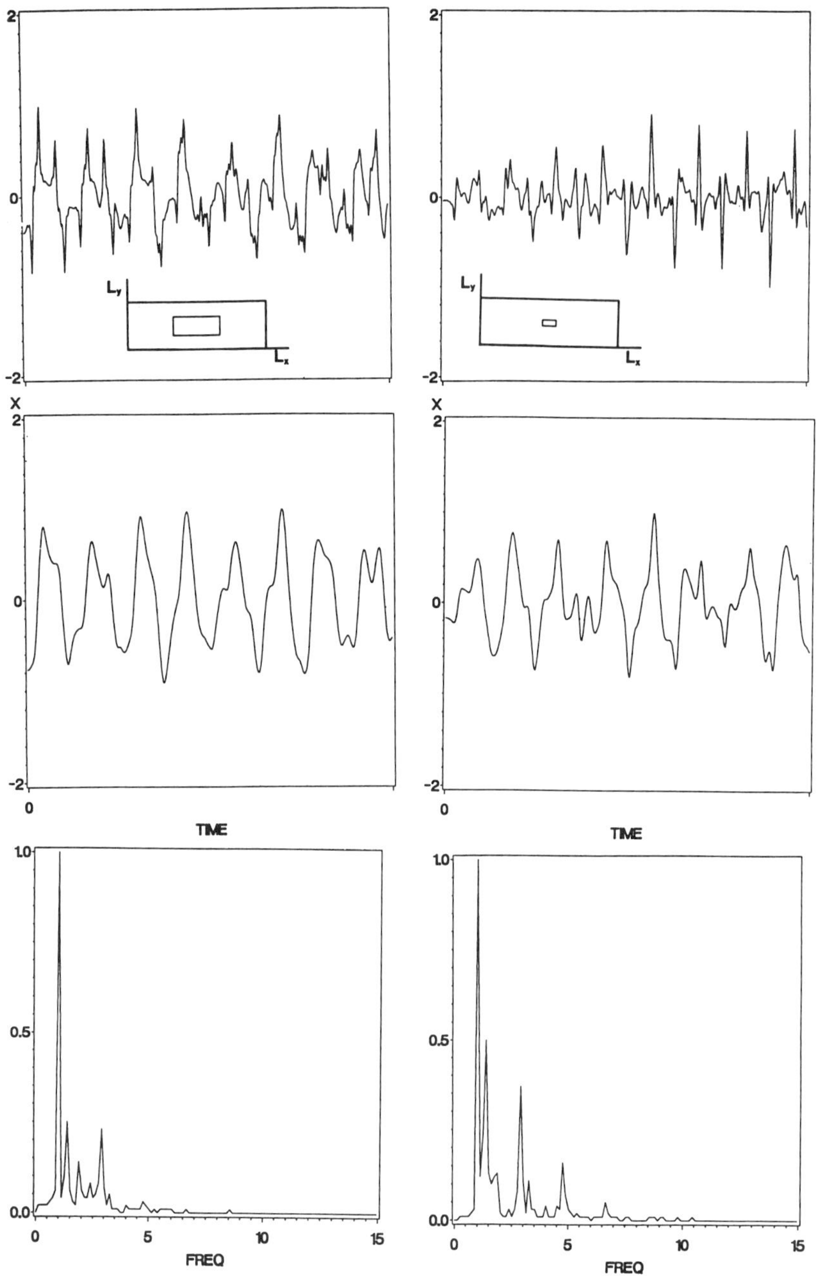

Figure 9-9. Comparison of actual waveforms $\Psi(x_1, y_1, t)$ of rectangular membrane (*first row*) and spatially filtered waveform $\hat{\Psi}(x_1, y_1, t)$ (*second row*), together with amplitude spectra of filtered data (*lower row*). The unfiltered waveforms are two of those shown in Figure 9-5. The modes were filtered by multiplication by the factor e^{-kD} with $D = 0.5/k_{11}$ in this case. This filtering might occur because of limitations of an experimental sensor.

lations can complicate this prediction, as discussed in Chapter 11. To illustrate how this general type of effect might occur, we will consider again the rectangular membrane system of Figures 9-4 and 9-5. Suppose we observed the oscillations of this membrane with an imperfect sensor, such as one in which spatial frequencies k are attenuated by a factor proportional to e^{-kD} (Nunez, 1981), where D is some characteristic distance (perhaps the distance of the sensor above the plane of the membrane). This is qualitatively similar to the spatial filtering of EEG between cortex and scalp. A comparison of an actual waveform $\Psi(x_1, y_1, t)$ with the corresponding spatially filtered waveform $\hat{\Psi}(x_1, y_1, t)$ is shown in Figure 9-9. Because the membrane motion is composed of waves, spatial filtering causes the temporal filtering shown by a comparison of waveforms in the two upper rows of Figure 9-9 or comparison of filtered and unfiltered spectra (Figure 9-5 compared with Figure 9-9). Similar phenomena apparently occur in EEG.

The Core Conductor Model of Membrane Diffusion

Biological membranes selectively pass some ions more readily than others. The resulting concentration gradients produce diffusion currents that are balanced by Ohmic currents when the membrane is in electrochemical equilibrium, that is, when no net current flows across the membrane. The equilibrium potential difference across the membrane is typically about 70 mV negative inside with respect to the outside. When an external current source $v(\mathbf{r}, t)$ is applied (either synaptic or electrode input), the change of the transmembrane potential from equilibrium along the surface $\Psi(\mathbf{r}, t)$ is of interest. The vector $\mathbf{r}$ generally locates a specific portion of the membrane along some branch of axon or dendrite. When the input $v(\mathbf{r}, t)$ is sufficiently small (its magnitude at the initial segment of the axon is much less than the threshold for action potential propagation), the core conductor model of the neuron provides a good prediction of the output $\Psi(\mathbf{r}, t)$. However, as the input approaches threshold, violations of Ohm's Law across the membrane become substantial. This range of subthreshold input for which nonlinear effects are evident may be called the quasi-linear range by analogy to similar effects observed in physical systems, as discussed in Chapter 10. When threshold is achieved, an entirely new phenomenon (not predictable by any linear or quasilinear theory) occurs, the propagation of the action potential.

The complicated geometry of neuron and extracellular conductor causes difficulties in the construction of accurate models; however, the core conductor model of the axon depicted in Figure 9-10 is a basis for more complex models. The core-

---

← For example, the sensor diameter might be large compared with short wavelengths in the motion or it might be placed a distance ~D above the membrane surface. This spatial filtering causes the temporal filtering shown in the middle and lower rows. The spectra in the lower row may be compared with those obtained in Figure 9-5 (*lower two rows*). Amplitudes shown in the middle rows have been renormalized to unit maxima.

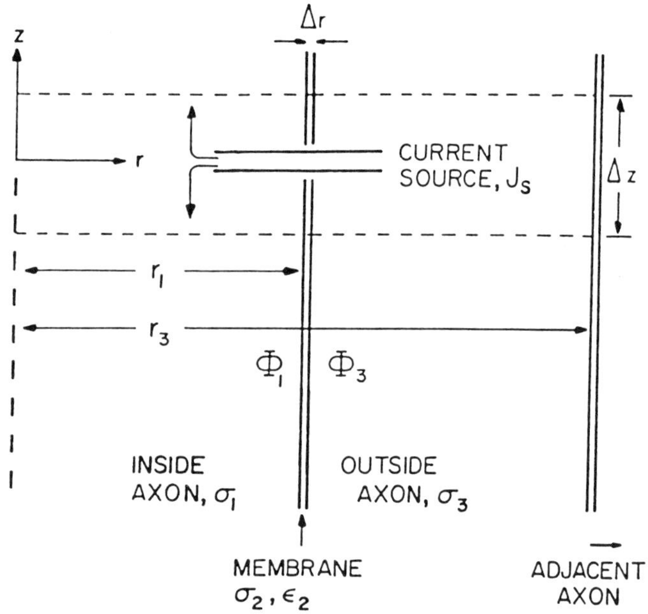

Figure 9-10. Cylindrical axon geometry. A current source disturbs the equilibrium potential difference across membrane ($\Psi = \Phi_1 - \Phi_3$). If the current source is turned off, Ψ will return to its original equilibrium value according to (9.23). This system is similar to the transmission line (Figure 9-7) except that tissue inductance is zero. (Reproduced with permission from Nunez, 1981.)

conductor model depends on the following assumptions that make it less general than Maxwell's equations from which it is derived (Plonsey, 1969; Nunez, 1981):

1. The nerve truck is cylindrical and infinite in extent and contains many axons that are uniformly spaced and have the same diameter.
2. The adjacent axons force the extracellular current to flow mainly in the axial direction and the current is approximately uniform in the space between cells. Also the intracellular current flows only in the axial direction.
3. The membrane thickness is much less than the space between axons.
4. The initial stimulus is symmetric with respect to the angular location on the circular cross-section of the axon.
5. The fibers are unmyelinated.
6. Inductive effects are negligible in tissue (an excellent approximation at relevant frequencies).
7. The membrane is linear in the conductive and dielectric senses.

As usually presented, the core-conductor model consists of an equivalent network with resistors representing intracellular and extracellular fluids and the resistors and capacitors representing the membrane. This circuit representation is similar to that of the transmission line in Figure 9-7, except that inductive effects are negligible in the neuron and consequently no wave propagation can result from the linear model. The equation for transmembrane protential $\Psi(x, t)$ may be obtained from either the lumped circuit of Figure 9-7 (Davis and Lorente de No, 1947), or directly from Maxwell's equations applied separately to the three regions of Figure 9-10, with appropriate boundary conditions at the interfaces (Scott, 1977; Nunez, 1981). With either approach, the basic partial differential equation of this chapter (9.1) may be rewritten here with standard symbols for the parameters:

$$\lambda^2 \frac{\partial^2 \Psi}{\partial x^2} - \tau \frac{\partial \Psi}{\partial t} - \Psi = -v(x, t) \tag{9.23}$$

Here $v(x, t)$ is proportional to injected membrane current density, λ is the space constant, and τ is the time constant of the membrane. The space constant is determined by the electric and geometric properties of the axon and surrounding nerve trunk, that is (Nunez, 1981)

$$\lambda^2 = \frac{r_1 \Delta r (r_3^2/r_1^2 - 1)\sigma_1/\sigma_2}{2(r_3^2/r_1^2 - 1 + \sigma_1/\sigma_3)} \tag{9.24}$$

The time constant depends only on the capacitive-resistive properties of the membrane, that is

$$\tau = \varepsilon_2/\sigma_2 \tag{9.25}$$

where ε_2 and σ_2 are membrane permittivity and conductivity, respectively. The subscripts 1, 3, and 2 refer to the intracellular, extracellular, and membrane media, respectively; r_1 is the radius of an axon, and $(r_3 - r_1)$ is the average extracellular space between axons. The time constant (9.25) is usually written in terms of the membrane capacitance and resistance, that is

$$\varepsilon = C\Delta r/A \qquad \sigma = \Delta r/AR \tag{9.26}$$

where C is capacitance and R is resistance for current flow across an area of cross-section A over a distance Δr (the thickness of the membrane). By substituting the above relations into (9.25), the usual expression for the membrane time constant is obtained

$$\tau = CR \tag{9.27}$$

Actually, (9.25) is perhaps a little more illuminating than (9.27) because it shows explicitly the independence of the time constant of axon geometry, whereas the space constant depends on geometry. The time constant is the characteristic time required for the transmembrane potential induced by an external stimulus to spread (diffuse) along the axial dimension to its equilibrium distribution. It is a measure of the time needed for membrane charge to redistribute in accordance with Maxwell's equations. Such "relaxation times" are short in good conductors and long in poor conductors. Laboratory measurements indicate the following approximate time constants: squid giant axon (1 millisecond), cortical pyramidal cell (8 milliseconds), and muscle fibers (30 milliseconds) (Lux and Poll, 1966). The subthreshold resistivity of a membrane can be estimated from (9.25) and the measured time constant because membrane capacity (or dielectric constant) is relatively constant over a wide variety of species (Cole, 1968). Recent measurements of axon magnetic fields have made possible more accurate estimates of cable properties (Woosley et al, 1985).

The space constant of the axon is approximately the spatial extent along the membrane's axial direction that will exhibit a substantial change in resting potential under the influence of an external stimulus. When membrane conductivity is very small, transmembrane potentials tend to spread over large distances along the axon. Myelinated axons have smaller average conductivity than do unmyelinated axons, thus their effective space constants are larger. Alternately, membranes with large conductivity tend to confine transmembrane potentials to local regions on the membrane surface. In this limit, charges in the membrane are more free to move and shield potentials, and the space constant becomes somewhat analogous to the Debye shielding distance for fluid conductors, as discussed later. When the extracellular space is large, $r_3 >> r_1$, the membrane space constant is proportional to the square root of fiber radius. Typically, λ is a few millimeters for large, unmyelinated axons, and several centimeters for myelinated fibers of the same diameter.

Synaptic Input to Branched Dendrites

The effect of synaptic input to dendrites on soma transmembrane potential obviously is critically important to neocortical dynamic function. Pyramidal cell dendrites have many branches that extend horizontally in the cortex, as shown in Figures 2-15 and 2-16. This complicated geometry makes theoretical analysis more difficult than the theory of the cylindrical axon of the previous section; however, appropriate theoretical and experimental studies have been performed and were reviewed by a principal contributor to the field of neuron cable theory (Rall, 1977). The approach to branching involves the mathematical transformation of a class of dendritic tree into an equivalent cylinder (Rall, 1962, 1967). For this particular class of tree (involving the manner in which dendrite diameter varies with branch number and distance from the soma and believed to be physiologically plausible), the basic cable equation (9.23) applies with the space constant λ replaced by an effective space constant for the tree. The effective space constant for the branched dendrites of the cortical pyramidal cell is about 0.2 mm (Jacobson and Pollen, 1968).

Several types of solution to the cable equation (9.23) are relevant, depending on input current source function v(x, t) and neuron boundary conditions. One is the transient solution due to a point current source (representing either electrode injection or synapse) $v(x, t) = \delta(x)\delta(t)$. The resulting transmembrane potential at distance x from a point source in a cylindrical axon is (Rall, 1977)

$$\Psi(x, t) = (\tau/t)^{1/2} \exp\left[-\frac{(x/\lambda)^2}{4(t/\tau)} - t/\tau\right] \quad t > 0 \qquad (9.28)$$

Transmembrane potential due to a source at distance x increases from zero to a maximum (postsynaptic potential [PSP] rise time) at time

$$(t/\tau)_{RT} = \frac{1}{4}\left(\sqrt{4(x/\lambda)^2 + 1} - 1\right) \qquad (9.29)$$

When the cable equation (9.23) is applied to a dendritic tree, the nondimensional distance (x/λ) must be replaced by an electrotonic distance X that accounts for the variation of local length "constant" $\lambda(x)$ with dendritic diameter (Rall, 1962, 1967), that is

$$X = \int_0^x \frac{dx'}{\lambda(x')} \qquad (9.30)$$

where $\lambda(x)$ represents the characteristic length constant that changes with branch diameter at each point of branching. Equation (9.30) is a generalization of the factor (x/λ) in (9.28). An important experimental observation is that the total electrotonic length X, obtained by calculating the integral in (9.30) from soma to the end of a representative dendritic terminal, is only one or two for a typical dendritic tree (Rall, 1977). This means that the functional distance of a dendritic synapse from the soma is often much less than its actual distance. Thus distant synapses on pyramidal cell dendrites can have relatively large effects on soma transmembrane potential, an idea important for models of neocortical dynamics that depend on the relative effectiveness of excitatory and inhibitory synaptic input (at different average distances from soma) in causing the firing of an output action potential. The solution (9.28) to the basic cable equation is qualitatively similar to the functional forms (8.30) and (8.31) used in Chapter 8 to match experimental data. All three functions are shown in Figure 8-9, with $x/\lambda = 2$ chosen in (9.28), and other parameters determined so that all three maxima coincide to produce equal PSP rise times and maxima.

The effects of end boundary conditions and branching may be accounted for with a lumped circuit or compartmental model of the dendrites, as shown in Figure 9-11 (Rall, 1967). The predicted soma transmembrane potential $\Psi(0, t)$ for the assumed input

$$v(x, t) = (t/t_p)e^{(1-t/t_p)}\delta(x - x_i) \qquad t > 0,\ t_p = 0.04\tau \qquad (9.31)$$

at three distances x_i from the soma to the remote region of the dendritic tree (end of equivalent cylinder) is shown in Figure 9-12 for a total electrotonic length of $X = 1.8$ or 0.2 per compartment (curves B, C, D). Also shown is uniformally distributed input over the dendric surface (A). The rise times predicted by the compartmental model are somewhat longer than those predicted by the elementary expression (9.28). For example, case D corresponds to input at compartment eight (an electrotonic length from the soma of $X = 1.4$ with rise time shown in Figure 9-12 of about $(t/\tau) \sim 0.7$. In comparison, if $(x/\lambda) = 1.4$ is used in (9.28), a rise time of $(t/\tau)_{RT} = 0.5$ is obtained. This discrepancy is, due however, in part to the longer time course $(\Delta t/\tau) \sim 0.1$ of the synaptic input function (9.31), shown

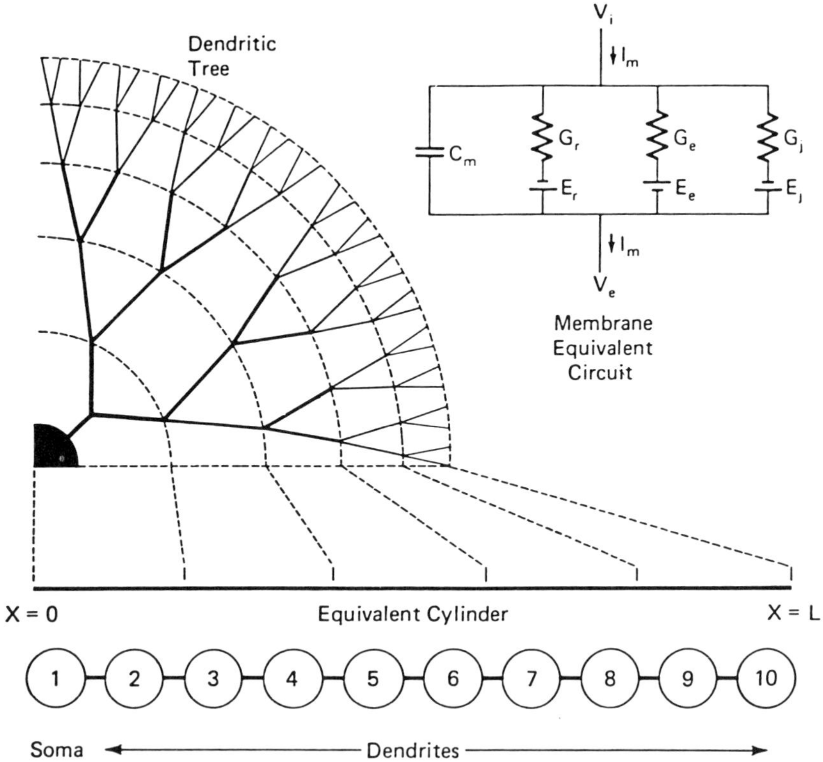

Figure 9-11. Electric equivalent circuit model of nerve membrane at the upper right. Branching dendritic tree at the upper left. Diagram indicates the mathematical transformation of a class of dendritic trees into an equivalent cylinder and into approximately equivalent chains of equal compartments. The chain of 10 compartments is shown in the lower figure. Compartment 1 represents the soma, and progressive electronic distance out into the dendrites is represented by compartments 2 through 10. This is an extension of the cylindrical axon model of Figure 9-10. (Reproduced with permission from Rall, 1967.)

in Figure 9-12 and assumed in the compartmental model computations. Thus, (9.28) gives a good semiquantitative approximation to the much more complicated computations of the compartmental model of the dendritic tree.

Another solution of the relevant cable equation (9.23) occurs when a spatial point and temporal sinusoidal input current source is applied to an infinite cylindrical fiber

$$v(x, t) = \cos(\omega t)\delta(x) \tag{9.32}$$

The resulting transmembrane potential at distance x from the source is expressed by Plonsey (1969)

$$\Psi(x, t) \propto \exp\left[-\sqrt{\frac{1}{2}(\sqrt{1 + \omega^2\tau^2} + 1)}\,\frac{x}{\lambda}\right]\cos(\omega t - \Theta) \tag{9.33}$$

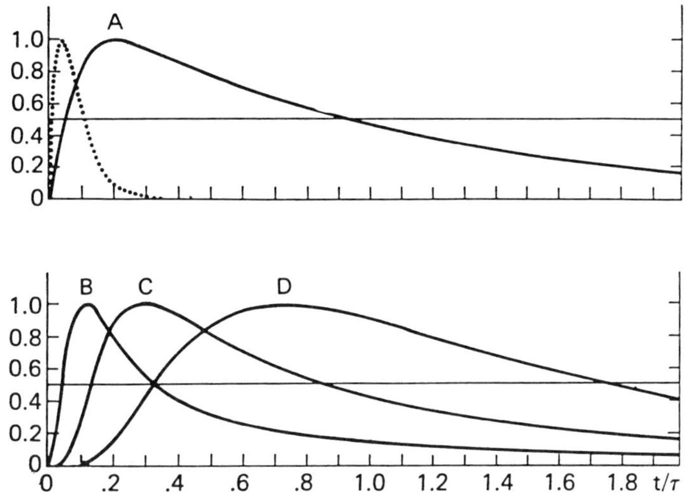

Figure 9-12. Comparison of four excitatory postsynaptic potential (ESPS) shapes computed for a chain of 10 compartments shown in Figure 9-11. Dotted curve shows the assumed excitatory conductance transient. Curve A shows the soma EPSP for equal input in all compartments, roughtly equivalent to uniformly distributed synapses. Curves B, C, and D show an EPSP in compartment 1 (the soma) for different cases of synaptic input restricted to 1 of the 10 compartments. For curve B, synaptic input was in compartment 1 only; for curve C, input was in compartment 4 only; for curve D, input was in compartment 8 only. Ordinate scale represents amplitudes relative to each peak amplitude. In each case, transmembrane potential peak occurred at some fraction of membrane time constant τ. These curves may be compared with the approximate solution shown in Figure 8-9c. (Reproduced with permission from Rall, 1967.)

where Θ is the phase difference between input and output. In the low-frequency limit ($\omega\tau << 1$), transmembrane potential decreases exponentially along the fiber with characteristic length λ, independent of frequency. At higher frequencies, transmembrane potential decreases more rapidly. Because any realistic input function $v(x, t)$ can be expressed in a Fourier series, (9.33) yields a reasonable semiquantitative example of low pass filter properties of dendrites. For example, $\Psi(x, t)$ is predicted by (9.33) to decay to the fraction F of its zero frequency amplitude when

$$\omega\tau = \sqrt{\left[2\left(1 - \frac{1}{X}\ln F\right)^2 - 1\right]^2 - 1} \tag{9.34}$$

where $X \sim x/\lambda$ is the total electrotonic length between source and location x. If cortical pyramidal cells have a membrane time constant $t \sim 8$ milliseconds and a total electrotonic length $X \sim 2$, the frequency $f = \omega/2\pi$ at which soma transmembrane potential due to remote dendritic sources is half its zero frequency value is, according to (9.34), $f \sim 48$ Hz. The choice of neocortical parameters in this example is, of course, somewhat arbitrary. Synaptic input is distributed over the dendritic surface and the value of electrotonic length X is only known approximately. Nevertheless, the low pass filter properties of neocortical dendrites appear quantitatively consistent with the observation that mammalian neocortical EEG is strongly attenuated at frequencies greater than 50 or 100 Hz. In humans, the high-frequency EEG cutoff for cortical EEG is probably about 15 to 50 Hz. Lower predictions of frequency cutoff result from larger electrotonic lengths; for example, the choice $X = 4$ in (9.34) leads to a soma amplitude of one half its zero frequency amplitude at $f \sim 29$ Hz. However, several other (and possibly more important) mechanisms may cause the dominance of the relatively low-frequency EEG observed in humans, as discussed in Chapters 2, 3, and 11.

Standing Waves in a Spherical Shell

To evaluate the idea that standing waves may exist in neocortex, a much simpler phenomenon, nondispersive standing waves on a closed surface, is considered here. The general ideas emphasized in this section do not require a surface of any particular shape, nor is it necessary that the surface be completely closed. Surface waves, rather than waves with radial dependence, are emphasized because of the many intracortical and corticocortical fibers (tangent to the neocortical surface), compared with radial fibers (thalamocortical projections), that connect midbrain to human neocortex, as discussed in Chapters 2 and 11. For traveling wave phenomena to exist on the surface, the surface medium must support a mechanism for signal propagation at finite velocity. That is, a disturbance at one location must occur at successively more distant locations at later times. Unlike the example of the stretched string fixed at both ends, no mechanism for wave reflection is required. Rather the surface is chosen to be at least partly closed so that waves traveling in different directions can coalesce to form standing waves. A one-dimensional example is the transmission line with ends connected to form a continuous closed loop, shown in Figure 2-3. In this case, an initial disturbance (caused perhaps by passing a magnet over a portion of the line) will lead to waves traveling around the loop of length L that form standing waves with wave numbers restricted to

$$k_n = n\pi/L \qquad n = 2, 4, 6 \ldots \tag{9.35}$$

where the requirement that both potential and its derivatives be continuous functions allows for only an integer number of spatial wavelengths (periodic boundary conditions). This result is in contrast to the case of the transmission line with both ends fixed at zero potential, boundary conditions that allow twice the number of wave numbers (that is, both odd and even n's), as indicated by (9.7). The normal mode frequencies for standing waves in the transmission line are obtained by combining (9.35) with the dispersion relation $\omega = \omega(k)$, which describes dominant wave properties of the wave medium, that is, (9.8) in the example of the transmission line.

Because the effects of nonelementary boundary conditions are of primary interest in this section, we should first consider a simple wave medium. Thus undamped, nondispersive, free oscillations are assumed on the surface so that our fairly general linear wave equation (9.1) is simplified to

$$\nabla^2\Psi - \frac{1}{c^2}\frac{\partial^2\Psi}{\partial t^2} = 0 \tag{9.36}$$

For example, we can imagine either electromagnetic waves or sound waves on the surface of a spherical metal shell. A known physical phenomenon involving standing electromagnetic waves in the spherical shell formed by the earth's surface and the bottom of the ionosphere (the "Schumann resonances" of Chapter 2) is considered in more quantitative detail at the end of this section. We assume here that the physical conditions are such that field interactions with any surrounding media (such as air or earth) are negligible. These and other complications of the boundary conditions, such as having holes in the surface or allowing the medium to be inhomogeneous $c = c(\mathbf{r})$ can, in principle, be accommodated. For example, we suggested in Chapters 3 and 13 that distributed circuits might act as multiple local regions of inhomogeneity. But in most of these cases, analytic solutions will not be possible and computer approaches such as finite element analysis will be needed. However, in all of these examples, the boundary conditions restrict the spatial shapes of surface potential (or other dependent variable, $\Psi(\mathbf{r}, t)$) distribution. These spatial shapes, called the eigenfunctions, are analogous to the eigenfunctions $\sin(k_n x)$ used in the transmission line, stretched string, or membrane examples. For potentials on a spherical surface due to any version of (9.1) (including volume conduction and diffusion problems), the appropriate eigenfunctions are the spherical harmonics (Jackson, 1975)

$$Y_{\ell m}(\theta, \phi) = \sqrt{\frac{2\ell + 1}{4\pi}\frac{(\ell - m)!}{(\ell + m)!}}\, P_\ell^m(\cos\theta)e^{jm\phi} \tag{9.37}$$

Here (θ, ϕ) are the usual spherical coordinates and the $P_\ell^m(\cos\theta)$ are called the associated Legendre functions. The standard spherical coordinate system is shown in Figure 9-13. If we imagine the z axis to pass through the north pole of the earth, the angle θ is latitude and the angle ϕ is longitude. A few examples of the spherical harmonic functions are shown in Figures 1-26, 1-27, 9-13, 9-14, and 9-15. The double indices (ℓ, m) are required because of the two spatial dimensions of the surface (analogous to the rectangular membrane with indices n and m). For the spherical harmonics to satisfy periodic boundary conditions and remain finite at all points on the surface, the indices can only assume the specific values

$$\ell = 0, 1, 2, 3 \ldots \text{ and } m = -\ell, -(\ell - 1), \ldots 0, \ldots (\ell - 1), \ell \tag{9.38}$$

in a manner analogous to allowing only discrete k_n's in rectangular systems. The

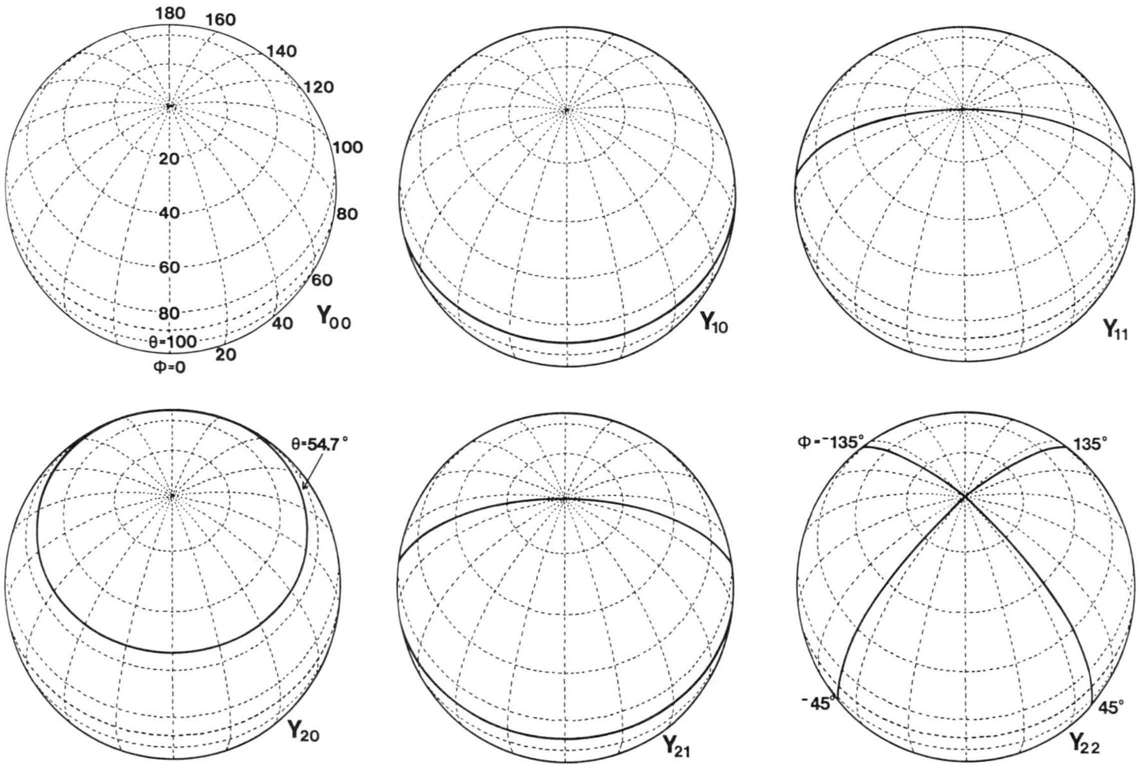

Figure 9-13. The standard spherical coordinate system is shown at the upper left. If we imagine the z axis passing through the earth's north pole, the angles θ and ϕ are latitude and longitude, respectively. The spherical harmonics $Y_{\ell m}(\theta, \phi)$ for various $\ell = 0$, 1 and 2 with $m = 0$ to ℓ are shown. Only the real parts of the $Y_{\ell m}(\theta, \phi)$ and nodal lines (where spherical harmonics change sign) are shown. These eigenfunctions occur as a result of spherical geometry and the Laplacian operator in (9.1). Potential distributions on a spherical surface are expressed as linear combinations of these spherical harmonics. These are analogous to eigenfunctions for rectangular membrane shown in Figure 9-4.

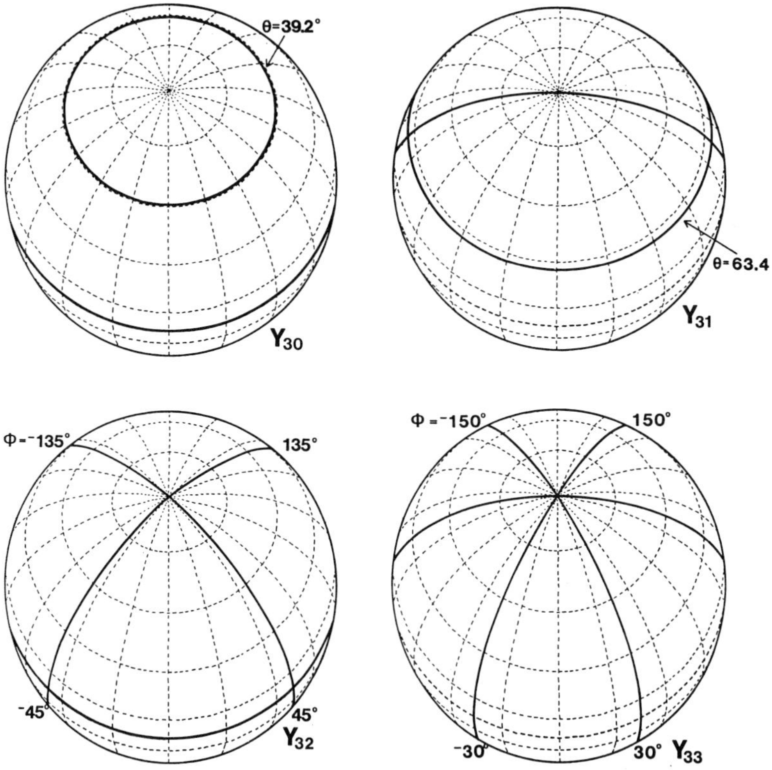

Figure 9-14. Higher ordered $Y_{\ell m}(\theta, \phi)$ that exhibit higher spatial frequencies in the θ and ϕ directions, depending on values of the indices ℓ and m. Here $\ell = 3$ with $m = 0$ to ℓ. Linear nondispersive waves on a spherical surface (such as the spherical shell between the earth's surface and the bottom of the ionosphere) produce higher temporal frequencies corresponding to higher spatial frequencies in a manner analogous to waves in the rectangular membrane as in Figure 9-4.

potential for surface waves on a spherical shell of radius R then may be expressed as

$$\Psi(\theta, \phi, t) = \sum_{\ell=0}^{\infty} \sum_{m=-\ell}^{+\ell} A_{\ell m} Y_{\ell m}(\theta, \phi) e^{j\omega_{\ell m} t} \tag{9.39}$$

which is analogous to its one-dimensional counterpart in the transmission line (9.6). The coefficients $A_{\ell m}$ depend on the initial conditions and possible inhomogeneity of the medium. For a homogeneous surface medium, the normal mode frequencies for the simple wave equation (9.36) are

$$\omega_{\ell m} = \sqrt{\ell(\ell + 1)}\, \frac{c}{R} \qquad \ell = 1, 2, 3 \ldots \tag{2.10}$$

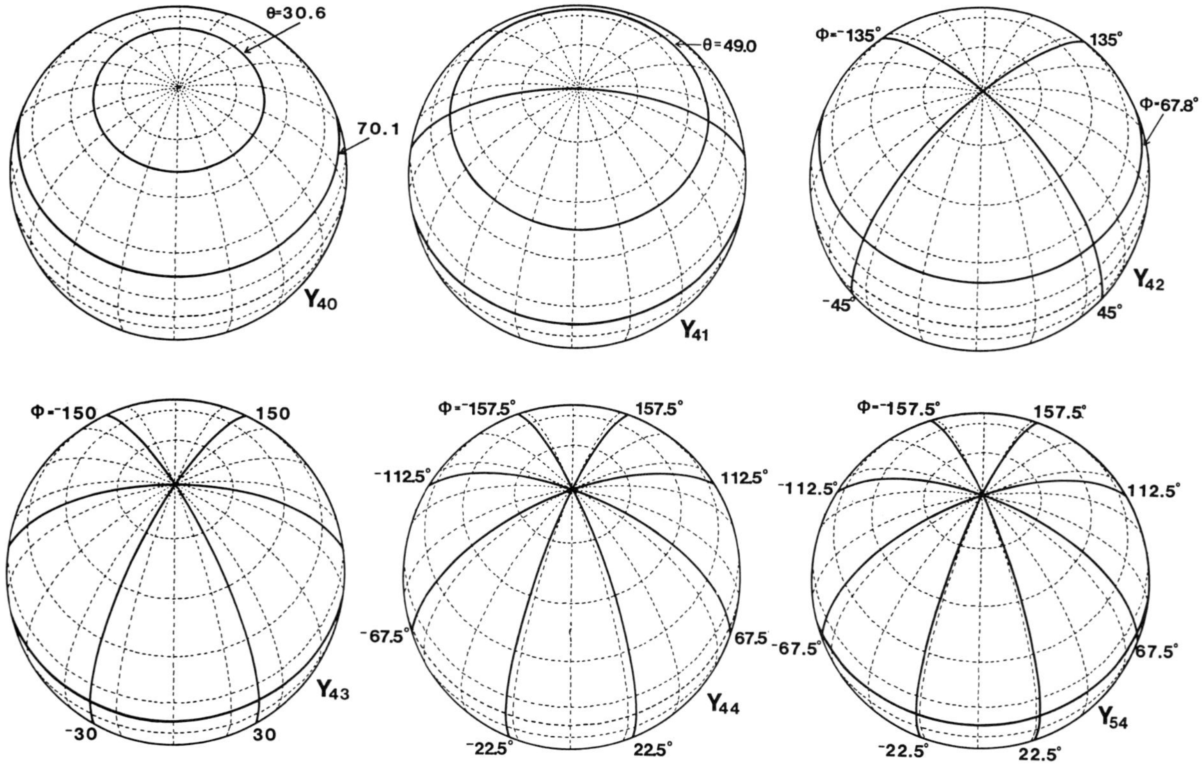

Figure 9-15. The spherical harmonics $Y_{\ell m}(\theta, \phi)$ for $\ell = 4$ and $m = 0$ to 4 are shown. $Y_{\ell m}(\theta, \phi)$ for $\ell = 5$ and $m = 4$ is shown at the lower right.

independent of the m index. That is, the eigenfunctions $Y_{\ell m}(\theta, \phi)$ for any fixed ℓ have the same normal mode frequency for each separate index m. These are called degenerate modes. However, as soon as the spherical symmetry is removed (such as by changing the shape of the surface or making the surface medium inhomogeneous), a splitting of the $\omega_{\ell m}$ modes occurs so that, for example, the $\ell = 3$ index may have different normal mode frequencies for each $m = 0, \pm 1, \pm 2, \pm 3$, corresponding to variations in eigenfunction shape in the ϕ coordinate. The terms "wave number" or "spatial frequency" usually are not used in spherical geometry; however, the general idea of high temporal frequencies occurring with high spatial frequencies, as in the dispersion relations (9.8) or (9.9) remains valid for waves on a closed surface. For complicated surfaces (for which the eigenfunctions are unknown), retaining the concept of wave number in some approximate manner may be useful. For example, the smallest wave number for waves in one dimension around the circumference of a sphere of radius R is $k = 1/R$. Thus the fundamental frequency for nondispersive waves in a closed loop is $\omega_1 = c/R$. In contrast, the fundamental frequency for nondispersive waves on spherical surface is $\omega_1 = \sqrt{2}c/R$.

To make the idea of surface standing waves more concrete, we should consider a specific physical phenomenon, the "Schumann resonance" (Jackson, 1975). These are standing electromagnetic waves in the spherical shell formed by the earth's surface and the bottom of the ionosphere. This geometry is the two-dimensional analog of the closed stretched string or transmission line. Because the thickness of the spherical shell is much smaller than the earth's radius, radial propagation is neglected and components of the electromagnetic field oscillate in tangential directions in the shell at resonant frequencies $\omega_{\ell m}$ given by (9.40), where, in this example, c is light velocity and R is the earth's radius. The simple wave equation (9.36) and corresponding dispersion relation (9.40) are easily derived from Maxwell's equations of electrodynamics if we assume that both the earth's surface and the bottom of the ionosphere are perfectly conducting boundaries. In this case, the field Ψ in (9.36) may represent any of the electric or magnetic field components E_r, E_θ, or B_ϕ. The oscillations are excited by lightning bolts containing a wide spectrum of frequencies, which act as sources of radial electric fields. The frequency components near the Schumann resonances are propagated preferentially because they are normal modes of the earth–ionosphere cavity. Using the physical constants $c = 3 \times 10^8$ m/second and $R = 6.4 \times 10^6$ m, the first seven ($\ell = 1, 7$) Schumann resonant frequencies are obtained from (9.40): $f_{\ell m} = \omega_{\ell m}/2\pi = 10.6$, 18.3, 25.8, 33.4, 40.9, 48.4, 55.8 Hz. These were predicted by Schumann (in 1952) and later observed (Basler and Wagner, 1960; Egeland and Larsen, 1967) with average frequency peaks given by 8, 14, 20, 26, 32, 37, 43 Hz and with progressively less power in the higher modes. The lack of precise agreement with theory is due to the somewhat inaccurate assumption of perfectly conducting boundaries. However, when the theoretical frequencies are multiplied by the constant correction factor 0.78, excellent agreement between the two sets is obtained thereby verifying the $[\ell(\ell + 1)]^{1/2}$ variation of resonant frequencies, as summarized in Figure 2-5.

That the fundamental ($\ell = 1$) Schumann resonance is so near the usual human alpha frequency is probably a coincidence, although it appears impossible to rule out subtle evolutionary coupling between the ambient electromagnetic field and human brains. The brain is exposed to a spatially constant 10-Hz magnetic field, which, unlike the electric field, is not attenuated by human tissue. However, the magnetic fields of the Schumann waves are very weak, that is, in the 10^{-12} Tesla range (Polk and Postow, 1986). For comparison, note that the earth's static magnetic field is about 3×10^{-5} Tesla and household appliances can produce local fields of about 10^{-4} Tesla. Human alpha rhythm sources produce a magnetic field in the 10^{-13} Tesla range near the scalp surface, which is about the same magnitude field as that produced by Schumann resonances.

The dispersion relation (2.10) applies to all linear, nondispersive waves in a spherical shell. Suppose that we reduce the physical medium to the size of the human brain, that is, replace the radius of the earth R by an effective neocortical radius (defined by the measured surface area). Can we imagine an analogous resonant phenomena in the brain? All that is required to produce standing waves is a surface partly closed on itself to allow superposition of traveling waves and some mechanism for finite propagation velocity of some field variable through the wave medium. The corticocortical fibers number about 10^{10} and interconnect all regions of neocortex. They carry action potentials that are mainly within a relatively narrow range of velocities, as shown in Figure 2-6. From these physiologic data, we can make a crude estimate of the predicted fundamental frequency in neocortex from (2.10), that is,

$$f_1 = \omega_{\ell m}/2\pi = \frac{\sqrt{2}}{2\pi} \, \frac{600 \text{ to } 900 \text{ cm/second}}{11 \text{ to } 18 \text{ cm}} \approx 7 \text{ to } 18 \text{ Hz} \tag{9.40}$$

where the values of parameters used in this estimate are suggested in Chapters 2 and 11. Of course, we have no a priori reason to suppose that neocortical waves are linear and nondispersive. The dispersion relation analogous to (2.10) must be derived from physiology and anatomy, an issue addressed in Chapter 11 and the Appendix. However, historically, it would have been reasonable to have made a tentative prediction of human EEG frequencies at about 10 Hz in the absence of experimental knowledge of EEG (as was the case before 1928), based only on the crude estimates of this section. But unlike the history of the Schumann resonances, EEG experiments preceded any such theory.

Surface Waves in a Prolate Spheroidal Shell

The degenerate modes obtained for surface waves on a sphere are somewhat less general than we would like in making the analogy to waves on the very complicated neocortical surface. Therefore we should investigate the splitting of the ℓ modes of nondispersive waves due to nonspherical geometry. This is just one of several ways in which wave degeneracy in an isolated, homogeneous sphere may be removed. Other possibilities include making the wave medium inhomogeneous or coupling the sphere to another system, such as the other half of the brain. Fourier transform of the nondispersive wave equation (9.36) yields the Helmholtz equation for the field $H(\xi, \eta, \phi)$ in prolate spheroidal coordinates

$$\nabla^2 H + \left(\frac{\omega}{c}\right)^2 H = 0 \tag{9.41}$$

where ξ = constant defines the surface of the prolate spheroid and (η, ϕ) are angular coordinates in the ranges $-1 \leq \eta \leq 1$ and $0 \leq \phi \leq 2\pi$. The factored solutions of the Helmholtz equation for surface waves (ξ = constant), which satisfy periodic boundary conditions in the index m, are (Morse and Feshbach, 1953)

$$H(\omega, \eta, \phi) = W_\omega(\eta)e^{jm\phi} \qquad m = 0, 1, 2 \ldots \tag{9.42}$$

Here the functions $W_\omega(\phi)$ satisfy the ordinary differential equation

$$\frac{d}{d\eta}\left[(1 - \eta^2)\frac{dW_\omega}{d\eta}\right] + \left[A(\omega) - \left(\frac{ae\omega}{c}\right)^2 \eta^2 - \frac{m^2}{1 - \eta^2}\right] W_\omega = 0 \tag{9.43}$$

where a and e are semimajor axis and eccentricity of the ellipse $\xi = 1/e$ = constant, respectively. The separation constant for surface waves of velocity c is restricted to

$$A(\omega) = \left(\frac{a\omega}{c}\right)^2 - \frac{e^2m^2}{1 - e^2} \tag{9.44}$$

The solution $W_\omega(\eta)$ to (9.43) may be expressed in terms of an infinite series of associated Legendre functions. The physical requirement that solutions be finite at both $\eta = \pm 1$ determines allowed eigenfunctions $W_{m\ell}(k, \eta)$ and corresponding eigenvalues given by (9.44) with $A(\omega) = A_{m\ell}(k)$, where the parameter $k = ae\omega/c$. In the limit $e \rightarrow 0$, $A_{m\ell} = \ell(\ell + 1)$, and (9.44) yields normal mode frequencies for nondispersive waves on the surface of a sphere with radius a given by (2.10). The separation constants $A_{m\ell}(k)$ can be obtained from existing tables (Stratton et al, 1941), and (9.44) can be solved for normal mode frequencies $\omega_{m\ell}$ by iteration. To make a very crude connection to neocortical dynamics, imagine that a single brain hemisphere is approximated by a prolate spheroid with semimajor axis a = 8.3 cm along the anterior-posterior direction, semiminor axis 5.0 cm, and eccentricity c = 0.81. This geometry is obtained by "inflating" the folded cortical surface so that the resulting free surface matches actual neocortical surface area (Nunez, 1981). If surface propagation velocity is assumed to be c = 645 cm/second (in the known range of action potential velocities in corticocortical fibers of 600 to 900 cm/second), the lowest normal mode frequencies in Hz are 10(ℓ = 1, m = 0), 11.6(ℓ = 1, m = 1), 17.2(ℓ = 2, m = 0), 18.1(ℓ = 2, m = 1), 21.2(ℓ = 2, m = 2), 24.1(ℓ = 3, m = 0), 24.8(ℓ = 3, m = 1), 27.2(ℓ = 3, m = 2), 30.6(ℓ = 3, m = 3), and so forth. The lower modes are plotted in Figure 2-11 along with the resonant response of the brain to sine wave-modulated light. Double-peaked alpha rhythms with peak separation typically in the 2-Hz range are observed and may represent closely spaced spatial modes (Nunez, 1981). The data used to generate Figure 1-21 has distinct peaks at 8.0 and 9.5 Hz, for example. Mode splitting due to nonspherical geometry, anisotropy, or inhomogeneity are also possible explanations of this effect, as is the existence of multiple branches of the dispersion relation, as discussed in Chapters 2, 3, 11, and 12.

Quantum Mechanical Waves

The nondispersive surface waves discussed in the previous two sections may have only minimal application in the physical sciences. However, with relatively minor complications, these ideas can be extended to encompass a field of immense practical importance, quantum mechanics. The Schrodinger wave equation describes the quantum mechanical wave function $\Psi(\mathbf{r}, t)$. The physical interpretation of this function in relation to a system of interacting particles is such that $|\Psi(\mathbf{r}, t)|^2$ is proportional to the probability of finding the system in a particular state. With a single particle of mass μ influenced by an electric potential $V(\mathbf{r})$, the Schrodinger equation is a special case of (9.1), that is

$$\nabla^2\Psi - \frac{2\mu}{\hbar^2} V(\mathbf{r})\Psi + j\frac{2\mu}{\hbar}\frac{\partial\Psi}{\partial t} = 0 \tag{9.45}$$

where $\hbar = h/2\pi$, h is Planck's constant, and $j = \sqrt{-1}$. For example, an electron of charge e in the hydrogen atom experiences a spherically symmetric potential $V(r) = -e/r$ (inverse square force). Application of an external field will cause removal of the spherical symmetry. In general, the solution to (9.45) is expressed in terms of the spherical harmonics $Y_{\ell m}(\theta, \phi)$, as the case of surface waves (9.39), except that the radial dependence of (9.45) causes the solution to contain an additional sum with corresponding index n and radial eigenfunction $f_{nl}(r)$, that is

$$\Psi(r, \theta, \phi, t) = \sum_{n=1}^{\infty}\sum_{\ell=0}^{\infty}\sum_{m=-\ell}^{+\ell} A_{n\ell m} f_{n\ell}(r) Y_{\ell m}(\theta, \phi) e^{j\omega_{n\ell m}t} \tag{9.46}$$

The three indices n, ℓ, m, which indicate the "spatial frequencies" of the wave function Ψ in the three spatial coordinates (r, θ, ϕ), are called the quantum numbers. Corresponding to each eigenfunction $f_{n\ell}(r)Y_{\ell m}(\theta, \phi)$ is an eigenvalue $\omega_{n\ell m}$ (or normal mode frequency). In the special case of the spherically symmetric potential in the hydrogen atom, the eigenvalues are

$$\omega_n = -\frac{\mu e^4}{2\hbar^2 n^2} \qquad n = 1, 2, 3 \ldots \tag{9.47}$$

Since these frequencies are independent of both indices ℓ and m, the corresponding normal modes are called doubly degenerate. Application of an external field will act to remove degeneracy so that, in general, each (n, ℓ, m) combination yields a different normal mode frequency $\omega_{n\ell m}$. The physical interpretation of the wave function frequency in the field of quantum mechanics is that it is directly related to the energy (E) of the electron, that is, $E = \hbar\omega$. Thus, (9.47) yields the allowed energy levels (quantized energy levels) for an electron in the hydrogen atom (negative energy indicates a bound electron). The ground state of the electron is E_1, and a quantum number of n greater than one indicates excited states. E_1 is the ionization energy, known from spectroscopy to equal 13.5 electron volts, a value in perfect agreement with (9.47). Of course, we can continue this discussion of the practical consequences of Schrodinger equation solutions and their physical interpretations for many volumes. Such discussion would probably include nuclear fusion and fission, lasers, integrated circuits, superconductivity, and the nature of the chemical bond.

The uncertainty principle of quantum mechanics places fundamental limits on our knowledge of even simple systems such as the hydrogen atom, that is, it indicates a fundamental information barrier. For example, a measurement of the energy of an electron performed during a time interval Δt must be uncertain by an amount ΔE, where the relation between the two uncertainties is $\Delta t \cdot \Delta E > \hbar$. If we recall that the energy of an electron is proportional to the frequency of its associated wave function, the uncertainty principle is seen as formally similar to a well-known property of Fourier series: If we measure a signal over the time interval Δt, we can only obtain a frequency resolution Δf given by $\Delta t \cdot \Delta f \sim 1$. Thus the position, velocity, and energy of an electron are uncertain. The wave function described by the linear equation (9.45) yields only the probability of finding the electron in a certain state. However, the wave function is itself entirely deterministic. Some nonlinear equations can yield deterministic, but chaotic solutions, as discussed in Chapter 10.

Collective Effects in Neocortex and Physical Systems

A critical issue in any theoretical description of interacting entities (such as electrons, persons, planets, neurons, or neocortical columns) concerns the typical number that interact simultaneously. To illustrate this point, we chose a particular physical system, hot plasma (ionized gas). Several phenomena occur in hot plasma that are normally absent in the relatively simple linear systems discussed in Chapter 8 and thus far in Chapter 9. A more important motivation for this section concerns the substantial number of apparent similarities between the interactions of charged particles in hot plasma and neocortical interactions, some of which are listed below.

Dominant Collective Interactions Occur in Both Systems

NEOCORTEX

Each cortical pyramidal cell interacts nearly simultaneously with about 10^4 local neurons through intracortical fibers and with more distant cortical neurons along corticocortical (association) fibers with important time delays. This dominance of collective interactions in neocortex is in marked contrast to serial activation of successive synapses that typically occur along a peripheral sensory pathway.

Hot Plasma

The adjective "hot" refers to the range of temperature and density of the plasma where the collective effects of interacting charged particles are more important to plasma properties than are the effects of close collisions. That is, the potential near a single test charge q placed in a plasma decreases with distance r according to

$$\Psi(r) = \frac{q}{r} e^{-r/R_D} \tag{9.48}$$

where R_D, the Debye shielding distance, depends on plasma density and temperature. Modification of the usual Coulomb's law (the q/r term) by the exponential factor is caused by other charges of opposite sign moving in to shield the field of the test charge, making R_D the effective interaction distance for the particles. The same effect occurs in electrolyte solutions. The field of the charged biological membrane is shielded in this same manner so that the external field due to an equilibrium membrane charge is essentially zero at macroscopic distances (a source of confusion in the electrophysiology literature). A typical laboratory plasma has a Debye length of $R_D \sim 10^{-3}$ cm, and a sphere of this radius contains about 10^5 charged particles that interact simultaneously. This is in marked contrast to interactions in a neutral gas, in which two-body interactions are predominant. Therefore, a large variety of new phenomena occur in plasma and thus plasma is often called "the forth state of matter."

Distinct Separation of Long- and Short-Range Interactions

Neocortex

Intracortical neural interaction lengths vary over about six orders of magnitude, ranging from the width of the synaptic cleft (10^{-6} cm) to the maximum spread of the pyramidal axon collaterals (~3 mm) and surface parallel intracortical system (6 to 8 mm). In contrast, corticocortical fibers in humans have an average length of a few centimeters, with the longest approximately 20 cm. Delays due to finite propagation velocity of action potentials along intracortical fibers are thought to be negligible compared with local delays (such as PSP rise and decay times). However, we suggest in Chapter 11 that such delays in corticocortical fibers may make important contributions to the production of EEG rhythms. There is considerable interest in a description of neocortical interaction at the hierarchical level of the modular column of diameter 0.3 mm and containing about 4×10^3 neurons. Each such column may interact with perhaps 50 or more similar columns through corticocortical fibers, and approximately 3×10^6 such modular columns are found in human neocortex.

Hot Plasma

In hot plasma theory, interactions between charged particles are separated into two parts: a short-range part called collisions and a long-range part due to the self-consistent electric field, that is, the macroscopic field generated by many particles acting together. Because a "collision" of charged particles is actually an interaction between microscopic electric fields, the distinction between these two types of interaction required detailed theoretical justification. As a result of such studies, a "collision" is considered an electric field interaction within a Debye radius R_D.

Statistical State Variables Are Appropriate

Neocortex

Of course, we cannot devise a theory that will predict the state of every cortical neuron, or even every cortical column. Thus one appropriate state variable for neocortex is the probability density function $f(\mathbf{r}, \mathbf{P}, t)$, which is defined to be proportional to the number of cortical columns (or, at lower hierarchical levels, number of neural masses) located between coordinates $\mathbf{r}$ and $\mathbf{r} + d\mathbf{r}$, and which have dipole moments per unit volume between $\mathbf{P}$ and $\mathbf{P} + d\mathbf{P}$ at time t. The cortical or scalp surface potential may be written explicitly in terms of this probability density function using Poisson's equation, as suggested in Chapter 1. A comprehensive nonlinear statistical approach to neocortex is taken in Chapter 14.

Hot Plasma

We cannot predict the position and velocity of all particles in a macroscopic volume of plasma. Thus an important state variable is the probability density function $f(\mathbf{r}, \mathbf{c}, t)$, which is defined to be proportional to the number of particles located between $\mathbf{r}$ and $\mathbf{r} + d\mathbf{r}$, which have velocities between $\mathbf{c}$ and $\mathbf{c} + d\mathbf{c}$ at time t. The self-consistent electric field in the plasma is directly related to this probability density function by Poisson's equation (9.51).

Multiple Branches of Dispersion Relations May Occur

Neocortex

The usual single-valued relations between frequency and wave number (that is, spatial frequency), $\omega = \omega(k)$, given in the previous examples of this chapter may become multivalued functions in complicated (although possibly linear) systems. In Chapter 11, we suggest that multiple corticocortical fiber systems (defined by having different spatial rates of decrease in numbers of fibers) may lead to multiple branches of dispersion relations for one-dimensional brain waves. The combined local-global theory also predicts multiple branches. Furthermore, two-dimensional brain waves on a closed surface can have multiple branches of the dispersion relation, even for a single corticocortical fiber system and with local effects neglected. That is, different types of brain wave that are predicted by a single theory can exist simultaneously, a general outcome also of the statistical theory of neocortical interactions outlined in Chapter 14.

Hot Plasma

Many kinds of wave phenomena can exist simultaneously in plasma: high and low frequencies, longitudinal and transverse waves, waves that travel along magnetic field lines, stable and unstable waves, and waves that experience collisionless damping dependent on wave number (Landau damping). These complications occur only because of the nature of the wave medium. That is, they occur in an infinite, linear plasma without the need for any of the additional complications caused by boundary conditions or nonlinearity.

Hot Plasma and Neocortex

Hot plasma theory is governed by a kinetic equation that describes the evolution of the plasma probability density functions $f_n(\mathbf{r}, \mathbf{c}, t)$ for each species of particle n as the result of some initial disturbance (transient solution) or as the result of an externally applied electromagnetic field (forced oscillations). The simplest practical example of the transient solution due to a disturbance in one spatial dimension in a plasma with no magnetic field in which close collisions are neglected is presented here (Montgomery and Tidman, 1964; Akheizer et al, 1967). One approach to forced oscillations is considered in Nunez (1971). Although the resulting kinetic equation is nonlinear (even with all of these simplifications), the limitation of small disturbances from the equilibrium density functions F_n (typically Gaussian in the velocity variable c) justifies use of linear equations for the perturbed density functions f_n, defined by.

$$f_n(x, c, t) \equiv F_n(c) + \mathit{f}_n(x, c, t) \qquad \frac{\partial \mathit{f}_n}{\partial c} << \frac{\partial F_n}{\partial c} \tag{9.49}$$

Plasma perturbations from equilibrium (analogous to small perturbations of a stretched string from its equilibrium position) are described by the Vlasov equations (also called collisionless Boltzmann equations) for the perturbations of electron f_e and ion f_i probability density functions

$$\frac{\partial \mathit{f}_{e,i}}{\partial t} + c\frac{\partial \mathit{f}_{e,i}}{\partial x} \pm \frac{e}{m_{e,i}}\frac{\partial \Psi}{\partial x}\frac{\partial F_{e,i}}{\partial c} = 0 \tag{9.50}$$

where e and $m_{e,i}$ are the charge and mass of the particles, respectively. $\Psi(x, t)$ is the local perturbation of electric potential in the plasma, and the positive sign is used when (9.50) applies to electrons. Much effort has been devoted to the study of this deceptively simple-looking partial differential equation. The principal difficulty is due to the fact that the probability density functions f_e and f_i affect the potential Ψ, which, in turn, interacts with the perturbed probability density functions. That is, the potential must be determined self-consistently from Poisson's equation

$$\frac{\partial^2 \Psi}{\partial x^2} = 4\pi e \rho_0 \int_{-\infty}^{+\infty} [f_e(x, c, t) - f_i(x, c, t)]\, dc \tag{9.51}$$

Poisson's equation (9.51) is coupled with (9.50) to form a set of integrodifferential equations. The total number density of electrons and ions (number per cubic centimeter) is assumed equal in a macroscopic volume of plasma (electroneutrality) and is given by ρ_0. Thus the right side of (9.51) is proportional to the net charge in a microscopic volume at location x at time t, because the integral simply sums the net charge contribution for particles with all possible velocities c.

Equations (9.50) and (9.51) were first solved by the Russian physicist, Landau. The perturbation of electric potential $\Psi(x, t)$ is expressed in terms of its Fourier transform, but the resulting dispersion relation for the case in which the equilibrium probability density function is Gaussian in the velocity variable c is most relevant to this discussion. The solution requires inversion of the Laplace transform with the contour integral (8.38). However, the singularities of the transfer function H(k, s) in the complex s plane are not limited to poles. A dispersion relation only exists in the asymptotic limit $t \rightarrow \infty$, a result in contrast to the usual macroscopic theories of wave phenomena in continuous media. In this limit, the complex frequency $\omega = \omega_R - j\gamma$ is expressed in terms of wave number for two frequency ranges (that is, two branches of the dispersion relation).

1. High-frequency electron waves, $|\omega_R/kc_e| >> 1$, where the electron thermal velocity c_e is related to the probability density function by

$$c_e^2 = \int_{-\infty}^{+\infty} c^2 f_e \, dc \tag{9.52}$$

The real part of the frequency is expressed by

$$\omega_R^2 \cong \omega_p^2 + 3k^2 c_e^2 \tag{9.53}$$

where

$$\omega_p^2 = \frac{4\pi e^2 \rho_0}{m_e} \tag{9.54}$$

is called the electron plasma frequency. Equation (9.53) is essentially the same dispersion relation that was obtained for the stiffened string or transmission line. These plasma waves are longitudinal waves due to bulk oscillation of the electrons around an approximately fixed background of ions (that is, the ions move much more slowly than the electrons). The waves have damping decrement that strongly depends on wave number (and frequency). That is

$$\gamma \cong -\left(\frac{\pi}{8}\right)^{1/2} \omega_p \left(\frac{\omega_p}{kc_e}\right)^3 \exp\left[-\frac{1}{2}\left(\frac{\omega_p}{kc_e}\right)^2 - \frac{3}{2}\right] \tag{9.55}$$

The Debye radius is expressed by

$$R_D = c_e/\omega_p \tag{9.56}$$

so that the exponential factor predicts large damping as (kR_D) approaches one. Thus the Debye screening length is a measure of the minimal wavelength for sustained high-frequency oscillations in the plasma. Interactions corresponding to shorter wavelengths are called "collisions." There is a loose analogy here to the neocortical medium in which the difference between excitatory and inhibitory synaptic action may determine the number of action potentials fired from within the neural mass. In the neocortical medium, with its multiple interaction lengths (somewhat analogous to the Debye distance), we might expect several preferred wave number ranges in which waves are more weakly damped.

2. Low-frequency ion waves, $|\omega_R/kc_e| << 1$ and $|\omega_R/kc_i| >> 1$, where c_i is the ion thermal velocity, defined similarly to (9.52). The real part of the frequency is expressed by

$$\omega_R^2 \cong \frac{\omega_i^2}{1 + (\omega_p/kc_e)^2} + 3k^2c_i^2 \tag{9.57}$$

where ω_i is the ion plasma frequency, defined similarly to (9.54), but with m_i replaced by m_e. These low-frequency oscillations of ions (in which the much faster electrons form a random background) can occur only in a plasma in which the electron temperature greatly exceeds the ion temperature. The ion wave damping decrement is expressed by a relation somewhat analogous to (9.55).

The results of this section illustrate several general features of wave phenomena that might be expected in media with complex properties, such as neocortex. These features may apply to the local theories described in Chapters 5 and 8 and to the global theory described in Chapter 11, because both approaches predict wave phenomena. In plasma, the following features are evident.

1. More than one branch of the dispersion relation can occur, as in the examples of (9.53) and (9.57). Electromagnetic oscillations in crystals also exhibit two branches of the dispersion relation, called the optical and acoustical branches.

2. The damping decrement γ is a function of wavelength. Disturbances with damping $|\gamma/\omega_R| > 0.5$ are overdamped and will not be observed. Thus the medium places restrictions on wavelengths in addition to the restrictions provided by boundary conditions.

3. Instabilities (that is, $\gamma > 0$) can occur in selective wavelength ranges. If we allowed the center of mass of the electrons to move relative to that of the ions in the above examples, streaming instabilities would be predicted in certain wave number ranges. Many instabilities have been studied in plasma. Instabilities are of great interest from a practical perspective (as in controlled nuclear fusion applications). Brain instabilities (the epilepsies) are also of practical im-

portance, and, in the future, may be studied with mathematical methods similar to those used in hot plasma and other complex physical systems. We will return to this subject several times in the remaining chapters.

4. Certain approximations apply to restricted time scales of the dynamics. For example, the high-frequency electron waves, described by the dispersion relation [(9.8) and (9.53)], are studied by assuming that the ions form a fixed background, although this is not strictly true. In contrast, the ion waves (9.57) may be studied on a much longer time scale, for which the electrons provide a background of random motion. Equations of neocortical dynamics also depend on time scale. For example, in Chapter 11 we treat certain control parameters in the global theory as constants, although they depend on neuromodulators that vary with time, but on a much longer time scale than EEG oscillation times. The issues of multiple time and space scales in neocortex are treated in Chapter 14.

Random Input to a Closed Transmission Line

In the last two sections of this chapter, we consider several additional solutions to the wave equation (9.1) that appear to be at least partly analogous to some EEG phenomena. Consider, for example, a closed transmission line (Figure 2-3) with a forcing function v(x, t) consisting of a series of random inputs (in both time and location along the line). This physical system was chosen because of the apparent existence of continual widespread input to the closed surface of neocortex in all physiologic states. This random input may obscure the possible wave-like behavior of EEG, so it is perhaps worthwhile to observe what happens in a relatively simple physical system. We chose a forcing function representing t_i monotonically increasing random times and x_i random locations with effective spatial extent of the forcing function given by Δx. That is,

$$v(x, t) = \sum_{i=1}^{I} C_i \exp\left[-\frac{(x - x_i)^2}{\Delta x^2}\right] \delta(t - t_i) \tag{9.58}$$

The corresponding solution to (9.1) is given by

$$\Psi(x, t) = \sum_{i=1}^{I} \sum_{n=1}^{\infty} \frac{1}{\omega_n} (a_{ni} \cos k_n x + b_{ni} \sin k_n x) \sin[\omega_n(t - t_i)] u(t - t_i) e^{-\alpha_n(t - t_i)} \tag{9.59}$$

Here $u(t - t_i)$ are unit step functions, which reflect the fact that the ith source does not contribute to $\Psi(x, t)$ until $t > t_i$. The Fourier coefficients are expressed by

$$\begin{aligned} a_{ni} &\cong C_i e^{-(k_n \Delta x/2)^2} \cos k_n x_i \\ b_{ni} &\cong C_i e^{-(k_n \Delta x/2)^2} \sin k_n x_i \end{aligned} \tag{9.60}$$

where the approximation is valid for inputs of relatively small spatial extent, that is, $\Delta x << L$. The periodic boundary condition of the closed wave medium restricts wave numbers to

$$k_n = 2n\pi/L \qquad n = 1, 2, 3, \ldots \tag{9.61}$$

and the normal mode frequencies are again expressed by (9.8).

Spatial shapes $\Psi(x, t)$ at successive times are shown in Figure 9-16, with the time interval in each column equal to one half of the period of the fundamental mode ω_1. These figures and (9.59) illustrate the following points concerning the transmission line potential $\Psi(x, t)$.

Random input causes the transmission line to act as a low pass filter for two separate reasons. First, the temporal behavior of the wave equation (9.1) is such that mode amplitudes are proportional to ω_n^{-1}. Second, when the spatial extent of the input Δx is not zero, the Fourier coefficients in (9.60) become very small for $k_n\Delta x > 2$ or so because input of width Δx is most efficient in exciting modes of spatial wavelength at least several times longer than Δx. Because long wavelengths typically occur with low frequencies in wave media, a second low pass (temporal) filter effect also occurs, as illustrated in Figure 9-5. Finally, more

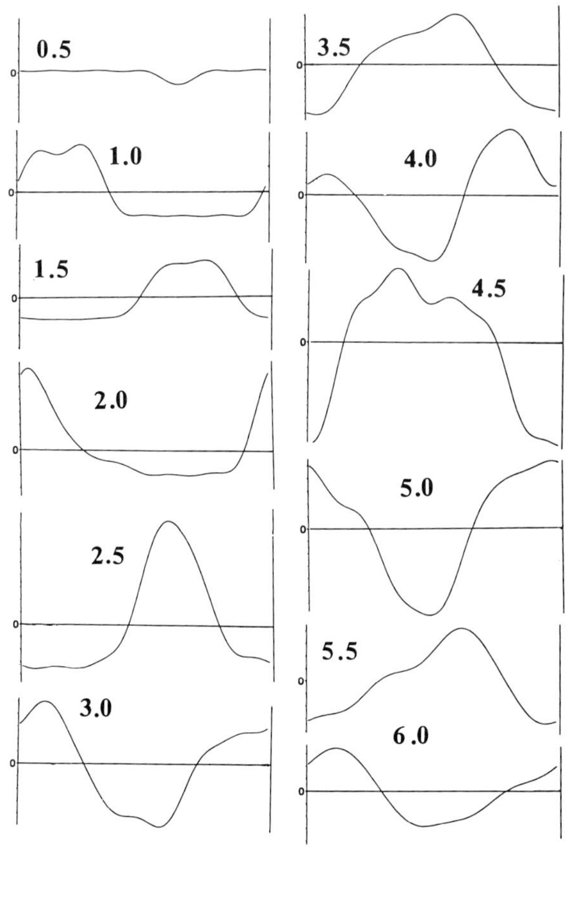

Figure 9-16. Spatial shapes of potential $\Psi(x, t)$ in the closed transmission line at successive times for random inputs with $\Delta x = 0.05$. Time intervals between plots in each column are one half the period of the fundamental frequency. Time is shown in each plot. Amplitudes (and their derivatives) at right and left ends of each plot must be equal because transmission line forms closed loop. For example, a wave packet traveling off the right end of a plot must appear on the left.

complex systems (but possibly also linear) may exhibit a complicated dependence of relative mode damping γ_n/ω_n on frequency. This later effect does not occur here but was discussed previously (see equation 9.55) in connection with plasma waves and again in Chapter 11 in connection with proposed brain waves.

A superficial look at the spatial properties of the potential (Figure 9-16) might suggest either traveling waves in a particular direction around the closed loop (such as $t = 1.0$ to 2.5) or standing waves (such as $t = 3.0$ to 5.0), depending on the specific time interval observed and the characteristics of the input, wave damping, and so on, as determined by the parameters in (9.59). Of course, (9.59) may be viewed as a combination of many traveling waves that partially combine to form standing waves. Whether a phenomenon is "really" composed of traveling or standing waves (as is often asked in the EEG field) is then seen to be a superficial question, because the answer tells us little about the wave medium. A better question in EEG is whether the field is really composed of waves. A two-dimensional version of the randomly driven transmission line, consisting of waves on the surface of a sphere, is described in Chapter 12 to make the analogy to EEG (waves on the closed cortical surface) more clear.

Suppose now we make a series of runs, that is solutions (9.59), with different sets of x_i and t_i for each run, except for a single input fixed at perhaps $t = 1$ and $x = 0.5$ over all runs. If we average over runs, the resulting waveform $\Psi(x, t)$ is somewhat analogous to a brain average evoked potential (averaged transient response). The time $t = 1$ is analogous to the arrival of evoked input to primary sensory cortex ($x = 0.5$). The averaged temporal waveforms $\Psi(0, t)$ for three example sets are shown in Figure 9-17, with differences due to changing the mode damping parameters α_n, $n = 1, 2, 3, \ldots$ or "width" of the input region Δx. In each case, the waveforms are composed of the underlying natural frequencies of the transmission line ω_n (plus some contribution from the random inputs); however, some frequencies may not be observed because of larger relative damping or because of the other low pass filter effects discussed above.

We do not suggest that brain evoked potentials can be modeled accurately by linear systems. However, in Chapter 11 a crude quasi-linear model is developed in which each mode k_n undergoes a separate, stable limit cycle oscillation, but the field analogous to $\Psi(x, t)$ is still given by a linear superposition of modes. In this manner, the amplitudes of each mode may grow or decay (depending on initial conditions) until settling into their appropriate limit cycle. Thus the maximum amplitude of the "evoked potential" need not occur close to the stimulus time, by contrast to the examples of Figure 9-17.

Regardless of whether we take a linear or nonlinear view of brain evoked potentials, much of the same brain tissue that generates spontaneous EEG probably also generates evoked potentials (except for very early components generated in brainstem and thalamus). In fact, the spectral content of evoked potentials is similar to that of spontaneous EEG. Furthermore, in a series of studies of several brain structures, several similarities were found between evoked and spontaneous EEG (Basar, 1980; Basar et al, 1987).

These ideas have important implications for experimental protocols used in

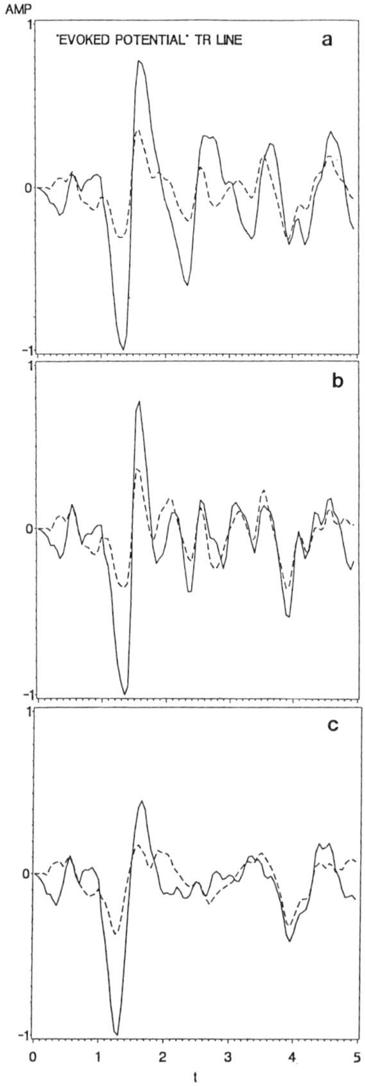

Figure 9-17. Averaged "evoked potentials" in the closed transmission line obtained from (9.59). Random input v(x, t) is used except that all waveforms used to construct averages contain fixed input at $t_s = 1$, $x_s = 0.5$ in (9.58), thereby making this example somewhat analogous to cortical evoked potentials with input arriving at a primary sensory cortical location x_s, with fixed latency from the stimulus t_s. Dashed lines are averages over 10 waveforms; solid lines are averages over 20 waveforms. Different waveforms occur because of different values of mode damping parameters α_n and different spatial extents of the input function (Δx). Larger Δx produces more low frequency content (**a**) than occurs with smaller Δx (**b**). Waveforms with larger damping are shown in (**c**). In this linear example, peaks in the averaged waveform occur just after the constant stimulus at $t_s = 1$. However, if modes follow limit cycles, peaks can occur at any time, as discussed in Chapters 10, 11, and 12.

evoked potential research. For example, attempts are sometimes made to filter evoked potentials to improve the signal-to-noise ratio. But procedures based on the common engineering assumption that the "noise" (mostly spontaneous EEG) is uncorrelated with the signal will probably fail, because such procedures just involve creating a new definition of the "evoked potential" (DeWeerd, 1981; McGillem and Aunon, 1987; Wright et al, 1990). That is, standard procedures that involve simple averages of the waveform over N trials define the "standard evoked potential." Changing this procedure only creates new waveforms, which may be no "better" than standard waveforms. The design of effective filters for cortical evoked potentials apparently requires more knowledge of brain dynamics than is available. At the very least, proposed filters for evoked potentials should be tested on several models of brain dynamics using computer simulations so the effects of different assumptions about brain mechanisms on final waveform can be better appreciated. We may speculate that much of the information in evoked potentials results from nonlinear interactions between stimulus and background EEG. Most of this information may be lost using simple averaging.

Inhomogeneities in the Wave Medium

Here we consider a simple, inhomogeneous physical system, the stretched string (or transmission line) having different properties in two regions of the independent variable x. The inhomogeneity might, for example, be due to increased mass density of the string in the region $a < x < b$, which causes decreased wave propagation velocity in this region. Alternately, the string might be undamped in one region and damped in another. We have two motivations for including this example. (1) Some EEG phenomena, such as the normal awake alpha rhythm, appear to have both local and global aspects. For example, we can interpret the spatial properties of alpha rhythm in terms of spatially dependent damping of waves in parts of frontal cortex. (2) A relatively simple "bottom-up" interaction is illustrated here. That is, when the properties of part of the wave medium are altered, mode frequencies, damping, and eigenfunctions for the entire system are changed.

The displacement of the inhomogeneous string is governed by (9.1) and can be expressed (Morse and Ingard, 1968) by a solution similar to (9.6). That is,

$$\Psi(x, t) = \sum_{n=1}^{\infty} A_n H_n(x) e^{-\gamma_n t - j\omega_n t} \tag{9.62}$$

where the eigenfunctions $H_n(x)$ and mode frequencies ω_n may be determined numerically as solutions to a coupled set of integral equations. However, if the perturbation parameter characterizing the region where string properties are altered is small (that is, if the string is not too inhomogeneous), approximate analytic expressions may be obtained. In this case, the eigenfunctions are perturbations of the usual homogeneous eigenfunctions

$$H_n(x) \cong \sin k_n x + \sum_{m \neq n} D_{mn} \frac{\sin k_m x}{m^2 - n^2} \tag{9.63}$$

Here the complex coefficients D_{mn} are expressed in terms of physical parameters of both regions of the string. The mode frequencies ω_n are reduced if propagation velocity $c(x)$ is reduced in the region $a < x < b$, but they are selectively reduced. That is, some mode frequencies are altered more than others, depending on the relative locations of altered medium ($a < x < b$) and nodes of the eigenfunctions. Similarly, if the altered medium produces damping, the mode damping coefficients γ_n are selectively altered. For example, if the altered region is small ($b \to a$) and located at one of the nodes of mode n, the damping of the nth mode γ_n will be unaffected by the inhomogeneity. An example of this effect is described by Nunez (1981).

A common characteristic of simple wave phenomena is the direct correspondence between frequency and wave number. However, the introduction of a region of inhomogeneity in the string causes each mode frequency ω_n to be associated with a range of wave numbers k_m, including the k_n associated with ω_n in the homogeneous case, as shown by (9.63). Another way to view this is to consider the inhomogeneity as an internal boundary condition that alters the eigenfunctions in a manner somewhat analogous to that which occurs when the usual external boundary conditions are changed. This type of effect generally occurs in inhomogeneous wave media of all sorts; that is, the introduction of inhomogeneity may be similar to changing the geometry of the medium.

Examples of string waves incident on localized inhomogeneities of different kinds are shown in Figure 9-18. In these examples, some of the incident wave energy is transmitted through the point load and some energy is reflected. With waves of synaptic action in neocortex, there is no mechanism for wave reflection and no obvious analogy to energy conservation. However, theories of neocortical dynamics predict increased wave damping in regions where control parameters

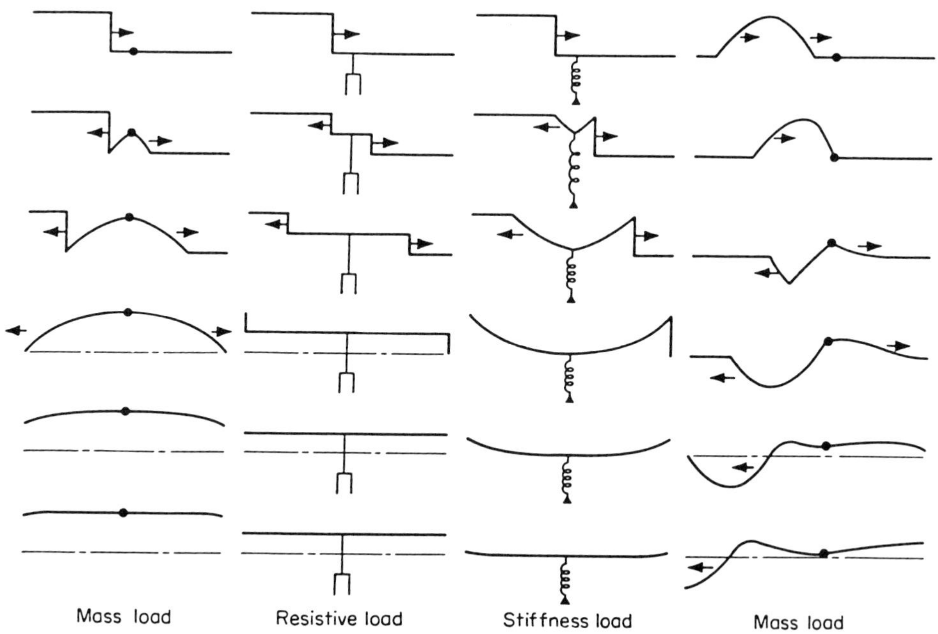

Figure 9-18. Reflection and transmission of waves at a point load on a string. The first three example sequences are for the case of an incident-step function wave. The last sequence is for a half sine wave. (Reproduced with permission from Morse and Ingard, 1968.)

effect a net strengthening of inhibitory or a weakening of excitatory neurotransmitter actions. These neurotransmitters may allow the continual creation of functional local and regional circuits in the brain which process information as discussed in Chapters 3 and 13.

References

Akheizer, A.L., Akheizer, I.A., Polovin, R.V., Sitenko, A.G., and Stepanov, K.N. *Collective Oscillations in a Plasma*. Cambridge, MA: MIT Press, 1967.

Basar, E. *EEG Brain Dynamics: Relations Between EEG and Evoked Potentials*. New York: Elsevier, 1980.

Basar, E., Basar-Erogul, C., Roschke, J., and Schutt, A. The EEG is a quasi-deterministic signal anticipating sensory-cognitive tasks. In: *Brain Dynamics*. (E. Basar and Bullock, T.H., Eds.) Berlin: Springer-Verlag, pp. 43–71, 1987.

Basler, M. and Wagner, C.A. Observations of earth-ionosphere cavity resonances. *Nature* 188:638–641, 1960.

Cole, K.S. *Membranes, Ions and Impulses*. Berkeley, CA: University of California Press, 1968.

Davis, L., Jr., and Lorente de No, R. Contribution to the mathematical theory of the electrotonus. In: *A Study of Nerve Physiology*. New York: Rockefeller Institute for Medical Research, 131:442–496, 1947.

De Weerd, J.P.C. Facts and fancies about a posteriori "Wiener" filtering. *IEEE Trans. Biomed. Eng*. 28:252–257, 1981.

Egeland, A. and Larsen, T.R. *Physica Norvegica*. 2:85–97, 1967.

Jackson, J.D. *Classical Electrodynamics*. 2nd Ed. New York: Wiley, 1975.

Jacobson, S. and Pollen, D.A. Electrotonic spread of dendritic potentials in feline pyramidal cells. *Science* 161:1351–1353, 1968.

Lux, H.D. and Pollen, D.A. Electrical constants of neurons in the motor cortex of the cat. *J. Neurophysiol*. 29:207–220, 1966.

McGillem, C.D. and Aunon, J.I. Analysis of event-related potentials. In: *Handbook of Electroencephalography and Clinical Neurophysiology*. (Revised series). (A.S. Gevin and Remond, A., Eds.) New York: Elsevier, pp. 131–169, 1987.

Montgomery, D.C. and Tidman, D.A. *Plasma Kinetic Theory*. New York: McGraw-Hill, 1964.

Morse, P.M. and Feshbach, H. *Methods of Theoretical Physics*. Vols. 1 and 2. New York: McGraw-Hill, 1953.

Morse, P.M. and Ingard, K.U. *Theoretical Acoustics*. New York: McGraw-Hill, 1968.

Nunez, P.L. Longitudinal wave propagation in a plasma containing an external time-dependent electric field. *The Physics of Fluids*. 14:633–639, 1971.

Nunez, P.L. *Electric Fields of the Brain: The Neurophysics of EEG*. New York: Oxford University Press, 1981.

Nunez, P.L. Spatial filtering and experimental strategies in EEG. In: *Statistics and Topography in Quantitative EEG*. (D. Samson-Dollfus, Ed.) Paris: Elsevier, pp. 196–209, 1988.

Plonsey, R. *Bioelectric Phenomena*. New York: McGraw-Hill, 1969.

Polk, C. and Postow, E. *CRC Handbook of Biological Effects of Electromagnetic Fields*. Boca Raton, FL: CRC Press, 1986.

Rall, W. Theory of physiological properties of dendrites. *Ann. N Y Acad. Sci.* 96:1071–1092, 1962.

Rall, W. Distinguishing theoretical synaptic potentials computed for different soma-dendritic distributions of synaptic input. *J. Neurophysiol.* 30:1138–1168, 1967.

Rall, W. Core conductor theory and cable properties of neurons. In: *Handbook of Physiology. Vol. 1. The Nervous System.* (E.T. Kandel, Ed.) Bethesda, MD: American Physiological Society, pp. 39–97, 1977.

Rush, S. and Driscoll, D.A. Current distribution in the brain from surface electrodes. *Anesthesia Analgesia.* 47:717–723, 1968.

Rush, S. and Driscoll, D.A. EEG electrode sensitivity: An application of reciprocity. *IEEE Trans. Biomed. Eng.* 16:15–22, 1969.

Scott, A.C. *Neurophysics.* New York: Wiley, 1977.

Stratton, J.A., Morse, P.M., Chu, L.J., and Hunter, R.A. *Elliptic Cylinder and Spheroidal Wave Functions*, New York: Wiley, 1941.

Woosley, J.K., Roth, B.J., and Wikswo, J.P. Jr. The magnetic field of a single axon: A volume conductor model. *Mathematical Bioscience* 76:1–36, 1985.

Wright, J.J., Sergejew, A.A., and Stampfer, H.G. Inverse filter computation of the neural impulse giving rise to the auditory evoked potential. *Brain Topography.* 2:293–302, 1990.

10

Nonlinear Phenomena and Chaos

PAUL L. NUNEZ

The separation of linear systems into discrete and continuous systems, described in Chapters 8 and 9, respectively, is also appropriate for nonlinear systems. This introductory treatment, however, emphasizes simple, discrete nonlinear systems, that is, systems with only a few degrees of freedom (and corresponding dependent variables) in which time is the only independent variable. A few continuous nonlinear systems are also considered, quasi-linear methods are applied to neocortex in Chapter 11, and a full nonlinear approach to neocortical dynamics is presented in Chapter 14. As with linear systems, studies can be separated into two parts: the analysis of known systems, and the characterization of experimental data as output from unknown systems, with or without known input.

Methods for analyzing known systems are separated further into classical methods, applicable primarily to quasi-linear systems, and modern methods, which nearly always involve computer solutions. Studies of unknown systems as black boxes are separated further into systems with known input and output, in which nonlinear transfer functions or kernels are estimated from experimental data, and into systems with unknown input in which other measures of dynamic properties of the system are sought from the measured output. Examples of the latter are the usual power spectra and correlation functions, or in cases of suspected chaotic behavior, Lyapunov exponents and fractal dimensions, discussed briefly in the section New Experimental Measures of System Dynamics. Because of space limitations, kernels are not considered here.

Renewed interest in nonlinear phenomena has paralleled the development of fast computers that make possible the solutions of many practical problems by the ordinary researcher, problems that have been far too difficult for the best mathematicians and physicists of several decades past. Another reason for current interest in nonlinear systems is a new appreciation for the complexity and richness of behavior of systems with only a few degrees of freedom. Many such systems can exhibit chaotic behavior, a class of motion (that is, dynamic behavior) characterized by complexity and exquisite sensitivity to the initial state of the system.

New studies of nonlinear electrical and mechanical systems appear each month

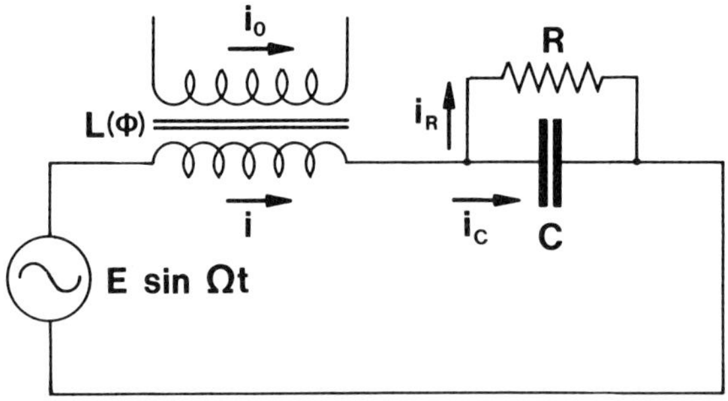

Figure 10-1. Electric circuit with ac generator, inductor, capacitor, and resistor. The input voltage is v(t) = E sin Ωt. The outputs are currents and voltages across each element. The inductor has a secondary winding and may be nonlinear.

in the physics and engineering literature. These include theory and experiments, and excellent agreement between the two is common. An historical account of chaos (Gleick, 1987), well-written books emphasizing engineering (Moon, 1992) or physics (Tabor, 1989) applications, a special issue of the *Proceedings of the IEEE* on chaotic electrical systems (published in August 1987), more than a decade's worth of articles in *Physica D* and *Physical Review*, and a new journal *Chaos: An Interdisciplinary Journal of Nonlinear Science* all provide background information. This chapter will cover a very small part of this literature, with more emphasis on general nonlinear effects than on those that are specifically chaotic. The reason for such emphasis is that although nonlinearity is critically important to neocortical dynamics, the importance of chaos in the field is not established.

A wide range of mechanical, electrical, and biologic systems behave nonlinearly. Mechanical vibrations, fluid flow, acoustics, circuits with diodes or transistors, magnetically levitated vehicles, feedback control devices, and nearly all neural network models are just a few examples of nonlinear systems that have been studied. Most of these systems also behave chaotically for certain ranges of system parameters. To obtain a qualitative "feel" for some of the additional complexity associated with nonlinearity, consider a system with input v(t) and outputs i(t), $i_R(t)$ and $i_C(t)$, as shown in Figure 10-1. If the system is linear, only the frequency components present in the input function can appear in the outputs, regardless of the exact nature of the system. In particular, consider the electric circuit of Figure 10-1. If the inductor, capacitor, and resistor are all linear elements, that is, if all obey the usual linear relations between current and voltage, the circuit is linear. Thus all currents and voltages forced by the ac generator with frequency Ω are sinusoidal oscillations of frequency Ω, but with generally different phases determined by the usual methods of elementary circuit analysis.

Consider the example of the electric circuit of Figure 10-1, in which the inductor is nonlinear (has a saturable core). A secondary winding with a constant dc current i_0 is provided to bring asymmetry to the nonlinear problem. The magnetic flux in the core of the inductor satisfies a form of the Duffing equation,

$$\frac{d^2\Phi}{dt^2} + 2\alpha \frac{d\Phi}{dt} + \omega_0^2\Phi + \beta\Phi^3 = B \cos \Omega t + B_0 \tag{10.1}$$

if hysteresis is neglected. Equation (10.1) is identical to the elementary equation (8.1) of linear systems except for the additional terms B_0 to account for the dc current i_0 and the term $\beta\Phi^3$ from the inductor core saturation curve. The addition of the linear term B_0 is of minor consequence to the original linear system. However, the nonlinear term $\beta\Phi^3$ apparently makes it impossible to find a general analytic solution. This term also causes a variety of system responses that could never be anticipated with linear systems analysis. This nonlinear circuit has been studied in some depth, experimentally and with an analog computer, by Hayashi (1953).

The inductor current i(t) and voltages across the inductor $v_L(t)$ and capacitor $v_C(t)$ are the system outputs followed by Hayashi. These output waveforms depend closely on system parameters, particularly the magnitudes of the input voltage (proportional to B) and dc current (proportional to B_0), and especially on whether this forcing function is symmetric ($B_0 = 0$). This study focused on the relative

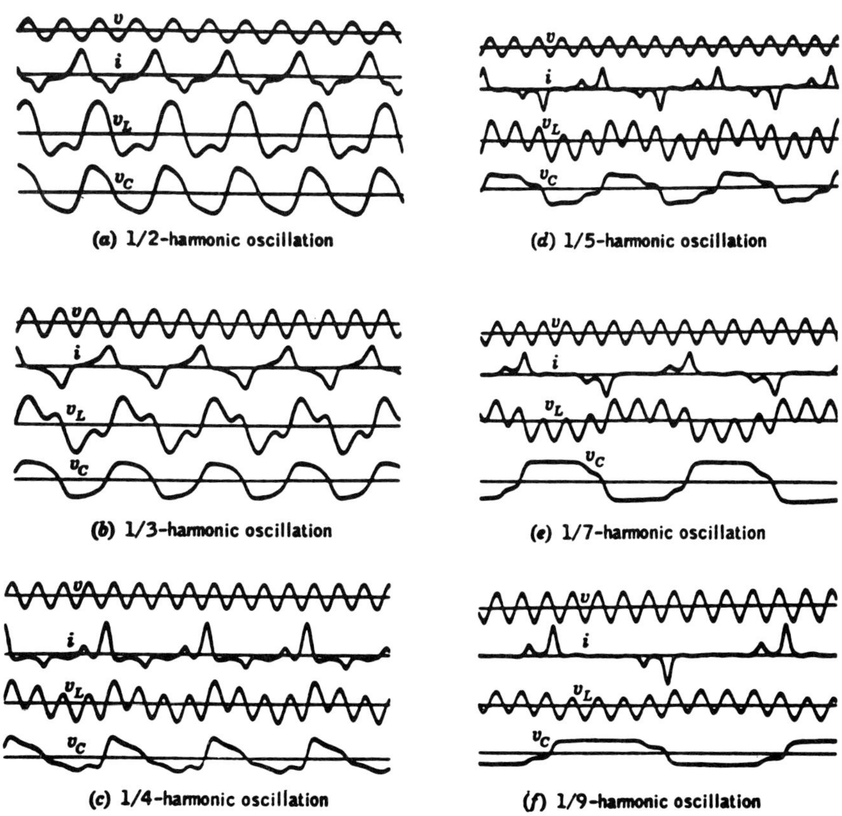

Figure 10-2. Input v(t) and outputs from the circuit of Figure 10-1 when the inductor is nonlinear. The outputs i(t) and $v_L(t)$ are inductor current and voltage, respectively; $v_C(t)$ is capacitor voltage. The waveforms correspond to different parameters B and B_0 in (10.1). (Reproduced with permission from Hayashi, 1964.)

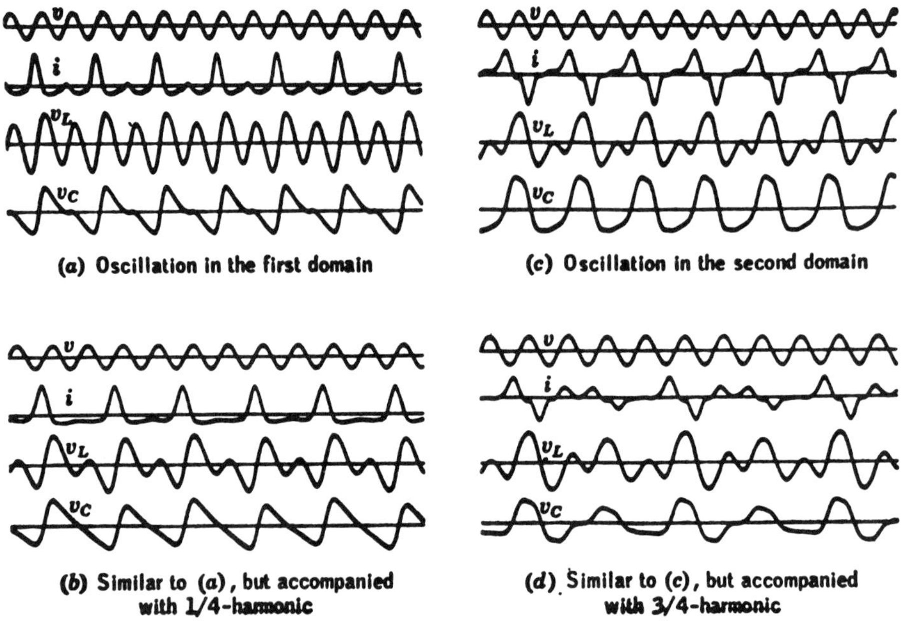

Figure 10-3. More waveforms from the circuit of Figure 10-1 for different domains of the B, B_0 parameter space. (Reproduced with permission from Hayashi, 1964.)

magnitudes of subharmonics of the input voltage, that is, on the relative magnitudes of frequency components $n\Omega/m$, where n and m are relatively prime integers in the outputs i(t), $v_L(t)$ and $v_C(t)$. We are not especially interested in the details of these results. However, the variety of output waveforms obtained for combinations of the parameters B and B_0, as shown in Figure 10-2 and 10-3, suggests the complexity of behavior possible in even apparently simple nonlinear systems. The addition of the single cubic term to the left side of (10.1) made possible all the behavior shown in these figures. Without this simple term due to the nonlinear properties of the inductor, all of Figures 10-2 and 10-3 would consist of sine waves of the same frequency Ω. In fact, more waveform complexity, including chaotic behavior, is possible in this circuit, as indicated in the section Periodic and Chaotic Behavior in a Duffing System.

Types of Behavior Exhibited by Time Series

The output X(t) of a deterministic system, that is, one without noise, generally can be classified according to one of the following four types with examples indicated.

1. Equilibrium: An initial disturbance of a mechanical or electrical oscillator decreases to zero amplitude as a result of damping.

2. Periodic: The steady-state oscillations of linear electrical or mechanical systems caused by sinusoidal input, or limit cycle motion in nonlinear systems.

3. Quasiperiodic: Linear oscillations in systems with more than one degree of freedom. Behavior of some nonlinear systems.

4. Chaotic: Complex oscillations in nonlinear systems that exhibit relatively broad frequency spectra and sensitivity to initial conditions and system parameters.

The first three categories are associated with linear systems, but all four may occur in nonlinear systems. These four types of behavior are, in the modern language of dynamic systems, called attractors. That is, after initial transients damp out, these distinct types of steady-state dynamic behavior may occur; the motion may be attracted to one of the listed states.

The distinctions between different types of attractors are most obvious when applied to systems with relatively few degrees of freedom and large signal-to-noise ratio. With electroencephalographic (EEG) data, the first of these conditions is highly unlikely, whereas the second may or may not hold. Thus considerable care must be exercised in extrapolating ideas developed for the simple systems discussed in this chapter to neocortical dynamics. For example, complex systems may have multiple attractors, so that the steady-state motion depends on the initial conditions. However, knowledge of simple systems is required as a basis for studying complex systems. Consider first systems that have periodic motion.

Periodic signals repeat themselves at regular intervals, that is,

$$X(t) = X(t \pm kT) \qquad k = 1, 2, 3, \ldots \tag{10.2}$$

where T is the period. A Fourier series approximation can be obtained for nearly any X(t), that is

$$X(t) \cong a_0 + \sum_{n=1}^{N} a_n \cos(\omega_n t - \theta_n) \tag{10.3}$$

where $\omega_n = 2n\pi/T$, and large values of N yield a closer approximation to the actual X(t). The approximation to the function X(t) is forced by (10.3) to be periodic with period T. When expressing a block of experimental data of length T as a Fourier series, we define the data to be periodic with period T. We are free to apply this definition because the original data are defined only on the interval T. In contrast to (10.3), a function of the form

$$X(t) = \sum_{m=1}^{M} b_m \cos(\omega_m t - \theta_m) \tag{10.4}$$

where the frequencies ω_m are arbitrary, generally is not periodic. It is periodic only when the ratios of all possible pairs of frequencies form rational numbers (commensurate frequencies). For example,

$$X(t) = b_1 \cos(3t + \theta_1) + b_2 \cos(7t + \theta_2) + b_3 \cos(17t + \theta_3) \tag{10.5}$$

is periodic with period $T = 2\pi$. In contrast, the function

$$X(t) = b_1 \cos(3t + \theta_1) + b_2 \cos(7t + \theta_2) + b_3 \cos(\pi t + \theta_3) \tag{10.6}$$

is not periodic because the frequency $\omega_3 = \pi$ is incommensurate with ω_1 and ω_2. Functions such as those of (10.6) are called quasi-periodic (although they may not be close to periodic), to distinguish them from chaotic behavior.

Four types of plot generally are used to illustrate the behavior of nonlinear system dynamics: (1) the usual $X = X(t)$ plots; (2) power (or amplitude) spectra; (3) phase plane plots; and (4) Poincaré maps.

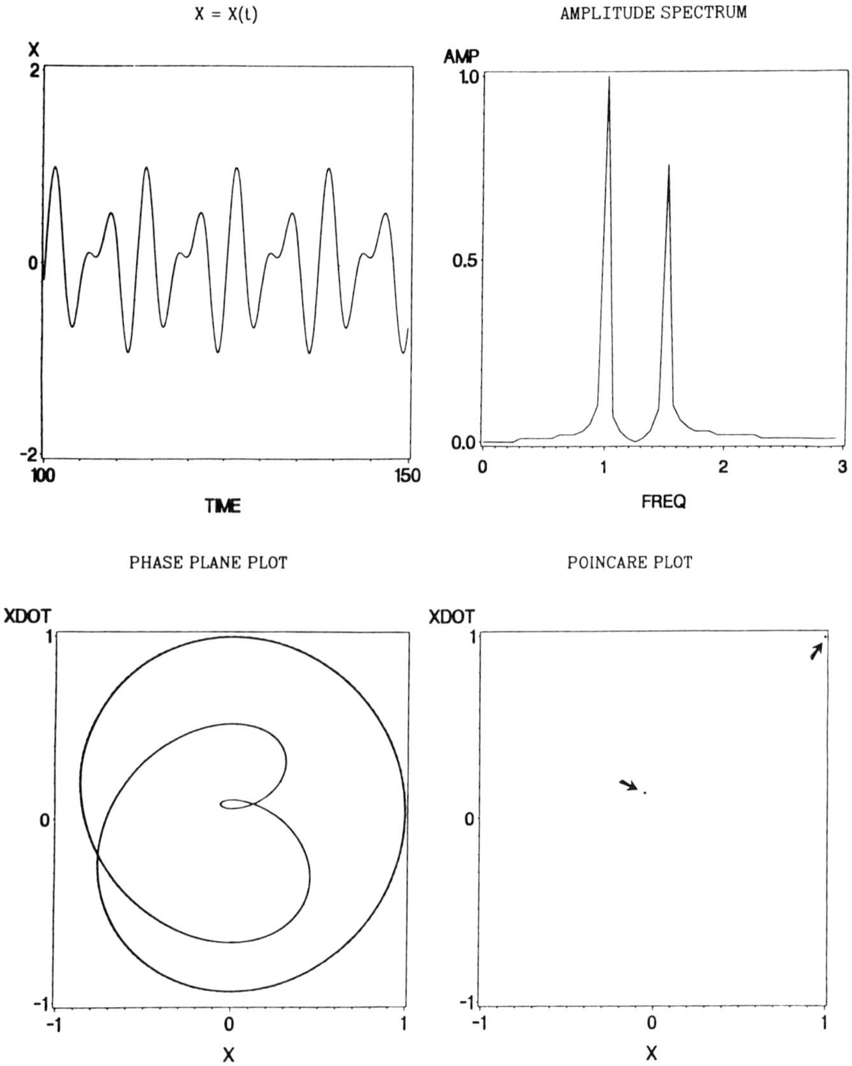

Figure 10-4. Four types of plot used to represent the dynamics of linear or nonlinear systems. In this example, the waveform consists of two commensurate frequencies 1.0 and 1.5 (arbitrary units). Waveform is periodic. Amplitude versus time (*upper left*), amplitude spectrum (*upper right*), phase plane (*lower left*), and Poincaré plot (*lower right*).

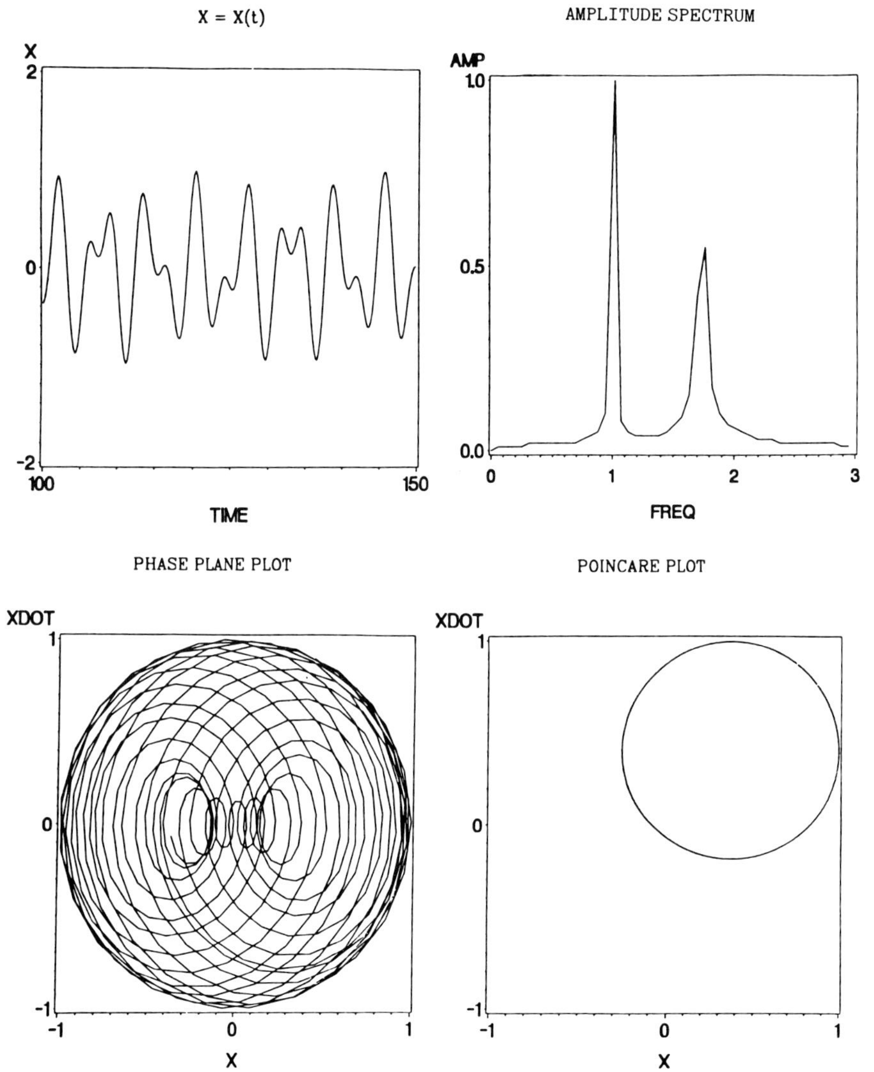

Figure 10-5. Four types of plot representing a waveform consisting of two incommensurate frequencies, 1.0 and $\sqrt{3}$. The phase plane plot resembles a ball of string since the waveform is not periodic.

All four types are shown in Figure 10-4 for a signal composed of two commensurate frequencies. The amplitude spectrum shows peaks at these frequencies, $\omega_1 = 1.0$ and $\omega_2 = 1.5$ (arbitrary units). The phase plane plot is constructed by plotting X(t) versus dX/dt, for example, position versus velocity or capacitor voltage versus current. Periodic behavior is evidenced by a phase plane orbit that traces out a closed curve as time increases. The Poincaré map is constructed in the same phase plane, but sampling of X(t) and dX/dt only occurs at times $t_n = nT + t_0$,

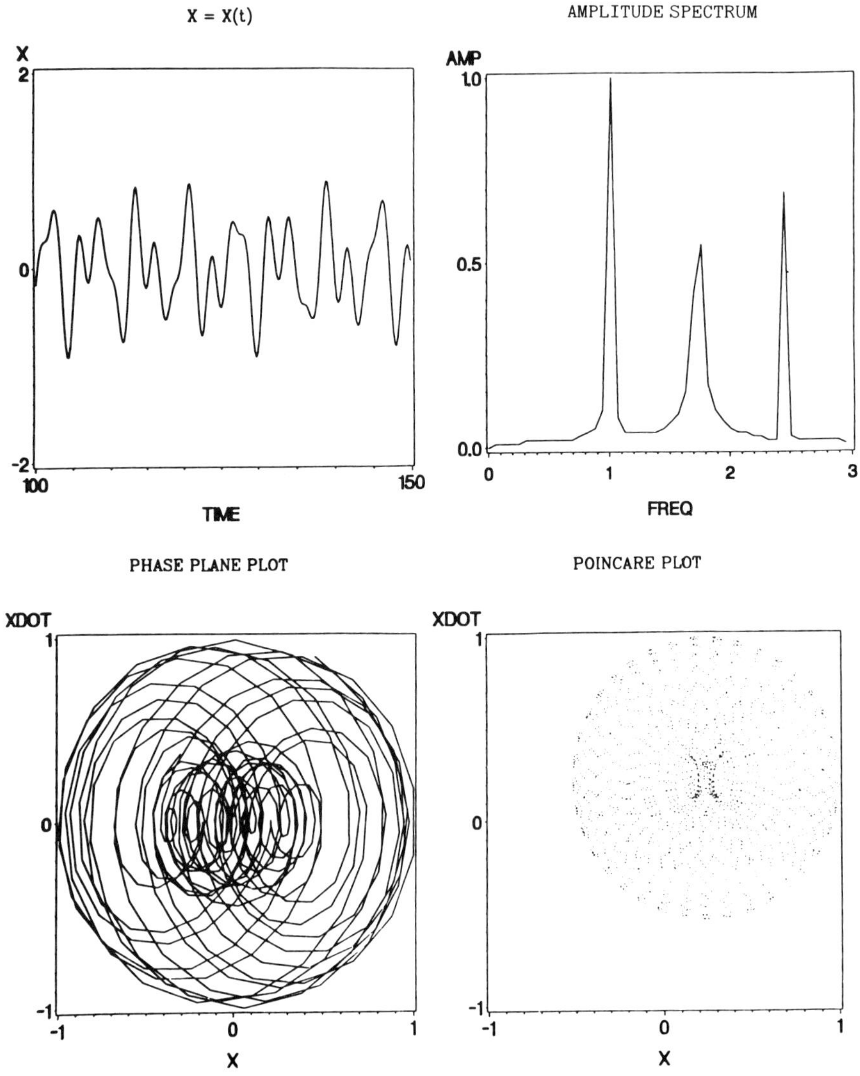

Figure 10-6. Four types of plot shown in Figure 10-4, but here representing a waveform consisting of three incommensurate frequencies 1.0, $\sqrt{3}$, and $\sqrt{6}$. Waveform is not periodic.

where T is based on a characteristic frequency of the system. For example, with the forced oscillator represented by (10.1) and Figures 10-2 and 10-3, we would normally choose $T = 2\pi/\Omega$, that is, the period of the voltage generator. The computer places a dot at the appropriate location in the phase plane each time X(t) and its derivative are sampled. The result, after many samples of a function with period T, is a single point in the phase plane because each dot is placed on top of the preceding one. Subharmonics of the forcing frequency appear on the

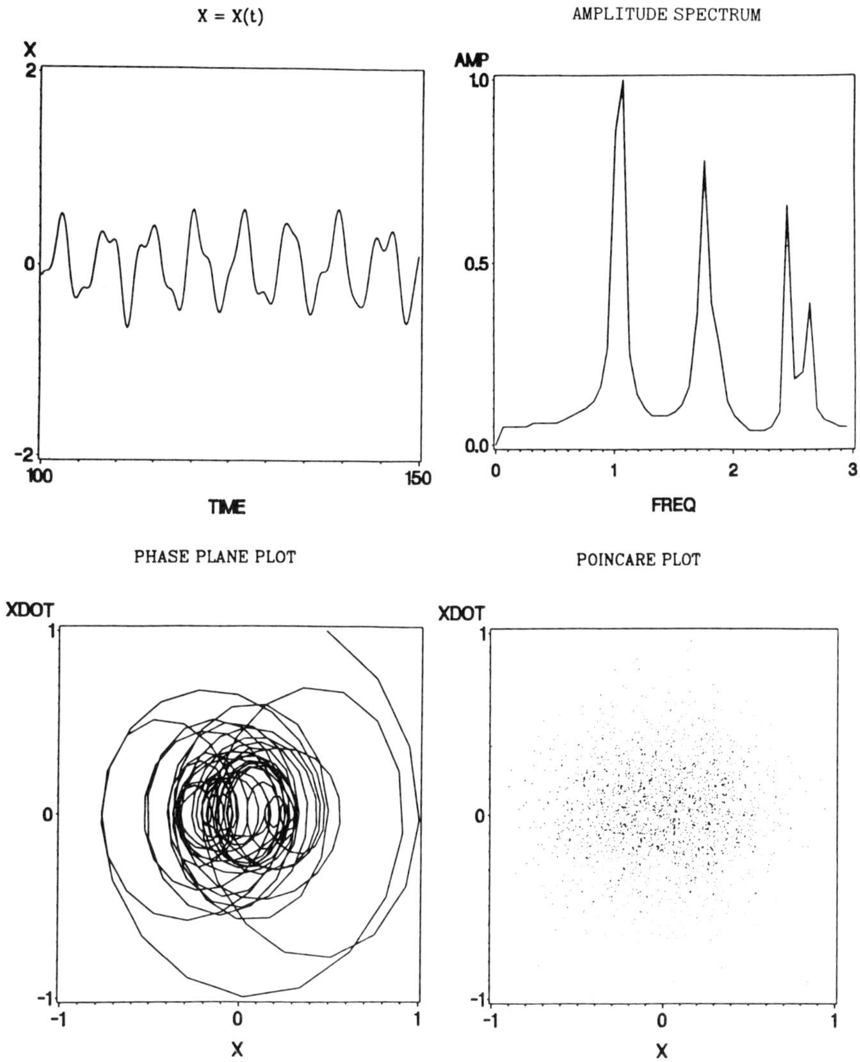

Figure 10-7. Four types of plot representing a waveform consisting of nine frequency components: two near 1.0, three near $\sqrt{3}$, and four near $\sqrt{6}$. This might result, for example, from the linear oscillations of the prolate spheroidal shell, as discussed in Chapter 9.

Poincaré map as additional isolated points that the system "visits" less often than a point associated with the forcing frequency.

Plots for a signal composed on two incommensurate frequencies are shown in Figure 10-5 and for three incommensurate frequencies in Figure 10-6. In contrast to the signal of Figure 10-4, these signals are not periodic and the phase plane plots do not form closed curves. The Poincaré plot consists of many points, which in Figure 10-6 exhibits an interesting pattern. A more complicated pattern occurs in Figure 10-7, which was obtained by simulating the oscillations of the prolate spheroidal shell discussed in Chapter 9. This is similar to the case shown in Figure 10-6, except that the modes (ℓ = 1, 2, 3) have been split (m = 0, ℓ) so that the waveform in Figure 10-7 consists of nine separate frequency components. The differences in m modes are mostly too small to appear in the spectrum with the resolution obtained here. In this example, the phase plane plot is complicated, and the Poincaré plot consists of apparently nearly random points, even though the underlying system is linear.

Several points must be emphasized about the signals depicted in Figures 10-4 through 10-7. First, all can be outputs from linear systems. In fact, by increasing the number of degrees of freedom, the degree of apparent complexity can be increased to arbitrary levels. For example, large electric circuits and mechanical systems with hundreds or thousands of degrees of freedom are common in engineering practice. The Schumann resonances discussed in Chapter 9 provide a physical example of a linear system with many degrees of freedom. Contrary to the apparent impression of some EEG researchers, complexity and nonlinearity are not synonymous. Another point is that in second-order systems with N degrees of freedom, the phase space has 2N dimensions (with autonomous systems). In such cases, the phase plane and Poincaré plots of Figures 10-4 through 10-7 may be viewed as projections of the motion (or flow) of the system on the (X, $\dot{X}$) plane. In nonautonomous systems, such as when time occurs explicitly as in the case of forced oscillations, time is treated as an additional dimension of the phase space.

A related concept is pseudo-phase space, in which experimental data, perhaps from a single channel, are analyzed. Given the single time series X(t), the axes of the M-dimensional pseudo-phase space are X(t), X(t + τ), X(t + 2τ), . . . X[t + (M + 1)τ]. In such applications, the time increment and space dimension M must be chosen as the result of data studies because the dynamics of the system, including the number of degrees of freedom, is not known a priori (Packard et al, 1980; Abarbanel et al, 1993). This is an area of active research and is discussed further later.

Limit Cycles in an Electric Circuit

An important class of nonlinear phenomena are self-excited oscillations or limit cycles. These oscillations occur in systems without external periodic forcing functions. Typically a balance is obtained between a damping mechanism and some external source of energy. For example, a variety of aeroelastic vibrations exist in which steady flow of a fluid past a solid object on elastic restraints produces steady-state oscillations (Moon, 1992). Important mechanical systems with these characteristics are power lines and airplane wings, for example. Limit cycles also may occur in ecologic systems and neural networks.

A famous example of limit cycle oscillations is the vacuum tube circuit in which the external energy source is a dc voltage, and damping is due to resistive losses.

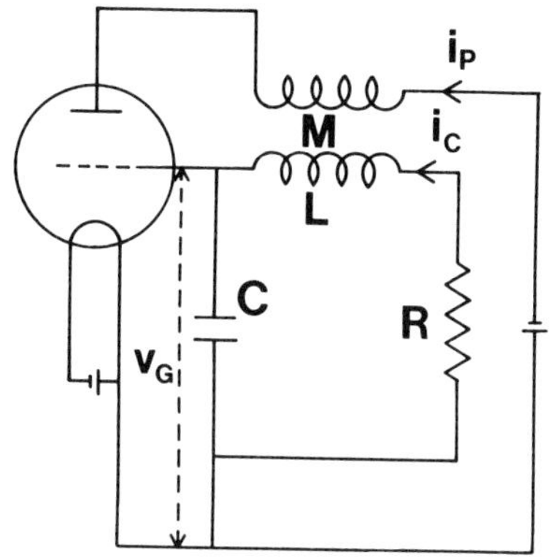

Figure 10-8. The famous Van der Pol oscillator circuit. The inductors, capacitor, and resistor are all linear. There is also a linear, mutual inductance M between the inductors. The circuit is nonlinear because of the nonlinear relation between plate current i_p and grid voltage v_G in the vacuum tube. Similar nonlinear relations occur in modern circuits, such as in transistors.

This circuit, the Van der Pol oscillator, is shown in Figure 10-8. The circuit equations include Kirchhoff's voltage law, applied to the inner loop

$$Ri_C + L\frac{di_C}{dt} - M\frac{di_p}{dt} + v_G = 0 \tag{10.7}$$

where i_C, i_p, and v_G are capacitor current, plate current, and grid voltage, respectively. Capacitor current is expressed by the usual linear relation

$$i_C = C\frac{dv_G}{dt}$$

The circuit is nonlinear because of the nonlinear relation between plate current and grid voltage

$$i_p = Dv_G\left(1 - \frac{v_G^2}{B}\right)$$

where D and B are constants. Equations (10.7) through (10.9) yield the Van der Pol equation

$$\frac{d^2v}{dt^2} - A(1 - v^2)\frac{dv}{dt} + \omega_0^2 v = 0 \tag{10.8}$$

where the normalized grid voltage is defined by

$$v \equiv \left[\frac{3MD}{B(MD - RC)}\right]^{1/2} v_G$$

The parameter in (10.8) associated with damping is

$$A \equiv \frac{MD - RC}{LC}$$

and the oscillation frequency for the linear limiting case is

$$\omega_0 = \left(\frac{1}{LC}\right)^{1/2} \tag{10.9}$$

If neither damping nor an external energy source were present in (10.8), the parameter A would be zero, and the voltage would oscillate with frequency ω_0 and amplitude determined by the initial conditions. The addition of the term A dv/dt provides negative damping (that is, energy input) for small voltages, which causes the grid voltage to increase with time. However, when the normalized voltage increases to greater than 1, damping becomes positive and voltage decreases. In this manner, a self-excited oscillation or limit cycle is created. The oscillation is depicted by the phase plane plots of Figure 10-9. If the initial voltage and voltage derivative are inside the limit cycle trajectory, the motion v(t) spirals out to the closed asymptotic trajectory or limit cycle. Initial conditions outside the limit cycle spiral into it. Thus the amplitude of the "motion" for large t (the steady-state or asymptotic solution) is independent of initial conditions. For values of the parameter $A << 1$, the limit cycle is a circle with a radius 2 in the phase plane with a frequency ω_0 equal to that of the corresponding linear system, that is

$$v(t) \sim 2\cos(\omega_0 t) \tag{10.10}$$

Larger values of A change the shape of the limit cycle and reduce the fundamental frequency. Also, larger values of A introduce odd harmonics $3\omega_0$, $5\omega_0$, and so on into the voltage, as shown in Figure 10-9. However, because they are true harmonics of the fundamental, the steady-state solution (attractor) remains periodic.

We are particularly interested in the relation between amplitude and frequency in the Van der Pol limit cycle because of its possible similarity to human EEG; that is, large-amplitude EEG occurs mainly at low frequencies. The following computer procedure was performed to study amplitude and frequency relations. Steady-state solutions of (10.8) (on the limit cycle) were obtained numerically for many values of $0 \leq A \leq 20$. The fundamental frequency was defined as the largest peak in the spectrum. The maximum magnitudes of v and dv/dt on the limit cycle were obtained. From these values, the maximum currents i_C and i_G and the maximum voltage v_G on the limit cycle were calculated by assuming that increasing values of the parameter A occur because of decreasing resistance R, whereas all other circuit parameters are constant. The results are presented in Figure 10-10, which shows how each of the maximum amplitudes increased as the fundamental frequency decreased.

Limit Cycles in Ecologic Systems

A second example of limit cycle behavior is taken from an entirely different field, theoretical ecology. When several populations of plant or animal species interact such that generations completely overlap, the dynamics of this interaction may

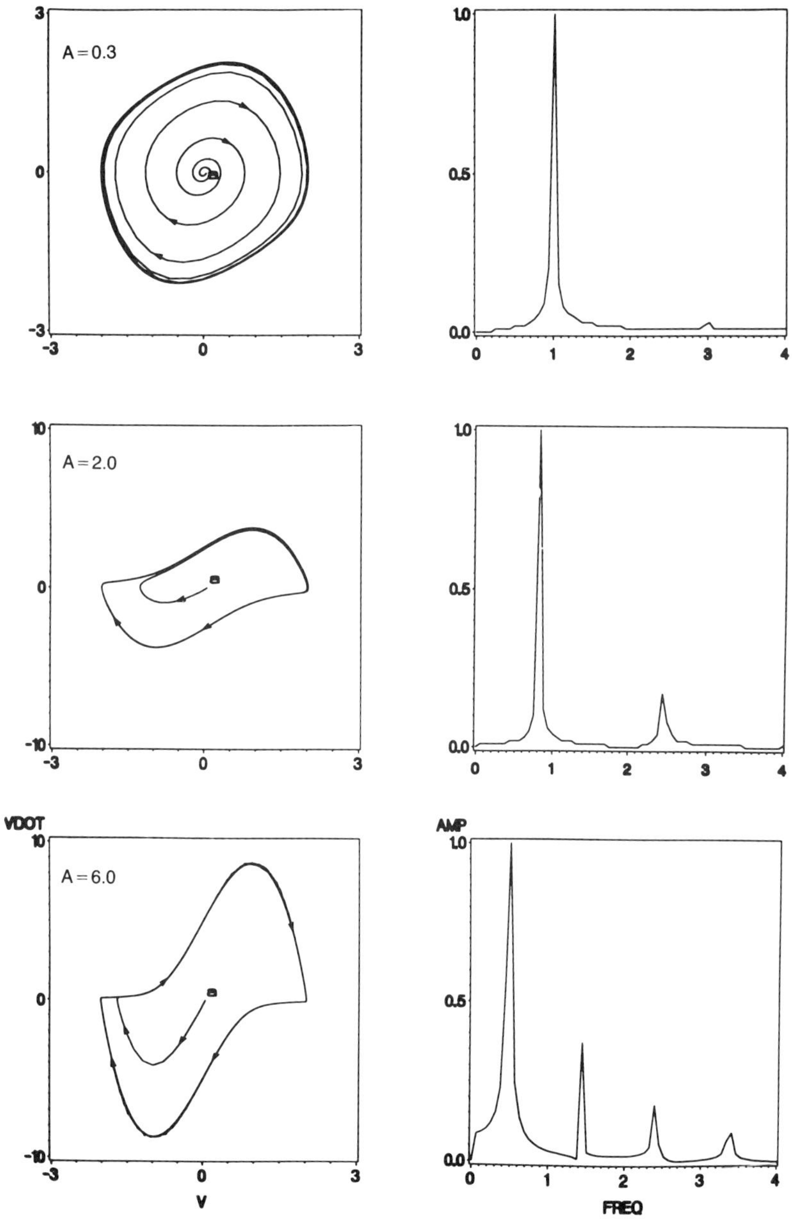

Figure 10-9. Phase plane plots and corresponding spectra for normalized grid voltage oscillations for different values of the parameter A, which determines the strength of the nonlinearity in the Van der Pol oscillator. All example solutions are limit cycles.

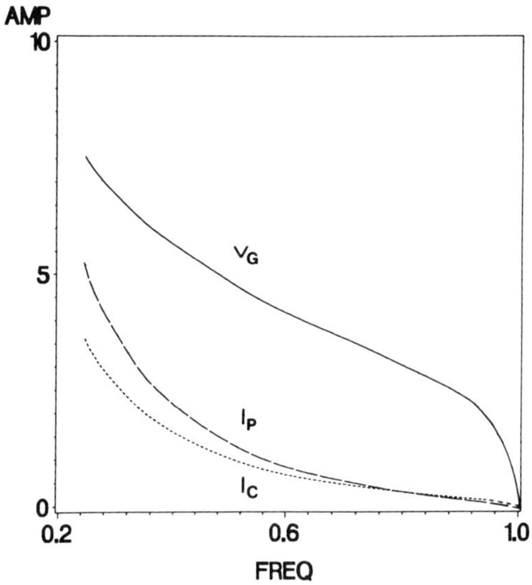

Figure 10-10. Changes in the amplitude of oscillations of grid voltage (v_G), plate current (i_p), and capacitor current (i_C) with fundamental frequency as the nonlinear parameter A is changed. Large A corresponds to low frequencies. Plots were obtained from multiple numerical solutions of (10.8).

be modeled by differential equations. For example, one model of predator–prey dynamics consists of the coupled set of differential equations (May, 1981)

$$\frac{dX}{dt} = X(1 - X/A) - XY/(X + 1) \tag{10.11}$$

$$\frac{dY}{dt} = (Y/B)(1 - Y/CX) \tag{10.12}$$

The numbers of (perhaps) rabbits and foxes are proportional to X and Y, respectively, and the time variable t is defined as the product of the intrinsic rabbit growth rate parameter with actual time. The parameter B is the ratio of intrinsic growth rate of rabbits to foxes, determined by how fast they each multiply in the absence of external constraints. The parameter A is the effective carrying capacity of the environment for rabbits (determined by the amount of grass available, for example). The parameter C allows for additional effects such as saturation in the foxes' capacity to take advantage of increasing rabbit density.

Equations (10.11) and (10.12) include critical negative feedback effects. For example, although the number of rabbits would increase exponentially in the absence of external constraints (that is, $dX/dt = X$), growth rate in the absence of foxes becomes negative when the population exceeds A because of environmental limitations. In addition, growth rate is decreased when some rabbits are eaten, an effect that is proportional to the number of foxes as described by the far right term in (10.11). Similarly, the population of foxes would increase exponentially in the absence of external constraints (that is, $dY/dt = Y/B$); however, fox growth rate becomes negative when the number of foxes Y becomes larger than CX. The presence of negative feedback in this ecologic system allows possible out-of-phase oscillations in the populations of rabbits and foxes that continue indefinitely (that is, limit cycles). In fact, a mathematical theorem for two-degree of freedom autonomous systems of differential equations (the Poincaré–Bendixson theorem) has been used to show that nearly all predator–prey models have steady-state solutions that are either stable equilibrium points or stable limit cycles (May, 1981).

A simple example of a system with a stable equilibrium is obtained for a single species, such as the population of rabbits in the absence of foxes. In this case, rabbit population is expressed by the solution to (10.11) with Y = 0, that is

$$X(t) = \frac{A}{1 + e^{t_0 - t}} \tag{10.13}$$

where the parameter t_0 is defined by the number of rabbits present at t = 0. As t becomes large, the asymptotic solution is $X(t) \rightarrow A$, where A is the equilibrium point or carrying capacity of the rabbit environment. Equation (10.13) is the logistic curve, which we will see again in studies of neocortical dynamics.

Phase plane plots of numerical solutions to the system described by (10.11) and (10.12) are shown in Figure 10-11 for different environmental capacities A when the ratio of growth rate of rabbits to foxes is fixed at B = 5. Rabbit and fox populations oscillate with limit cycle amplitudes that decrease as environmental carrying capacity is decreased to about A = 8. Further reductions in carrying capacity cause the solution to spiral into an equilibrium point, that is, population levels of foxes and rabbits that then remain forever fixed, as shown in Figure 10-11 (upper row). Further reductions in carrying capacity cause a more rapid approach to equilibrium at lower population levels. The general behavior of the system as changes are made in parameters A and B is shown in Figure 10-12.

We are not especially concerned about how well these equations model real ecologic systems. The main point is that this model has several features that are relatively easy to understand and that may have relevance to other complex systems such as neocortex. For example, when the number of excitatory action potentials in a mass of neural tissue increases, a corresponding increase in inhibitory firings occurs with some time delay, that is, there is negative feedback. Although the system represented by (10.11) and (10.12) is somewhat more complicated than the simplest predator–prey systems (such as the classical Lotka–Volterra system), there are many idealizations. Most obvious perhaps is uncoupling the rabbit–fox system from the rest of the environment. That is, several external influences are included with the parameters A, B, C, but no feedback of, for example, rabbit population to grass density, fox to human population, foxes to disease agents, and so on, is modeled. Each coupling with other species adds another equation and new parameters to the system. Perhaps the most difficult aspect of creating realistic models of complex systems is determining where to truncate potentially large sets of equations. The choice of when to stop adding additional complications to a basic theory is a judgment decision and depends on how well the additional parameters are known and on the underlying motivations

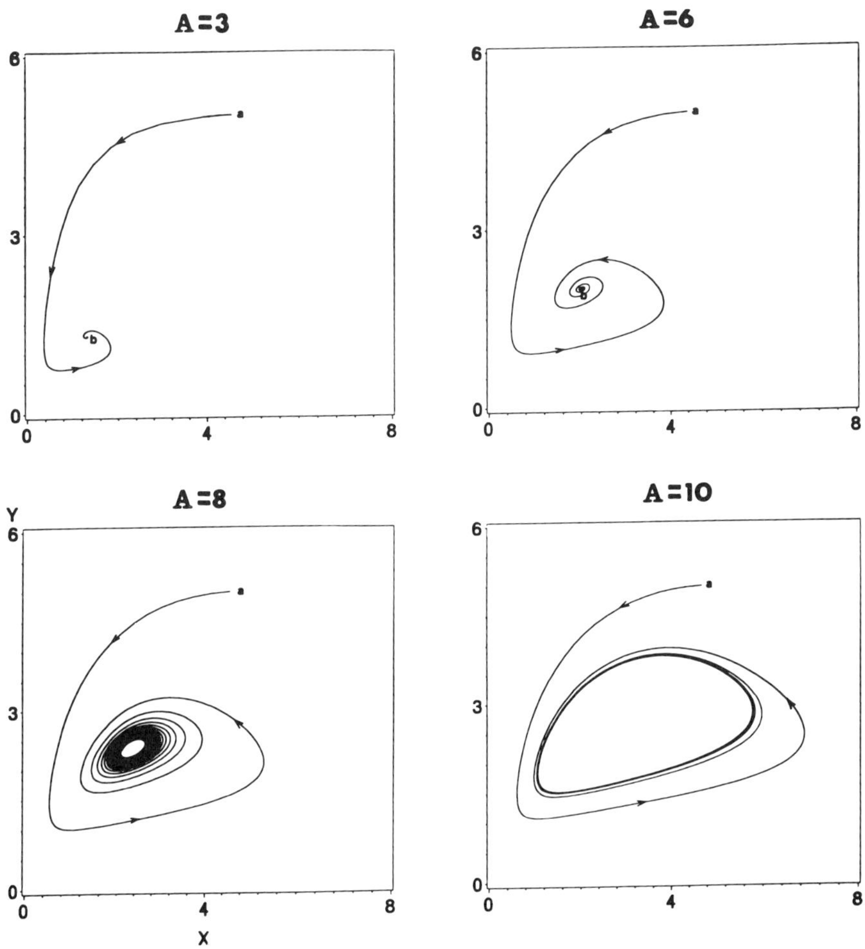

Figure 10-11. Numerical solutions to the predator (Y)–prey (X) equations (10.11) and (10.12). The phase plane plots are shown for different environmental carrying capacities of the prey, determined by the magnitude of parameter A. The parameters B = 5 and C = 1 are constant. The steady-state solution changes from a stable point to a stable limit cycle when A ~ 8. This type of change of system dynamics is called a Hopf bifurcation. In the examples with parameter A < 8, the system evolves to a point where the numbers of (perhaps) foxes (Y) and rabbits (X) are forever fixed. In contrast, if the parameter A > 8, the system evolves to a limit-cycle attractor, in which both X and Y forever oscillate but out of phase.

for constructing the theory. This is a central issue in the theoretical studies of neocortical dynamics of Chapters 11 and 14.

Given the availability of modern computers, we are not generally concerned with computing limitations on obtaining solutions to models involving many coupled equations if the number of parameters is fewer than two or three. However,

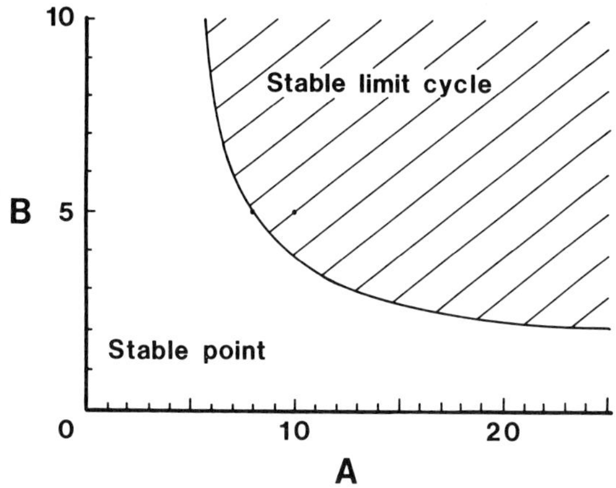

Figure 10-12. Two types of steady-state solution exhibited by (10.11) and (10.12) depend on parameters A and B for fixed C = 1. The dots correspond to four solutions shown in Figure 10-11. (Reproduced with permission from May, 1981.)

each time another equation is added to the model, additional parameters that determine the degree of coupling are also added. These parameters may be known only approximately, or perhaps not at all. The number of computer runs necessary to investigate numerically a system with n parameters that take on N discrete values is N^n. For example, a system with two parameters, each of which can assume 100 discrete values, requires 10,000 computer runs to study numerically by "brute force." If five parameters are present, the same coverage (N) of each parameter requires 10^{10} computer runs, generally an impossible task even with today's fast computers. Of course, it is often possible to use both analytical methods and parameter knowledge to limit the required scope of numerical studies, especially for nonchaotic attractors.

More complex systems can have multiple limit cycles. In this case, the initial conditions determine which limit cycle attracts system dynamics. The region of phase space for which the initial conditions produce a steady-state solution on a particular attractor (such as a particular limit cycle) is called the basin of the attractor. Usually this set of points in phase space is connected and forms a continuous subspace. This implies that when the input parameters are away from a boundary in phase space, small uncertainties in the parameters will not affect the behavior of the system. In such cases, we can reduce the number of values (N) assigned to each parameter because small to moderate changes may not cause substantial changes in dynamic behavior (at least for certain parameter ranges). However, in many nonlinear systems, boundaries are not smooth, that is they may be fractal. In this case, small uncertainties in either initial conditions or system parameters can introduce such profound changes in the evolution of observed dynamics that predicting the motion becomes impossible. The number of parameter values N required to cover all possible dynamic outcomes may increase without limit. Such dynamic systems are said to have fractal basin boundaries and strange attractors.

Forced Oscillations

To illustrate some salient characteristics of forced nonlinear systems, consider again the Duffing equation (10.1) with $B_0 = 0$. This equation describes the oscillations of magnetic flux in the core of the nonlinear inductor of the circuit shown in Figure 10-1 with the dc current $i_0 = 0$. It also describes the oscillations of the simple mass on a spring system shown in Figure 8-1b for a spring with a nonlinear restoring force. In nonlinear studies, it is useful to rewrite (10.1) as two first-order equations

$$\frac{dX}{dt} = Y$$

$$\frac{dY}{dt} = -2\alpha Y - \omega_0^2 X - \beta X^3 + B \cos \Omega t \qquad (10.14)$$

where the symbols Φ and $d\Phi/dt$ have been replaced by X and Y, respectively. This system differs from the Van der Pol and ecologic systems described previously in that the explicit time-dependent term ($\cos \Omega t$) occurs. In the language of nonlinear dynamics, this system is called nonautonomous because of the addition of this new term.

When the nonlinear term βX^3 is absent, this system exhibits classical linear resonance behavior. That is, all parameters except the forcing frequency Ω are fixed, and this frequency is varied from values less than to values greater than the natural frequency of the system ω_0. The amplitude of the response, that is, X(t) averaged over half a cycle, is maximum when $\Omega = (\omega_0^2 - 2\alpha^2)^{1/2}$, and the resonance curve contains a sharp peak for small damping, $\alpha << \omega_0$, as shown in Figure 8-2 and (8.15).

The inclusion of a small nonlinear effect ($\beta > 0$; hard spring for nonlinear spring systems) changes the linear resonant curve in the manner shown in Figure 10-13 (Stoker, 1951; Minorsky, 1962). Thus, if we begin by increasing the forcing frequency from Ω_1, the amplitude of oscillation steadily increases by following the curve 1-2. For a frequency slightly greater than Ω_2, the amplitude decreases suddenly to the lower branch 4-5, yielding the much smaller amplitude at point 3. Further increases in Ω toward point 4 result in a gradual reduction in amplitude. If the forcing frequency is then reduced, the amplitude follows the curve 4-3-5; however, at point 5 an abrupt change occurs as the amplitude increases from point 5 to 6. Further decreases in Ω follow the curve 6-1. This jump phenomenon is often called hysteresis, even though it may have minimal relation to the usual hysteresis effects in magnetic materials.

Jump phenomena are, of course, qualitatively different from those associated with linear resonance, in which there is a unique relation between amplitude and forcing frequency. We can imagine the confusion that jump phenomena might cause in laboratory experiments if not anticipated by theoretical analysis. For example, such experiments might appear not to be reproducible. The analogous effect for a radio or television tuner (which involves a resonant circuit or filter)

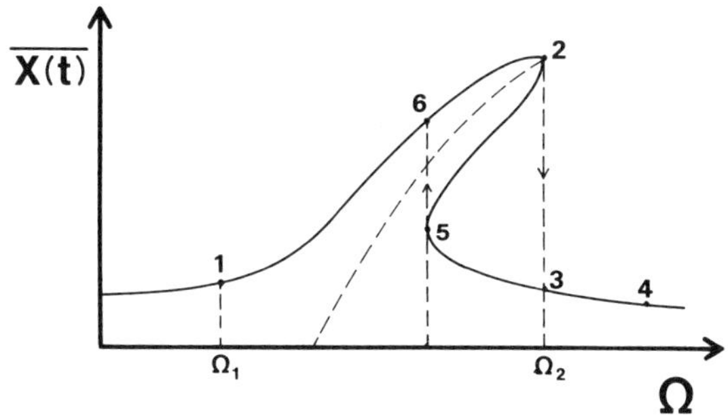

Figure 10-13. Resonance curve for a nonlinear, forced oscillator illustrating jump phenomena. Vertical axis is amplitude of oscillation. Horizontal axis is frequency (Ω) of the forcing function. This particular curve corresponds to resonance in the Duffing equation, such as oscillations of a mass connected to a nonlinear (hard) spring. The amplitude of the resonance in response to a change in driving frequency depends on whether frequency is increasing or decreasing. See the text for more detail. (Reproduced with permission from Minorsky, 1962.)

would be when stations actually received at fixed points on the dial depend on the direction in which the dial is turned!

Nonlinear systems in general, and the Duffing equation in particular, can show a variety of periodic and nonperiodic behavior. To illustrate expected types of periodic solutions, we may write down the general solution to the usual, second-order system with zero damping, that is, (10.1) or (10.14) with $\alpha = \beta = 0$. The solution is expressed as the sum of free and forced oscillations

$$X(t) = \left(A + \frac{B}{\Omega^2 - \omega_0^2}\right) \cos \omega_0 t - \frac{B}{\Omega^2 - \omega_0^2} \cos \Omega t \qquad (10.15)$$

where A is the initial condition X(0), and $\dot{X}(0) = 0$ is assumed. As argued by Stoker (1950), all possible types of periodic motion may be obtained from (10.15). The solutions are periodic only if one of the following occurs:

1. $C = A + B/(\Omega^2 - \omega_0^2) = 0$. The free oscillation does not occur. The motion is called a harmonic oscillation with frequency Ω, and amplitude depends on the frequency.
2. $\omega_0 = \Omega/n$. Here n is any integer except 1 and $C \neq 0$. The motion is called a subharmonic oscillation. That is, X(t) is composed of the forcing frequency plus a subharmonic frequency of order n.
3. $\omega_0 = m\Omega$. Here m is any integer except 1 and $C \neq 0$. The motion may be called an ultraharmonic oscillation.
4. $\omega_0 = (m/n)\Omega$. Here m and n are relatively prime integers and $C \neq 0$. The motion may be called an ultrasubharmonic oscillation.

Because all real systems have some damping, which involves multiplication of the first term of (10.15) by a negative exponential, cases 2 through 4, which require the coexistence of free and forced oscillations, normally will not be observed in actual practice. (For linear systems with very small damping, these cases may be approximated over a limited time interval.) However, in nonlinear systems, all four cases may occur even when damping is present. A variety of solutions (both periodic and chaotic) to the forced Duffing equation are presented in the section Periodic and Chaotic Behavior in a Duffing System.

Chaotic Dynamics

Throughout this book we have considered several physical and biologic systems. Implicit in these discussions has been the general idea that simple systems, that is, systems with few degrees of freedom, behave simply. Certainly this idea is justified for linear systems; however, with nonlinear systems, qualitatively new phenomena have been described that are entirely unpredictable by linear theory, such as limit cycles, jump phenomena, subharmonics, action potentials, and so forth. Despite these complexities, there has been no reason to anticipate any fundamental limitations on the study of simple systems. Thus, until recently, many investigators believed that with modern, fast computers all simple systems, and indeed many complex systems, could be solved. That is, given the initial state of some simple system, all future states of the system can be predicted.

We have long known that complex systems, that is systems with many degrees of freedom, can show apparently random behavior even though the governing equations of motion are fully deterministic. The recent revolution in the field of nonlinear dynamics occurred because of a wider appreciation of the fact that even simple systems, if nonlinear, can exhibit very complex, seemingly random behavior. The modern term for this phenomenon is chaos, a class of dynamic behavior that is very sensitive to initial conditions. That is, chaotic systems quickly "forget" their initial states. This loss of information may be pictured using the phase plane plot shown in Figure 10-14 (Moon, 1992). For example, suppose the position X and velocity Y of some part of a mechanical system are known at arbitrary time t_0 with accuracies ΔX and ΔY, respectively. If the phase plane (or 2N-dimensional phase space, if the system has N degrees of freedom) is divided into areas (or N-dimensional volumes) of size $\Delta X\,\Delta Y$, the system initially occupies the shaded area of Figure 10-14a. In chaotic systems, this uncertainty increases exponentially with time, that is, the area or volume is expressed by

$$V = V_0 e^{h(t-t_0)} \quad t \geq t_o \tag{10.16}$$

where $V_0 = \Delta X\,\Delta Y$ in a system with one degree of freedom. The exponent h measures the rate of information loss and is related to "entropy" in information theory. The exponent h is also related to the Lyapunov exponents, which are measures of the rate at which nearby phase space trajectories of a system diverge.

A very simple example of a nonlinear dynamical system that can exhibit chaotic behavior is the difference equation

$$X_{n+1} = \lambda X_n(1 - X_n) \tag{10.17}$$

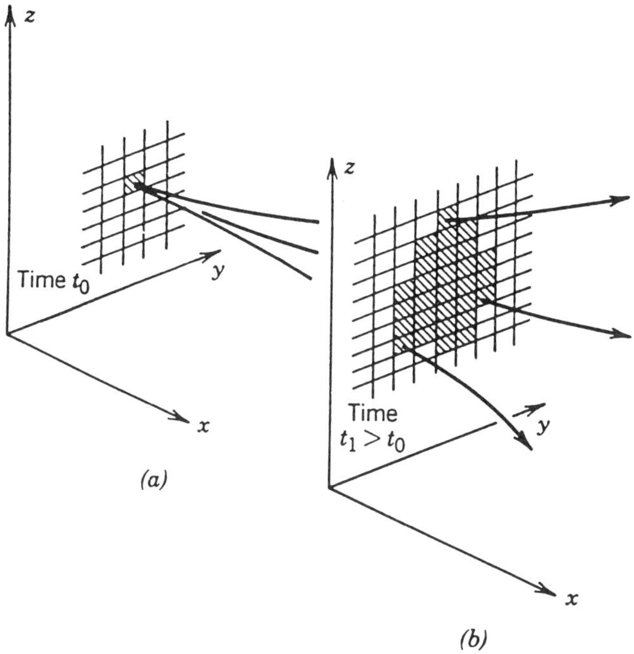

Figure 10-14. Divergence of system trajectories in phase space. Chaotic systems are defined by exponential divergence of such trajectories. (Reproduced with permission from Moon 1992.)

called the logistic map (May, 1976). This equation has been used as a model for population growth of a single, isolated species in which there is no overlap between successive generations and thus population growth occurs in discrete steps. Examples are provided by many temperate-zone anthropods, such as cicadas (May, 1981). Equation (10.17) provides the opposite extreme to the case of completely overlapping generations considered previously. Here X_n is the normalized population of the species at generation n, which lies in the range $0 < X_n < 1$, and λ is a parameter that determines the strength of the nonlinearity.

In the continuous case (of completely overlapping generations), the population simply grows or decreases to some equilibrium value, the carrying capacity of the environment as indicated by (10.13). We might expect qualitatively similar behavior in the discrete case of nonoverlapping generations, described by (10.17). In fact, for values of the parameter $\lambda < 1$ or $\lambda > 4$, the population always decreases to zero. For $1 < \lambda < 3$, almost all initial populations eventually evolve to the equilibrium population $X = (\lambda - 1)/\lambda$, thereby confirming qualitative expectations based on the continuous case. However, as λ is increased between 3 and 4, remarkable changes occur in the system dynamics, as shown in Figure 10-15. For $\lambda = 2.99$, the population evolves to a fixed state; however, for $\lambda = 3.1$, the fixed point has become unstable so that the population evolves to a steady state in which population alternates between two values $X \sim 0.5$ and 0.8 (in a manner

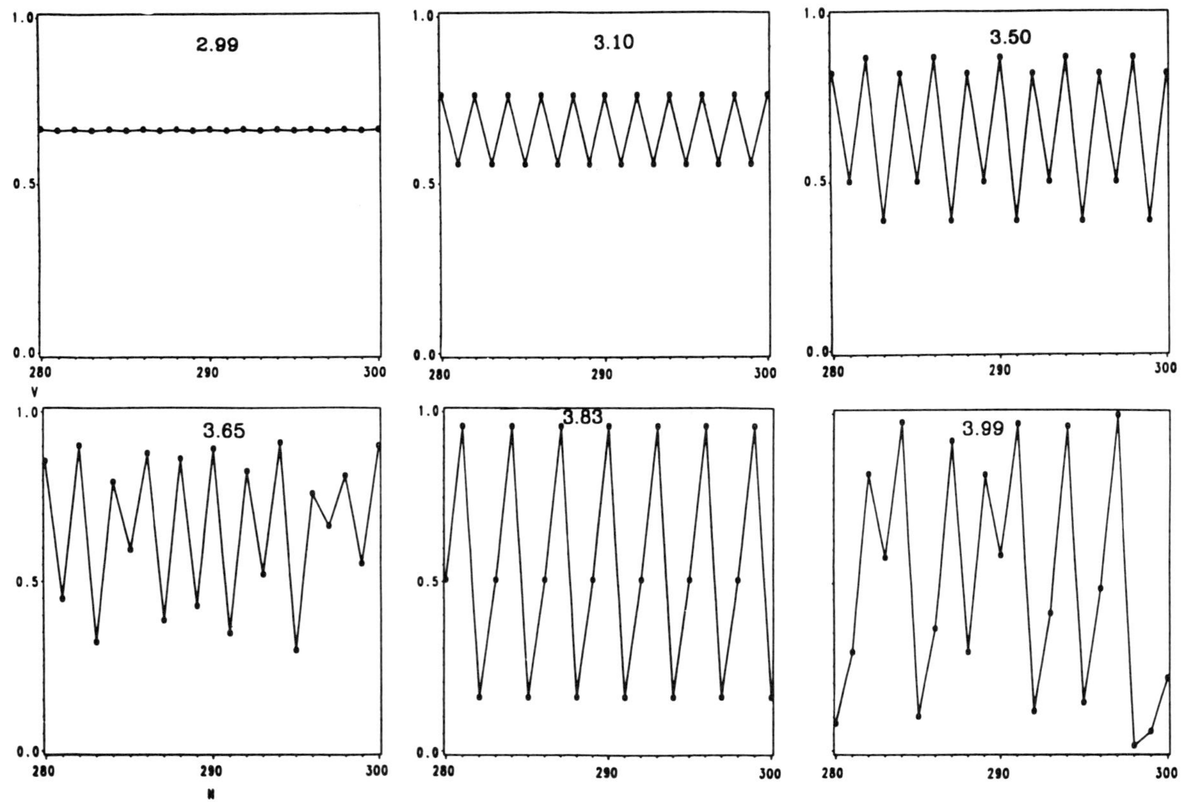

Figure 10-15. Steady-state solution for the logistic map (10.17) for several values of the nonlinear parameter λ. The vertical axis X_n might, for example, represent normalized species populations at the nth generation (horizontal axes). The steady-state solution changes from a constant value (λ = 2.99) to oscillation between two states (λ = 3.10) to oscillation between four states (λ = 3.50) to chaos (λ = 3.65) to oscillation between three states (λ = 3.83) and again to chaos (λ = 3.99).

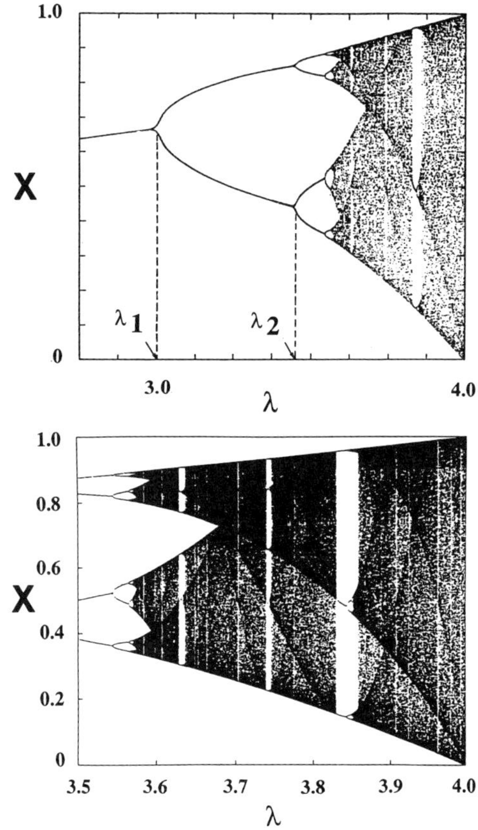

Figure 10-16. Bifurcation diagram for the logistic map (10.17). Plots show the occurrence of states X_n (steady-state solution, that is large n) as a function of nonlinear parameter λ. Top. First- and second-period doublings are shown at λ_1 and λ_2, respectively. Bottom. More detail is shown in chaotic and periodic regions. (Reproduced with permission from Jensen, 1987.)

somewhat analogous to a limit cycle). This is called a period 2 cycle because X_n is periodic with a period of $n = 2$ generations. For somewhat larger values of λ, the period 2 cycle becomes unstable and is replaced by a period 4 cycle, in which the population alternates between four different levels. As λ is increased further but only slightly, the steady-state dynamics become period 8, period 16, and so on, finally becoming a motion of infinite period or chaos at $\lambda \sim 3.57$. The asymptotic (long time) behavior of the system as the parameter λ is increased between 1 and 4 is displayed in Figure 10-16.

The bifurcation diagrams of Figure 10-16 are created as follows. At many large values of n such that steady state is obtained in each case, a mark is placed corresponding to the computed value of X and the parameter λ. For values of λ less than about 3.57, the system can be in only a certain number of discrete states, which follow the plotted lines for increasing values of λ. The first bifurcation occurs at $\lambda = 3.0000$; successive bifurcations occur as λ is increased toward the chaotic region that forms most of the region $\lambda > 3.5700$. Within the chaotic region, many values of X are possible but with unequal probabilities, which explains the patchy appearance of Figure 10-16. However, also within this mostly chaotic region are narrow bands in which periodic motion returns. For example, the broadest of these bands begins at $\lambda = 3.8284$, where a period 3 cycle begins (May, 1976).

As the parameter λ is increased, the probability density function $P(X)$ of the steady-state motion spreads vertically (except in the periodic regions). In particular, when $\lambda = 4$, $P(X)$ is a continuous function on the interval $0 \leq X \leq 1$ and is expressed by (Ulam and von Neumann, 1947)

$$P(X) = [X(1 - X)]^{1/2} \tag{10.18}$$

Equation (10.18) is qualitatively similar to the probability density for the continuous function $X(t) = 1/2(1 + \sin \omega t)$, that is, points in the bifurcation diagram are continuously distributed but more dense near $X = 0$ and 1. In contrast, the probability density functions in the periodic regions are sums of delta functions. The nature of $P(X, \lambda)$ is also indicated by the dark streaks that crisscross the chaotic domains in Figure 10-16. These regions of local ridges in $P(X, \lambda)$ were discovered "experimentally" by displaying hundreds of thousands of iterations of the logistic map. Once discovered, their explanation was simple. The intersections of dark streaks in Figure 10-16 correspond to crises in the chaotic dynamics, where disjoint intervals of chaotic orbits collide to form larger regions. Similar crises are a current topic of research in physical systems (Jensen and Meyers, 1985; Jensen, 1987).

Several general concepts exhibited by the logistic map and other systems discussed here are actually observed in many physical systems and may eventually prove to be important in studies of neocortical dynamics.

1. Bifurcations: Changes in the qualitative steady-state behavior of system dynamics to multiple branches occur when some parameter or set of parameters is varied. Examples are jump phenomena in nonlinear resonance, the transition from stable point to limit cycles (Hopf bifurcation), and the period-doubling bifurcations of the logistic map.
2. Routes to chaos: The logistic equation illustrates one important way in which chaotic behavior may emerge in system dynamics. In this case, it is the period doubling route to chaos. That is, the range of the parameter λ over which a single cycle is stable decreases quickly as the period of the cycle increases so that there is a rapid accumulation of cycles with larger and larger periods. The intervals over which a cycle is stable decrease at a fixed geometric rate (Feigenbaum, 1983). This and other features of the period doubling sequence occur in a variety of physical systems, including some turbulent fluids, oscillating chemical reactions, electric circuits, and ring lasers (Feigenbaum, 1980, reviews by Thompson and Stewart, 1986; Moon, 1992; Jensen, 1987). For example, in one experimental study of a nonlinear semiconductor circuit with an ac voltage generator with frequency Ω, the diode voltage (analogous to X of the logistic equation) showed bifurcation subharmonics of the driving frequency $\Omega/2^n$ to $\Omega/16$ as the amplitude of the driving frequency (analogous to λ of the logistic equation) was increased (Testa et al, 1982). Measured values of intervals for cycle stability agree with those predicted by theory, and a bifurcation diagram similar to Figure 10-16 is obtained. Thus many systems undergo an orderly and quantitatively predictable transition to chaos. Another possible route to chaos includes parameter changes leading to two or more Hopf bifurcations so that three si-

multaneous coupled limit cycles occur. This may be called the quasi-periodic route to chaos. Still another route involves long periods of periodic motion with bursts of chaos. As a parameter is changed, the bursts become more frequent and have longer duration. This behavior is called intermittency.

3. Statistical properties: The logistic map shares an important property with many nonlinear physical and biological systems; it exhibits apparently random behavior even though the equations of motion are fully deterministic. An alternate approach to following individual trajectories, such as the variable X, is to follow probability density functions. This is the approach of the theory of stochastic processes. The prime example is the classical theory of statistical mechanics, which accurately describes macroscopic properties of a gas, for example, in terms of velocity integrals over the probability density function $f(\mathbf{r}, \mathbf{v}, t)$, described in Chapter 9. In complex systems, a statistical approach is often appropriate (and usually necessary) regardless of whether microscopic chaos in the X variables is present. Typically we do not measure the X variables but rather macroscopic variables at coarser spatial–temporal scales. In such cases, the macroscopic significance of microscopic chaos may not be clear.

Periodic and Chaotic Behavior in a Duffing System

Following the work of Ueda (1980), we consider the dynamics represented by the nonlinear electric circuit or mechanical system described by

$$\frac{d^2X}{dt^2} + k\frac{dX}{dt} + X^3 = B\cos t \tag{10.19}$$

This is a somewhat simplified version of the Duffing equation (10.1) or (10.14), in which the number of parameters has been reduced to two (k, B) so a comprehensive study of system dynamics is more practical using analog and digital computation. Ueda's results are summarized in Figure 10-17, in which different kinds of steady-state solutions occur in regions of the parameter space (k, B) shown. The Roman numerals I, II, II′, II″, III, and IV indicate regions of periodic motion at the frequency ($\Omega = 1$) of the forcing function, that is, harmonic oscillations. The fractions m/n (m = 1, 3, 4, 5, 6, 7, 11; n = 2, 3) indicate regions in which subharmonic and ultrasubharmonic periodic motions are sustained.

Two types of chaotic regions are shown. In the dotted regions, chaotic motion always occurs; in the shaded regions, chaotic motion occurs only with certain initial conditions. Basins of attraction indicating which initial conditions lead to chaotic behavior are not shown. Also not all parameter details have been included in Figure 10-17. For example, ultrasubharmonic motions of higher orders (n = 4, 5, . . .) occur, but are not shown, and some details of small regions near the origin are omitted. Also different types of harmonic motion occur within each of the regions I, II, and so forth. Jump phenomena occur on the boundaries of regions I, II′, and III.

To obtain waveforms and spectra for solutions to the modified forced Duffing equation (10.19), we reproduced some of Udea's results using a standard fourth

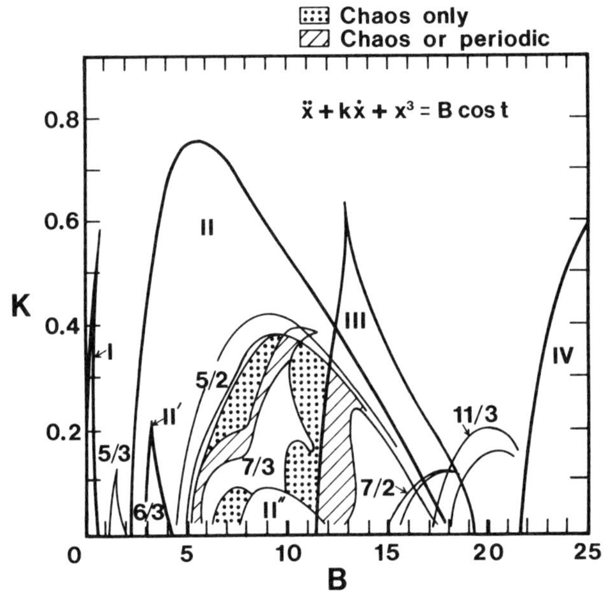

Figure 10-17. Types of steady-state solutions obtained from modified, forced Duffing equation (10.19) for different values of the parameters k and B. Periodic solutions of different types are obtained in all but dotted regions, where chaotic solutions occur independent of initial conditions. In shaded regions, chaos occurs only for certain initial conditions. Fractions indicate dominance of different ultrasubharmonics in periodic solutions. (Adapted with permission from Ueda, 1980 and Moon, 1992.)

or fifth order Runge-Kutta algorithm (IMSL program DIVPRK) with a step size of $\Delta t = 0.05$ (about 126 points per cycle of the driving frequency) to integrate (10.19) from $t = 0$, 150 (3,000 steps). Waveforms and spectra for $k = 0.1$ and various values of the parameter B are shown in Figure 10-18. As B is increased, the steady-state solution (shown for $50 \leq t \leq 150$) is first periodic with ultraharmonics $n = 2, 3, 4$, and so on (a), then chaotic with various harmonics and spectral broadening (b), and again periodic with ultraharmonics $n = 3, 5, 7$, and so forth (c). Similarly, in Figure 10-19, the line $k = 0.22$ is followed for increasing B. Case (d) is close to the chaotic boundary, case (e) is inside the chaotic region, and case (f) is apparently periodic but with many harmonics. Phase plane plots for all six examples are shown in Figure 10-20. The periods shown are for times $50 \leq t \leq 150$ except for case (f), which is shown for times $150 \leq t \leq 300$. The plot (f) for the earlier period is similar but contains small effects of the initial conditions. The orbits shown in the phase plane are attractors, either periodic attractors (cases a, c, f) or chaotic attractors (b, d, e). The terms chaotic attractor and strange attractor are often used interchangeably, although there are technical differences between the two.

In these examples, the difference between periodic and chaotic solutions appears clearly in the phase plane plots. The spectral plots also show a clear distinction,

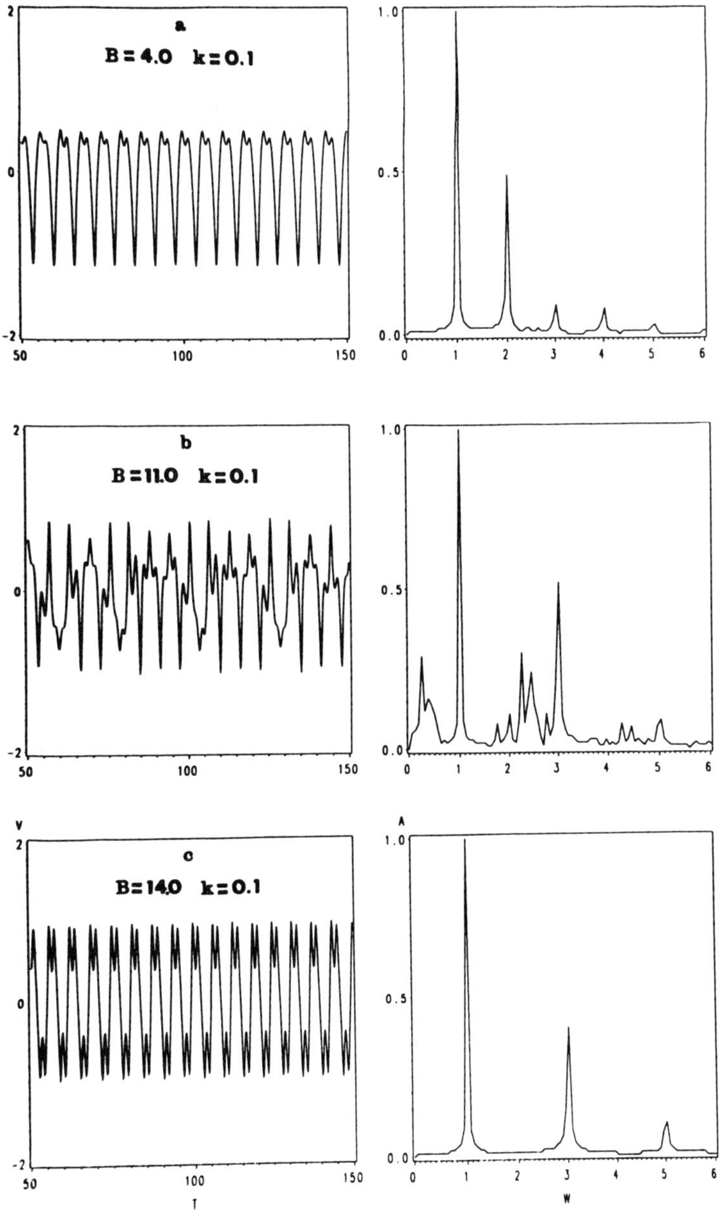

Figure 10-18. Steady-state solutions X(t) and corresponding amplitude spectra to modified, forced Duffing equation (10.19) for k = 0.1 and increasing values of control parameter B. Numerical solutions were obtained with International Mathematical and Statistical Library, Houston (IMSL) program DIVPRK, which uses the Runge-Kutta-Verner fifth- and sixth-order method. As predicted by Figure 10-17, the solution is first periodic (B = 4.0), then chaotic (B = 11.0), and again periodic (B = 14.0).

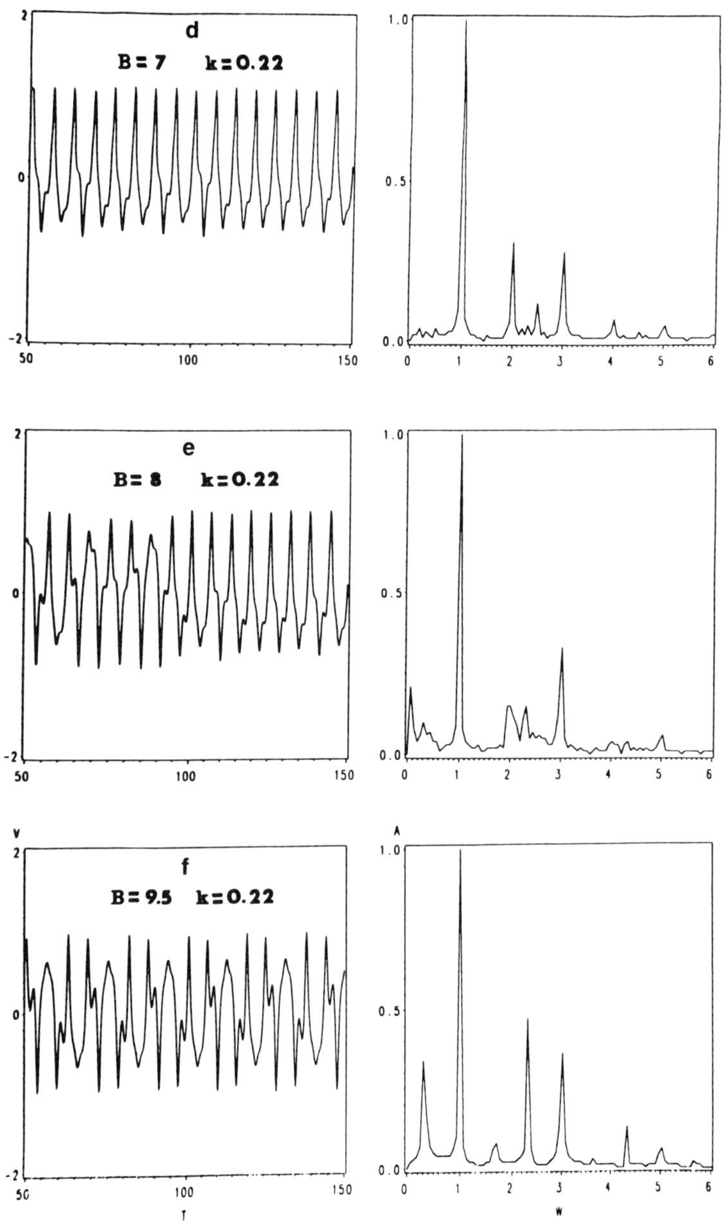

Figure 10-19. Solutions to (10.19) for k = 0.22 and increasing values of B. Weak chaos is evident in the first two cases (B = 7.0, 8.0). The case B = 9.5 exhibits a subharmonic at ⅓ the driving frequency, ultraharmonics at 3 and 5 times the driving frequency and ultrasubharmonics at the following fractions of the driving frequency: 5/3, 7/3, 11/3, 13/3, and 17/3. See the section Forced Oscillations for definitions of these terms.

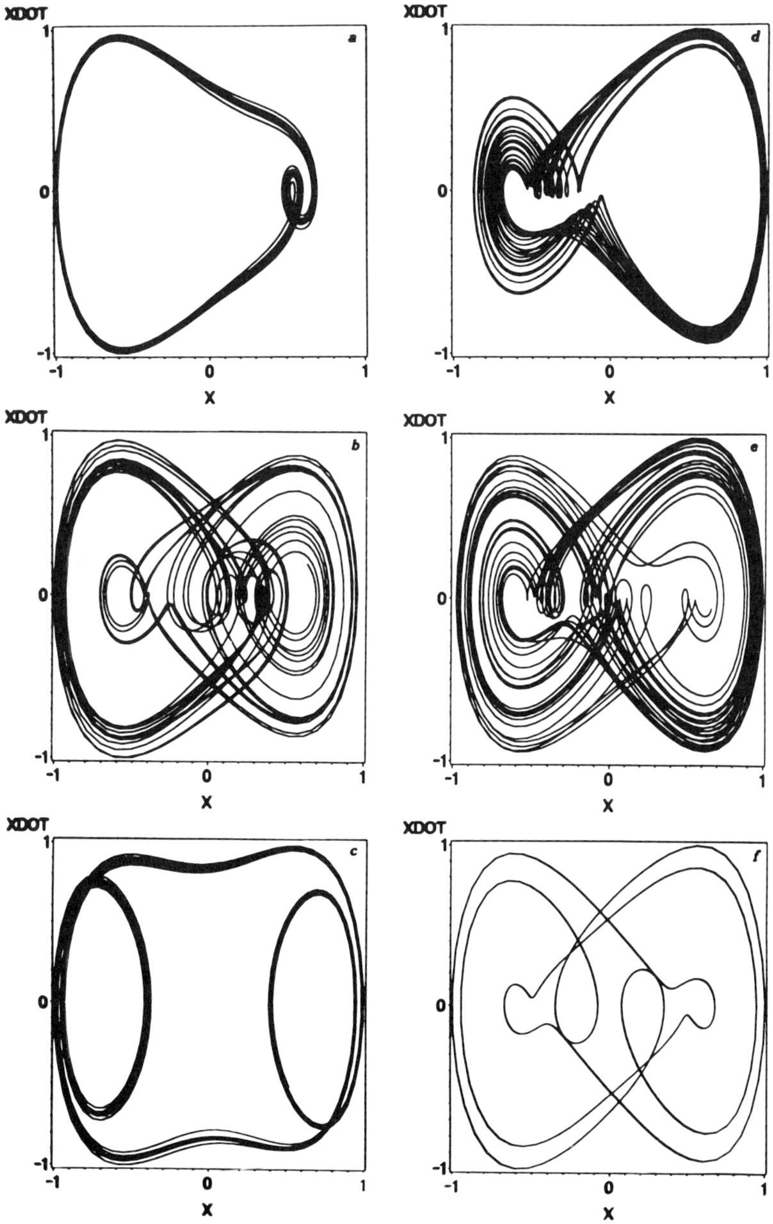

Figure 10-20. Phase plane plots for the six solutions of (10.19) shown in Figures 10-18 and 10-19. Periodic solutions occur in three cases (*a*, *c*, *f*) with the parameters k, B given by 0.1, 4.0; 0.1, 14.0; and 0.22, 9.5.

except perhaps for case (f), which contains many harmonics. From these results, we could draw the erroneous conclusion that identifying chaotic behavior in an unknown system is easy. In fact, it is usually difficult to identify chaos in unknown systems using only experimental data. There are at least two reasons for this. First, the number of degrees of freedom is unknown. In second-order systems with more than one degree of freedom, the resulting quasi-periodic behavior can be complicated in all types of plot. Second, the addition of noise to a signal of finite length can make the identification of chaos practically impossible in unknown complex systems.

Chaotic and Quasi-Periodic Behavior in Autonomous Systems

Nonautonomous systems (such as forced oscillators) involving two simultaneous first-order ordinary differential equations can produce chaotic behavior. Examples are the forced Duffing equation (10.19) and the forced Van der Pol oscillator. In autonomous systems, in which no driving term occurs, at least three simultaneous first-order equations are required to produce chaos. As an example autonomous system, consider the coupled system of two masses that move only in the horizontal direction, as shown in Figure 10-21. The spring on the left is assumed to have a cubic nonlinearity, whereas the other two springs are considered linear. The equations of motion for the displacements X and Y of the two masses are expressed by

$$
\begin{aligned}
\frac{dX}{dt} &= V_X \\
\frac{dV_X}{dt} &= -\omega_X^2 X - \beta X^3 + c_1 Y - d_1 V_X \\
\frac{dY}{dt} &= V_Y \\
\frac{dV_Y}{dt} &= -\omega_Y^2 Y + c_2 X - d_2 V_Y
\end{aligned}
\tag{10.20}
$$

Here V_X and V_Y are velocities of the two masses, ω_X, ω_Y are individual oscillation frequencies that occur if one mass is fixed, that is, $\omega_X^2 = (k_X + k)/m_X$ and $\omega_Y^2 = (k_Y + k)/m_Y$. The coupling constants are $c_1 = k/m_X$ and $c_2 = k/m_Y$. A small amount of damping ($d_1 = d_2 = 0.001$) is included to improve convergence of numerical solutions. In the linear case ($\beta = 0$), all oscillations are some linear combination of the two normal mode frequencies. This mixture of normal mode frequencies depends on how the masses are set in motion. With zero damping in the linear system, the two normal mode frequencies are (Morse and Ingard, 1968)

$$\omega^2 = \frac{1}{2}(\omega_X^2 + \omega_Y^2) \pm \frac{1}{2}[(\omega_X^2 - \omega_Y^2)^2 + 4c_1c_2]^{1/2} \tag{10.21}$$

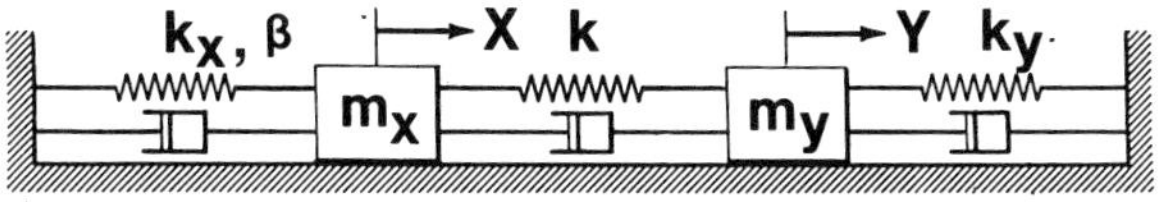

Figure 10-21. Two masses connected to three springs are assumed to undergo one-dimensional motion. The left-most spring has a cubic nonlinearity (k_x, β); the other two springs are linear (k and k_y). In the linear case ($\beta = 0$), the motion is expressed by some linear combination (depending on initial conditions) of the two normal mode frequencies (10.21). Example nonlinear solutions are shown in Figures 10-22 and 10-23. (Modified with permission from Sato, 1964.)

Numerical solutions of (10.20) for different values of the parameters are shown in Figures 10-22 (very strong coupling $k = 11$) and 10-23 (moderate coupling $k = 1$). For small values of the nonlinear parameter β (first column), the late time solutions are approximately those of the linear system, that is peaks in the frequency spectrum occur at the two frequencies given by (10.21). Because these two normal mode frequencies are incommensurate, the motion is quasi-periodic, as indicated by the phase plane plots. For $\beta = 4.5$ (second column of Figure 10-22), the spectrum broadens around each peak, a characteristic of weak chaos. The phase plane plot begins to look like a more tangled ball of string, also characteristic of chaos. Because these equations contain a little damping and there is no mechanism for energy input to the system, the oscillations eventually must cease, that is converge to an equilibrium point at the origin. However, the period studied here ($150 < t < 250$) occurs before substantial damping effects become apparent. No attempt is made to provide a comprehensive study of the coupled oscillators of Figure 10-21. Early studies of similar systems of two coupled nonlinear oscillators have shown they can exhibit chaotic behavior (Henon and Heiles, 1964).

The classic example of chaos in an autonomous system is the Lorenz system that tries to model thermal convection in a fluid (Lorenz, 1963). The original numerical study of these equations yielded unexpected results, that is random-like behavior by a deterministic system. This work ignited recent interest in chaotic systems. Although considerable doubt exists about how well this system describes the actual fluid mechanics, it has been studied extensively because of its interesting mathematical properties. The Lorenz system is described by the following set of equations:

$$\frac{dX}{dt} = A(Y - X)$$

$$\frac{dY}{dt} = -XZ + BX - Y \tag{10.22}$$

$$\frac{dZ}{dt} = XY - CZ$$

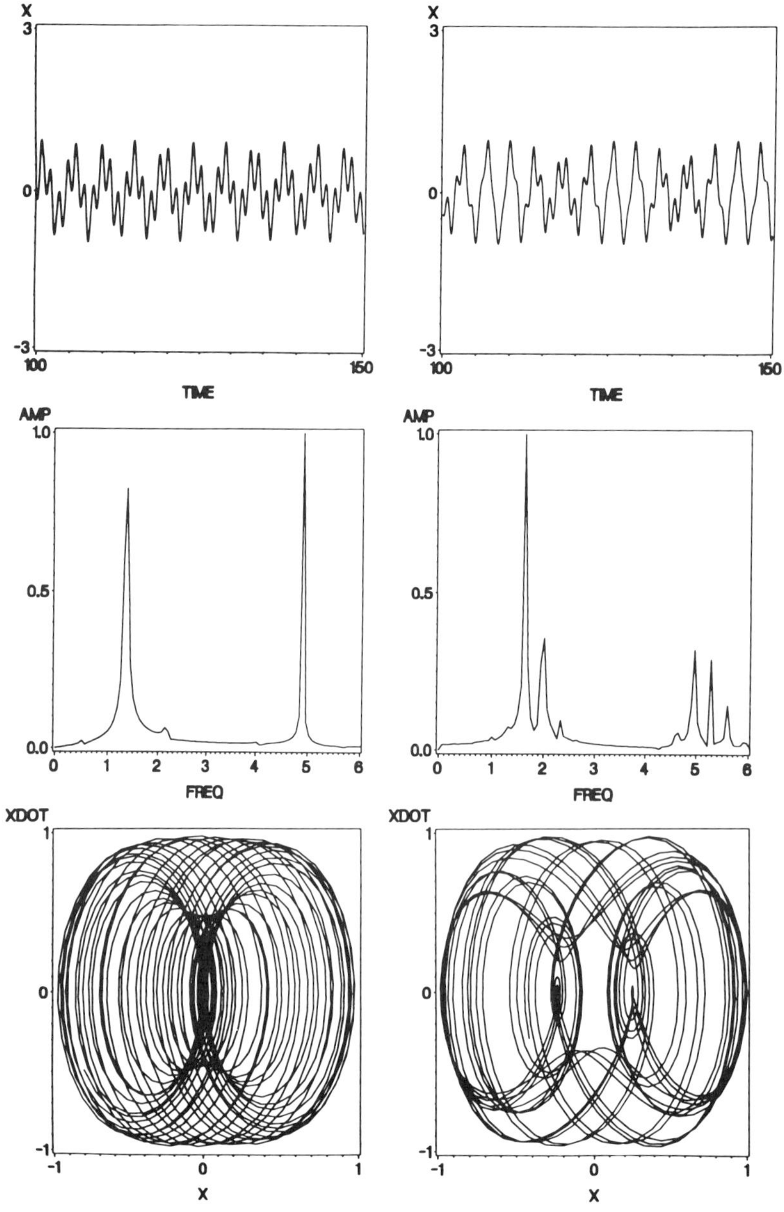

Figure 10-22. Steady-state solutions X(t), amplitude spectra, and phase plane plots for spring mass system of (10.20) and Figure 10-21. In all cases, the masses $m_x = m_y = 1$, and the damping $d_1 = d_2 = 0.001$. Strong coupling between the two masses ($k = 11$) is illustrated here for weak ($\beta = 3$, column 1) and stronger ($\beta = 4.5$, column 2) nonlinearity. For weak nonlinearity, principal peaks in spectra are expressed by (10.21) and the solution is close to periodic. Weak chaos is evident for stronger nonlinearity in the second column.

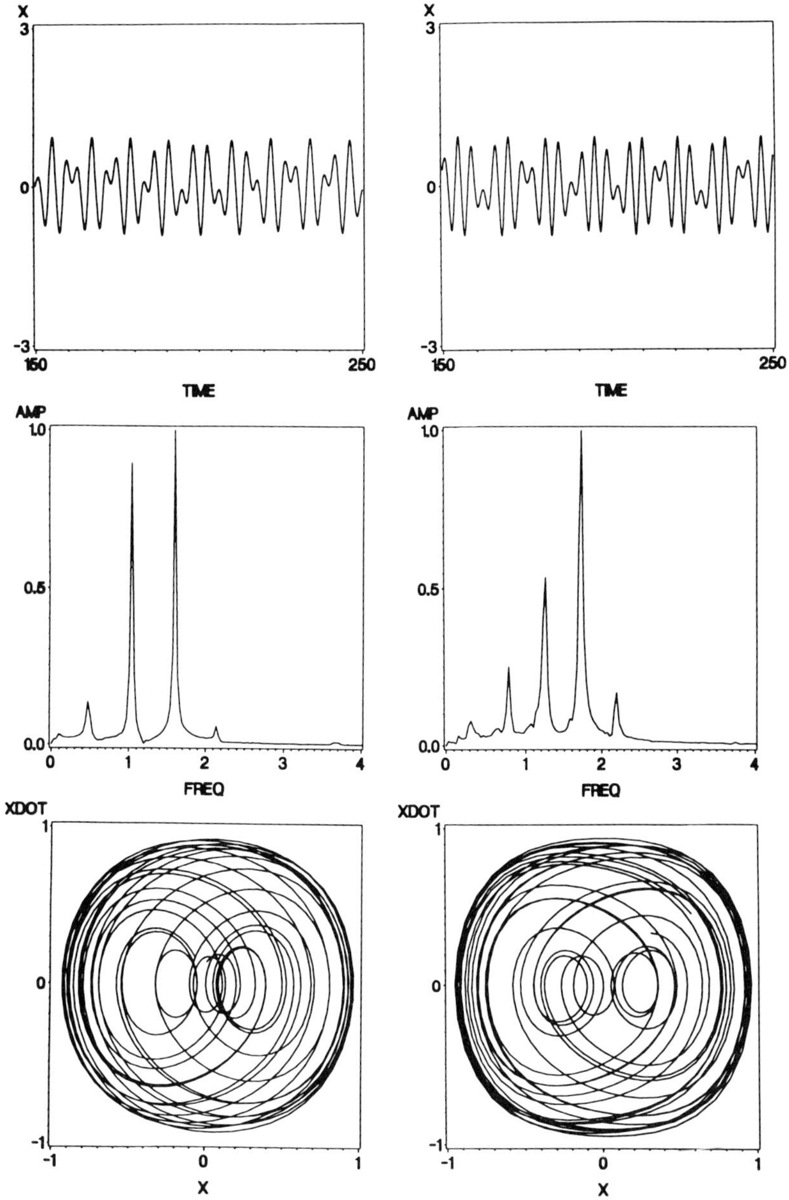

Figure 10-23. Steady-state solutions X(t), amplitude spectra, and phase plane plots for the spring-mass systems of (10.20) and Figure 10.21. Moderate coupling between the masses (k = 1) is illustrated for weak (β = 3, column 1) and stronger (β = 7, column 2) nonlinearity. Numerical solutions were obtained using IMSL program DIVPRK.

where X, Y, and Z are spatial Fourier coefficients of the stream function and temperature field. The nondimensional time t is inversely proportional to the depth of the tank squared. A, B, and C are Prandtl number, normalized Rayleigh number, and geometric factor dependent on the ratio of length to depth of the tank, respectively, which indicate the "background state" of the fluid system. With the choice of parameters A = 10 and C = 8/3 (following Lorenz), the behavior of the system has been examined as the control parameter B is varied. The numerical solution becomes chaotic, that is the dynamics becomes "turbulent" for $B > 24.74$. With very large B values, alternating regions of chaotic and periodic (limit cycle) behavior occur. Transitions from limit cycles to chaos occur through different types of intermittency (Bergé et al, 1984; Tabor, 1989) rather than through the period-doubling route expected of real physical turbulence.

The physical Lorenz fluid system is actually described by a complicated coupled set of nonlinear partial differential equations in the stream function Ψ and temperature T. To obtain the Lorenz equations (10.22) from this complicated system, these dependent variables are expanded in the spatial Fourier series

$$\Psi(x, y, t) = \sum_{m=1}^{\infty} \sum_{n=1}^{\infty} a_{mn}(t) \sin k_m x \sin \eta_n y$$
$$T(x, y, t) = \sum_{m=0}^{\infty} \sum_{n=1}^{\infty} b_{mn}(t) \sin k_m x \sin \eta_n y \qquad (10.23)$$

The dependent variables X, Y, and Z in (10.22) are the Fourier coefficients a_{11}, b_{11}, and b_{02}, respectively. To obtain the Lorenz system, all other coefficients in (10.23) are set to zero, that is only the very lowest modes (low spatial frequencies k_m and η_n) are included in the solution. This extreme truncation has no general mathematical justification (Tabor, 1989; Srinivasan and Nunez, 1993). That is, with linear systems (such as a vibrating membrane) we can choose initial conditions such that only selected modes occur in the motion. However, this is no longer generally true for nonlinear systems in which the modes are coupled. Equations (10.23) have been studied by retaining more modes (Curry, 1978). Rich dynamic behavior, including strange attractors, is obtained; however, the most sensitive parameter determining the motion is the number of modes retained in the truncation of the original fluid equations. This suggests that small-mode truncations of nonlinear partial differential equations generally will not yield reliable pictures of the actual behavior of systems in which many spatial scales are physically significant (Tabor, 1989). Such distinctions between interesting mathematical systems and real physical systems that they may or may not accurately describe are critical. This issue is addressed again in this chapter and in Chapter 11 in connection with neocortical dynamics.

Dynamics of Complex Systems

Many discrete systems with N degrees of freedom (in which time is the only independent variable, as described in Chapter 8) are governed by the set of N first-order ordinary differential equations

$$\frac{dX_i}{dt} = F_1(X_1, \ldots, X_N, t) \qquad i = 1, N \tag{10.24}$$

where the F_i are generally nonlinear functions of the independent variables X_i. For example, the two-mass spring system described previously involves motion only in one dimension. Because the equations of motion are second order, the system consists of $N = 2 \times 2 = 4$ first-order differential equations. If the two-mass system moved in a plane, the number of equations would have been $N = 8$. Equations (10.24) might also result from some approximation of continuous systems described by partial differential equations (such as the Lorenz system), but there is always a question of the validity of the truncation, discussed previously, when applied to nonlinear systems. Another system generally described by (10.24) is the classical three-body problem of mechanics, such as motion of a planet in a binary star system. General three-dimensional motion is, in this example, governed by $N = 18$ first-order equations (nine nonlinear), with dependent variables being the three positions and three velocities for each of the three bodies. This is a problem of enormous complexity involving motion in 18-dimensional phase space. Its notorious insolubility has been appreciated at least since the time of the famous mathematician Poincaré (1952) who studied it.

Comprehensive study of even moderately large systems may be impractical, even with combined analytic and computer methods, especially if the nonlinear functions contain more than two or three unknown parameters. For example, much effort has been devoted by more than a few researchers to examining the general nature of solutions to the Lorenz system, which involves only three equations and three parameters. Later in this chapter we will examine alternate ways to characterize dynamical systems, that is, methods that do not require precise knowledge of the motion of each of the dependent variables X_i.

One issue of current theoretical interest involves the criteria for chaos. There are good reasons to distinguish between local and spatio-temporal chaos, although it may be difficult to establish quantitative measures of the boundary between the two (Tabor, 1989). Local chaos is characterized by the behavior of trajectories X(t) in N-dimensional phase space. That is, closely neighboring chaotic trajectories, having slightly different initial conditions, diverge exponentially, as suggested by (10.16) and Figure 10-14, whereas nonchaotic trajectories separate only linearly with time. Local chaos can occur with regular spatial structure. By contrast, spatio-temporal chaos involves complex, changing spatial patterns such as occurs in turbulent fluids (Moon, 1992).

The rate of trajectory divergence is quantified in terms of the Lyapunov exponents, which measure the mean rate of exponential separation of neighboring trajectories. They provide a useful way to characterize known dynamical systems. Positive Lyapunov exponents indicate chaos and have been calculated for some systems. For example, when plotted against the parameter λ in the logistic equation (10.17), the first Lyapunov exponent is positive only in the chaotic regions shown in the bifurcation diagram of Figure 10-16 (Moon, 1992). Calculation of exponents for N-dimensional flows (differential equations) rather than maps (difference equations) is more difficult. Computer algorithms also have been developed to estimate Lyapunov exponents using only experimental data (Wolf et al, 1985). However, these methods are not robust when applied to noisy data or systems of high dimension having many degrees of freedom. Thus, when faced with an unknown and very complex system (such as the human brain), it may be difficult to identify chaos using only experimental data, such as EEG. We will return to this issue later.

An area of active research concerns the prediction of when local chaos first occurs and when local chaos changes to spatio-temporal chaos when parameters in (10.24) are changed (Tabor, 1989). Different types of dynamical systems have greater and lesser degrees of randomness, a measure that may be related closely to the extent that chaos is present. For example, the term Lagrangian turbulence has been used to characterize phase space chaos exhibited by individual fluid–particle trajectories, as described by (10.24). These systems exhibit only temporal chaos. In contrast to Lagrangian turbulence, the term turbulence in fluid mechanics refers to the observed state of widespread or spatio–temporal chaos in which the fluid exhibits chaos at all spatial and temporal scales (also called Eulerian turbulence). The transition from laminar to turbulent flow in a pipe, for example, or at the surface of an airplane wing occurs at a characteristic Reynolds number, as fluid velocity is increased above a certain point. Although motion of a fluid satisfies a set of partial differential equations (the Navier–Stokes equations), no known solution of these equations satisfactorily describes the turbulent state of a fluid. We have only minimal understanding of possible connections between "turbulence" related to local chaos and described by (10.24) and the observed fluid turbulence that is (apparently) inherent in the full Navier–Stokes equations. Any such description probably involves wave–wave coupling, that is, interaction of spatial Fourier coefficients of different modes, an effect largely neglected in the derivation of the Lorenz system, for example.

In the study of genuine complex systems (rather than mathematical models), in which we try to match mathematics with experiment, many important questions remain. For example, how important is the occurrence of local chaos in submacroscopic variables X_i to macroscopically measurable quantities? That is, macroscopic variables typically involve a coarse graining in space or time or both of submacroscopic variables. Local chaos in the variables X_i may be, in practice, indistinguishable from noise. How sensitive are macroscopic variables to the operations of space and time averaging of chaotic variables? Are tests for local chaos really important in systems with many degrees of freedom in which the motion is very complex? These questions probably will be formulated in many contexts and in many fields in the near future.

Linearization in Complex Systems

There are several possible motivations to study linear versions of complex systems, such as the systems described by (10.24). Some systems are weakly nonlinear so that a good idea of the general behavior of the nonlinear system can be obtained using a linear approximation. For example, the fundamental oscillation frequency of the Van der Pol circuit can be estimated by that of an equivalent linear circuit when the parameter A is sufficiently small. A linear analysis of the Van der Pol equation would, of course, not reveal the existence of limit cycles, jump phenomena (for the forced system), and so on; however, we might obtain some important information using only a linear approach.

Another linear approach is that of perturbation theory, in which we search for solutions to the system of equations (10.24) in the form

$$X_i(t) = X_{i0}(t) + \varepsilon X_{i1}(t) + \varepsilon^2 X_{i2}(t) + \cdots \qquad i = 1, N \tag{10.25}$$

where the small parameter ε multiplies nonlinear terms in (10.24). A classic example is the treatment of the motion of the earth around the sun, in which the influence of Jupiter may be treated as a perturbation of the two-body problem. Truncation of the series (10.25) leads to a coupled set of linear equations. For systems with more than one degree of freedom, perturbation theory presents formidable problems associated with convergence of perturbation series. However, an important breakthrough occurred in the period 1954 to 1963 with the development of the KAM mathematical theorem (named after its developers Kolmogorov, Arnold, and Moser). Perturbation theory and its many variants is now a valuable tool and active area of research (Tabor, 1989).

A third linear approach to (10.24) is stability analysis, which concerns the behavior of the solution near the fixed points (or equilibrium points) in phase space, where all time derivatives of X_i are zero. With autonomous systems, the fixed points are obtained as solutions to the set of simultaneous equations

$$F_i(X_1, X_2, \ldots X_N) = 0 \qquad i = 1, N \tag{10.26}$$

The functions F_i are expanded in Taylor series about each of the fixed points, that is, for each fixed point (10.24) are replaced by a different set of linear equations that describe (approximately) the behavior of the system when it is close to the appropriate fixed point. The solution to the linearized version of (10.24) is

$$X_i(t) = \sum_{n=1}^{N} C_{in}\, e^{j\omega_n t} \qquad i = 1, N \tag{10.27}$$

where the N frequencies (at each fixed point) have real and imaginary parts, that is,

$$\omega_n = \omega_{Rn} - j\gamma_n \qquad n = 1, N \tag{10.28}$$

and are easily obtained from the standard methods of linear systems analysis. Stability near each fixed point is determined by the signs of the γ_n, as discussed in Chapter 8, that is all γ_n's equal to zero or negative indicates a stable, fixed point. If any γ_n is positive, the fixed point is unstable. Phase plane trajectories that approach an unstable fixed point will be repelled by it. They will be attracted to stable, fixed points, provided, of course, that the flow (dynamic behavior) brings the system sufficiently close to the fixed point where the linearized equations are valid approximations. When all $\gamma_n = 0$, the flow is a locally pure rotation about the fixed point, called a center in this case. Other names associated with fixed points are node, saddle point, and spiral point, depending on the local shape of the phase space trajectory.

With linear stability analysis of nonlinear equations, we try to construct an approximate idea of the "global" (in all of phase space) nature of the system dynamics by creating linearized solutions that are valid only in the neighborhoods of the fixed points. This approach has serious limitations when applied to systems with more than a few degrees of freedom (Hayashi, 1964) and probably is most useful when combined with numerical methods. Linear approximations typically require some understanding (either physical or mathematical) of the full nonlinear problem to specify regions where linear approximations are valid.

To gain some understanding of complex systems, consider the coupled oscillations of a loaded string similar to that in Figure 8-6. When each mass is connected only to masses on either side (nearest-neighbor interactions), the equations of motion for small displacement are expressed by (8.24). This is a special case of (10.24), in which each of the functions F_i depend on at most three X_i, and the nonlinear equations (for large displacement) have been linearized. Consider the case in which more distant neighbors are also coupled by elastic strings with identical properties. This problem is of interest in part because of the importance of long-range (corticocortical) interaction in neocortex. Because coupling between more distant masses involves longer strings, the vertical restoring forces due to distant coupling weaken progressively. For example, with nearest- and next-nearest neighbor coupling, the equations of motion are

$$\frac{d^2X_i}{dt^2} = \frac{T}{ma}\left[X_{i-1} + X_{i+1} - 3X_i + \frac{1}{2}(X_{i+2} + X_{i-2})\right] \qquad i = 1, N \qquad (10.29)$$

which is analogous to (8.24). Solutions to (10.29) or string systems with more distant coupling are given by (10.27), with all $\gamma_n = 0$. If suitable boundary conditions are applied (such that each mass has the same number of attached strings), the normal mode frequencies ω_n are obtained by substitution of (10.27) into (10.29) (or similar equation for more distant coupling) and solution of the resulting linear, algebraic equations obtained (Morse and Ingard, 1968).

Results for 100 masses on the string (N equal to 200 degrees of freedom) and coupling to nearest neighbors, nearest and next-nearest neighbors to nearest through 32nd nearest neighbors are shown in Figure 10-24. In each case, 100 real, normal mode frequencies (positive and negative ω_n occur in pairs) are plotted versus mode number. The actual motion of the system, obtained by including effects of the coefficients C_{in} in (10.27), depends on the manner in which the oscillation is started. Normal mode frequencies are normalized so that the lowest modes ω_1 are equal in each of the three cases (by adjusting the string tension T, mass m, or mass separation a). The effect of more distant coupling is then a compression of the range of the normal mode frequencies, that is, frequency ratios are $\omega_{100}/\omega_1 = 64.3$ (nearest neighbor), 39.5 (nearest and next-nearest neighbor), and 5.03 (nearest neighbor through 32nd nearest neighbor). Thus, as the system be-

Figure 10-24. The normal modes of a loaded string system similar to that of Figure 8-5 with 100 discrete, equal masses m, separated by equal distances. Non-local interactions may occur, that is the masses may be connected by more than one string to distant masses. Nearest-neighbor, nearest- and next-nearest neighbor, and so on interactions may occur. The normal mode frequencies ω_n (n = 1,100) are shown for the case of nearest-neighbor interactions only (1), nearest- and next-nearest neighbor interactions (2), and interactions from nearest neighbor through 32nd nearest neighbor (32). System parameters in (10.28) or similar equations have been adjusted so that the fundamental frequency ω_1 is the same in all three cases. More distant coupling, that is longer interaction lengths, compresses the range of normal mode frequencies, that is, simpler motion occurs.

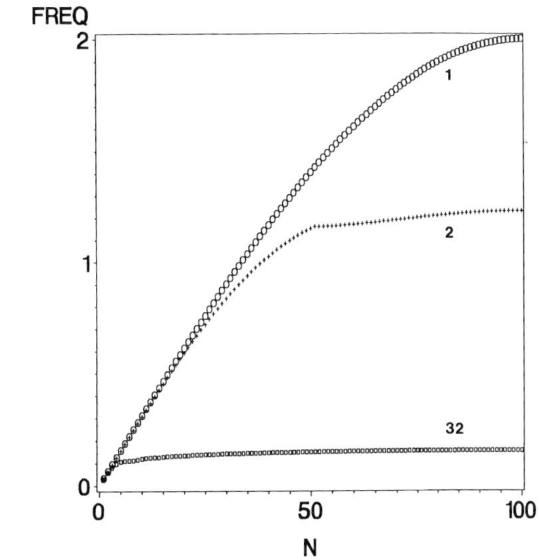

comes more strongly coupled by long-range interactions, it behaves more like a system with fewer degrees of freedom. Furthermore, the loaded string system contains a memory that is both distributed and local. That is, information about the initial state of the system is coded in the coefficients C_{in} of (10.27), where the i index represents a local property (amplitude of mass X_i), and the n index denotes a global property (amplitude associated with each normal mode). Phase plane plots for cases of nearest-neighbor and more distant coupling are obtained from (10.27) and shown in Figure 10-25. Initial conditions for these examples were chosen so the coefficients $|C_{in}|$ decrease as $1/\sqrt{n}$. As expected, inclusion of more distant coupling between masses leads to simpler motion, that is motion with fewer effective degrees of freedom.

Inclusion of the linear loaded string example under the category of "complex systems" might elicit objections. After all, the motion expressed by (10.27) is easily obtained for arbitrarily large N if computer memories are not exceeded. However, suppose we try to obtain experimental data from an unknown system, such as neocortex. In this case, neither the degree of linearity nor the number of degrees of freedom of the system are known a priori. Experimental data are typically sampled at some fixed rate (limiting high-frequency content that can be observed in the spectrum) and over a finite time period (thereby limiting the lowest frequencies that can be observed). Furthermore, real data contain noise with statistical properties that usually are not well known. We may in fact, obtain only

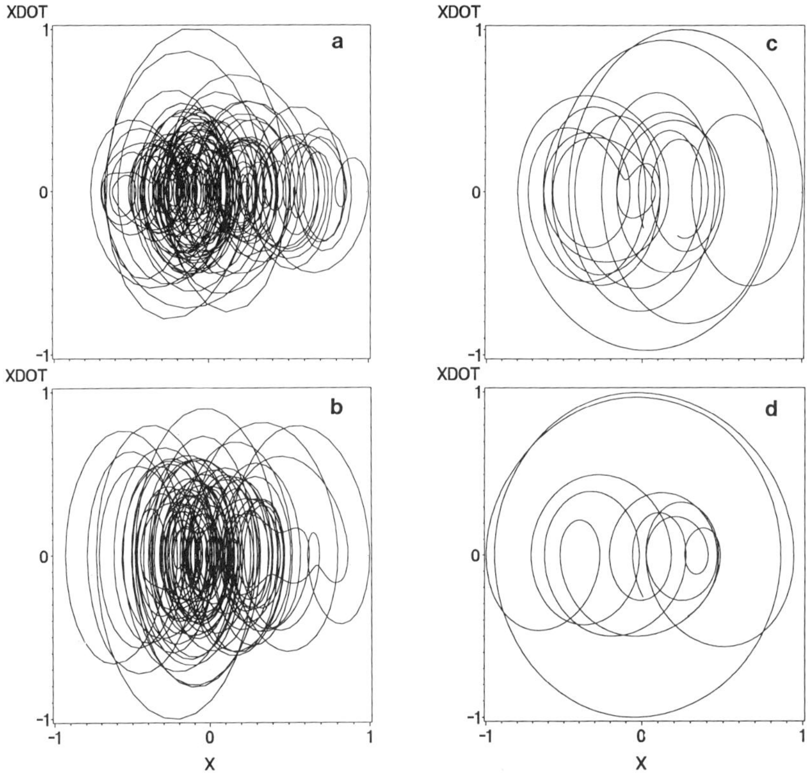

Figure 10-25. Motion in the phase plane of one of the masses $X_i(t)$ of the loaded string system, expressed by (10.27), with N = 100 normal mode frequencies. The amplitude associated with each mode C_{in} is arbitrarily chosen to decrease as $n^{-1/2}$. In each case, the time shown is t = 400 (arbitrary units). (**a**) nearest-neighbor interactions only. (**b**) nearest- and next nearest-neighbor interactions. (**c**) nearest- and up to 16th nearest-neighbor interactions. (**d**) nearest- and up to 32nd nearest-neighbor interactions. The dimension of the attractor (that is, the effective number of degrees of freedom) decreases as the interaction distance increases. A similar process may occur in neocortex, for example in epilepsy and anesthesia.

minimal information about the underlying nature of an unknown system with many degrees of freedom, given only a finite length of noisy data, other than to characterize the system by the usual statistical measures, such as power spectra. Therefore, we should examine carefully claims of chaotic behavior in neocortex when the only evidence is provided by an EEG waveform. Even linear systems can produce very complex waveforms.

Continuous Nonlinear Systems and Solitons

Relatively simple nonlinear systems can exhibit complex behavior. In contrast, let the number of degrees of freedom N become infinite so that our medium is treated as a continuum, as in the transition from Chapter 8 to Chapter 9. Thus we might replace the set (10.24) by a simple partial differential equation for the dependent variable $\Psi = \Psi(x, t)$, which replaces all the dependent variables X_i, and the spatial variable x replaces the index i (indicating local variables). We would expect the behavior of such systems to be even more complex than those with moderate numbers of degrees of freedom. Although this is often the case, such as with spatio-temporal chaos, there are also many important cases in which the behavior is regular. The propagation of an action potential along a nerve axon is, of course, the classical example of such regular but highly nonlinear behavior in the field of neurophysiology. There are, in addition, several important phenomena that are adequately described by quasi-linear theories, in which systems in some sense are close to linear.

An important class of strongly nonlinear waves in physical media are soliton waves, which remain stable as they propagate. Observation of a soliton was first reported 150 years ago by a Scottish engineer in the form of a water wave produced by a boat in a narrow channel. As he described it, the boat stopped and the wave

> rolled forward with great velocity, assuming the form of a large solitary elevation, a rounded, smooth and well defined heap of water, which continued its course along the channel apparently without change of form or diminution of speed. I followed it on horseback and overtook it still rolling on at a rate of some eight or nine miles an hour, preserving its original figure some thirty feet long and a foot to a foot and half in height. Its height gradually diminished and after a chase of two miles I lost it in the windings of the channel (Russel, 1844).

This moving "heap" of water had a different appearance and behavior than the usual deep water waves propagating from the bow of a moving boat, and its existence was at first doubted. However, theoretical support for the phenomena has since been obtained, that is, long wavelength, shallow water wave propagation can be approximated by the "KdV equation" (Gibbon, 1985; Tabor, 1989)

$$\frac{\partial \Psi}{\partial t} + \beta \Psi \frac{\partial \Psi}{\partial x} + \frac{\partial^3 \Psi}{\partial x^3} = 0 \tag{10.30}$$

Here β is the nonlinear parameter and the dependent variable $\Psi(x, t)$ is a transformed wave amplitude. The time (t) and distance (x) also have been transformed to incorporate the relevant physical parameters, that is depth of channel, gravitational constant, surface tension, and density of the liquid.

A ubiquitous property of nonlinear waves is that they steepen and eventually break as they propagate. This property is observed, for example by surfers, as deep water ocean waves approach a shore; steepening is caused by influence of the sea bottom. Wave steepening caused by nonlinearity also occurs in shock formation by sound waves. Strong electromagnetic waves in material media also may show similar behavior. For example, the field of nonlinear optics has become increasingly important with the advent of more powerful lasers. The middle term of (10.30) leads to water wave steepening; however, the right-most term leads to wave dispersion, a linear phenomenon that causes the wave packet to spread out spatially. The existence of stable solitary water waves generally is due to a balance between nonlinearity and dispersion. The study of solitons is an active area of research, for example, in the case of nonlinear plasma waves with possible application to controlled fusion.

Another nonlinear partial differential equation being studied is the driven, damped sine-Gordon equation

$$\frac{\partial^2 \Psi}{\partial t^2} + 2\alpha \frac{\partial \Psi}{\partial t} - c^2 \frac{\partial^2 \Psi}{\partial x^2} + \beta^2 \sin \Psi = B(x) \sin \Omega t \tag{10.31}$$

If $\beta = 0$, this is the one-dimensional version of the wave equation (9.1), which is linear and describes, for example, the forced vibration of a stretched string or voltage oscillations in a transmission line. In this linear case, the solution $\Psi = \Psi(x, t)$ is expressed by (9.13). The (nonlinear) sine-Gordon equation occurs in studies of relativistic field theory, in Josephson-type transmission lines, and in certain oscillations of changed particles.

Before addressing the nonlinear problem, we should first consider the case in which the wave amplitude Ψ is small so that $\sin \Psi$ may be approximated by Ψ. If (10.31) is then solved with periodic boundary conditions, such as in a transmission line of length L closed on itself, both the dependent variable $\Psi(x, t)$ and driving amplitude $B(x)$ can be expanded in Fourier series, that is,

$$B(x) = \sum_{n=1}^{\infty} b_n \sin(k_n x) \tag{10.32}$$

$$\Psi(x) = \sum_{n=1}^{\infty} V_n(t) \sin(k_n x) \tag{10.33}$$

where the wave numbers (spatial frequencies) k_n are restricted by the boundary conditions to

$$k_n = \frac{n\pi}{L} \tag{10.34}$$

and the allowed eigenvalues n depend on whether the system has fixed ends (all integer n's) or periodic boundary conditions (closed loop, even n's with cosine terms included in the Fourier series). The temporal parts of the solution satisfy the uncoupled, ordinary differential equations

$$\frac{d^2 V_n}{dt^2} + 2\alpha \frac{dV_n}{dt} + (\omega_n^2 + \beta^2) V_n = b_n \sin \Omega t \tag{10.35}$$

Although this is a set of differential equations, one for each of the spatial Fourier coefficients $V_n(t)$, they are uncoupled because of the linearity of the original partial differential equation. In contrast, nonlinearity generally leads to coupling between equations representing different spatial modes k_n. The linear solution is given by (9.13) with ω_n^2 replaced by $\omega_n^2 + \beta^2$, and each $V_n(t)$ has a peak in its resonance curve when

$$\Omega = (\omega_n^2 + \beta^2 - 2\alpha^2)^{1/2} \qquad \omega_n = ck_n = \frac{n\pi c}{L} \tag{10.36}$$

Thus each spatial mode is maximally excited by a different driving frequency, and the dynamic motion Ψ is linear combination of spatial modes (10.33).

We cannot obtain an analytic solution to (10.31) for arbitrary amplitude $\Psi(x, t)$; however, numerical studies (Bishop et al, 1983) have shown several interesting results that are generic to other physical systems governed by nonlinear partial differential equations. In particular, the standing waves predicted by (10.31) have the following properties:

1. With flat initial conditions, that is $\Psi(x, 0) = 0$ for $0 \leq x \leq L$, there are parameter ranges with periodic behavior and ranges with temporal chaotic behavior, as would be expected from studies of the forced Duffing equation and similar systems.
2. When spatial structure is introduced into the initial conditions, that is $\Psi(x, 0) = f(x)$, an interesting symbiosis of temporal and spatial structures occurs. Spatial patterns inhibit the temporal chaos that occurs in the absence of spatial structure, but the competing tendencies of temporal versus spatial structure can lead to a rich intermittency in space and time.
3. Typically the spatial structure of the soliton-like waves tends to be coherent, that is they exhibit just a few well-defined spatial modes k_n. Perhaps most importantly, this spatial coherence can be maintained even when the temporal behavior of individual modes $V_n(t)$ becomes chaotic.

In strongly nonlinear systems, we would expect considerable spatial mode (or wave–wave) coupling, such as waves of wave number k_1 and k_2 combining to produce waves $k_1 \pm k_2$, which then produce more waves, and so on until spatial–temporal chaos occurs. That persistent coherent spatial structures can occur in strongly nonlinear systems, even in the presence of temporal chaos, is a very important finding. Known examples in other physical systems include dislocations in fluid flow between parallel walls (Couette flow), clumps in turbulent plasmas, and large-scale structures in turbulent fluids, such as Jupiter's giant red spot. The work of Walter Freeman and colleagues, cited in Chapters 2 and 8, suggests that spatially coherent chaos may also occur in the olfactory bulb. Studies by Lopes da Silva and colleagues suggest that some epileptic phenomena are temporal chaos (Chapter 5). When we first introduced the concept of chaos, we found that simple nonlinear systems sometimes displayed complex behavior. Now we find that complex systems sometimes display behavior that is, in some sense, much simpler than expected.

Stochastic Systems

Many, if not most, important physical and biological systems have many degrees of freedom. In such cases, a statistical approach is required if a general understanding is to be gained. With chaotic phenomena, a statistical approach may be required for prediction even when the number of degrees of freedom is small. Consider, for example, the problem of predicting the final state of a roulette system (consisting of ball and roulette wheel), given initial positions and velocities of the ball and wheel. Although it may not be practical (or even possible) to predict the exact slot in which the ball falls, such exact prediction is not required to "beat" the game. It is only necessary to gain enough information about the final state to overcome the inherent statistical advantage of the "house." For example, if the resting slot could be accurately predicted to fall into a certain three-quarter portion of the wheel, the player would have such a large advantage over the house that he or she could quickly bankrupt the house. This idea has been applied in Las Vegas casinos with some success by at least two groups of scientists separated in time by two generations. The first approach was strictly experimental, that is it involved a search for a biased roulette wheel. Amazingly, one was found with sufficient bias so that quick profits were made—until the house changed the wheel (Wilson, 1965). The second group developed a specialized computer to be placed in the shoe of one player. Initial conditions were signaled by a second player. The computer apparently was moderately successful, although it was beset by practical problems in the noisy casino environment (Bass, 1985).

The roulette wheel example is not so different from important scientific systems as might first appear. For example, it graphically demonstrates that exact solutions at microscopic levels (such as predicting the exact slot in which the ball will fall) are often not required in applications. A coarse-grained solution is often sufficient. In the roulette example, coarse graining in space simply means treating a certain predetermined number of adjacent slots as a single state. Such methods are common to the theory of stochastic processes, whether the randomness is believed to be fundamental (as in quantum systems and classical chaos) or simply due to our inability to model complex systems accurately. A comprehensive discussion of the modern theory of stochastic processes with its many variants and applications would require several large volumes. A nonmathematical but highly provocative treatment of the second law of thermodynamics with implications for complex physical, chemical, biological, and social systems is given by Prigogine and Stengers (1984). An introduction to nonequilibrium phase transitions and self-organization in physics, chemistry, and biology is given by Haken (1983). The modern theory of critical phenomena in physical systems, which is applicable to media having multiple-length scales for interaction between the functional units of the media, is presented in Ma (1976). An excellent popular account of the essence of this subject is given by Wilson (1979). Multiple interaction lengths is, of course, a critical issue in the neocortical medium, as we have emphasized throughout this book.

This section is limited to a few examples from the literature that should convey some of the flavor of the subject and provide some background for statistical approaches to neocortex. Quantum mechanical methods that are required in condensed matter physics are omitted. Rather we focus on systems of low density (such as neutral gasses and plasmas) in which classical forces between interacting particles provide an accurate description. However, complex systems share many generic features. These general features are observed and similar mathematical techniques are required, although the specific features of the interactions between functional units of the media differ, such as differences of quantum and classical forces between interacting entities (electrons and molecules, for example) or differences between physical and neocortical interactions.

An important example of these general features taken from physics are phase transitions. These are transitions between different aggregate states of a medium, which originate as a new ordering at microscopic levels but are manifested as qualitatively different macroscopic properties. Descriptions of such processes is a primary goal of theoretical physics, that is to explain macroscopic properties of a medium that are subject to experimental measurement in terms of microscopic behavior. Examples of phase transitions are the change of a ferromagnet from unmagnetized to magnetized, the sudden vanishing of electric resistance in a semiconductor, the gas to water to ice transitions, and the transition from laminar to turbulent fluid flow. In all these examples, energy input to the system causes a phase transition, which occurs at critical temperatures in the first three examples, or a critical fluid velocity in the last example. Thus temperature and velocity serve as control parameters. Also, in these examples, energy input leads to an abrupt transition from macroscopic order to disorder.

In other systems, energy input may cause transition from macroscopic disorder to order, as in the example of the transition of a laser's output from incoherent to coherent light at some critical input power. This latter example may be more characteristic of biological processes. Energy fed randomly into a system may result in the system forming a few well-defined macroscopic modes, that is a spatially coherent organization. Such systems are self-organizing. An example from the physical sciences is the soliton-like behavior in the sine-Gordon system, discussed previously. Self-organization is also observed in fluid and chemical systems. An interesting example from the social sciences in urbanization due to local positive feedback effects at population centers. Life on our planet is apparently a supreme expression of self-organization (Prigogine and Stenger, 1984). Phase transitions in neocortex also result from external input. For example, the transition from the sleeping to awake state occurs when electric or chemical input (or both) from the midbrain changes, as discussed in Chapters 3, 4, 5, and 13.

Two simple examples of self-organizing systems are illustrated in Figure 10-26, which consists of grids with 2940 units at successive time intervals. The units might represent many things, such as columns of neocortex, at arbitrary scale. The state of each unit is determined in part by simple rules; that is, a positive unit (such as upward current flow) tends to create either negative (a) or positive (b) units in the eight nearest-neighbor units. Example (a) is analogous to the phenomenon of inhibitory surround (of an excitatory region) in neocortex due to local synaptic inhibition of pyramidal cells. Initially positive and negative cells are distributed randomly throughout the grid. However, as time progresses, two kinds of self-organization occur: (a) regions of vertical or horizontal organization or (b) islands of positive and negative units, according to the corresponding local inter-

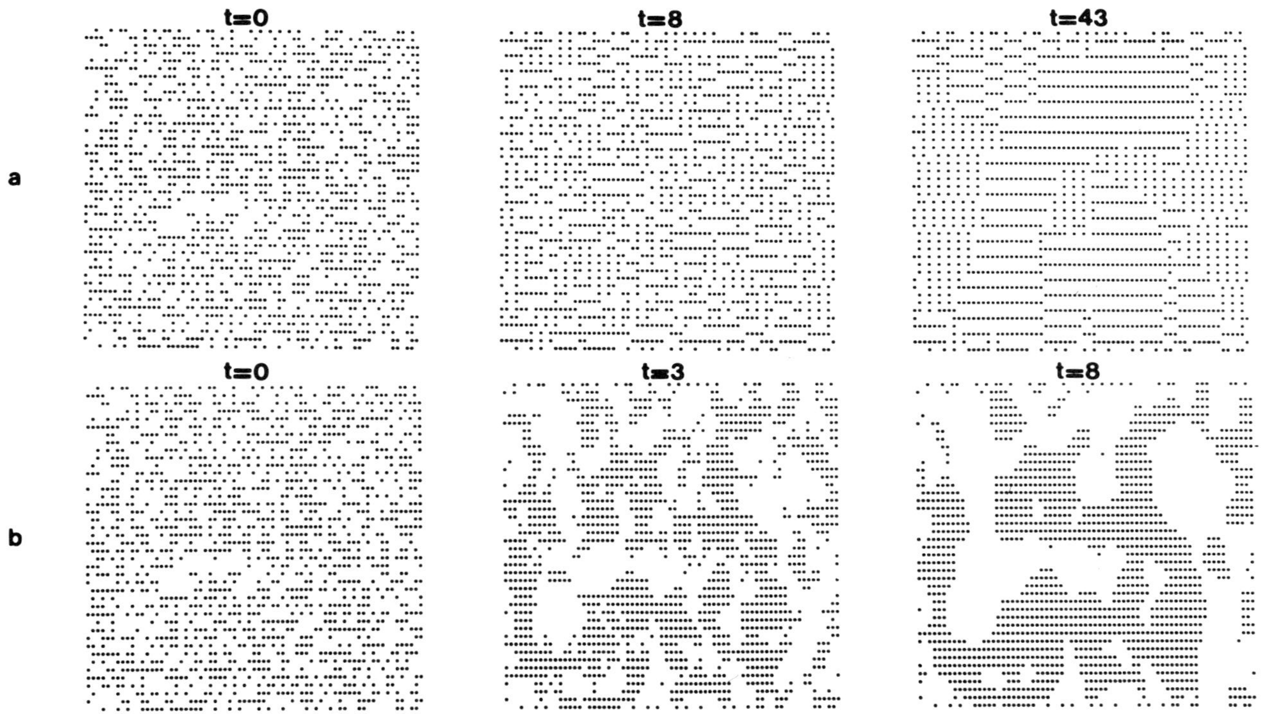

Figure 10-26. Self-organization due to nearest-neighbor interactions in a 70 × 42 grid, representing, for example, neocortical columns. Each unit in the grid has a value $p_i(t)$, such as a dipole moment. A positive value of $p_i(t)$ is indicated by a filled space, a negative value by an empty space. At t = 0, the p_i are randomly distributed. They evolve according to the simple rule $p_i(t) = Ap_i(t - 1) + B \sum_{k=1}^{8} p_k(t - 1)$, where the sum is over the eight nearest-neighbor cells. In this simulation, the calculation progresses row by row from the upper left corner to the lower right corner of the grid at each iteration, t. The parameters are (*a*) A = 0.5, B = −0.0625 ("inhibitory surround") or (*b*) A = 0.5, B = +0.0625 ("excitatory surround").

action rule. More complex rules in physical systems are, of course, often expressed as partial differential equations.

To understand the quantitative methods used in stochastic theories, we begin with the coupled set of nonlinear, ordinary differential equations (10.24). Define the probability density function $P(X_1, X_2, \ldots X_N, t)$, which is simply a measure of how likely we are to find the system trajectory in the phase space volume element $\Delta V = \Delta X_1 . \Delta X_2 \ldots \Delta X_N$ at time t. For example, when $N = 2$, the phase plane plots shown in this chapter yield a qualitative picture of $P(X_1, X_2, t)$. Equilibrium is defined as a time when $\partial P/\partial t = 0$. The probability density function of the motion in N-dimensional phase space satisfies the linear, partial differential equation (Haken, 1983)

$$\frac{\partial P}{\partial t} + \nabla_{\mathbf{X}} \cdot (P\mathbf{F}) = 0 \qquad (10.37)$$

which is Liouville's theorem in the field of classical statistical mechanics (Tolman, 1938). The vector notation $[\mathbf{F}(\mathbf{X}, t) = F_i(X_1, X_2, \ldots X_N, t), i = 1, N]$ represents the known functions on the right side of (10.24). The operator $\nabla_{\mathbf{X}}$ is just the usual vector gradient operator expressed in N-dimensional space

$$\nabla_{\mathbf{X}} \cdot (P\mathbf{F}) = \frac{\partial(P\mathbf{F}_{X1})}{\partial X_1} + \frac{\partial(P\mathbf{F}_{X2})}{\partial X_2} + \ldots + \frac{\partial(P\mathbf{F}_{XN})}{\partial X_N} \qquad (10.38)$$

When $N = 3$, (10.37) is in the standard form of the continuity or conservation equation; for example, it expresses the conservation of mass in a fluid flow (one of the Navier-Stokes equations) or the conservation of charge (inherent in Maxwell's equations). P is then analogous to a density (mass or charge), **F** to a velocity, and the product (P**F**) assumes the role of a flux, such as fluid mass flow or current density. Thus we started with a system of deterministic equations (10.24), but our statistical description (10.37) is a conservation of probability in phase space. Also we started with nonlinear equations in the N dependent variables X_i and showed that the same system satisfies a linear equation in P. However, the number of independent variables was increased from one (t) to $N + 1$, and the new number of degrees of freedom is infinite.

Many systems contain a mixture of deterministic and random interactions. The classic example is Brownian motion, in which small but macroscopic particles immersed in a liquid are moved by the random action of molecular collisions. The deterministic force in this example is fluid friction, proportional to particle velocity. Another example occurs in a hot plasma, in which interactions between charged particles are separated in the theory between the macroscopic, smoothly varying electric field (due collectively to many charged particles) and random collisions. Of course, collisions are just interactions of electric fields, but a distinction is made between coherent and incoherent electric fields. Each particle in the plasma or similar system then undergoes motion described by the equations

$$\frac{d\mathbf{X}}{dt} = \mathbf{F}(\mathbf{X}, t) + \mathbf{R}(t) \qquad (10.39)$$

which is the same set as (10.24) except that the random forces $\mathbf{R}(t)$ are added. Given some rather general statistical properties of the random forces R_i, $i = 1, N$, the probability density function for the motion (dynamics) obeys the Fokker-Planck equation

$$\frac{\partial P}{\partial t} + \nabla_{\mathbf{X}} \cdot (P\mathbf{F}) = \frac{1}{2} \sum_{i=1}^{N} \sum_{j=1}^{N} Q_{ij} \frac{\partial^2 P}{\partial X_i \partial X_j} \tag{10.40}$$

which also may be written

$$\frac{\partial P}{\partial t} + \sum_{i=1}^{N} \frac{\partial}{\partial X_i} \left(F_i P - \frac{1}{2} \sum_{j=1}^{N} Q_{ij} \frac{\partial P}{\partial X_j} \right) = 0 \tag{10.41}$$

Here the Q_{ij} are diffusion coefficients that are proportional to correlation functions between the stochastic interaction forces $R_i(t)$ and $R_j(t)$ at zero lag, that is, the derivation assumes that correlations decrease rapidly with lag time. Thus (10.40) or (10.41) describe a flow (dynamics) in N-dimensional phase space in which probability is no longer conserved because of the influence of random forces. Adding this diffusion process "smears" otherwise well-defined orbits. The F_i terms in (10.24) and (10.37) through (10.41) are called drifts.

The quantitative statistical methods just described are rather formal, that is they provide the beginnings of a theoretical framework to study complex systems, but, by themselves, they are of minimal help in making actual calculations. That is, the Liouville and Fokker-Planck equations are intractable, as formulated above, for large N. In a neutral gas or plasma consisting of M particles, P is proportional to the joint probability of finding particle 1 at location $\mathbf{x}_1$ and velocity $\mathbf{v}_1$, while particle 2 is at location $\mathbf{x}_2$ with velocity $\mathbf{v}_2$, and so on, and finally particle M is at location $\mathbf{x}_M$ with velocity $\mathbf{v}_M$. To generalize to other systems, we use the symbols X_i in the formalism to represent the three position and velocity coordinates for each particle so that the number of degrees of freedom of the system is $N = 6M$.

The formalism of the Liouville equation depends only on the validity of the system of nonlinear, ordinary differential equations (10.24). Thus, for example, it is applicable to an ecologic system with N interacting species. The outside influence of additional species, which might be treated stochastically because the appropriate coupling parameters are not known, could be included with the diffusion term and multivariate drifts, that is the Fokker-Planck equation. In neocortex, the X_i might represent L internal states of M synapses (such as the concentrations of L different chemicals at each synapse) so the number of coupled equations (10.24) or phase space dimensions would be $N = LM$. At higher levels of description, X_i might represent $L = 3$ dipole moments (three components of the polarization vector) of M cortical columns (at any scale) so the number of phase space dimensions would be $N = 3M$.

In more complex systems, such as neocortex studied in Chapter 14, the variables X_i are generalized to a field, denoted by $M^G(X_i, t)$ for a set of G variables called order parameters in the parlance of modern statistical field theories. The order parameters may be continuous or discrete functions of space and time. The

Fokker-Planck equation (10.41) also may contain a potential term VP when applied to some systems. Furthermore, boundary conditions should be considered an integral part of these partial differential equations; their effects sometimes may be included in the potential.

The next step in our stochastic description is crossing hierarchical levels. For example, we may want to construct a probability density function P at the level of the neocortical column from a more microscopic P at the level of smaller columns or at the synaptic level. Ultimately we want to express macroscopic variables, such as surface potentials, in terms of more microscopic variables. This is essentially the approach taken in Chapter 14, in which a theory of multiple scales of statistical physics of neocortex is developed. Here we return to the less complex example of a gas, which provides several parallels and analogs that should clarify approaches to statistical theories of neocortex.

An important macroscopic variable, entropy, is simply related to the phase space probability density. Entropy is a measure of the "disorder" of complex systems. The entropy S of a system is expressed by the multiple (N) phase space integrals

$$S = -k \iint \ldots \int P \log P \, dX_1 \, dX_2 \ldots dX_N \tag{10.42}$$

With a neutral gas, k is Boltzmann's constant. The second law of thermodynamics (as applied in practical engineering systems or in statistical mechanics) is a quantitative statement of the minimum possible increase in the entropy of a system, given a certain amount of thermal energy input. In closed systems, that is those with no input, entropy (or disorder) can only increase. Thus the system must become more disordered as time passes. Information about initial states or "memory" in the system is lost. The second law is derived directly from the ideas of classical statistical mechanics (Tolman, 1938). As far as we know, it is a fundamental law of nature, not just a practical limitation (Prigogine and Stengers 1984). Of course, most real systems are not closed; the concept of a closed system, that is one without external influences, is an idealization that can be approached only in actual physical or biological systems. In open systems, self-organization is possible, that is entropy can decrease and the system may become more ordered as the result of energy input. "Entropy" can have different meanings, depending, for example, on the scale at which P is defined.

The kinetic theory of a neutral gas or plasma involves a coarse graining of the probability density function $P(X_1, X_2, \ldots X_N, t)$. This joint probability over all phase space is averaged to obtain the one particle probability density function $f(\mathbf{x}, \mathbf{v}, t)$ discussed in Chapter 9, that is,

$$f(X_1, \ldots X_6, t) = \iint \ldots \int P \, dX_7 \, dX_8 \ldots dX_N \tag{10.43}$$

where the integrals are over the entire volume of phase space, excluding the first six coordinates, X_1 through X_6, which here represent the position $\mathbf{x}$ and velocity $\mathbf{v}$ of a single particle. The product $f(\mathbf{x}, \mathbf{v}, t)\, d^3x\, d^3v$ is the total number of particles that occupy the phase space volume element $d^3x\, d^3v$, that is the total number of particles in the physical volume d^3x, which also have velocities in the range d^3v. With M noninteracting particles, P may be expressed as the product of M statistically independent density functions, that is,

$$P(\mathbf{x}_1, \ldots \mathbf{x}_M, \mathbf{v}_1, \ldots \mathbf{v}_M, t) = P(\mathbf{x}_1, \mathbf{v}_1, t) \cdots P(\mathbf{x}_M, \mathbf{v}_M, t) \tag{10.44}$$

and the Vlasov or collisionless Boltzmann equation, discussed in Chapter 9, obtained from the Liouville equation (10.37) (Montgomery and Tidman, 1964). When local interactions (collisions) are included, Fokker-Planck terms are added to the resulting equation for the evolution of the one-particle density function $f(\mathbf{x}, \mathbf{v}, t)$.

In a plasma or neutral gas, macroscopic variables are expressed directly in terms of velocity integrals over the one-particle probability density function. For example, the local number density of particles is

$$\rho(\mathbf{x}, t) = \rho_0 \int f(\mathbf{x}, \mathbf{v}, t)\, d^3v \tag{10.45}$$

The bulk velocity of the fluid flow $\mathbf{u}$ at any location $\mathbf{x}$ is just the average velocity of all the particles,

$$\mathbf{u}(\mathbf{x}, t) = \frac{\rho_0}{\rho(\mathbf{x}, t)} \int \mathbf{v} f(\mathbf{x}, \mathbf{v}, t)\, d^3v \tag{10.46}$$

and the local temperature is

$$T(\mathbf{x}, t) = \frac{m\rho_0}{3k\rho(\mathbf{x}, t)} \int w^2 f(\mathbf{x}, \mathbf{v}, t)\, d^3v \tag{10.47}$$

where $\mathbf{w}$ is the random velocity of a particle, that is $\mathbf{w} = \mathbf{v} - \mathbf{u}$, m is the particle mass, and ρ_0 is the total number of particles. Similar expressions can be obtained for the pressure tensor (including viscous forces), heat flux vector, and so forth. Thus the success of the classical kinetic theory of gasses (and to a somewhat lesser extent, hot plasma theory) is in obtaining the theoretical connection between microscopic variables and measurable, macroscopic variables. Modern theories have added considerably to this early success, such as in the area of predicting phase transitions in a variety of media. Similar relations between "microscopic" variables in neocortex and more macroscopic variables are described throughout this book. However, with the neocortical medium, many hierarchical levels of description are possible, the terms "microscopic" and "macroscopic" are insufficient. Rather we must adopt more quantitative descriptors of hierarchical level at several scales. The need for intermediate scales (between micro and macro) appears to be a general trademark of nonequilibrium systems (see Chapter 14).

New Experimental Measures of System Dynamics

The standard methods of time series and spatial analysis, long used in physical science applications, have been applied successfully to EEG data. Such methods have been described extensively (Nunez, 1981, 1990; Niedermeyer and Lopes da Silva, 1987), and a three-volume revised set of the *Handbook of Electroencephalography and Clinical Neurophysiology* (Gevins and Remond, 1987; Lopes da Silva et al, 1986; Picton, 1988) is available. Some of the principal results of this work, as it applies to neocortical dynamics, were presented in Chapters 1 to 7 of this book. The recent increase in interest in nonlinear dynamics with application to many fields prompted the development of new methods for time series analysis. These methods were recently applied to EEG data (see Chapter 5). The new methods are being developed so rapidly that popular algorithms and instructions for their use may be outdated by the time this book is published. Furthermore, at this time it is not clear that the new methods are of practical use in EEG. Nevertheless, a brief description of general features is presented here because we have little doubt that many such studies of experimental nonlinear dynamics of EEG will be published soon, if only as a consequence of development of the new theoretical contributions. Consider first the following possible motivations for an experimental EEG study. (1) To establish robust relations between the physiologic or clinical state of the brain and quantitative measures of EEG. Such information is, of course, of great scientific and practical interest, although, by itself, it may tell us little or nothing about neocortical dynamics. (2) To test theories of neocortical dynamic function. For example, to test predictions of critical parameter changes that lead to bifurcations or phase transitions. (3) To measure quantitative features of attractors, such as Fourier spectra, Lyapunov exponents, probability density functions, or fractal dimensions of the EEG.

Of course, these goals are strongly related. The success of modern science is due largely to a marriage of theory and experiment. With complex systems, we cannot develop meaningful theory without substantial data or easily design good experiments without some theoretical construct on which to base experimental methods. This is especially true of human brains, systems in which data may be obtained in a variety of physiologic states, which may show considerable variations among different brains in the "same" physiologic state, and which may produce nonstationary data even within the "same" physiologic state.

A way to avoid some of these complications might be to use general information about system dynamics (approach 3) to develop better theoretical models, which then may be tested (approach 2). This idea is based in part on some recent mathematical developments, which are summarized in general terms by Theiler (1990), Rapp and coworkers (1989), and Arbarbanel and associates (1993). This mathematical work is applicable to complex systems (such as neocortex) with many dependent variables $X_i(t)$, which might, for example, represent the data from different EEG channels. The mathematical theorems suggest that if any one of these variables, perhaps $X_1(t)$, is measured with sufficient accuracy (low noise), with a sufficiently high sampling rate, and over a sufficiently long period, quantitatively meaningful inferences can be made about the dynamic behavior of the entire system from the behavior of the single variable $X_1(t)$ using appropriate methods of data analysis, such as estimation of Lyapunov exponents or fractal dimensions. These new forms of analysis may be able to provide a richer description of system dynamics than can traditional methods of time series analysis. However, this potential has not, at this time, been realized in the field of EEG. The new methods may prove more useful simply to supplement traditional methods to quantify EEG state (approach 1), at least for now.

Much experience with the field of EEG and evoked potentials has shown that although it is easy to obtain data, it is far more difficult to conduct a meaningful and robust experimental program. The difficulties often can be more severe in EEG than in the physical sciences partly because of the complexity of the system being studied and partly because of the inherently interdisciplinary nature of the work, which requires that the scientist be knowledgeable in several fields (Nunez, 1981, 1990; Gevins and Remond, 1987; Regan, 1989). Historically, the extent of such difficulties has not been fully appreciated in EEG. Thus EEG scientists commonly have been careful in their own areas of expertise but somewhat sloppy outside them. As a result, many published EEG works are candidates for the *Journal of Irreproducible Results*. Unfortunately a real danger exists that the new methods of nonlinear system dynamics may be misapplied to EEG with similar adverse results. Many popular algorithms are readily available to estimate correlation dimension (for example), and formally implementing the cookbook procedures is simple. However, much more knowledge of the underlying theory and experimental limitations is required to produce good science. Rather than duplicate descriptions of the details of different methods here, it would be more useful to list some of the probable pitfalls, while remembering that further research may produce more knowledge of EEG dynamics and more sophisticated applications of the new methods to EEG.

One important quantitative measure of the dynamics of a system is its dimension. For example, if the system is described by the N differential equations for the dependent variables $X_i(t)$, the system is "contained" in the N-dimensional phase space. That is, we can completely specify states of the system with multiple points in this space. The steady-state motion or attractor might be simple, such as a limit-cycle (in the phase plane) or limit-toris (the higher dimensional analog). But the dimension of a system on a limit cycle attractor is equal to one because only a single coordinate (such as an angle measured from some fixed location in the phase plane) is required to locate the system on its limit cycle. Thus the dimension of an attractor is a measure of its geometric complexity in phase space. Complex systems (with large N) sometimes have states that exhibit simple behavior, as in long-range interactions between mechanical oscillators, charged particles in a hot plasma, or neocortical columns. In these examples, simple behavior is possible regardless of whether the underlying interactions are linear or nonlinear. Thus a system trajectory in an N-dimensional phase space can be contained in a subspace of some lower dimension D, which is the effective or active number of degrees of freedom (for a particular background state or phase of the system).

The fractal is an important concept for modern methods to study complex systems. Fractals can be physical objects such as coastlines or neocortical structure that, because of their highly irregular form, are not easily characterized by conventional measures such as length, area, or volume; see the review and beautiful pictures of fractals in Barnsley and coworkers (1988). Fractals have statistical self-similarity at different length scales. For example, a magnified view of a small part of a mountain range, forest, or possibly neocortical macrocolumn does not precisely reproduce the original picture, but it has a similar qualitative appearance. The geometric complexity of the object may be quantified by a dimension that generally is not an integer. The fractal dimension determines the relative amount of detail or irregularities at different spatial scales. For example, several surfaces, such as mountain ranges of height denoted by the function $z_D = z_D(x, y)$, have dimensions in the range $2 \leq D < 3$, with $D = 2$ indicating a smooth surface, and larger dimensions indicating progressively rougher surfaces. Alternately, another physical variable, such as temperature, might vary in three-dimensional space as $T = T(x, y, z)$ and have a fractal dimension in the range $3 \leq D < 4$, depending on the irregularity of the function. The general fractal concept appears to be tailor made to describe the geometric complexity of biological systems, especially neocortex.

Given the geometric interpretation inherent in a phase space description of dynamical systems, the natural extension of the general fractal concept from physical objects to phase space trajectories is central to studies of complex systems. Thus the dimension D (effective number of degrees of freedom of an attractor) provides a measure of system complexity (determined by the size of D), and motion complexity (partly determined by whether D is an integer). Attractors with noninteger dimensions D are called strange attractors. Most known strange attractors are also chaotic attractors, that is they exhibit an exponential divergence of adjacent phase space trajectories. Whereas conservative dynamical systems (Hamiltonian systems in which energy is conserved) can exhibit chaos, apparently only dissipative dynamical systems (in which energy lost through frictional forces is provided by external input, for example) can have strange attractors.

These discussions suggest that if we are sufficiently clever and have enough "good" (relatively artifact free) EEG data, we can use this mathematical foundation to extract important information about neocortical dynamics from even a single EEG channel. For example, the following questions might be asked experimentally. (1) Approximately how large is the EEG dimension D corresponding to a fixed physiologic or clinical state, to a specific spatial scale of the recorded data, or both? (2) Is D a noninteger, that is does the EEG follow a strange attractor? (3) Is one of the Lyapunov exponents positive, that is does the EEG follow a chaotic attractor?

The application of these ideas to real data is, in the understated parlance of physicists and mathematicians, "nontrivial." For detailed background, note that several practical issues for application to low-dimensional electric and mechanical systems are discussed by an experimentalist experienced with chaotic behavior (Moon, 1992). Summaries of mathematical and practical issues for general data are given by Theiler (1990) and Abarbanel and associates (1993), and specifically for EEG data by Rapp and colleagues (1989, 1990). Some of the issues raised in these publications (plus a few others) can be applied to EEG analysis.

1. Embedding strategies. The dimension D of an attractor (for example the D associated with a particular physiologic state of the brain) typically is estimated by expressing the data from a single EEG channel in an M-dimensional pseudo-phase space. That is, M successive values of potential $X_1 = X(t)$, $X_2 = X(t + \tau)$, . . . $X_M = X[t + (M - 1)\tau]$ are used as the coordinates of this space. Here M is called the embedding dimension and τ is the time increment, which is either equal to or some other integral multiple of the digital sampling interval. A single point in this space is then located by the vector $\mathbf{R}_1(t) = (X_1, X_2, \ldots X_M)$. The next location of the system "point" is given by the vector $\mathbf{R}_2(t) = (X_2, X_3, \ldots X_{M+1})$ and so on. Thus, in a time series consisting of K measured values, $\mathbf{R}(t)$ can assume $L = K - M + 1$ discrete values in the embedding space. If the embedding dimension M is chosen to be larger than $2D + 1$, it is theoretically possible to estimate D. However, these issues are complicated by the fact that several types of fractal dimensions have been introduced, including correlation dimension, information dimension, Hausdorff dimension, and so forth. Also different algorithms may be used to estimate a single type of dimension. Often there is confusion about the relations between these different definitions and algorithms.

When the dimension of an attractor is large, the practical problems of estimating the dimension D from noisy data of finite length may be severe. For example, a guess for the minimum number of points L required to obtain a reasonable estimate of D can be obtained from the heuristic formula (Theiler, 1990)

$$L = A^D \tag{10.48}$$

Here the parameter A is generally not known, but Theiler suggests that A is perhaps of the order of ten. For example, if $L = 10^4$ points were required to estimate a dimension $D = 4$, $L = 10^D$ time points would be required to estimate a dimension of D. This L is only a guess, but it is consistent with some EEG experiments. For example, see Roschke and Basar (1988). Suppose we also assume a τ of 10 milliseconds, which is a typical time interval for noticeable EEG changes and is also the approximate membrane time constant of cortical pyramidal cells. In this case, an EEG dimension of $D = 4$ and $L = 10^4$ points corresponds to about 100 seconds of data. However, a dimension $D = 10$ and $L = 10^{10}$ points corresponds to more than 3 years of continuous data. We are not allowed to shorten this period by making τ arbitrarily small because of the effects of autocorrelation, that is data points that are too close together are essentially the same point. Other work by Essex and Nerenberg (1991) suggest that although data requirements are substantial, they may not be as severe as implied by these arguments, especially if moderate errors in the estimated correlation dimension are acceptable. However, the minimal data set is at least

$$L = 10^{D/2} \tag{10.49}$$

Published estimates of the dimensions of human EEG data range from about 2 to 10 (Rapp et al, 1989). Although some of this variation is due to differences of participant and physiologic state, much of the variation appears due to the use of different experimental protocols (filter settings on the EEG machine, amount of artifact removal, bipolar versus reference records, and so on) (Nunez and Srinivasan, 1993). Thus fractal dimensions have not yet proved a robust measure when applied to EEG with the possible exception of epileptic data. An often-overlooked point, which may partly explain this lack of robustness, is that the standard correlation algorithm does not efficiently compute system dimension when the attractor is nonchaotic (Theiler, 1990). Because there is no obvious theoretical support for chaotic EEG, the correlation algorithm may not obtain the appropriate measure of system dynamics.

2. Temporal filtering. Temporal filtering of the data generally changes the estimated dimension of a time series. All EEG data are low pass filtered (60 Hz, for example) and high pass filtered (0.5 Hz, for example). Low pass filtering can increase dimension estimates (Badii et al, 1988).

3. Nonstationarity of EEG. We know that EEG is somewhat nonstationary even when generated in a "fixed" physiologic state. For example, the resting alpha rhythm typically exhibits a frequency drift of perhaps 0.5 Hz during several minutes (Nunez, 1981). Thus any measure of system dynamics must refer to an average over the recording period. With very high dimensional attractors, the required recording period may be too long to obtain values approximating a fixed physiologic state.

4. Spatial filtering. All EEG recordings involve space averages of neocortical source activity. With scalp recordings, the active neural tissue contributing to a single EEG record typically contains from 10^8 to 10^{10} neurons (Nunez, 1981). We must be careful in interpreting system dynamics when the contributing data have been severely coarse grained. For example, as indicated in Chapter 2, spatial filtering of EEG implies temporal filtering because of the nature of the dynamics (Nunez and Srinivasan, 1993).

5. Spatial properties of EEG. Many of the interesting properties of EEG, that is those that are at least moderately correlated with physiologic or clinical state, involve spatial properties: distributions of amplitude, coherency, correlation function coefficients, and so on. The new methods for analysis described here have been limited to time series analysis. Obviously, this approach involves ignoring much of the available data in a given experiment. If the new approaches can be viewed as useful measures of EEG system dynamics, spatial and temporal properties should be incorporated into the methods. The study of spatial–temporal chaos is an area of active research (Abarbanel et al, 1993; Chapters 12 and 14).

6. Fuzzy system boundaries. Neocortex (or even the entire nervous system) is not a closed system, that is, it is not autonomous. Even in the most controlled environment, it receives external input with generally unknown statistical properties. Any dynamic measure of the system must partly depend on this input.

7. Comparison with filtered noise. A minimum test for data suspected to exhibit low dimensional chaos involves a test of the algorithm on filtered noise (Theiler, 1990). Noise is filtered to have the same autocorrelation function as the actual data. The algorithm then is applied to filtered noise and the actual data. But can we tell the difference? That is, is there evidence for rejecting the null hypothesis that the signal consists of autocorrelated noise? Only a few of the published papers claiming chaos in EEG have applied this simple test. This issue is discussed in Chapter 5 and reviewed by Pijn and coworkers (1992).

Although the theory of Fourier series was developed in the early seventeenth century, practical algorithms to obtain spectral estimates from experimental data came much later. In fact, refinements in spectral methods continue to be published. We would expect that new methods of time and space series analysis of nonlinear systems would also develop over a long period. However, this caveat should not discourage immediate application of these new methods to EEG if the problem of proper interpretation of results is fully appreciated.

References

Abarbanel, H.D., Brown, R., Sidorowich, J.J., and Tsiming, L.S. The analysis of observed chaotic data in physical systems. *Reviews Modern Physics* 65:1331–1392, 1993.

Badii, R., Broggi, G., Derighetti, B., Ravani, M., Ciliberto, S., Politi, A., and Rubio, M.A. *Physical Rev. Lett.* 60:979–982, 1988.

Barnsley, M.F., Devaney, R.L., Mandelbrot, B.B., Peitgen, H., Saupe, D., and Voss, R.F. *The Science of Fractal Images.* New York: Springer-Verlag, 1988.

Bass, T.A. *The Eudemonic Pie: or Why Would Anyone Play Roulette without a Computer in His Shoe?* Boston: Houghton Mifflin, 1985.

Bergé, P., Pomeau, Y., and Vidal, C. *Order Within Chaos.* Paris: Hermann, 1984.

Bishop, A.R., Fesser, K., Lomdahl, P.S., and Trullinger, S.E. Influence of solitons in the initial state or chaos in the driven, damped sine-Gordon system. *Physica.* 7D:259–279, 1983.

Curry, J. A generalized Lorenz system, *Communications in Mathematical Physics* 60:193–204, 1978.

Essex, C. and Nerenberg, M.A.H. *Proc. R. Soc. London.* 435:287–292, 1991.

Feigenbaum, M.J. Universal behavior in nonlinear systems, *Los Alamos Scientific Laboratory Report*, pp. 4–27, Summer 1980.

Feigenbaum, M.J. Universal behavior in nonlinear systems, *Physica.* 7D:16–39, 1983.

Gevins, A.S. and Remond, A. *Handbook of Electroencephalography and Clinical Neurophysiology (Revised series). Vol. 1. Methods of Analysis of Brain Electrical and Magnetic Signals.* Amsterdam: Elsevier, 1987.

Gibbon, J.D. A survey of the origins and physical importance of soliton equations. *Philos. Trans. R. Soc.* London (A) 315:335–365, 1985.

Gleick, J. *Chaos: Making a New Science.* New York: Viking, 1987.

Haken, H. *Synergetics: An Introduction to Nonequilibrium Phase Transitions and Self-Organization in Physics, Chemistry.* Berlin: Springer-Verlag, 1983.

Hayashi, C. *Forced Oscillations in Nonlinear Systems.* Osaka: Nippon, 1953.

Henon, M. and Heiles, C. The applicability of the third integral of motion: Some numerical experiments. *Astronomy Journal.* 69(1):73–79, 1964.

Jensen, R.V. Classical chaos. *Am. Sci.*, 75:168–181, 1987.

Jensen, R.V. and Meyers, C.R. Images of critical points of nonlinear maps. *Physical Rev.* 32:1222–1224, 1985.

Lopes da Silva, F.H., Storm van Leeuwen, W., and Remond, A. *Handbook of Electroencephalography and Clinical Neurophysiology (Revised Series). Vol. 2. Clinical Applications of Computer Analysis of EEG and other Neurophysiological Signals.* Amsterdam: Elsevier, 1986.

Lorenz, E.N. Deterministic non-periodic flow. *Journal of Atmospheric Science.* 20:130–141, 1963.

Ma, S.K. *Modern Theory of Critical Phenomena*. Reading, MA: Benjamin/Cummings, 1976.

May, R.M. Simple mathematical models with very complicated dynamics. *Nature*. 261:459–467, 1976.

May, R.M. Models for two interacting populations. In: *Theoretical Ecology. 2nd Ed.* (R.M. May, Ed.) Oxford: Blackwell Scientific Publications, 1981.

Minorsky, N. *Nonlinear Oscillations*. Princeton: Van Nostrand, 1962.

Moon, F.C. *Chaotic and Fractal Dynamics*. New York: Wiley, 1992.

Montgomery, D.C. and Tidman, D.A. *Plasma Kinetic Theory*. New York: McGraw-Hill, 1964.

Morse, P.M. and Ingard, K.U. *Theoretical Acoustics*. New York: McGraw-Hill, 1968.

Niedermeyer, E. and Lopez da Silva, F.H. *Electroencephalography: Basic Principals, Clinical Applications and Related Fields*. Second ed. Munich: Urban & Schwarzenberg, 1987.

Nunez, P.L. *Electric Fields of the Brain: The Neurophysics of EEG*. New York: Oxford University Press, 1981.

Nunez, P.L. Physical principles and neurophysiological mechanisms underlying event-related potentials. In: *Event Related Potentials: Basic Issues and Applications*. (J.W. Rohrbaugh, Parasuraman, R., and Johnson, R., Ed.) New York: Oxford University Press, 1990.

Nunez, P.L. and Srinivasan, R. Implications of recording strategy for estimates of neocortical dynamics with electroencephalography. *Chaos* 3:257–266, 1993.

Packard, N.H., Crutchfield, J.P., Farmer, J.D., and Shaw, R.S. Geometry from a time series. *Physical Review Letters*. 45:712–716, 1980.

Picton, T.W. *Handbook of Electroencephalography and Clinical Neurophysiology. (Revised Series) Vol. 3. Human Event Related Potentials*. Amsterdam: Elsevier, 1988.

Pijn, J.P., Van Neerven, J., Noest, A., and Lopes da Silva, F.H. Chaos or noise in EEG signals: dependence on state and brain site. *Electroencephal. Clin. Neurophysiol.* 79:371–381, 1992.

Poincaré, H. *Science and Method*. New York: Dover, 1952.

Prigogine, I. and Stengers, I. *Order Out of Chaos: Mans New Dialogue with Nature*. Toronto: Bantam Books, 1984.

Rapp, P.E., Bashore, T.R., Marinerie, J.M., Albano, A.M., Zimmerman, I.D., and Mees, A.I. Dynamics of brain electrical activity. *Brain Topography*. 2:99–118, 1989.

Rapp, P.E., Bashore, T.R., Zimmerman, I.D., Martinerie, J.M., Albano, A.M., and Mees, A.I. Dynamical characterization of brain electrical activity. In: *The Ubiquity of Chaos*. New York: American Association for the Advancement of Science. 1990.

Regan, D. *Human Brain Electrophysiology: Evoked Potentials and Evoked Magnetic Fields in Science and Medicine*. New York: Elsevier, 1989.

Roschke, J. and Basar, E. The EEG is not simple noise: Strange attractors in intracranial structures. In: *Dynamics of Sensory and Cognitive Processing by the Brain*. (E. Basar, Ed.) Berlin: Springer-Verlag, pp. 203–216, 1988.

Russel, J.S. Report on waves. In: *Report of the 14th Meeting of the British Association for the Advancement of Science*. London: John Murry, London, pp. 311–390, 1844.

Seto, W.W. *Theory and Problems of Mechanical Vibrations*. New York: Schaun Publishing, p. 51, 1964.

Srinivasan, R. and Nunez, P.L. Neocortical dynamics, EEG standing waves and chaos. In: *Nonlinear Dynamical Analysis for the EEG*. London: World Scientific, pp. 310–355, 1993.

Stoker, J.J. *Nonlinear Vibrations*. New York: Interscience, 1950.

Tabor, M. *Chaos and Integrability in Nonlinear Dynamics*. New York: Wiley, 1989.

Testa, J., Pérez, J., and Jeffries, C. Evidence for universal chaotic behavior of a driven nonlinear oscillator. *Physical Rev. Lett.* 48:714–717, 1982. (Comments in 49:1054–1055, 1982)

Theiler, J. Estimating fractal dimension. *J. Opt. Soc. Am.* 6:1055–1073, 1990.

Thompson, J.M.T. and Stewart, H.B. *Nonlinear Dynamics and Chaos*. Chicester, Wiley, 1986.

Tolman, R.C. *The Principals of Statistical Mechanics*. New York: Oxford University Press, 1938.

Ueda, Y. Steady motions exhibited by Duffing's equation: A picture book of regular and chaotic motions. In *New Approaches to Nonlinear Problems in Dynamics*. Philadelphia: SIAM, pp. 311–322, 1980.

Ulam, S.M. and von Neumann, J. *Bull. Am. Math. Soc.* 53:1120, 1947.

Wilson, A.N. *The Casino Gambler's Guide*. New York: Harper & Row, 1965.

Wilson, K.G. Problems in physics with many scales of length. *Sci. Am.* 241:158–179, 1979.

Wolf, A., Swift, J.B., Swinney, H.L., and Vastano, J.A. Determining Lyapunov exponents from a time series. *Physica* 16D:285–317, 1985.

11

Global Contributions to EEG Dynamics

PAUL L. NUNEZ

In contrast to the work presented in Chapters 5 and 8, this chapter is concerned primarily with a global view of electroencephalographic (EEG) dynamics. The word global was chosen to emphasize that, in this view, important features of EEG generation cannot be understood at the level of the cortical column, regardless of spatial scale. Rather delays due to the finite velocity of action potentials in corticocortical fibers together with global boundary conditions partly determine EEG frequencies and damping. Thus the global theory may be viewed as a "top-down" approach to EEG dynamics, in contrast to the "bottom-up" approaches of the local theories considered in Chapters 5 and 8. This chapter provides physiologic and quantitative support for many of the ideas outlined in Chapters 2 and 3.

No claim is made by the global theory that local circuit properties are generally unimportant to neocortical dynamics and EEG phenomena. However, several salient properties of spontaneous EEG and some evoked potentials are predicted by the purely global theory, suggesting that the global theory may describe physiologically realistic limiting cases. The section Marriage of Local and Global Theories shows that the global theory combines naturally with local theories, such as the one described in Chapter 5. Thus the local-versus-global argument, which is central to more general studies of brain function, is expressed explicitly for EEG in quantitative terms. That is, the relative importance of local and global contributions to neocortical dynamics is determined by physiologic control parameters that may change with brain state. Therefore, local properties may be dominant in some physiologic states, whereas global properties are more important in other states.

An extension of this idea, which has the experimental support outlined in Chapters 3, 12, and 13, is that the purely global theory is most applicable to EEG states of minimal cognitive processing, that is, sleep, anesthesia, coma, and perhaps to a lesser extent, the awake alpha rhythm. Such states are probably critically important to studies of cognition and EEG, if only because of their relative simplicity. That is, one way to approach the complex neocortical dynamics of cognitive processing is first to try to understand the relatively simple (at large scales), near-sinusoidal, spatially coherent EEG generally associated with minimal cognitive processing. Later modifications of the model then may lead to some understanding of cognition. In addition, global effects may play a direct role in cognition, even if their most obvious manifestations (such as standing waves) may not be observed easily during demanding mental activity.

The purely global theory predicts standing waves of synaptic action density in neocortex with oscillation frequencies similar to those observed in human EEG (within a factor of perhaps two). It also says something about relations between spatial and temporal properties of EEG; these predictions have experimental

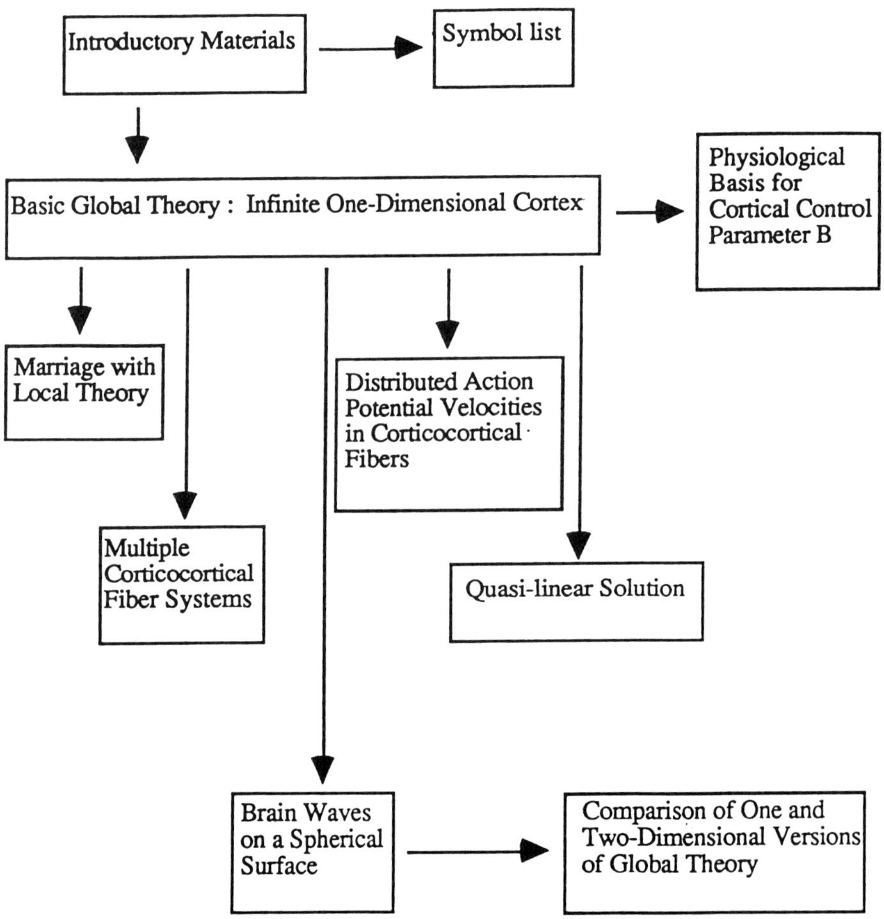

Figure 11-1. Overview of the theoretical methods of the global EEG theory in which complications of the basic one-dimensional version are examined individually. The robustness of general predictions of the theory to different mathematical approximations is evaluated in this manner.

support in Chapter 12. Before addressing the physiologic and mathematical details of the global theory, it would be worthwhile to test the general intuitive idea of standing waves in neocortex. Thus, in the next section, we will examine several physical phenomena that are well understood and somewhat similar to EEG. Of course, even the highly simplified EEG theory presented in this chapter includes complexities not usually observed in simple mechanical and electric systems. That is, our model brain, which is far less complex than the real brain, has a level of complexity comparable to standard models of more complex physical systems, such as hot plasma or complex fluid systems. These models typically represent oversimplifications of real physical systems. That is, model oversimplification of complex systems is nearly always required in physics and engineering just as in biology.

This chapter is partly concerned with deriving plausible dispersion relations for neocortical waves, and thus we emphasize the one-dimensional theory, with boundary conditions applied post hoc. This general kind of approach has proved successful in studies of complex physical systems, and is verified for brain waves later in the chapter. That is, when studying a complex medium, of which neocortex is an extreme example, it is often appropriate to begin with the simplest plausible models based on genuine physiology, that is, models with only potentially measurable parameters. Descriptions or models containing free parameters or those that base conclusions on analogies to physical systems are often useful for communication but are not here afforded the status of "theory." In other sections of this chapter, the effects of different complications on the basic theory (Basic Global Theory) are studied separately. The additional complications are combination with local theories, inclusion of multiple corticocortical fiber systems (and alternate functional forms for corticocortical fiber distribution), effects of distributed propagation velocities in corticocortical fibers, quasi-linear effects, and neocortical waves on a spherical surface. A later section compares results obtained with one and two-dimensional theories. A list of symbols and dimensions is given in the last section, and an overview of the chapter is provided in Figure 11-1.

The Usual Ways of Waves

The general concept of a wave is one of the most profound ideas in all of science. Many of the observed properties of waves, such as propagation velocity and dispersive characteristics, depend only on the wave medium, independent of boundary and initial conditions. Thus, for example, important properties of the wave packet produced in a large swimming pool by a diver are, at great distances from its source, independent of the size, shape, velocity, and entry angle of the diver. Important properties of light or sound waves depend only on the wave medium, independent of wave guide geometry, and so on. This is also partly true of the wave of compound action potential in which the dispersive characteristics are determined by the medium, that is by the specific mixture of axons of different diameter, as depicted in Figure 11-2. The mathematical basis for separating source

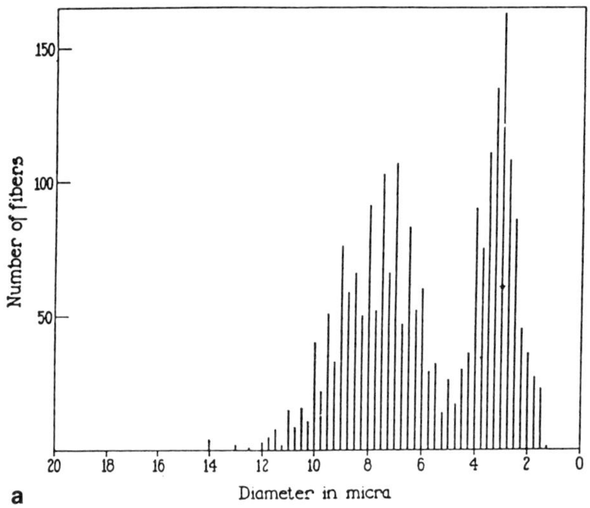
Number of fibers
150
100
50
20
18
16
14
12
10
8
6
4
2
0
Diameter in micra

a

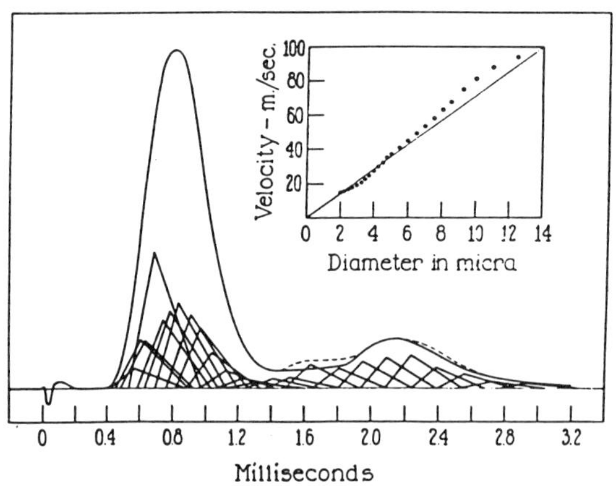
Velocity - m./sec.
100
80
60
40
20
0
2
4
6
8
10
12
14
Diameter in micra
0
0.4
0.8
1.2
1.6
2.0
2.4
2.8
3.2
Milliseconds

b

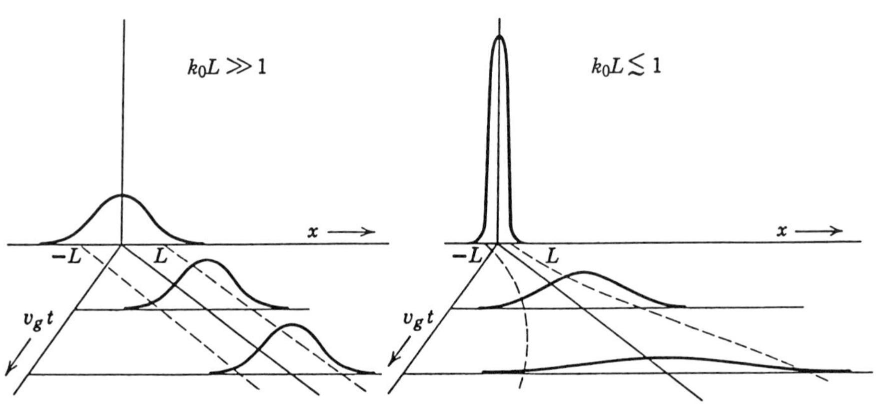
$k_0 L \gg 1$
$k_0 L \lesssim 1$
$x \longrightarrow$
$-L$
L
$v_g t$

c

and medium contributions to waves described by linear, partial differential, or integral equations is described in Chapter 9.

Wave propagation is nature's way of transmitting energy and information over relatively long distances with minimal energy loss and little permanent distortion of the intervening medium. Thus sound waves, ocean waves, seismic waves, electromagnetic waves, waves in mechanical structures, probability waves of quantum mechanics, and (as proposed here) macroscopic brain waves share important characteristics and may be studied from a somewhat similar prespective. That is, once a phenomenon is identified as a wave, important aspects of the phenomenon can be predicted, although details of wave generation and transmission are poorly understood. The connection between disparate wave phenomena is most obvious with linear waves; however, as discussed in Chapter 10, such similarities also apply to certain nonlinear wave phenomena, such as solitons.

A classic example of successful "analysis by analogy" for linear waves is provided by light. That is, once the wave nature of light was realized, many important consequences were identified, long before its electromagnetic nature was realized. Similarly, the identification of EEG as a wave phenomenon (perhaps linear or quasilinear in certain limiting cases) can greatly improve our understanding of EEG and neocortical dynamics, even in the absence of detailed knowledge of the underlying physiologic process. Of course, the local theory of Chapter 5, the global theory of this chapter, and the statistical approach of Chapter 14 all predict waves as limiting cases. The waves may have a different character depending, for example, on whether corticocortical interactions are included in the theory. However, the physiologic parameters of the global theory are the best known of all the neural parameters, which facilitates comparison with EEG experiments.

For wave propagation to occur, the wave medium must possess some underlying mechanism for signal propagation at finite velocity. Thus a disturbance of the medium at one location is not felt immediately at distant locations but rather only after some medium-dependent time delay. For example, the speed of sound in a gas is proportional to the mean thermal speed of molecular motion. The underlying velocity for waves in a stretched string is $[(\text{string tension})/(\text{mass per unit length})]^{1/2}$. With electromagnetic waves in a vacuum, the medium is empty space, which is understood (as a result of the theory of relativity) to have fundamental physical properties, including a finite, fixed value for the speed of light. When

←

Figure 11-2. **a.** Distribution of axons according to size in the saphenous nerve of the cat. **b.** Relation of axon diameter to propagation velocity of simple action potential (inset). Shape of compound action potential (in either space or time) depends on the mixture of nerve axons. Compound action potential propagates as a dispersive wave. (Reproduced with permission from Gasser and Grundfest, 1939; Freeman, 1975.) **c.** A wave pulse (packet) is confined to the region $-L < x < +L$ at $t = 0$. The dominant wave number in the wave packet is k_0, but the packet contains multiple wave numbers spread over the range $\Delta k \sim 1/2L$. Changes in the shape of the pulse as it travels in the x direction are shown. The time axis is scaled by the group velocity v_g. The broad pulse containing many wave lengths ($k_0L >> 1$) shows small distortion as it travels with the group velocity. The narrow pulse ($k_0L < 1$) broadens rapidly. (Reproduced with permission from Jackson, 1975.)

an electromagnetic wave packet passes through a physical medium, its propagation velocity is reduced and its shape altered by the medium. Furthermore, the medium may allow the propagation of only certain kinds of waves, and only waves in restricted wave number and temporal frequency ranges. Such restrictions are expressed quantitatively by the damping constant of the wave, as discussed in Chapter 9.

In the neocortical medium, signals are transmitted by intracortical and corticocortical fibers. The former may be too short to produce substantial time delays due to action potential propagation velocity; in this case delays are strictly local, such as postsynaptic potential (PSP) rise and decay times. In contrast, the myelinated corticocortical fibers have lengths up to about 20 cm and carry action potentials with typical speed of about 6 to 9 m/second (Figure 2-6), thereby producing time delays between neocortical regions as large as 30 milliseconds. In addition, many long fibers (myelinated and nonmyelinated) apparently carry action potentials with even slower velocities. Thus delays due to action potential propagation between distant cortical regions can be substantially longer than PSP rise times in cortical neurons, which appear to be only a few milliseconds. Whether corticocortical interactions may be neglected in theories of neocortical dynamics and EEG is then determined in part by the relative strengths of interaction effected by intracortical and corticocortical fibers. Although the interaction strengths are not well understood, human neocortex is interconnected by 10^{10} corticocortical fibers, as indicated in Figure 2-19 and Figures 11-9 through 11-13. This number is sufficiently large so that every cortical column with a diameter of several millimeters (such as macrocolumns) would, in the limiting case of perfectly homogeneous and isotropic fibers systems, be connected to a considerable fraction of other similar columns, as discussed in Chapter 2. The number of synapses of corticocortical axons is apparently approximately equal to those of intracortical axons, at least in mouse cortex (Braitenberg and Schuz, 1991). Thus no justification is apparent for neglecting corticocortical interactions in EEG theories; that is, the purely local theories of Chapters 5 and 8 should be viewed as limiting cases in the same way that we view the purely global theory of this chapter.

When waves interact, interference phenomena occur. That is, interacting linear waves, when in phase, add amplitudes to produce a wave amplitude equal to the sum of individual amplitudes (constructive interference). In contrast, waves that are exactly out of phase combine to produce zero amplitudes (destructive interference). An interference pattern in a two-dimensional medium is shown in Figure 11-3, in which waves from two separate sources combine. This example might represent any type of linear wave phenomenon, such as water waves caused by two rain drops in a pond, sound waves having two point sources, EEG waves with two epicenters, and so forth. The regions of zero amplitude in Figure 11-3 usually do not indicate zero field (that is, pressure, synaptic activity, and so on) but rather only zero perturbation of the field. That is, many waves are linear only when they have "small" amplitudes, that is, if the wave field is a small perturbation of some background field. For example, the usual sound waves involve small negative and positive changes from the ambient pressure. Their linearity allows

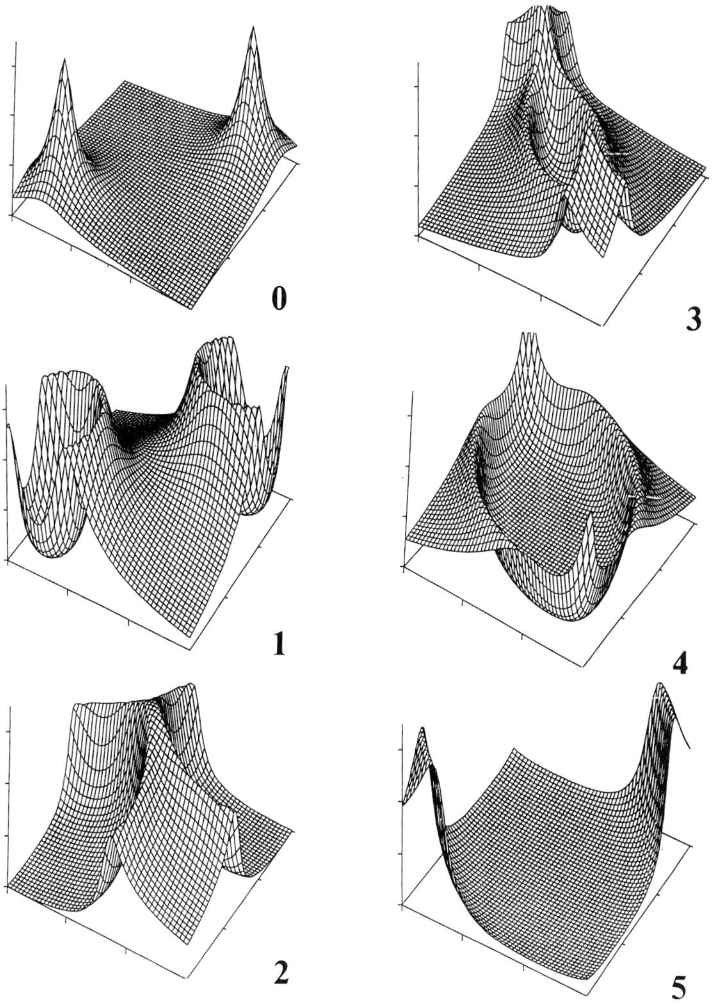

Figure 11-3. Linear wave interference phenomenon in a two-dimensional medium. Two isolated disturbances ($t = 0$) spread in radial directions from their respective origins. Substantial interference between the two wave packets occurs for the approximate time period $2 < t < 3$. At later times, the wave packets have mostly passed through each other. The wave amplitude often refers to a small perturbation of some background field, such as small pressure changes in sound waves or modulation of synaptic action in brain waves. Linearity of wave phenomena often depends on small amplitude changes of the background field. Large perturbations may cause nonlinear waves.

the waves produced by two speakers to pass through each other undistorted so that normal conversation within groups of persons is possible. In contrast, shock waves are highly nonlinear sound waves that may be severely distorted by their interaction. The EEG waves proposed by local and global theories are perturbations of some neocortical activity. In the global theory, the activities followed are the perturbations of synaptic action density (that is, fluctuations in the numbers of active excitatory or inhibitory synapses per unit volume). Small perturbations of synaptic action from the background activity in a neural mass may produce linear or quasi-linear waves. This idea has theoretical and experimental support, as discussed in Chapters 11 through 14.

Standing waves occur in closed systems because of interference of many waves traveling in different directions. With a stretched string, waves are reflected by fixed supports and combine as shown in Figure 9-2. With a closed surface (such as the spherical shell formed by the earth's surface and the bottom of the ionosphere), interference occurs when waves traveling on the surface meet waves traveling in other directions. The resulting standing wave patterns on the surface (the eigenfunctions and their linear combinations) are determined by the specific shape of the surface that provides periodic boundary conditions for the wave equation describing the wave medium. In summary, the nature of linear standing waves on a surface (that is, normal mode frequencies and eigenfunctions) depends on two separate properties of the wave medium. (1) The physical material that serves as the wave medium and is described by the appropriate wave equation. The Fourier transformed wave equation then yields the dispersion relation, which indicates how a wave packet distorts and spreads as it propagates in the material (such as water, air, plasma, vacuum, or neocortex). The dispersion relation also may restrict the ranges of temporal and spatial frequency that can be observed as a result of heavy wave damping in some ranges. (2) The size and shape of the surface, that is the global boundary conditions. These provide specific restrictions on the spatial frequencies that are allowed to persist due to interference of waves traveling in different directions that coalesce to form standing waves. The resulting spatial patterns associated with each normal mode frequency are called the eigenfunctions. Thus the surface medium acts as a multiple band pass spatial filter.

When the material and geometric properties of the medium are combined, the normal mode frequencies are obtained. For example, when the transmission line is closed on itself (Figure 9-7c), the wave equation (9.1) yields the dispersion relation

$$\omega_\ell^2 = \omega_0^2 + c^2 {k_\ell}^2 - \alpha^2 \tag{9.8}$$

independent of the geometry of the line. The one-dimensional, closed line of length L results in sinusoidal eigenfunctions and restricts wave numbers (or spatial wavelengths) to the discrete values

$$k_\ell = \ell\pi/L \qquad \ell = 2, 4, 6, \ldots \tag{9.35}$$

When these last two equations are combined, the medium acts as a multiple band pass spatial and temporal filter. Standing waves are allowed only for the discrete (normal mode) frequencies

$$\omega_\ell^2 = \omega_0^2 + (\ell\pi c/L)^2 - \alpha^2 \qquad \ell = 2, 4, 6, \ldots$$

Of course, continual stimulation of the medium by external forcing functions generally causes traveling waves over broad frequency ranges. However, the waves of frequency given by (9.8) are generally dominant because the medium acts as a multiple band pass filter as a result of interference phenomena. In addition, even with fixed wave medium and boundary conditions (that is, fixed normal mode frequencies), a variety of oscillatory motion is possible, as determined by the nature of the input (that is driving) or initial conditions. These determine the manner in which field energy is distributed over the normal modes (the eigenfunctions and associated Fourier coefficients), as in the example of the variety of sound that may be produced by a musical instrument, even one with fixed boundary conditions.

With waves on a closed surface, the basic ideas outlined for one-dimensional media are not changed, except the eigenfunctions are no longer sinusoidal spatial functions but rather functions characteristic of the particular geometry, such as the spherical harmonics $Y_{\ell m}(\theta, \phi)$ for a spherical surface. For example, the normal mode frequencies for waves on the surface of a prolate spheroidal shell of small eccentricity e are expressed approximately by

$$\omega^2_{\ell m} = \frac{c}{R}\left[\ell(\ell + 1) + (\mathrm{Rem}/b)^2\right]$$

$$\ell = 1, 2, 3, \ldots \qquad m = -\ell, -(\ell + 1), \ldots 0, \ldots (\ell - 1), \ell$$

where R and b are the semimajor and semiminor axes of the ellipse (and the prolate spheroid), respectively, and c is a velocity parameter determined by the nature of the wave medium. See Chapter 9 for more details.

If eccentricity is small, the eigenfunctions are closely approximated by the spherical harmonics. Oscillations in a prolate spheroidal shell (similar to the Schumann resonances in a spherical shell) are depicted in Figure 2-12. The spatial patterns are linear combinations of spherical harmonics associated with each normal mode frequency. The normal mode frequencies are determined here for a prolate spheroidal shell of large eccentricity, approximately matching the shape of one brain hemisphere, with medium propagation velocity in the range of corticocortical action potential velocities. The resulting temporal oscillations are linear combinations of normal mode frequencies, but weighted according to the spatial properties of the forcing function, which may be due to lightning in the case of Schumann resonance, or subcortical synaptic input in the case of EEG waves. This characteristic relation between spatial and temporal properties also occurs in the global theory of EEG, but with some important modifications possibly unique to neocortex.

Basic Global Theory

In contrast to local theories, the basic global theory neglects local delays but includes delays due to finite velocity of action potential propagation along the corticocortical fibers (Nunez, 1972, 1974a, 1974b, 1981a, 1981b, 1981c, 1988, 1989a,

1989b). Intracortical interactions are excitatory and inhibitory; corticocortical interactions are exclusively excitatory (Braitenberg, 1978). Because surface EEG represents space-averaged neural activity, the global macroscopic theory follows the excitatory $h_E(\mathbf{r}, t)$ and inhibitory $h_I(\mathbf{r}, t)$ synaptic action densities (number of active synapses per unit volume at time t) at macroscopic scales (such as macrocolumn to regional scales; Table 2-2). These columns are not restricted in size other than being limited to sizes sufficiently large to contain enough synapses so that the approximations discussed here are valid. The equations linking synaptic activity to action-potential firings $g(\mathbf{r}, t)$ then follow directly from the basic idea that synaptic action in a mass of neural tissue is due to action potentials fired from some other location, generally at earlier times, as indicated in Figure 11-4, that is

$$h_E(\mathbf{r}, t) = u(\mathbf{r}, t) + \int_0^{\infty} dv \int_S R_E(\mathbf{r}, \mathbf{r}_1, v) g\left(\mathbf{r}_1, t - \frac{|\mathbf{r} - \mathbf{r}_1|}{v}\right) d^2r_1 \qquad (11.1)$$

$$h_I(\mathbf{r}, t) = u_0 + \int_S R_I(\mathbf{r}, \mathbf{r}_1) g(\mathbf{r}_1, t)\, d^2r_1 \qquad (11.2)$$

In these integral equations, $u(\mathbf{r}, t)$ represents excitatory input to the cortex and corticocortical fiber system from the midbrain. For convenience, any midbrain inhibitory input u_0 is assumed to be constant during a fixed physiologic state; the results are not sensitive to this assumption. These equations express the idea that action potential firings $g(\mathbf{r}_1, t)$ at cortical location $\mathbf{r}_1$ cause synaptic activity at location $\mathbf{r}$ at later times, depending on separation distance $|\mathbf{r} - \mathbf{r}_1|$ and action potential velocities v, as depicted in Figure 11-4. Equations (11.1) and (11.2) follow directly from these ideas and should not be controversial, except that the distance $|\mathbf{r} - \mathbf{r}_1|$ is not, in general, a Euclidean distance but rather some appropriate measure related to the geodesic distance between neocortical surface points. This ambiguity does not pose major theoretical difficulties, but does introduce some uncertainty in numerical estimates of normal mode frequencies, as discussed in more detail in later sections.

All the complications of intra- and intercortical connections are combined in the functions R_E and R_I. That is, the number density of corticocortical fibers connecting locations $\mathbf{r}_1$ with $\mathbf{r}$, which also have propagation velocity v, is described by the probability density function $R_E(\mathbf{r}, \mathbf{r}_1, v)$. Propagation velocities of action potentials leading to inhibitory synapses (intracortical) are effectively infinite because the time delay over short distances is apparently much less than local delays. Thus the decrease in number density with distance is described by $R_I(\mathbf{r}, \mathbf{r}_1)$, that is, inhibitory delays are only local; such delays are included in the combined global-local theory presented later. The surface integrals in (11.1) and (11.2) sum the contributions of corticocortical input to a cortical column from the entire cortex.

The neglect of feedback circuits between cortex and thalamus in this model is based primarily on the numeric dominance of the corticocortical fibers, as discussed by Braitenberg (1978) and Katznelson (1981) and in Chapter 2. However, we must also consider the relative "strengths" of input by corticocortical and thalamic systems. That is, synaptic inputs close to somas are expected to have

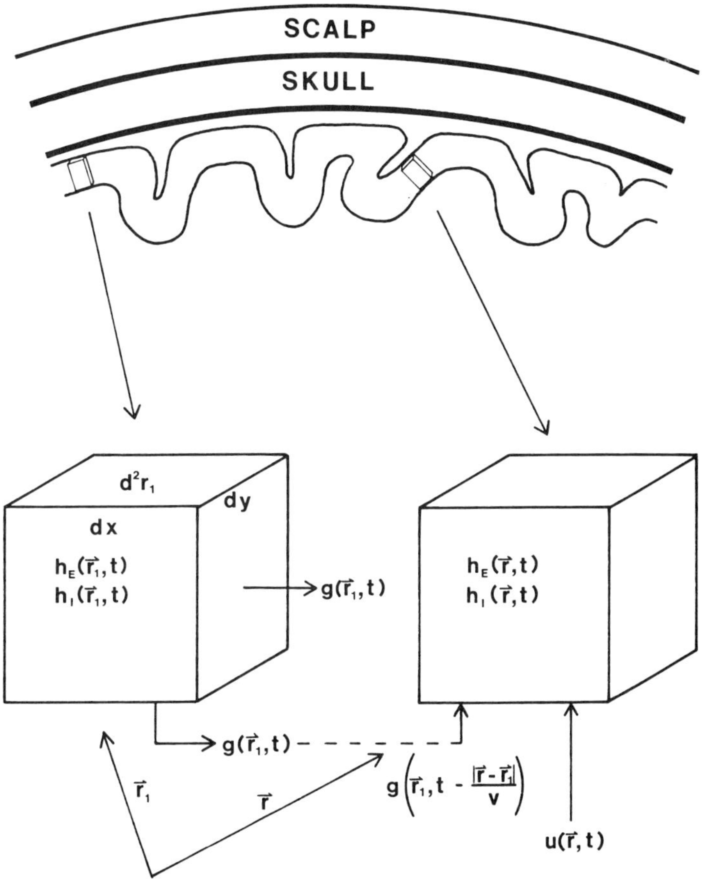

Figure 11-4. Neocortical column at location $\mathbf{r}_1$ produces action potentials $g(\mathbf{r}_1, t)$, which cause synaptic input $h_E(\mathbf{r}, t)$ at location $\mathbf{r}$, at later times $|\mathbf{r} - \mathbf{r}_1|/v$, depending on separation distance between the columns $|\mathbf{r} - \mathbf{r}_1|$ and propagation velocity of action potentials v. Separation distance is measured along the mentally "inflated" cortical surface (that is the equivalent smooth cortex). In general, corticocortical fiber synaptic connections and action potential velocities are distributed and described by the distribution function $R_E(\mathbf{r}, \mathbf{r}_1, v)$, which also includes intracortical excitatory connections. Time delays due to action potential propagation velocity in short excitatory fibers and all inhibitory (all intracortical) fibers are believed to be much shorter than local delays; propagation velocity is effectively infinite in such cases. Thus the distribution function for inhibitory fibers is $R_I(\mathbf{r}, \mathbf{r}_1)$, independent of velocity v. Equations (11.1) and (11.2) follow directly from this figure. That is, integrated action potential input from the entire cortical surface integral S at earlier times produces synaptic action h_E at time t and location $\mathbf{r}$. Mental inflation of the cortical surface does not pose fundamental problems for the theory but does introduce some uncertainty in the numeric estimates because some corticocortical fibers follow the original surface, whereas others cut across fissures and sulci (see the text).

more influence on firing rates of postsynaptic neurons. The corticocortical fibers (the total number is about 10^{10}) terminate mainly on the dendritic spines and shafts of pyramidal and stellate cells and relatively few on soma (Scheibel and Scheibel, 1970; Garey, 1979). The specific thalamocortical fibers (total number is about 10^6) terminate mainly in layer IV and provide disproportionate inputs to cell bodies and proximal dendritic locations of pyramidal cells (Szentagothai, 1979). In contrast, the nonspecific thalamocortical fibers (total number is about 10^8) apparently terminate mainly on more distal dendrites of pyramidal cells (Purpura, 1972; Creutzfeldt, 1974; Scheibel and Scheibel, 1970). Furthermore, studies by Rall (1977), discussed in Chapter 9, suggest that functional distances of dendritic synapses from soma often are much less than actual distances, due to variations in dendrite diameter in dendritic branches. The end of a typical dendritic terminal may be only one or two effective length constants from the soma. Thus remote synaptic input can have relatively large effects on soma transmembrane potential. The neglect of thalamocortical feedback appears justified based on available data. If new data suggest that such feedback loops should be included in the theory, this can be accomplished without great difficulty as shown in the Appendix.

Because the cortex is treated as a continuum of columns of arbitrarily large size, (11.1) and (11.2) involve surface integrals rather than volume integrals over surface and cortical depth. Thus synaptic delays due to action potential firings from within the same column (mostly in directions normal to the cortical surface) are neglected in this approximation but included as part of local circuit effects in the section Marriage of Local and Global Theories and the Appendix.

The number density of action potentials $g(\mathbf{r}, t)$ fired from within a cortical column depends on a synaptic input $h_E(\mathbf{r}, t)$ to the column. Thus, (11.1) and (11.2) form a coupled set of integral equations, which are generally nonlinear. The two equations contain three unknowns, g, h_E, and h_I, and thus a third equation is required. The expected qualitative relation between action potentials and synaptic input for zero local delays is illustrated by the sigmoid functions in Figure 11-5. However, the predictions of the linear theory are independent of the exact shapes of these curves. That is, these curves simply express the idea that very low levels of excitatory input to a neural mass cause minimal or zero action potential firing and a sufficiently large input causes saturation of the mass (Rall, 1955a, 1955b; Wilson and Cowan, 1973; Freeman, 1975; Nunez, 1981a), as may occur in epilepsy. This situation is modified later in this chapter with the inclusion of local delays in the global model. If fluctuations about some local equilibrium g_0 are small, as might be expected in a fixed physiologic state, the modulation of action potential activity δg may be followed (Nunez, 1974a; Katznelson, 1981). That is

$$\delta g = \frac{\partial g}{\partial h_E} H_E + \frac{\partial g}{\partial h_I} H_I \tag{11.3}$$

where the definitions $H_E = \delta h_E$ and $H_I = \delta h_I$ are used to simplify notation. Furthermore, the positive definite "cortical excitability" control parameters are

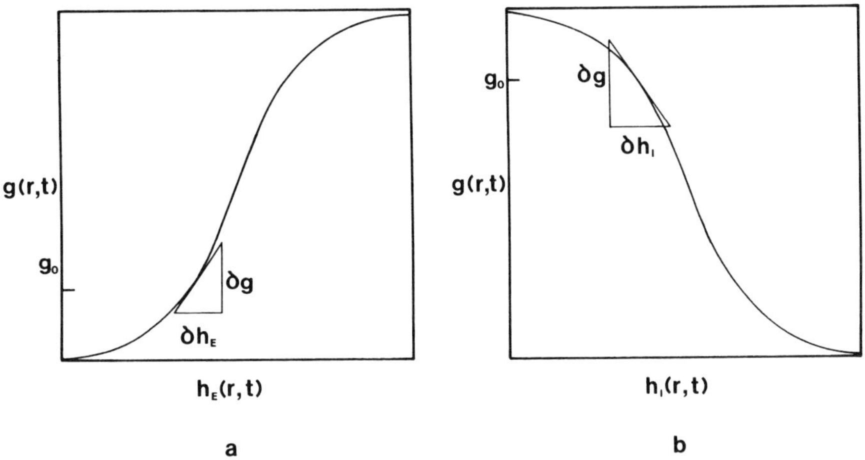

Figure 11-5. Assumed qualitative relation (at fixed time t) between number density of action potential firings g(**r**, t) in a neural mass (such as a cortical column) and the excitatory (**a**) or inhibitory (**b**) input to the mass denoted by $h_E(\mathbf{r}, t)$ and $h_I(\mathbf{r}, t)$ respectively. Predictions of the linear global theory of EEG do not depend on the shapes of these curves, but only assume the equations may be linearized around a fixed mathematical state denoted by g_0, which may correspond to a fixed physiologic state. The control parameter B, denoted by (11.12) and only weakly dependent on spatial frequency k for long wavelength waves, depends on the local derivatives shown here. For example, if in the fixed state g_0, the addition of 100 excitatory inputs to a neural mass is required, on the average, to increase by one the number of action potentials fired, and 50 inhibitory inputs reduce the number of action potentials by one, the local derivatives are $Q_E = (\partial g/\partial h_E) \sim 0.01$ and $Q_I = (\partial g/\partial h_I) \sim 0.02$. In the proposed model, the magnitude of diffuse excitatory and inhibitory input (electric, chemical, or both) from the midbrain determines the background excitability of the cortex. This input may go directly to cortical pyramidal cells or involve excitatory input to interneurons which, in turn, inhibit pyramidal cells. Thus reduction of inhibitory influences changes the state g_0 and increases the control parameter B. As B approaches a critical value $(2k_m/\lambda_E)$, the frequency of the k_m mode decreases abruptly in a manner that suggests the transition from the awake to sleeping state. These suggested input-output relations for the neural mass are modified in the combined local and global theory to account for time delays in local neural circuits. That is, in the local-global theory, the number of action potentials fired at time t depends on synaptic input integrated over earlier times. The sigmoidal curves are used in the Appendix to obtain a crude quasi-linear solution to the brain wave equations.

defined

$$Q_E = \left(\frac{\partial g}{\partial h_E}\right)_{g=g_0} \qquad Q_I = -\left(\frac{\partial g}{\partial h_I}\right)_{g=g_0} \tag{11.4}$$

which indicate the responsiveness (in terms of action potentials fired or not fired) of cortical columns with excitatory and inhibitory input. Linearization about a fixed state g_0 in (11.1) and (11.2) yields two coupled equations for the modulation of excitatory and inhibitory activity, H_E and H_I, respectively, that is

$$H_E(\mathbf{r}, t) = U(\mathbf{r}, t) + \int_0^\infty dv \int_s R_E(\mathbf{r}, \mathbf{r}_1, v) \left[Q_E H_E \left(\mathbf{r}_1, t - \frac{|\mathbf{r} - \mathbf{r}_1|}{v} \right) - Q_I H_I \left(\mathbf{r}_1, t - \frac{|\mathbf{r} - \mathbf{r}_1|}{v} \right) \right] d^2 r_1 \quad (11.5)$$

$$H_I(\mathbf{r}, t) = \int_s R_I(\mathbf{r}, \mathbf{r}_1)[Q_E H_E(\mathbf{r}_1, t) - Q_I H_I(\mathbf{r}_1, t)]\, d^2 r_1 \quad (11.6)$$

where $U(\mathbf{r}, t) = \delta u(\mathbf{r}, t)$ is the modulation of midbrain excitatory input to the cortex about some mean value.

Equations (11.5) and (11.6) are a coupled set of (linear) Fredholm integral equations in the dependent variables (unknowns) H_E and H_I. For purposes of relative simplicity, solutions to the one-dimensional version of these "brain wave equations" in an infinite medium are first considered in this section. Solutions for a finite, one-dimensional loop and for waves on a spherical surface are presented in the Appendix. Dynamic neural interaction is assumed here to produce spatial–temporal patterns of synaptic activity along a strip of cortex in some direction x (such as the anterior-posterior direction of one hemisphere), forming a neocortical circumference. Action potential and synaptic action densities then refer to space averages over the width of the strip and depth of cortex. This solution corresponds to a limit of extreme anisotrophy in which corticocortical fibers run only in the anterior-posterior and posterior-anterior directions. The one-dimensional probability density function for corticocortical connections is assumed to be of the form

$$R_E(x, x_1, v) = \frac{1}{2} \sum_{n=1}^{N} \rho_n \lambda_n f_n(v) e^{-\lambda_n |x - x_1|} \quad (11.7)$$

That is, corticocortical connections are assumed to be composed of N overlapping fiber systems. The anatomic basis for this functional form is considered later in this chapter. Within each fiber system n, the number density of connections decreases with characteristic distance λ_n^{-1}, and the distribution of propagation velocities expressed by the functions $f_n(v)$. The number of synapses per neuron associated with each excitatory fiber system is given by ρ_n. The spatial distribution of corticocortical fibers for an example case of two systems ($N = 2$) with $\lambda_2/\lambda_1 = 3$ is illustrated in Figure 11-6. Equation (11.7) is sufficiently general to account for intracortical excitatory fibers, relatively short corticocortical fibers of about 1 cm, and long corticocortical fibers (as long as 20 cm) that are part of the superior longitudinal bundle, uncinate fasciculus, and other prominent corticocortical systems.

The intracortical fiber connection density function is approximated by

$$R_I(x, x_1) = \frac{1}{2} \rho_I \lambda_I e^{-\lambda_I |x - x_1|} \quad (11.8)$$

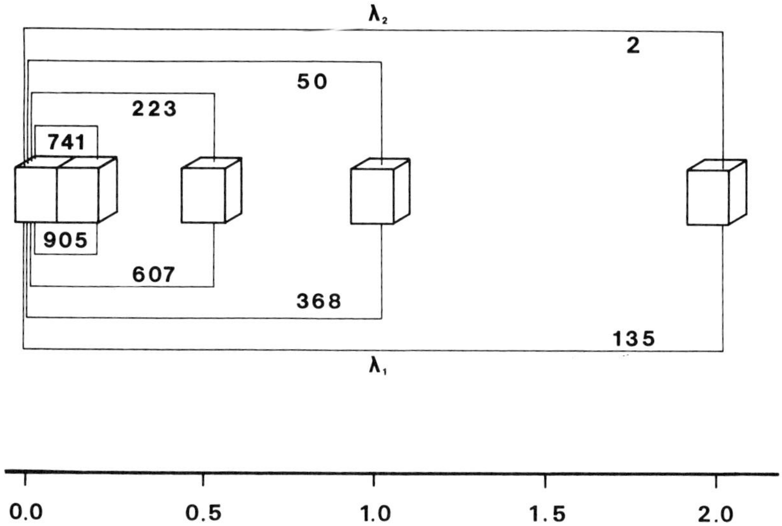

Figure 11-6. Assumed form of the distribution R_E in (11.7) of excitatory synapses of corticocortical fibers between neural masses for the special case of two fiber systems (N = 2) with $\lambda_2/\lambda_1 = 3$. The numbers shown are proportional to number of synapses and indicate that fiber system two (n = 2) exhibits a faster decrease in connectivity with separation distance $|x - x_1|$ than does fiber system one (n = 1). Actual magnitudes of numbers have no meaning here because actual number of synapses of corticocortical fibers connecting cortical columns depends on size of columns, and neocortex is treated as a continuum. Intracortical synaptic connections (not shown) are both excitatory and inhibitory and short range; corticocortical synaptic connections are only excitatory. With many excitatory fiber systems (large N), the assumed distribution function (11.7) is general. The longest fibers appear to be dominant in determining the dispersion relation for weakly damped "brain waves" recorded from the scalp.

which is based on data obtained for stellate cells and basal dendrites in the motor and visual cortices of the cat and mouse for which $\lambda_I \sim 350\ \text{cm}^{-1}$ (Sholl, 1956). Somewhat longer effective length constants (smaller λ_I's) apply to surface parallel connections, as discussed in Chapter 2. We have neglected possible delays due to finite propagation velocity in these surface parallel systems. Some of these fibers are branches of corticocortical fibers, in which case the theory need not be altered by their inclusion, except that some of the global delays suggested here should be longer, especially if the ends of the fibers are unmyelinated over 6 to 8 mm, for example. We have neglected possible effects of delays due to propagation in strictly intracortical fibers. Based on the theoretical results of this chapter, delays in short fibers appear to contribute primarily to waves of short wavelength, perhaps too short to be measured on the scalp. However, the main reason for their neglect here is that we have no quantitative information on the possible importance of these fibers.

Note that λ_I is essentially parameter d used in the local theory of Chapter 5 and in a later section of this chapter. Using (11.7) and (11.8), (11.5) and (11.6) have been solved (Nunez, 1981a, 1989a); the Appendix contains solutions for cortical strips of infinite length and finite length. The relation between the Fourier transforms of the cortical input function U(k, ω) and the excitatory synaptic firing density $H_E(k, \omega)$ is then given by

$$H_E(k, \omega) = \frac{U(k, \omega)}{D_G(k, \omega)} \tag{11.9}$$

where $T_G(k, \omega) = D_G^{-1}(k, \omega)$ is the global transfer function for the entire cortex and corticocortical fiber system. Under reasonable assumptions, the modulation of extracellular potential, averaged over the width and depth of the cortical column, is approximately proportional to modulation of synaptic firing density (Nunez, 1981a; also see Chapter 1). Thus D_G is analogous to (5.1) obtained in the local circuit model of Chapter 5.

As shown in the Appendix, the dispersion relation for brain waves in the global theory is obtained as a solution of (11.5) and (11.6). With waves in an infinite loop, that is for waves of wavelength short compared with the circumference of the loop, we obtain

$$D_G(k, \omega) = 1 - \frac{Q_E}{Q_I} \sum_{n=1}^{N} \frac{\rho_n}{\rho_I} \int_0^{\infty} \frac{\lambda_n^2 v^2 + j\omega\lambda_n v}{(\lambda_n v + j\omega)^2 + k^2 v^2} f_n(v)\, dv = 0 \tag{11.10}$$

We should consider first the case in which all fiber systems but one (n = 1 or n → E) have effectively infinite propagation velocity (negligible global delays). Equation (11.10) then yields

$$1 - B(k) \int_0^{\infty} \frac{\lambda_E^2 v^2 + j\omega\lambda_E v}{(\lambda_E v + j\omega)^2 + k^2 v^2} f_E(v)\, dv = 0 \tag{11.11}$$

where the control function B(k) is only weakly dependent on wave number k for waves of relatively long wavelength, and is expressed by

$$B(k) = \frac{\dfrac{Q_E \rho_E}{Q_I \rho_I}}{1 - \dfrac{Q_E}{Q_I} \displaystyle\sum_{n \neq E} \frac{\rho_n}{\rho_I} \left(1 + \frac{k^2}{\lambda_n^2}\right)^{-1}} \tag{11.12}$$

Here the sum is over all excitatory systems (both inter- and intracortical) that have negligible delays due to action-potential propagation.

For long wavelengths, B(k) → B evidently may be considered a control parameter independent of k, which partly determines the physiologic state of the cortex. For a highly peaked corticocortical velocity distribution at $v = v_E$, which is approximately consistent with the experimental data summarized in Figure 2-6

$$f_E(v) = \delta(v - v_E) \tag{11.13}$$

In this limiting case, (11.11) yields expressions for wave frequency (ω_R) and damping decrement (γ), as shown in Nunez (1989a) and in the Appendix

$$\omega_R^2 = v_E^2[k^2 - \lambda_E^2 B^2(k)/4] \tag{11.14}$$

$$\gamma = -\lambda_E v_E[1 - B(k)/2] \tag{11.15}$$

If the number of synapses associated with the longest fibers ρ_E is small compared with the number of inhibitory synapses ρ_I, the condition $0 < B(k) < 5$ may apply over a wide range of the ratio Q_E/Q_I. An estimate of lowest modes to be expected in finite cortex can be obtained from (11.14) by assuming an effective "circumference" of the cortex, which may be defined as the circumference of sphere having the same surface area as that of the neocortex. Reported surface areas vary from about 1600 to 4000 cm^2, corresponding to "circumferences" L ~ 35 to 56 cm.

However, the anterior-posterior circumference is of most interest here because it is longest and provides for the standing wave of lowest frequency. Furthermore, the longest corticocortical fibers follow this general direction. Thus, in the following numeric estimates, we take L ~ 50 to 100 cm as a reasonable first guess (Nunez, 1981a, 1989a) given the additional uncertainty in this parameter depending on the degree to which corticocortical fibers cut across fissures and sulci. Discrete wave numbers for standing waves in a homogeneous, closed strip of cortex are forced by periodic boundary conditions, thereby requiring both synaptic action and its derivatives to be continuous functions of x, that is

$$k_m = \frac{2\pi m}{L} \qquad m = 1, \infty \tag{11.16}$$

This wave number restriction is required for synaptic action variables or potentials in a closed isotropic and homogeneous strip. Such variables must be continuous functions of location around the strip, as in the example of the closed coaxial cable discussed in Chapters 2 and 9. With neocortex, only a continuous path needs to be followed along the surface without leaving regions with substantial corticocortical connections. For example, multiple closed strips might be formed that weave through different lobes, with side boundaries either fixed due to corticocortical fiber systems or variable due to local inhomogeneous inhibitory mechanisms. This general condition seems realistic given the very high density of these fibers in all regions of the neocortex. No other restriction on the corticocortical fibers is implied other than a limit on the length of the longest fibers to less than half a cortical circumference. Equations (11.14) and (11.15) then yield an estimated frequency for the lowest mode (m = 1) when B is small

$$f_1 \approx \frac{k_1 v_E}{2\pi} \approx 6\text{–}18 \text{ Hz} \tag{11.17}$$

This estimate shows that predicted frequencies of the lowest few modes are generally consistent with awake EEG rhythms for small B. As B approaches a critical value ($2k_m/\lambda_E$), there is an abrupt decrease in the frequency of the kth mode in a manner suggestive of the transition from the awake to sleeping state. This change in B might be caused by a reduction in the diffuse inhibitory input from the brainstem known to be required to maintain the awake state, thereby changing the value of g_0 in Figure 11-5 and increasing the corresponding ratio Q_E/Q_I. The apparent lowest mode $k_1 \sim 0.06$ to $0.12\ cm^{-1}$, assuming λ_E represents long corticocortical fibers with $\lambda_E^{-1} \sim 5$ to 15 cm, corresponds to a threshold value of $B(k_1)$ in the range 0.6 to 3.6. However, when $B(k_m) = B_{\ell u}(k_m) = 2$, (11.15) predicts unstable oscillations so that the range of $B(k_m) < 2$ is emphasized in this section. In the next section, an estimate of B, based on fundamental anatomy and physiology, is obtained, suggesting that B is of the order of one. In the section Quasi-linear Effects, we consider the case of $B > 2$ and resulting limit cycle oscillations of each spatial mode. For small B, weakly damped waves occur if

$$\frac{\gamma}{\omega_R} \approx \frac{\lambda_E}{k_m} << 1 \tag{11.18}$$

If we use the parameter ranges noted above, this ratio appears to be about 0.2 to 3.0 for the lowest modes, $m = 1, 3$. Damping is further decreased as λ_E decreases (longer fibers) or B increases (more "excitable" cortex). Although the appropriate neural parameters are not known with sufficient accuracy for close quantitative comparison, the theoretical predictions of this section appear qualitatively consistent with observed spatial and temporal properties of much spontaneous EEG. That is, the predicted frequency range is approximately correct, and standing waves of long wavelength (spatially coherent over large regions of scalp) are expected.

The simple analytic solution just outlined is based on several assumptions that require further examination: the existence of only a single long-range fiber system with exponential decrease of connection density, the neglect of spreads in the velocity distribution functions $f_n(v)$, the linear approximation, and the choice of an infinite, one-dimensional cortex. Relaxation of each one of these restrictions yields new insights about and variations in the predicted behavior of EEG; however, the approximate semi-quantitative results of this section appear valid under the microscopy of more exact mathematics, as shown in the following sections.

Physiologic Estimates of the Control Parameter B

The relation between different neuromodulators and the control parameter B expressed by (11.12), is evidently complex. One complication is that most cortical neurons operate under the influence of a dozen or more neuroactive substances (see Chapters 5 and 13). Despite the many difficulties, it is valuable to obtain a crude estimate of B in the anticipation that more accurate estimates will be possible in the future. The sum in (11.12) is over all excitatory fiber systems with negligible global delays, that is, $|\omega/\lambda_n v_n| << 1$. If these are all intracortical fiber systems, such as recurrent collaterals of pyramidal cells or surface parallel systems (see

Chapter 2), $\lambda_n > 1\ \text{cm}^{-1}$ so that $k/\lambda_n << 1$ for all waves of long wavelength. With this approximation

$$B(k) \sim B = \frac{\dfrac{Q_E \rho_E}{Q_I \rho_I}}{1 - \dfrac{Q_E}{Q_I} \displaystyle\sum_{n \neq E} \frac{\rho_n}{\rho_I}} \tag{11.19}$$

In this case, the cortical control parameter B is independent of wave number k.

Table 11-1 summarizes some of the anatomic studies of Braitenberg and Schuz (1991). A simplified cortex, composed of 85% pyramidal cells and 15% stellate cells, is proposed by these anatomists as a reasonable first approximation. Two kinds of synapses, called type I and type II, have been identified according to their appearance in electron micrographs. They are believed to correspond to excitatory and inhibitory functions, respectively. Excitatory synapses are distributed mainly over dendritic shafts and spines, whereas inhibitory synapses focus primarily on cell bodies and the initial segment of axons. From Table 11-1, the ratio of excitatory to inhibitory synapses is estimated to be

$$\frac{\displaystyle\sum_n \rho_n}{\rho_I} \sim \frac{85\%}{15\%} \sim 6 \tag{11.20}$$

A reasonable guess (for mouse cortex) is that about one half of the excitatory synapses occur on intracortical axons and one half occur on corticocortical axons (Braitenberg and Schuz, 1991). However, it has been suggested that the fraction of excitatory synapses on corticocortical fibers in humans is much higher, perhaps 80% (Wright and Liley, 1994). For the crude approximations of this section, we consider all $n = E$ fibers to be corticocortical and all $n \neq E$ fibers to be intracortical. This idea is reconsidered later in this chapter. If the fraction of corticocortical excitatory fibers is in the range of 0.5 to 0.8

$$\frac{\displaystyle\sum_{n \neq E} \rho_n}{\rho_I} \sim 1 \text{ to } 3 \tag{11.21}$$

The cortical excitability parameters Q_E and Q_I are defined by (11.4). Because

Table 11-1 Types of Synaptic Connections in Neocortex*

Synaptic Connection	Percentage	Location
Pyramidal to pyramidal cell	72	Type I on spines
Pyramidal to stellate cell	13	Type I mainly on dendritic shafts
Stillate to pyramidal cell	13	Type II on cell bodies
Stillate to stellate cell	2	Type II mainly on dendritic shafts

*Type I synapse believed to be excitatory and type II synapse believed to be inhibitory. (Reproduced with permission from Braitenberg and Schuz, 1991.)

excitatory synapses are located on spines and dendritic shafts, whereas inhibitory synapses occur mainly on cell bodies, we expect

$$Q_E/Q_I < 1 \tag{11.22}$$

However, we have no quantitative estimate for the relative "local strengths" of excitatory and inhibitory transmitters. Given the many transmitters affecting each neuron, the difference of locations of synaptic input to the neuron, and other complicating factors, we are not now able to obtain a good estimate for the ratio Q_E/Q_I. However, we can illustrate these ideas with an example. Suppose that an addition of 1,000 synchronous excitatory synaptic inputs to a macroscopic mass of neocortex causes an additional 30 neurons to fire action potentials, as estimated by Abeles (1982). A assumed ratio of $Q_E/Q_I = 0.2$ would cause a further input of 200 inhibitory synaptic inputs to return the neural mass to its original firing rate. If we assume that Q_E/Q_I is about 0.1 to 0.3 and that the synaptic ratio given by (11.21) is correct, the resulting estimate of the control parameter is

$$B \sim 0.4 \text{ to } 9.0 \tag{11.23}$$

As Q_E/Q_I approaches the value $\rho_I \Big/ \sum_{n \neq E} \rho_n$, the control parameter (11.19) becomes large and we expect a breakdown of the linear approximation (11.3). This issue is considered further in connection with the quasi-linear approach later in this chapter.

We have treated the distinction between synchronous and moderately asynchronous synaptic input superficially in this section because of application of the linear approximation (11.3) at fixed time points, for example, local delays have been neglected. This procedure amounts to coarse graining over a time approximately equal to the rise and fall of PSPs. The effects of these local delays are included in an approximate manner in the next section. Abeles (1982) estimated that about 30 simultaneous presynaptic spikes are needed to bring the average membrane potential to threshold. In contrast, the number of asynchronous synaptic inputs is estimated to be more like 300. In this context, Q_E might be uncertain by a factor of 10 or more, depending on the degrees of asynchrony. However, the control parameter B depends only on the ratio of Q_E/Q_I, so a wide range of estimates of Q_E or Q_I does not necessarily result in large changes in the corresponding estimate for B if Q_E and Q_I are estimated consistently.

Marriage of Local and Global Theories

In the combined local-global theory, input to the cortex consists of the modulating afferent input from the midbrain $U(k, \omega)$ (the driving "force") and input $H_E(k, \omega)$ from other (perhaps distant) cortical regions through the corticocortical fibers, as indicated in Figures 11-4 and 11-7. Thus the basic input – output relation, obtained with the local theory of Chapter 5, is replaced by

$$V(k, \omega) \approx \frac{U(k, \omega) + H_E(k, \omega)}{D_L(k, \omega)} \tag{11.24}$$

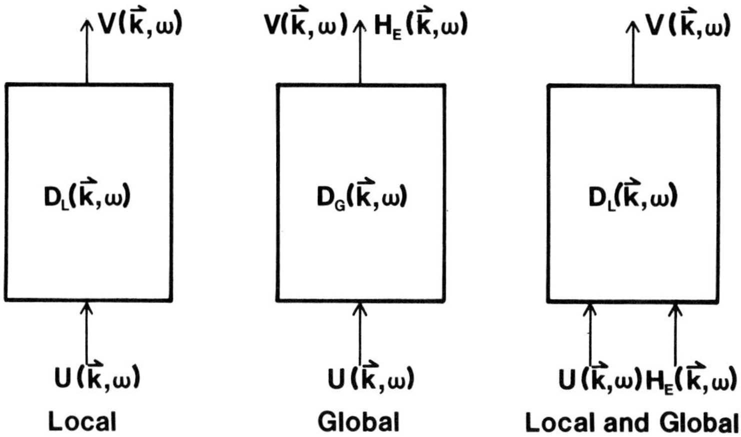

Figure 11-7. Input-output relations for local, global, and combined local-global theories. $U(\mathbf{k}, \omega)$ is the spectral density function for midbrain input to the cortex-corticocortical fiber system. $D_L^{-1}(\mathbf{k}, \omega)$ and $D_G^{-1}(\mathbf{k}, \omega)$ are local and global transfer functions, respectively. In the combined local-global theory, modulation of synaptic action from remote cortical regions provides an additional input to local columnar circuits (right-most box). In each case $V(\mathbf{k}, \omega)$ refers to the modulation of synaptic action at macroscopic scales. See the Appendix for more information.

where $D_L(k, \omega)$ is the local dispersion function (5.1), and $V(k, \omega)$ is the total output from a neocortical mass due to midbrain and nonlocal cortical input. With this approach, the linearized relation between synaptic and action potential activity (11.3) is modified to account for local delays that are neglected by using (11.3) at fixed time.

The input–output relation for the cortex, which may include inhibitory and excitatory feedback from the local theory and excitatory corticocortical interactions from the global theory, is obtained in Nunez (1989a) and in the Appendix (using a different approach). That is, modulation of cortical synaptic firing density $H_E(k, \omega)$, which is believed to be approximately proportional to modulation of extracellular potential, is expressed by

$$H_E(k, \omega) = \frac{[D_L(k, \omega) + BF(k, \omega)]U(k, \omega)}{D_L(k, \omega) - BF(k, \omega)} \tag{11.25}$$

where the function $F(k,\omega)$ is defined by

$$F(k, \omega) \equiv \sum_{n=1}^{N} \frac{\rho_n}{\rho_E} \int_0^{\infty} \frac{\lambda_n^2 v^2 + j\omega\lambda_n v}{(\lambda_n v + j\omega)^2 + k^2 v^2} f_n(v)\, dv \tag{11.26}$$

and B is the global control parameter determining background excitability. The local–global dispersion relation is then given by

$$D(k, \omega) = D_L(k, \omega) - BF(k, \omega) = 0 \tag{11.27}$$

The complex roots of (11.27) then yield oscillatory frequencies ω_{Ri} to be expected in a cortex with the local and global properties outlined in this chapter. The following limiting cases are of interest:

1. Waves of relatively long spatial wavelength, that is, $k << c$ and d, where c^{-1} and d^{-1} are characteristic lengths for the decrease of intracortical excitatory and inhibitory connections. This limit applies to all potentials measured with large electrodes and all scalp electrodes. The local dispersion function (5.1) is then given by $D_L(k, \omega) = D_L(0, \omega)$.

2. Short excitatory and inhibitory postsynaptic potential rise times a^{-1} and b^{-1}, respectively, that is, $|\omega| << a$ and b. In this limit, $D_L(0, \omega) = 1$, and the dispersion relation (11.27) is due only to global delays, as indicated by (11.10) or (11.11).

3. Short global delays (infinite propagation velocity along cortocortical fibers), that is, $|\omega/\lambda_n v_n| << 1$ for all long-range systems $n = 1, N$. In this limit (11.27) becomes

$$D(k, \omega) = D_L(k, \omega) - B \sum_{n=1}^{N} \frac{\rho_n/\rho_E}{1 + k^2/\lambda_n^2} = 0 \qquad (11.28)$$

This limit does not fully reduce to the local theory of Chapter 5, because no corticocortical interactions are included in this local theory. In the strictly local theory with the EPSP and IPSP rise times assumed here, instability occurs when the local control parameter $Q = 4.5$. When the corticocortical interactions in (11.27) are included, this value is reduced.

4. Waves of long wavelength, case (1), with a single corticocortical fiber system ($n \rightarrow E$), and long local and global delays. The dispersion relation (11.27) with approximation (11.13) then reduces to

$$D(k, \omega) = \frac{(j\omega + b)^2(j\omega + a)^2 + Qa^2b^2}{(j\omega + b)^2(1 + Q)a^2} - B \frac{\lambda_E^2 v_E^2 + j\omega\lambda_E v_E}{(\lambda_E v_E + j\omega)^2 + k^2 v_E^2} = 0 \qquad (11.29)$$

The combined local-global dispersion relation (11.29) yields a sixth-degree polynomial in ω corresponding to three branches of the dispersion relation ($i = 1, 3$). The results of numerical solutions of (11.29) are summarized in Figure 11-8, in which real frequencies ω_{Ri} and damping decrements γ_i are plotted as a function of normalized wave number k/λ_E for waves of long wavelength. In all three examples, only the two branches of the dispersion relation with weak to moderate damping are shown. The parameters chosen for Figure 11-8a correspond to short EPSP and IPSP rise times (2 and 4 milliseconds, respectively) or $a = 500$ second^{-1}, $b = 250$ second^{-1}, and moderate global delays $\lambda_E v_E = 30$ second^{-1}. The results are essentially those of the pure global theory (the local mode f_2 occurs at higher frequencies than can be shown on this scale). In Figure 11-8b, the opposite limit is illustrated with $a = 100$ second^{-1}, $b = 50$ second^{-1}, and $\lambda_E v_E = 300$ second^{-1}, so that the principal contribution to the low-frequency EEG range occurs as the result of local delays. This corresponds to a solution to (11.28) with $N = 1$.

In the example of Figure 11-8c, both local and global delays are in the range

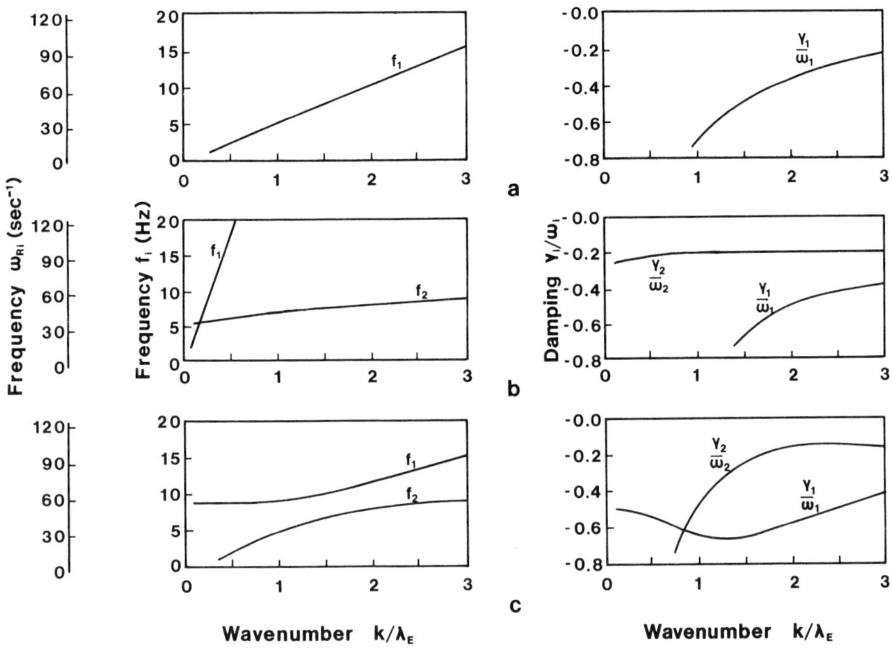

Figure 11-8. Real frequencies (ω_{Ri}, left column) and corresponding relative damping decrements (γ_i/ω_{Ri}, right column) are plotted as functions of normalized wave number (k/λ_E) for three sets of the physiologic parameters in the local-global dispersion relation (11.29). This sixth-degree polynomial yields six complex roots corresponding to three branches (i = 1, 2, 3) of the dispersion relation (complex roots occur in pairs with positive and negative real frequencies). Only the two branches (i = 1, 2) with weak to moderate damping are shown; the third branch is overdamped. Different branches of the dispersion relation correspond physiologically to the simultaneous existence of different types of brain waves (in a manner analogous to the simultaneous existence of optical and acoustic wave branches in crystals and plasmas, for example). (**a**) Frequency and damping of branch 1 in the limit of very short local delays; the results essentially are those of the pure global theory. The second branch corresponding to local phenomena occurs at high frequencies off the scale. (**b**) Frequency and damping for branches 1 and 2 in the opposite limit of very short global delays; the results essentially are identical to those of the purely local theory. (**c**) Frequency and damping for branches 1 and 2 when both local and global delays are in the range required to produce characteristic EEG frequencies. In closed systems, wave numbers (k) are restricted by boundary conditions, that is, such systems act as spatial filters. Because frequencies are restricted by the dispersion relation, the combination of dispersion relation and boundary conditions produces the characteristic frequencies observed in the system.

required to produce low frequencies. The local control parameter Q = 2.0 chosen in all examples of Figure 11-8 is about one half the value at which local instability occurs (the threshold value is 4.5 when the global parameter is B = 0). As Q is increased toward this threshold, the frequencies of the f_2 branch of the dispersion relation increase and the damping γ_2 decreases. The global parameter B = 0.5

chosen in the examples of Figure 11-8 is about one fourth the value required to produce a global instability (the threshold for instability is 2.0 when $D_L(\omega, k) = 1$). As B is increased, the frequencies of the f_1 branch of the dispersion relation are unchanged until B is close to the critical value $(2k_m/\lambda_E)$, at which point the frequencies of modes (k_m) decrease sharply, in a manner that suggests the transition from the awake to sleeping state, as described in (11.14) and (11.15). Also, as B is increased, the damping γ_1 of the branch decreases.

Because the damping of all branches depends on the magnitudes of control parameters Q and B, we cannot predict which of the two branches shown in Figure 11-8c is most likely to be observed without knowing the magnitudes of these parameters. Here the local control parameter Q is closer to the value that results in local instability than is the global control parameter B to the value that results in global instability. Thus, for these choices of parameters Q and B, the local mode f_2 is more weakly damped for wave numbers in the range shown $(0 < k/\lambda_E < 3)$, and is more likely to be observed in the EEG. A variety of neuromodulators may selectively alter control parameters Q and B so that EEG dynamics can switch between more local and more global operation in this manner. The roles of different neuromodulators in effecting such changes between local and global operation in neocortex are discussed in Chapter 13.

Effects of Multiple Long-Range Fiber Systems

The dispersion relations obtained in previous sections depend on the assumption of a single long-range corticocortical fiber system. That is, axon connection density for all axons having finite action potential velocities was assumed to obey (11.7) with the $n = 1$ fiber system. Here we examine the case $N = 2$, depicted in Figure 11-6, for the purely global theory. With a choice of sufficiently large N's, we can expect (11.7) to match nearly any functional decrease in connection density with distance. However, the accuracy of results obtained with small N are subject to more critical scrutiny. Thus we first consider the available experimental evidence concerning decrease in corticocortical fiber connections with cortical separation distance, some of which is reviewed by Katznelson (1981, 1982).

Human cerebral cortex is strongly interconnected by approximately 10^{10} intercortical fibers. That is, nearly every pyramidal cell in neocortex sends an axon into the white matter. Most of these axons re-enter the cortex at a distant location. Axons that project to the same hemisphere are corticocortical fibers; projections to opposite hemispheres are mostly fibers through the corpus callosum. Some of the human corticocortical fibers near the lateral surface of the cortex are shown in Figure 11-9a. Deeper fibers of the lateral aspect appear in Figure 11-9b. Fibers in the medial aspect are shown in Figure 11-10. A horizontal section of the brain is shown in Figure 11-11. These pictures were constructed from detailed dissection studies (Krieg, 1963, 1973). The most superficial are the U-shaped fibers, which tend to connect adjacent gyri. Also shown are extensive fiber systems of varying geometry that allow direct signals between remote cortical locations. For example,

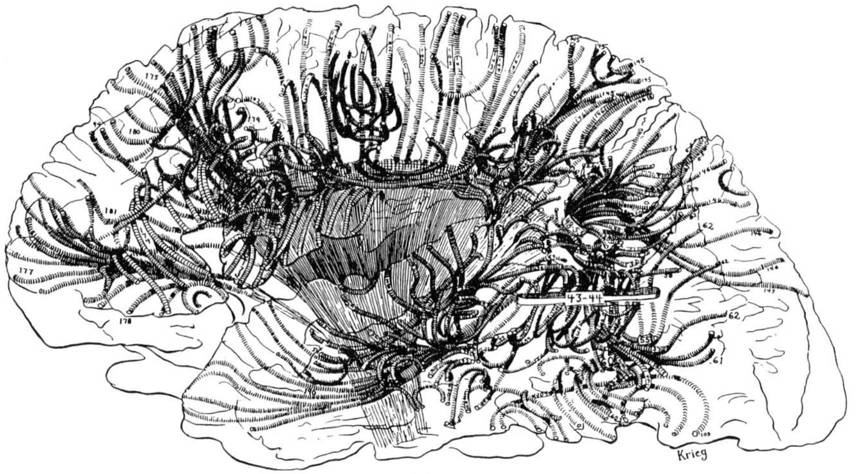

(a)

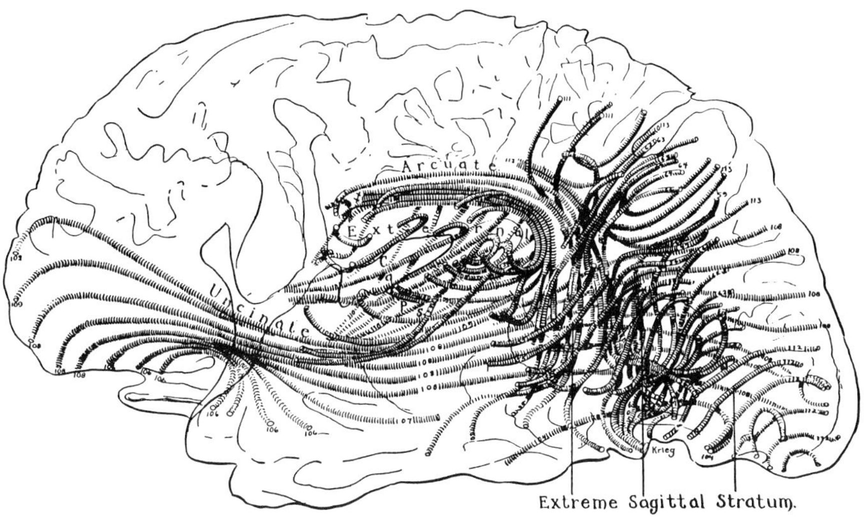

(b)

Figure 11-9. (**a**) Some of the more superficial corticocortical fibers of the lateral aspect of the cerebrum. This is a duplicate of Figure 2-19. (**b**) Some of the deeper corticocortical fibers of the lateral aspect of the cerebrum. For every fiber shown here, about 100 million are not shown. (Reproduced with permission from Krieg, 1963, 1973.)

fibers of the uncinate fasciculus run the entire length of the brain as shown in Figure 11-9b. By using the appropriate scale factor for one hemisphere, an estimate of 17 cm is obtained for the projection of these long fibers on the plane of the figure. Only a small fraction of corticocortical and callosal fibers are shown. For every axon shown in these figures, about 100 million are not shown.

Another type of study of corticocortical and callosal projections involves the

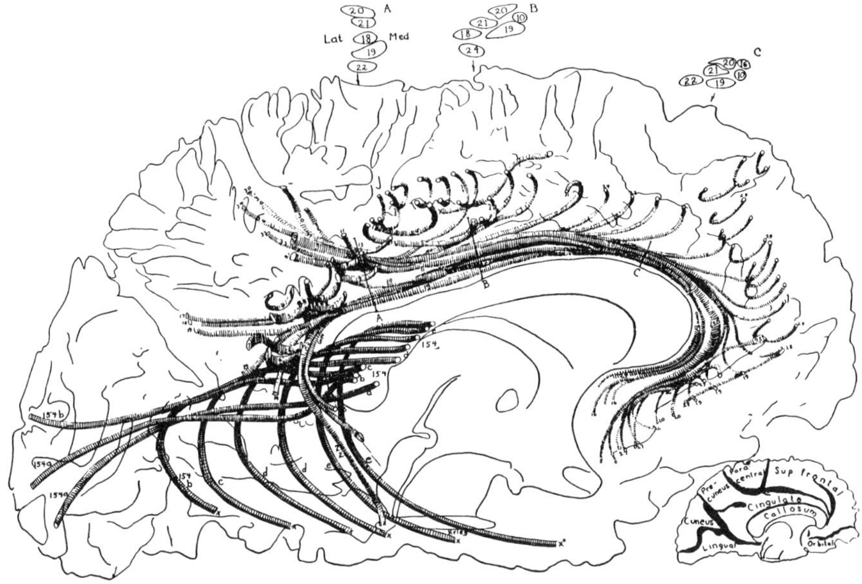

(a)

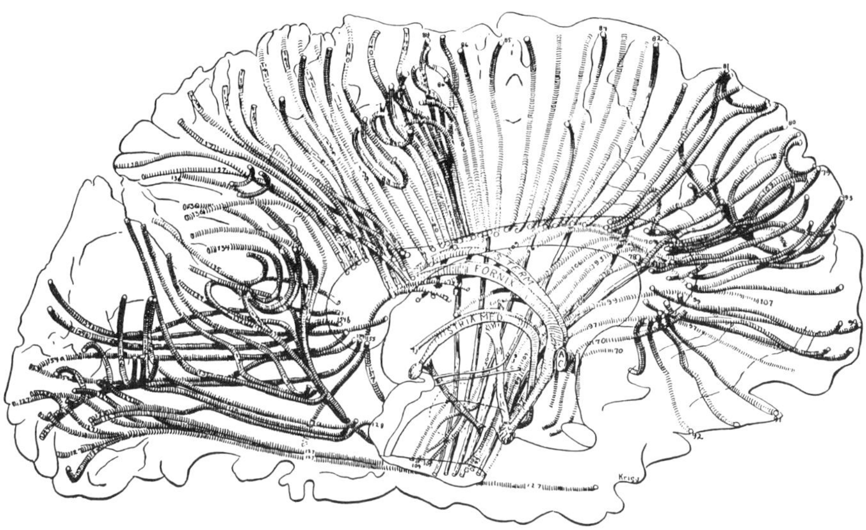

(b)

Figure 11-10. (**a**) Some of the deeper corticocortical fibers of the medial aspect of the cerebrum. Some of the longer fibers wrap around the corpus callosum. Also shown are some of the relatively short U fibers. (**b**) Fibers in the medial aspect of the cerebrum which are mainly radiations of callosal fibers with a few association (corticocortical) fibers also shown. (Reproduced with permission from Krieg, 1963, 1973.)

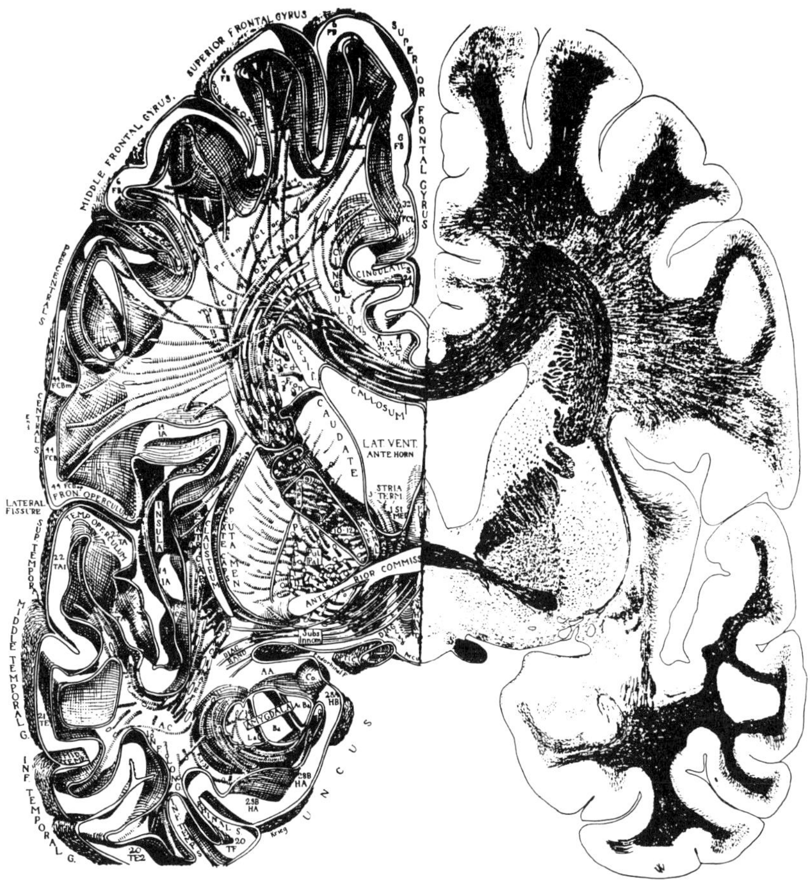

Figure 11-11. Horizontal slice through the human brain showing a few of the callosal and thalamocortical fibers. (Reproduced with permission from Krieg, 1963.)

injection of radioactive amino acids into the cortex of a monkey. The local cortical cells transport the amino acids to the ends of their axons. Some of the results of one such study are shown in Figures 11-12 and 11-13, in which injection sites were in motor and somatosensory cortex (Kunzle, 1978). The cortical regions of axon termination are characterized by homogeneous and heterogeneous grain arrangements concentrated in different cortical layers. The grain distribution is bilateral; however contralateral projections are less dense. For our purposes, an important issue is the general tendency for the number of connections to decrease with distance from the injection site. That is, although the anatomic literature on corticocortical fibers tends to emphasize specificity of connections, other studies suggest the simultaneous existence of specific connections at spatial scales below a few millimeters together with a relatively smooth decrease in connection density at centimeter scales, as suggested by Figure 11-14. The probability density func-

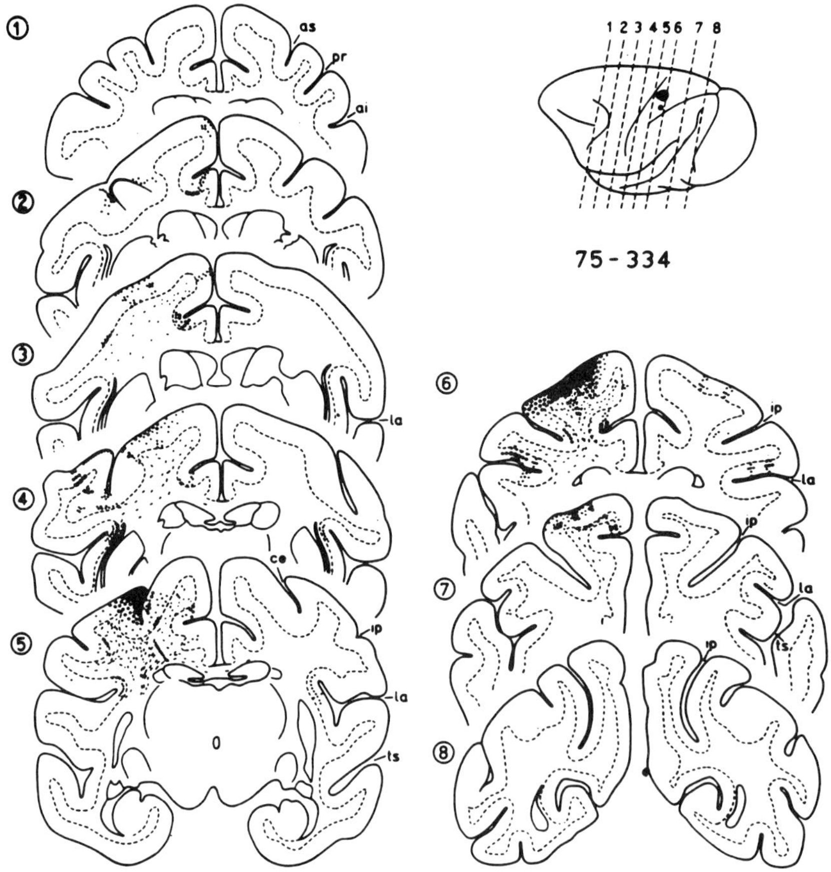

Figure 11-12. A study of corticocortical fibers using the injection of radioactive amino acids into monkey motor cortex at the position of the black spot shown on cortical surface. Local cells transport amino acids to the ends of their axons. A series of brain slices is shown with tracer concentration indicating that intrahemispheric connection density tends to decrease with distance from injection site. (Reproduced with permission from Kunzle, 1978.)

tion (11.7) is most accurate for these larger scales. However, with the assumption of multiple fiber systems $N > 1$, (11.7) can be made to fit many possible connection functions.

Including two long-range excitatory fiber systems (that is, systems in which action potential propagation velocity must be considered finite) in the dispersion relation (11.10) is straightforward. The parameters ρ_E, λ_E for one long-range system are replaced by ρ_1, λ_1 and ρ_2, λ_2, corresponding to two long-range systems. As in one such system, all other excitatory system parameters (n greater than 2) are

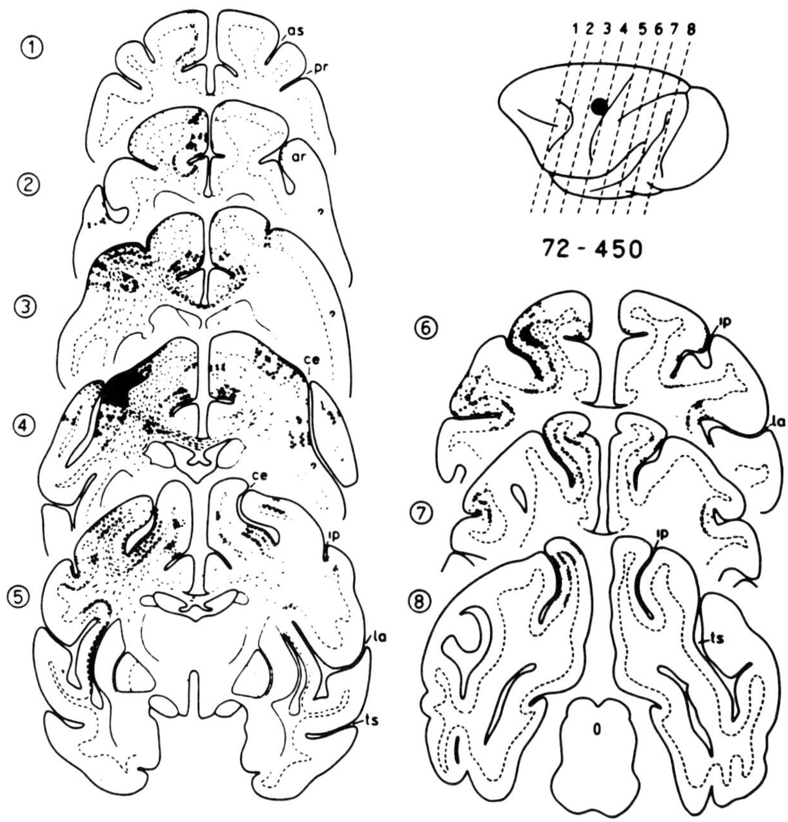

Figure 11-13. This figure is similar to Figure 11-12, except the injection site is the somatosensory cortex. (Reproduced with permission from Kunzle, 1978.)

combined in the control parameter B, expressed by (11.12) with the sum now over n = 3, N. If all long-range systems carry action potentials with the same delta function (peaked) velocity distribution, the dispersion relation (11.10) gives rise to a fourth-degree algebraic equation for frequency as a function of wave number, as shown in the Appendix.

We consider here the case of a single intracortical excitatory system (n = 3). Following the anatomic evidence outlined previously, we can take the ratio of total excitatory to inhibitory synapses to be $(\rho_1 + \rho_2 + \rho_3)/\rho_I = 6$, and an equal number of inter- and intracortical excitatory synapses $\rho_3 = \rho_1 + \rho_2$. This implies that the ratio of intracortical excitatory to inhibitory synapses is $\rho_3/\rho_I = 3$. Some electrophysiologic evidence shows that the ratio of excitatory to inhibitory synapses between neurons with very close soma (less than 0.1 m) is about 1.5 (Abeles, 1982). This result is consistent with a total intracortical ratio of $\rho_3/\rho_I = 3$ if the longer range intracortical fibers are mainly excitatory, which seems to be so (see

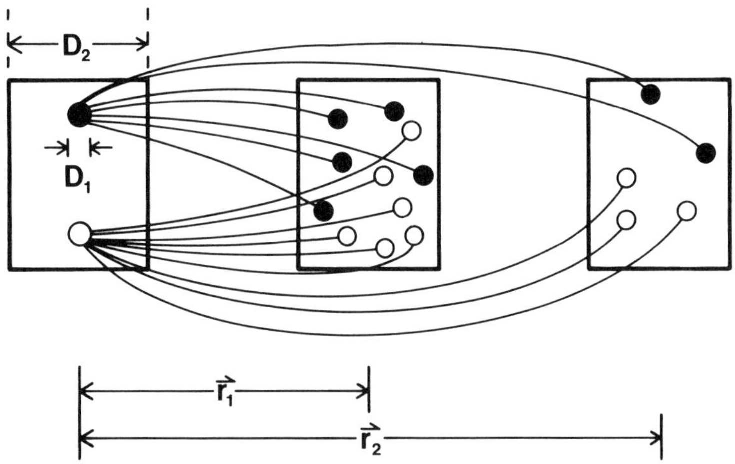

Figure 11-14. Symbolic representation of a system in which connection density is specific at small scales (D_1) and decreases monotonically with distance at large scales (D_2). This is consistent with corticocortical fiber connections if D_1 is less than a millimeter and D_2 is a few centimeters.

Chapter 2). With two long-range corticocortical fiber systems (n = 1 and 2) and one intracortical excitatory system (n = 3), the single control parameter of (11.19) is replaced by the two control parameters (B_1 and B_2):

$$B_{1,2} = \frac{\dfrac{Q_{1,2}\rho_{1,2}}{Q_I\rho_I}}{1 - \dfrac{Q_3\rho_3}{Q_I\rho_I}} \tag{11.30}$$

If we further assume that all excitatory synapses have equal strength (that is, $Q_1 = Q_2 = Q_3$) and that the number of synapses per neuron of the two long-range systems is equal (that is, $\rho_1 = \rho_2$), the range $Q_1/Q_I \sim 0.1$ to 0.3 yields the estimate

$$B_{1,2} \sim 0.2 \text{ to } 4.5 \tag{11.31}$$

Again these numerical estimates are only educated guesses, but they show that the parameters of this theory are physiologically based. Thus we can anticipate more accurate estimates in the future. The dispersion relation for two long-range excitatory fiber systems and representative physiologic parameters is plotted in Figure 11-15. Equation (11.10) gives rise to two branches of the dispersion relation; however, one is overdamped in the low-frequency range of interest in EEG. Another example is shown in Figure 11-16, in which the lower modes of the underdamped branch are substantially reduced in frequency as a result of an increase in the cortical control parameter B_1. Also the damping is reduced; in fact, waves exhibit negative damping or instability if B_1 is increased further. Such instabilities predicted by the linear theory perhaps lead to limit cycle oscillations,

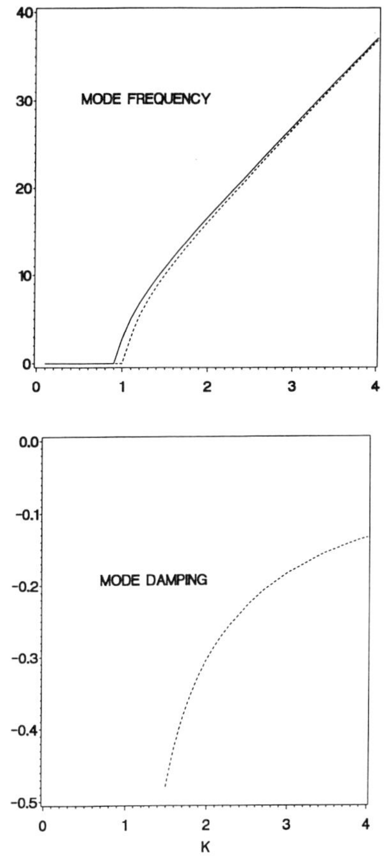

Figure 11-15. Dispersion relation (11.10) for a model cortex with two (n = 1, 2) long-range fiber systems. Fourth-degree polynomial yields two branches of the dispersion relation (solid and dotted lines). In the upper figure, frequency (Hz) is plotted versus normalized wave number $K = k/\lambda_1$. Parameters are $\lambda_1 = 0.1\ \text{cm}^{-1}$, $\lambda_2 = 0.3\ \text{cm}^{-1}$, $v_E = 600$ cm/second, $B_1 = 0.5$, and $B_2 = 0.8$. Damping is expressed as the nondimensional ratio γ_i/ω_{Ri}. Damping curve of one branch (solid line) lies below -0.5 over the range of K shown.

as suggested by the quasi-linear approximation discussed later. The change illustrated by the transition from Figure 11-15 to Figure 11-16 is qualitatively similar to the transition of EEG from the awake to sleeping state. That is, an increase in the "background" excitability level of the cortex (due perhaps to removal of inhibitory influence from the brainstem) causes a decrease in the frequencies of lower modes. At the same time, higher modes may be relatively unchanged.

The addition of each new long-range excitatory fiber system increases the degree of the polynomial dispersion relation by two. Underdamped solutions occur in pairs corresponding to positive and negative real frequencies, that is, underdamped solutions appear as complex conjugate roots to the polynomial dispersion relations. Thus the addition of each new long-range excitatory system adds a new branch to the dispersion relation. Some will be overdamped and some underdamped, depending on physiologic parameters. Although multiple fiber systems add some complications to the simple situation outlined in the section Basic Global Theory, semiquantitative conclusions, such as the general range of lower mode frequencies expected, are not substantially modified.

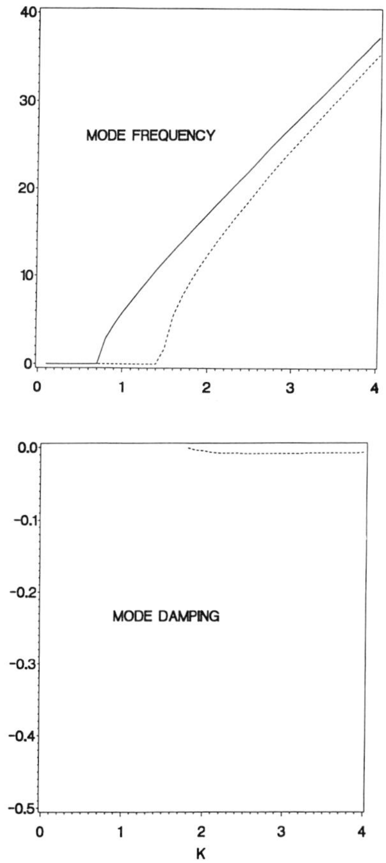

Figure 11-16. Dispersion relation (11.10) for a model cortex with two ($n = 1, 2$) long-range fiber systems. This is identical to Figure 11-15 except the first control parameter has a value $B_1 = 1.15$. The frequencies of modes with K near 1 decrease sharply and the damping of a wide range of modes approaches zero. Further increases in either B_1 or B_2 cause some modes to have positive values of γ_i, that is to become unstable in the context of the linear theory. Such modes may become limit cycles.

Alternate Functional Forms for Corticocortical Fiber Distributions

Little quantitative information on the distribution of corticocortical fibers appears in the literature. However, in a recent study of mouse cortex, a chemical substance used for retrograde axonal transport (horseradish peroxidase) was injected to many 1-mm^2 patches of cortical surface (Braitenberg and Schuz, 1991). Horseradish peroxidase travels along the axon toward the cell body, filling the cell and allowing it to be stained appropriately. The injection sites were chosen in 21 mouse brains to let the entire sample cover the whole dorsal surface of cortex as completely as possible. Cells with axons projecting to the injection site were localized in discrete patches of size about equal or smaller than the injection sites. More than one patch of remote cortex projected to the injection site. In some cases, as many as eight separate patches were distributed widely over the cortex. The distribution of measured distances between cell body and injection site (that is, the cortical termination point of the corticocortical axon) is shown in the histogram of Figure

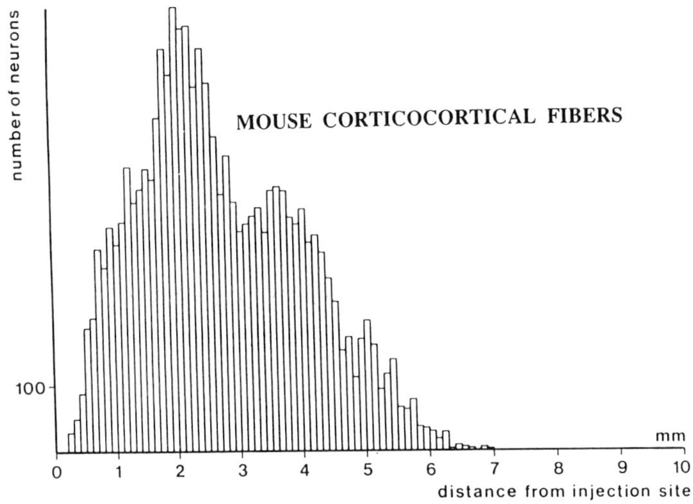

Figure 11-17. Distribution of the distances spanned by the corticocortical connections in many mouse brains obtained by the injection of horseradish peroxidase to about 1 mm^2 of cortical surface at different injection sites to cover the entire dorsal surface of cortex as completely as possible. Only homolateral connections are shown. The longest corticocortical fibers found in this study are about 7 mm. The peaks at 2 and 4 mm correspond to about 3 and 6 cm in the human brain if the linear scale factor of Table 2-1 is applied without correction for the disproportionate increase in human cortical surface area. The longest fibers found in mouse ~ 7 mm scale in this manner to 10 cm. The mouse has an unfolded cortex and folding of the human cortex increases the linear scale factor by a factor of about two. Thus we predict that the longest corticocortical fibers in humans are about 20 cm, which is approximately the correct value. If this same reasoning is applied to the peaks of the mouse histogram, human peaks at 6 and 12 cm would be predicted. However, no detailed human data on the distribution of corticocortical axon lengths are known. (Reproduced with permission from Braitenberg and Schuz, 1991.)

11-17. The average axon length is about 3 mm, with a maximum length of about 7 mm.

The distribution of corticocortical fiber lengths shown in Figure 11-17 is precisely the type of quantitative anatomic information required by global theory. However, these mouse data, which involve more than 10,000 length measurements, is apparently unique, that is, data approaching this degree of detail are not available for any other mammalian cortex. Thus in the short run we can only try to rescale the data to provide a first guess about the equivalent distribution in human brain. Two issues in such scaling are obvious: the linear scale factor of 1.0/0.07 ~ 14, based only on brain weight (Table 2-1) and the fact that mouse cortex has a smooth surface whereas human cortex is folded. The latter factor introduces an additional scale factor of about 2.2 to account for the increased distance along the folded surface (Nunez, 1981a).

The shorter corticocortical axons of the human brain must circumscribe fissures and sulci, whereas many of the longer fibers cut across some of these folds, as shown in Figure 11-9. Thus the shorter fibers of Figure 11-17 might be scaled by the factor 14 × 2.2 = 31, whereas the longest fibers may scale by a factor closer to 14. However, the longest fibers found in mouse brain were 7 mm. Application of the scaling factor 14 results in a prediction of longest human fibers of about 10 cm, whereas the scale factor 31 results in an equivalent prediction of about 22 cm. The later value is much closer to the real maximum for human brain, as shown in Figure 11-9. Given these arguments, we scaled the distribution of Figure 11-17 by the factor 31 and plotted both this rescaled data and the functional form

$$R_E(x, x_1, v) \sim (x - x_1)^2 e^{-\lambda|x-x_1|} \tag{11.32}$$

with $\lambda = 0.1$ cm in Figure 11-18. Alternately, if we rescaled the mouse data by the factor 14, the same fit would be obtained, but with $\lambda = (0.1 \times 31)/14 \sim 0.22$ cm^{-1}.

Substitution of the functional form (11.32) into (11.5), thereby replacing the simple exponential decrease of (11.7) creates a new dispersion relation for a single fiber system ($n = 1$) that replaces (11.14) and (11.15)

$$D_G(\omega, k) = \left[\left(1 + \frac{j\omega}{\lambda v_E}\right)^2 + (k/\lambda)^2\right]^3 - B\left[\left(1 + \frac{j\omega}{\lambda v_E}\right)^3 - 3(k/\lambda)^2\left(1 + \frac{j\omega}{\lambda v_E}\right)\right] = 0 \tag{11.33}$$

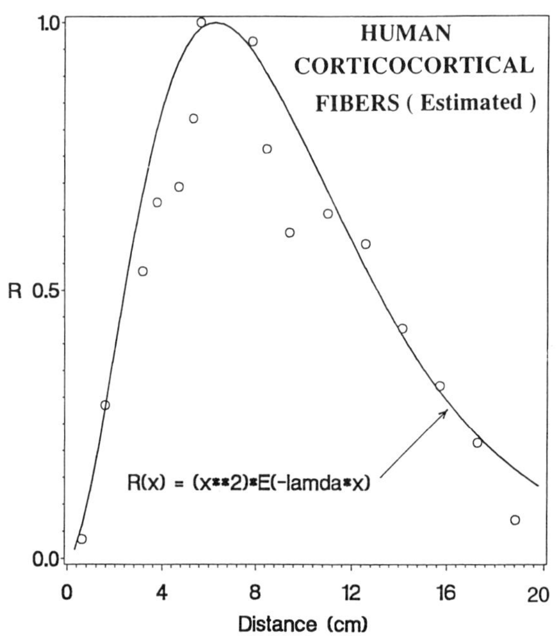

Figure 11-18. Scaled version of distribution of corticocortical fiber lengths in Figure 11-17, that is a guess of the distribution of human corticocortical fiber lengths. Horizontal scale is stretched based on linear brain scale (Table 2-1) multiplied by a stretching factor of 2.2 to account for the folding of human neocortex. Circles are samples taken from Figure 10-17. These data were then fit to the (normalized) function shown with $\lambda = 0.1\ \text{cm}^{-1}$. This same function fits all stretching factors but with different λ values.

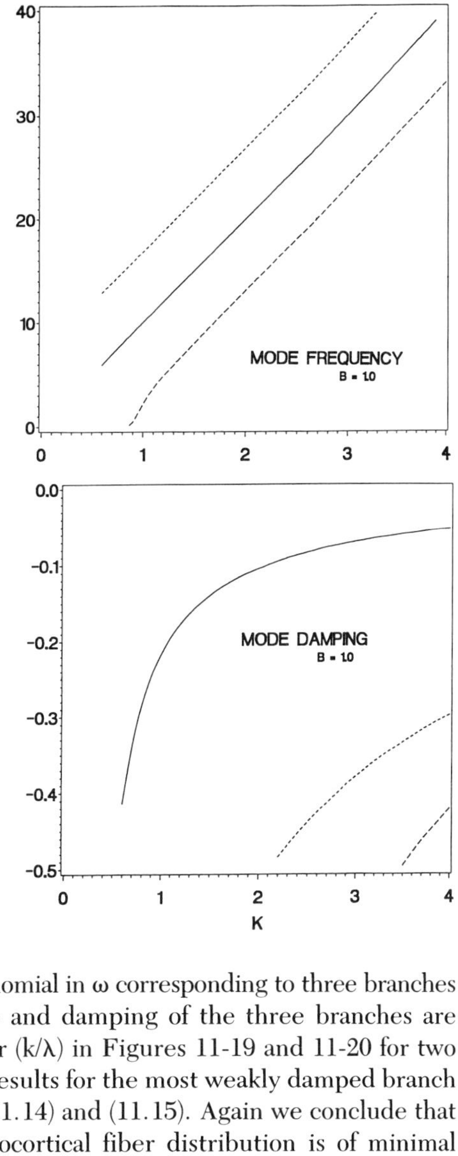

Figure 11-19. Dispersion relation (11.33) showing frequency versus normalized wave number $K = k/\lambda$ when the cortical control parameter $B = 1.0$. These results correspond to the assumed functional decrease in number of corticocortical fibers with distance given by Figure 11-18 and (11.32). The sixth-degree polynomial (11.33) yields three branches of the dispersion relation. One branch (solid line) is weakly damped at small wave numbers. Frequency is expressed in Hz based on $\lambda = 0.1\ \text{cm}^{-1}$ and $v_E = 600$ cm/second. Damping is expressed in terms of the nondimensional ratio γ_i/ω_{Ri}.

Equation (11.33) is a sixth-degree polynomial in ω corresponding to three branches of the dispersion relation. Frequencies and damping of the three branches are plotted versus normalized wave number (k/λ) in Figures 11-19 and 11-20 for two values of the control parameter B. The results for the most weakly damped branch are very similar to those predicted by (11.14) and (11.15). Again we conclude that the exact functional form of the corticocortical fiber distribution is of minimal consequence to important predictions of the global theory.

We also consider the case in which all long-range fibers are the same length. Although this is not physiologically realistic, it reflects the robustness of results obtained using different assumptions about corticocortical fiber distributions. When all fibers have the same length (s) and carry action potentials with the same velocity (v), weakly damped oscillations are predicted by (11.5) and (11.6) for frequencies near

$$\omega s/v = n\pi \qquad n = 1, 2, 3, \ldots \tag{11.34}$$

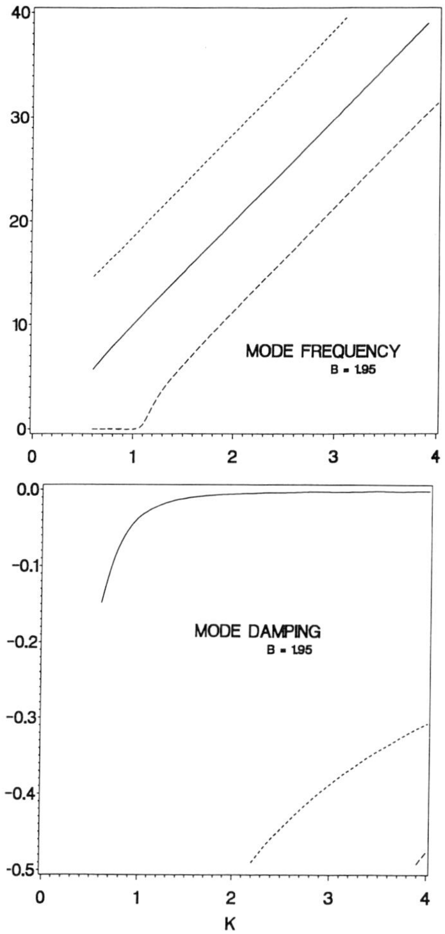

Figure 11-20. Dispersion relation (11.33), identical to Figure 10-19 except B = 1.95. Damping of most weakly damped branch is further reduced.

For a propagation velocity of v = 600 cm/second and fiber length s = 15 cm, (11.34) yields a lowest frequency of about 20 Hz. Predicted frequencies in the global model depend primarily on the number, average length, and action potential propagation velocity in the longest corticocortical fibers. Details of fiber length distribution are not critical to these general predictions.

Finally, there is the issue of fiber length in relation to the folded cortical surface. The short U-fibers appear to follow the folded surface so that a fiber of length (s) connects cortical regions separated by distance (s) within the cortex, except for a correction due to fiber pathways into the white matter layer and back to the cortex. In contrast, the longest corticocortical fibers typically appear to cut across fissures and sulci so that the effective fiber length (that is the corresponding cortical separation distance) is perhaps twice the actual length. In this case, the effective λ's are one half their actual values, and effective propagation velocities are twice their actual values. We can appreciate this by mentally inflating the cortex so that the surface becomes smooth. At the same time, corticocortical fibers that cut across fissures and sulci must be lengthened so that each fiber connecting two cortical locations before inflation connects the same two locations after inflation. Furthermore, to make frequency estimates, the transmission time between any two locations must be fixed so that effective velocity increases with cortical inflation. Because frequency estimates are obtained in terms of the nondimensional variable $\omega/\lambda v$, and the product λv remains constant, no change in the frequency estimates of this chapter are implied, regardless of whether fibers cut across fissures, if the wave number interpretation is consistent. Of course, different fiber systems may exhibit different geometric behavior with respect to cortical folding, which introduces additional uncertainty in numeric estimates. It appears that much of spontaneous EEG observed on the scalp is in a general wave number range of about $k/\lambda_1 = 0.5$ to 10, where λ_1 refers to the system with the longest fibers.

Effects of Spreads in Action Potential Velocity Distributions

To simplify calculations, we have assumed that the distributions of velocity of action potentials for long-range corticocortical fiber systems were highly peaked in previous sections, that is, they were delta functions. In this section, we examine the effects of spreads in the velocity density function $f_E(v)$ (for one long-range system) on frequencies and damping decrements. The $f_E(v)$ data originally reviewed by Katznelson (1981) are summarized in Figure 2-6. We also consider additional data. Experimental evidence of action potential velocities in human corticocortical fibers is available indirectly from several sources.

1. Diameter histograms of corticocortical, callosal, and pyramidal tract axons in humans. Information on the fraction of myelinated fibers was also obtained in these studies by Tomasch (1954), DeMeyer (1959), Bishop and Smith (1964), and Biedenbach and colleagues (1986).
2. Experimental data on the relation between axon diameter and propagation velocity in small myelinated axons, that is, axons with diameters of about 0.4 to 2 μm (Waxman and Bennett, 1972).
3. Experimental data on the relation between axon diameter and propagation velocity in small unmyelinated axons, that is, axons with diameters of about 0.1 to 1 μm (Lee et al, 1986; Swadlow et al, 1980).
4. Measurement of delay times between homologous regions of two cortical hemispheres in the monkey after direct stimulation of single neurons at the neocortical surface or corpus callosum (Swadlow et al, 1978, 1980).

Experimental results from several of these studies (in 1,2, and 4) were combined to form Figure 2-6, which shows the estimated velocity density function $f_E(v)$ for myelinated white matter fibers. Despite the fact that the data originate from different studies and different regions of white matter and are a mixture of human and monkey data, the agreement is good. Thus Figure 2-6 forms the basis for most of the corticocortical propagation velocity estimates in this book.

However, several important questions remain unanswered. For example, in one study of the brains of three men who died in their 50's from causes unrelated to the central nervous system, the percentages of unmyelinated fibers in the corpus callosum were 31%, 41%, and 45% (Tomasch, 1954). In another study of callosal fibers in the rabbit, 45% of the fibers were unmyelinated (Swadlow and Waxman, 1976). The callosal fiber data contrast with data on medullary pyramidal tract axons, which were reported to be 94% myelinated in humans (DeMeyer, 1959) and 88% myelinated in cats (Biedenbach et al, 1986). However, the data on callosal fibers apparently are more applicable to the global wave theory because unlike the pyramidal tract data, they involve connections between pairs of cortical locations. It is not entirely clear whether the callosal data imply a large fraction of unmyelinated fibers or incomplete myelination of fibers. For example, Krieg (1973) noted incomplete myelination in the longer corticocortical axons. If axons are incompletely myelinated or if many are unmyelinated, our velocity and frequency estimates would be decreased.

Little data have been found concerning the relation of propagation velocity in small unmyelinated fibers to fiber diameter. Studies of nonmyelinated callosal fibers in the rabbit have reported fibers as small as 0.1 μm and propagation velocities as slow as 0.3 m/second (Swadlow et al, 1980). In the feline medullary pyramidal tract nonmyelinated fibers as small as 0.5 μm were found (Biedenbach et al, 1986). Although clear evidence showed an increase in velocity with diameter, considerable data scatter was obtained and thus no simple mathematical function could be fit to the data. In another study (Lee et al, 1986), small unmyelinated axons with diameters of about 0.5 to 2.0 μm were measured; corresponding propagation velocities were about 0.2 to 1.1 m/second. The slope of the linear regression line for this data was about 0.44 m/second/μm, that is, the nonmyelinated axons had propagation velocities of about 10% of expected propagation velocities for myelinated axons of the same diameter. Other studies suggest that nonmyelinated axon propagation velocities are perhaps 20% of corresponding myelinated axon propagation velocities, and that propagation velocity is approximately proportional to the square root of the diameter. Finally, evidence suggests that propagation velocity in callosal axons varies with their short time history of action potential conduction; however, the changes are typically less than 10% (Swadlow et al, 1978).

If small, nonmyelinated axons occur in considerable numbers among the corticocortical and callosal axons, an important mechanism for signal propagation to distant cortical locations with very long time delays would be implied. An approximate idea of how these very "slow axons" combine with the myelinated axons may be obtained using a method similar to that used to study multiple fiber systems that have different characteristic length constants in a previous section. To illustrate this effect, two fiber systems with the same length constants ($\lambda_1 = \lambda_2$) were assumed. The velocity density functions $f_1(v)$ and $f_2(v)$ were assumed to be delta functions, peaked at $v = v_1$ (myelinated corticocortical fibers) and $v = v_2$ (nonmyelinated corticocortical fibers). These assumptions again result in two branches of the dispersion relation. Frequency and relative damping for the two branches are shown in Figure 11-21 for the specific case of $v_1 = 6$ m/second $= 10\ v_2$, B_1

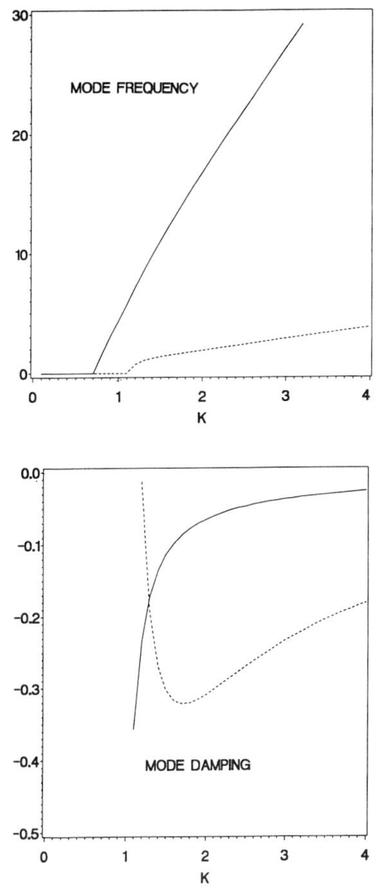

Figure 11-21. Dispersion relation (11.10) for a model cortex with two fiber systems, one myelinated and one nonmyelinated. Corticocortical propagation velocities are assumed to be peaked at $v_1 = 6$ m/second and $v_2 = 0.6$ m/second. Other parameters are $\lambda_1 = \lambda_2 = 0.1$ cm^{-1}, $B_1 = 1.8$, and $B_2 = 0.5$. Frequency is expressed in Hertz. Damping is denoted by the nondimensional ratio γ_i/ω_i for the two branches of the dispersion relation.

$= 1.8$, and $B_2 = 0.5$, corresponding to 22% nonmyelinated fibers with propagation velocities equal to 10% of myelinated fiber velocity. In this example, the two branches are moderately to weakly damped, but one branch has frequencies of approximately 10% of the other. Experimental studies of the human alpha rhythm (~10 Hz) often show substantial delta power (~1 Hz) in apparent agreement with these theoretical arguments (Nunez, 1981a). Unfortunately, it is difficult to distinguish these low brain frequencies from several artifacts that contribute to this part of the spectrum, such as electrocardiogram, muscle potentials, and movement of the head. Thus we cannot easily distinguish brain from nonbrain origins in this frequency range using only scalp recordings.

The more realistic case of distributed corticocortical velocities requires that we solve the dispersion relation in the form of an integral equation. With a single fiber system (that is, one λ or $N = 1$), the dispersion relation is expressed by (11.11). Because the dispersion relation is not a polynomial, singularities in the complex ω-plane appropriate for inversion of Fourier or Laplace transforms may no longer be poles. In fact, dispersion relations may no longer exist in the usual sense familiar in the fields of electrodynamics, acoustics, and so on (Montgomery and Tidman, 1964; Nunez, 1971). However, the predicted filter properties of the cortex still may be estimated through an approximate search for numerical solutions of (11.11), as indicated in the Appendix. The general approach involves the assumption that the probability density function for myelinated fibers is given by one of two functions.

In the first set of examples, the following functional form was chosen:

$$\begin{aligned} f_E(v) &= \text{constant} \qquad v_1 \leq v \leq v_2 \\ &= 0 \qquad\qquad \text{otherwise} \end{aligned} \tag{11.35}$$

where the constant is determined by the general requirement for normalization of probability density functions

$$\int_0^\infty f_E(v)\, dv = 1 \tag{11.36}$$

The assumed form for $f_E(v)$ in (11.35) has the advantage of relative simplicity. That is, the integral in (11.11) was calculated using the symbolic manipulation system MACSYMA for $f_E(v)$ given by (11.35) (Kowalski and Nunez, 1991). This procedure allowed for an independent check of numerical methods and study of the effects of spreads $\Delta v = v_2 - v_1$ in $f_E(v)$, with $\Delta v \rightarrow 0$ corresponding to $f_E(v) = \delta(v - v_E)$.

The second functional form chosen for the probability density function for corticocortical propagation velocity was

$$\begin{aligned} f_E(v) &= C_n v^n e^{-nv/v_E} \qquad v \geq v_{min} \\ &= 0 \qquad\qquad\qquad v \leq v_{min} \end{aligned} \tag{11.37}$$

This function peaks at $v = v_E \sim 7.5$ m/second, and is based on the experimental data summarized in Figure 2-6. Numerical studies were performed for n = 3, 4, 5. The constants C_n were chosen to satisfy the normalization condition (11.36). The minimum velocity below which no action potentials occur ($v_{min} \sim 0.4\, v_E$) was chosen to avoid singularities in the v integrand of (11.11). This assumption appears reasonably consistent with anatomy and physiology as we understand them; however, the results of future experiments may require a re-examination of these calculations, as discussed in the Appendix. Although the functional form (11.37) is more similar to the experimental estimates of Figure 2-6 than the form (11.35), an analytic expression for the integral in (11.11) was not found when $f_E(v)$ is expressed by (11.37). In this case, the integral in (11.11) was numerically integrated many times as part of the iterative procedure to solve the dispersion equation (11.11).

To illustrate the effects of spreads in the corticocortical velocity density function $f_E(v)$, we first show the dependence of frequency and damping on the control parameter B for the case of a peaked density function $f_E(v) = \delta(v - v_E)$. This is obtained directly from the simple dispersion relation of (11.14) and (11.15). The

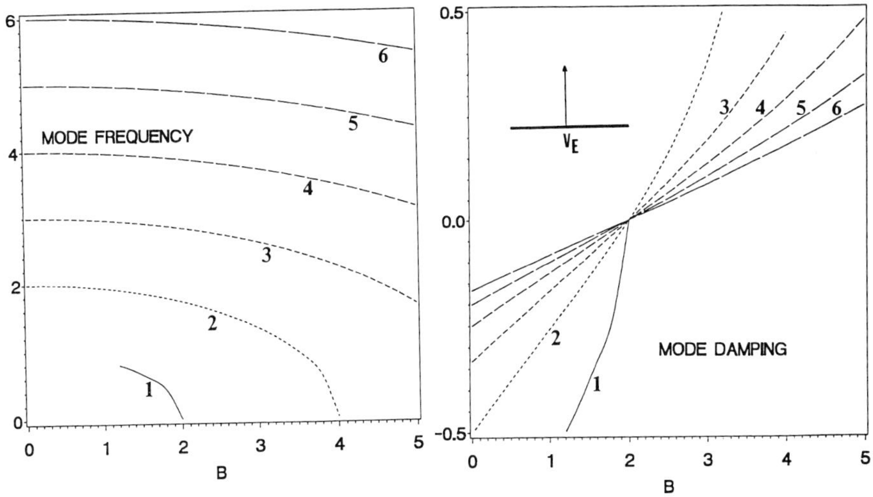

Figure 11-22. Normalized frequency ($\omega_R/\lambda_E v_E$) and damping (γ/ω_R) for the modes ($k_m/\lambda_E = 1, 6$) are plotted versus the control parameter B. The right inset shows the assumed form of the probability density function for corticocortical action potential velocity $f_E(v)$ in (10.11). In this case, $f_E(v) = \delta(v - v_E)$ so the plots were obtained from the analytic solution (11.14) and (11.15). Curves are shown only when weakly damped or unstable ($\gamma/\omega_R > -0.5$) oscillatory solutions were obtained. For example, no oscillatory fundamental mode ($k_1/\lambda_E = 1$) solution is obtained from (11.14) when $B > 2$. Furthermore, the fundamental mode is heavily damped for $B < 1.2$. The modes k_m correspond to those determined by the boundary condition of (11.16) for the choice of parameters $\lambda_E L/2\pi = 1$, such as $\lambda_E = 0.1\ \text{cm}^{-1}$, and effective brain "circumference" (such as in the posterior-anterior direction) of $L \sim 62$ cm, which appear to be physiologically realistic.

appropriate plot is shown in Figure 11-22 for the lower modes $k/\lambda = 1, 6$. The normalized frequency plots exclude regions of heavy damping $\gamma/\omega_R < -0.5$. For example, because the mode $k/\lambda = 1$ is heavily damped for $B < 1.2$, no frequency plot is shown in this parameter range to suggest that the corresponding oscillatory EEG activity will not be observed. Furthermore, the damping plot of the mode $k/\lambda = 1$ does not appear for $B > 2$ because no oscillatory solution of (11.14) is obtained in this parameter range.

The effect of a small (rectangular) spread in $f_E(v)$ was obtained by solving (11.11) with $f_E(v)$ given by (11.35) for $\Delta v = 0.4\ v_E$ ($v_1 = 0.8\ v_E$, $v_2 = 1.2\ v_E$). The principal effect of the spread in the velocity distribution is to low pass filter the predicted EEG for any fixed value of the control parameter B. For example, if $B = 1$, all modes k_m for $m \geq 2$ have weakly damped solutions when $f_E(v) = \delta(v - v_E)$, as shown in Figure 11-22. However, with the spread shown in Figure 11-23, only the modes $m = 2$ and 3 are weakly damped if $B = 1$. Weakly damped or unstable higher modes only occur in this example for larger values of the control parameter B.

The effects of a broader, nonsymmetric spread in $f_E(v)$ are shown in Figure

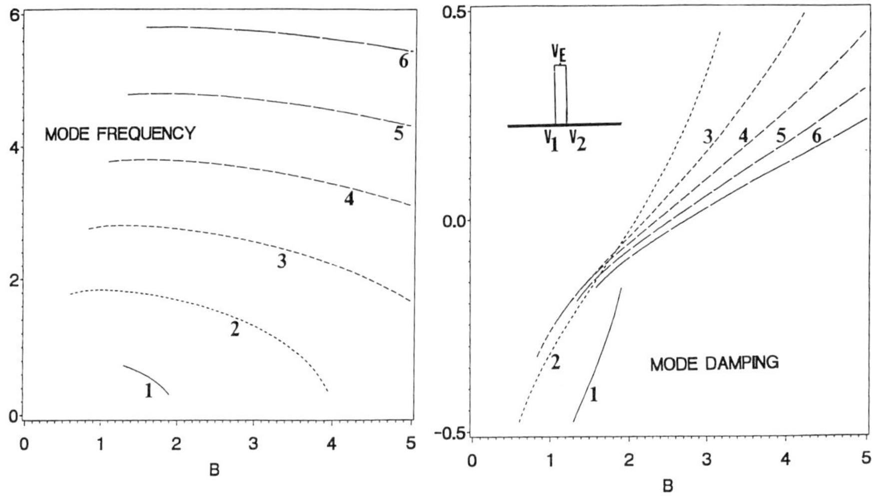

Figure 11-23. Normalized frequency ($\omega_R/\lambda_E v_E$) and damping (γ/ω_R) for the modes (k_m = 1, 6). This is similar to Figure 11-22 except for a small spread in corticocortical propagation velocities $f_E(v)$ given by (11.35) with $v_1 = 0.8\ v_E$ and $v_2 = 1.2\ v_E$, as indicated in the inset. Higher modes begin to disappear for small values of the control parameter B when compared with Figure 11-22. Solutions were obtained by solving integral equation (11.11).

11-24 for $v_1 = 0.5\ v_E$, $v_2 = 2.4\ v_E$. In this case, the only modes that have weakly damped or unstable oscillatory solutions over the wide range of control parameter $0 \leq B \leq 5$ are $k/\lambda_E = 1, 2, 3$. Furthermore, the effect of increasing the magnitude of B is to scan different modes. That is, for B less than about 1.7, no weakly damped oscillations are predicted. The mode $k/\lambda_E = 3$ appears for $B > 2.7$ and disappears again at a large value of $B > 5$ off the plot. Unstable modes have been included in the linear analyses because amplitudes of the synaptic action density could grow beyond the linear range and follow limit cycles, as in the example of the Van der Pol oscillator in Chapter 10 and the quasi-linear solution discussed in the next section.

The functional form for (11.37), which is the $f_E(v)$ based on the experimental data of Figure 2-6, is used in (11.11) to obtain the plots of Figure 11-25. As might be expected, the results are qualitatively similar to those of the rectangular distribution (Figure 11-24), except that in Figure 11-25, the modes $k/\lambda_E = 1, 3$ are more weakly damped for fixed values of B in the approximate range $B \sim 2$ to 3.

In summary, by including a spread in the velocity distribution for corticocortical propagation, (1) higher modes for any fixed value of the control parameter B are removed, and (2) more generally, a mode scanning mechanism is added in which certain ranges of the control parameter can produce only a few specific modes. A different mechanism for mode scanning is discussed later.

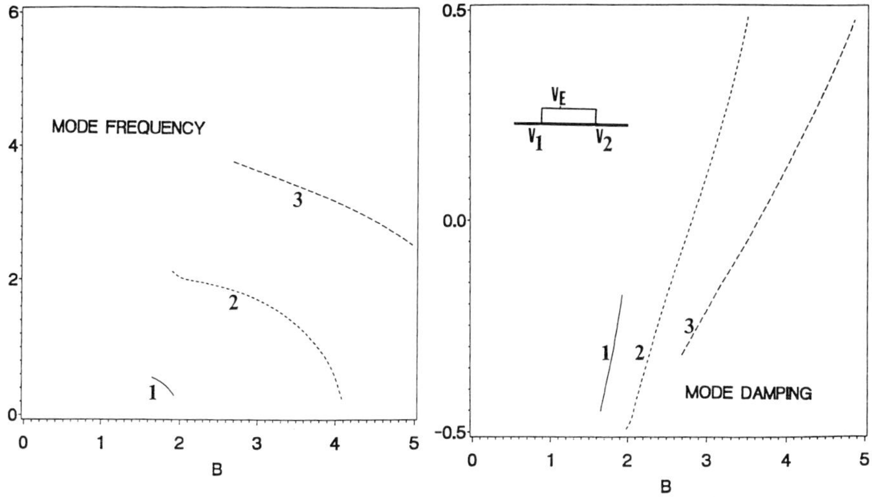

Figure 11-24. Normalized frequency ($\omega_R/\lambda_E v_E$) and damping (γ/ω_R) for the modes (k_m = 1, 6). This is similar to Figure 10-22 and 10-23, except for a large spread in $f_E(v)$ denoted by (11.35), with $v_1 = 0.5\ v_E$ and $v_2 = 2.4\ v_E$, as indicated in the inset. Only the modes $k_m/\lambda_E = 1, 3$ appear in this example. Furthermore, the system exhibits a mode scanning property in the sense that only certain modes can occur for certain values of the control parameter B.

Quasi-linear Effects

The results obtained in this chapter and in linear, local theories discussed in Chapters 5 and 8 predict overdamped neocortical activity when some cortical control parameter (B, in the purely global theory) is very small. As this parameter is increased, weakly damped oscillations are predicted. In this limited view, further parameter increases cause unstable oscillations, which prompts us to ask whether the cortex must operate in an unrealistically narrow parameter range to exhibit weakly damped but stable oscillations. To address this question, we again consider the assumed qualitative relation between the density of action potential firings and excitatory and inhibitory synaptic action, that is, $g = g(h_E, h_I)$, depicted in Figure 11-5 in two separate plots, one for the plane h_E = constant and one for the plane h_I = constant.

A three-dimensional plot representing a possible shape for the function $g = g(h_E, h_I)$ is shown in Figure 11-26. A crude quasi-linear solution to the basic brain wave equations (11.1) and (11.2) may be constructed if the derivatives of $g(h_E, h_I)$ defined by (11.4) undergo small changes about a background stage g_0. Thus (A.12) may be replaced by

$$G(k, \omega) = Q_E[H_E(k, \omega)]H_E(k, \omega) - Q_I[H_I(k, \omega)]H_I(k, \omega) \qquad (11.38)$$

The Appendix suggests that the spatial modes $H_E(k, t)$ (modulation of excitatory

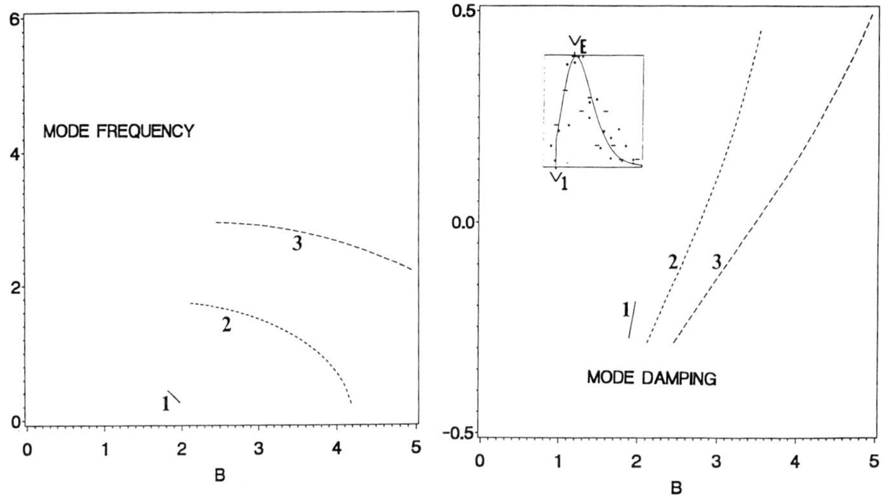

Figure 11-25. Normalized (k_m = 1, 6) frequency ($\omega_R/\lambda_E v_E$) and damping (γ/ω_R) for the modes (k_m/λ_E = 1, 6) plotted versus the control parameter B. This is similar to Figures 10-22 through 10-24, except the more realistic form for the probability density function $f_E(v)$ is used, that is, (11.37) with n = 4 and v_{min} = 0.4 v_E. Results are similar to those obtained in Figure 11-24 except for lower damping over the approximate range B ~ 2 to 3.

synaptic action) are described approximately by the nonlinear differential equations

$$\frac{d^2H_E}{dt^2} + \lambda_E v_E[2 - B_{kt}(H_E, H_I)] \frac{dH_E}{dt} + [(\lambda_E^2 + k^2)v_E^2 - \lambda_E^2 v_E^2 B_{kt}(H_E, H_I)]H_E = 0 \quad (11.39)$$

Here the control parameter B is replaced by the functions $B_{kt}[H_E(k, t), H_I(k, t)]$ which are determined by the instantaneous derivatives (in k space) of the function

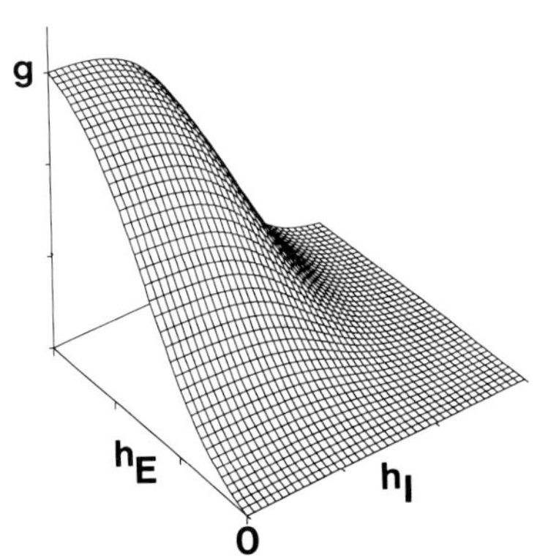

Figure 11-26. Symbolic representation of the postulated relation g = g (h_E, h_I) between the number of action potentials (g) fired at a fixed time from within a neural mass and the excitatory (h_E) and inhibitory (h_I) synaptic input to that neural mass. This is a two-dimensional version of Figure 11-5. See the Appendix for modification of the relationship by local circuit delays.

$g = g(h_E, h_I)$ shown symbolically in Figure 11-26. If the B_{kt} are constant, temporal Fourier transform of (11.39) yields the linear dispersion relation (A.13). In the quasi-linear approximation, the mode equations (11.39) are generally coupled through the functions B_{kt}.

For illustrative purposes, we consider an example in which derivative changes along the h_I axis of Figure 11-26 are neglected so that the B_{kt} are only functions of H_E. To keep the presentation simple, we also assume that the B_{kt} have isolated maxima as indicated by point (b) of Figure 11-27. This assumption is consistent with the sigmoid functions $g = g(h_E)$ shown in Figures 11-5 and 11-26; however, the general results of this section do not depend on the details of the B_{kt} functions. If the functions B_{kt} are expanded about their background states B_{kb}, (11.39) yields Van der Pol-like equations for the spatial modes $H_E(k, t)$, which are uncoupled in this approximation. The solutions are point attractors for $B_{kb} < 2$. If $B_{kb} > 2$ the higher modes $k >> \lambda_E$ have limit cycle solutions for each k mode given approximately by

$$H_E(k, t) \cong 2 \left[\frac{2(B_{kb} - 2)}{-\left(\dfrac{\partial^2 B_{kt}}{\partial H_E^2} \right)_b} \right]^{1/2} \cos(k v_E t) \tag{11.40}$$

where the second derivatives of B_{kt} are negative at the maxima (b).

Limit cycle solutions also occur if $g = g(h_E)$ is a sigmoid function and point (a) of Figure 11-27 is chosen as the background state. An example is shown in Figure 11-28. The quasi-linear approach implies that the modulation of synaptic action $H_E(x, t)$ in a strip of cortex may be approximated by a linear combination of spatial modes

$$H_E(x, t) = \sum_{m=1}^{\infty} H_E(k_m, t) \sin k_m x \tag{11.41}$$

where some modes $H_E(k_m, t)$ might be limit cycles (11.40), but others could be chaotic, due, for example, to coupled versions of (11.39). Synaptic action on a

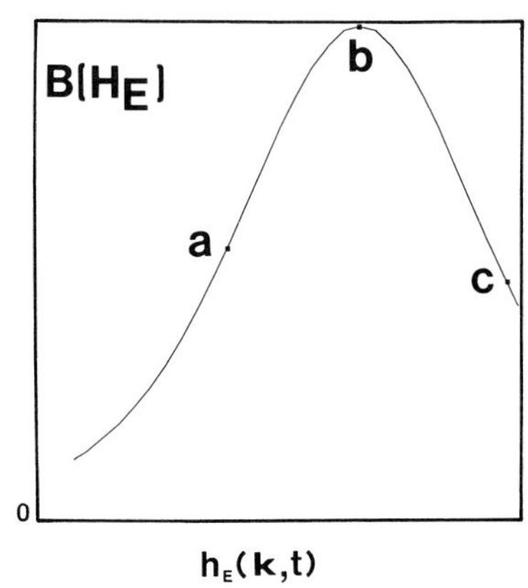

Figure 11-27. The function $B(H_E)$ derived from the sigmoidal function $g = g(h_E)$ when h_I is constant. A single maximum occurs at $H_E = H_b$ corresponding to the maximum slope of $g = g(h_E)$. The plot of B versus the modulation H_E is identical except for a shift to the left determined by the particular background state of neocortex (a, b, or c, for example). Since these curves are symbolic only, we can apply them to either $h_E(k, t)$ or $h_E(k, \omega)$. The functional form changes, but general results of this section do not require knowledge of exact functions.

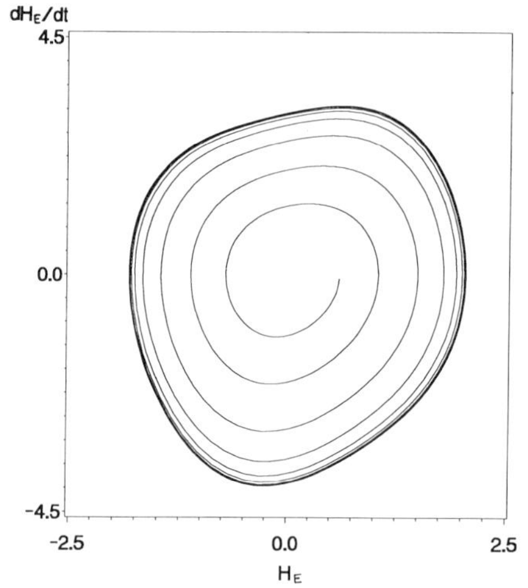

Figure 11-28. Numerical solution of (11.39) for $k/\lambda_E = 2$ with $B = B(H_E)$ given in Figure 11-27. Phase plane plot (dH_E/dt versus H_E) shows classic limit cycle behavior with frequency not very different than that predicted by the linear theory (11.14).

sphere satisfies a relation analogous to (11.41), but with the single sum replaced by a double sum over ℓ and m modes. Changes in control parameters analogous to the B_{kb} could cause bifurcations of selective modes, as suggested in Chapter 12. Although details of these limit cycle oscillations cannot be regarded too seriously because of the approximations and arbitrary choice of parameters, this preliminary study of possible global quasi-linear behavior has the following implications, which may be relatively independent of the magnitudes of realistic physiologic parameters.

1. When a cortical control parameter exceeds its threshold value for stability in a linear theory, unstable behavior (such as epilepsy) is not necessarily implied. Rather stable limit cycle oscillations are possible.
2. The frequencies of EEG global limit cycles may be in the same general range as frequencies predicted by linear theories. Amplitudes depend on cortical control parameters.
3. If the control function $B(H_E)$ has multiple maximum values, multiple limit cycles are possible. The specific limit cycle followed by each $H_E(k, t)$ then depends on initial conditions or forcing functions or both (due to sensory input, for example).
4. In the very crude theory outlined here, each mode $H_E(k, t)$ undergoes its own separate limit cycle. Linear superposition of different modes k is valid, as in the linear theory, that is no wave–wave coupling is predicted. For example, in Figure 11-29, a waveform of $\widetilde{H}_E(t)$ composed of several different k modes (which might be forced by global boundary conditions) is shown. A corresponding phase plane plot is also shown. This is a quasi-periodic oscillation composed of several limit cycle modes. However, use of apparently more realistic forms for the function $g(k, t) = g[h_E(k, t), h_I(k, t)]$ may result in a coupled set of equations similar to (11.39), that is two equations for each spatial mode. In this case, mode coupling occurs as is generally expected in nonlinear global systems.
5. As indicated in Chapter 10, the undriven Van der Pol equation cannot exhibit chaotic behavior. However, in more accurate theories, it may be coupled

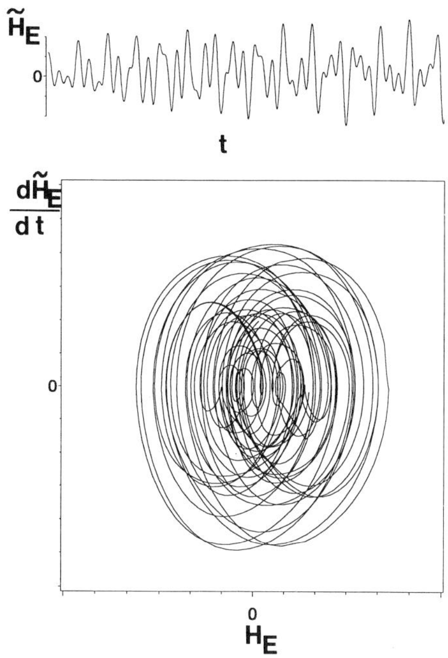

Figure 11-29. Linear combination of three limit cycle modes $k_m/\lambda_E = 1.3, 2.0,$ and 2.7. Each limit cycle is obtained by numerical solution of (11.39). $\tilde{H}_E(t) = \Sigma A_n H_E(k_n, t)$ is plotted at the top; the coefficients A_n were chosen arbitrarily. The corresponding phase plane plot is shown at bottom. The linear combination of modes $\tilde{H}_E(t)$ is quasi-periodic and may be difficult to distinguish from chaos when the experimental times series is the only available information about the underlying dynamics.

to similar equations involving different k values. Alternately, it might contain a driving term, perhaps corresponding to driving the visual system with sine wave modulated light. In either of these cases, the resulting equations for $H_E(k, t)$ might exhibit chaotic behavior for certain parameter ranges. Also some modes k might be chaotic whereas others follow limit cycles. Persistant coherent spatial structures might occur, even in the presence of temporal chaos. Physical phenomena that exhibit this general type of behavior were described in the section Continuous Nonlinear Systems and Solitons in Chapter 10.

Brain Waves on a Closed Surface

The one-dimensional solutions to the brain wave equations outlined in this chapter are relatively simple. That is, we added the complications to the basic theory discussed in previous sections individually, thereby gaining a semi-quantitative understanding of each separate effect with minimal mathematical difficulty. However, most solutions were obtained for an infinite, one-dimensional medium, with boundary conditions applied post hoc. Although this type of approach has clear precedent in the physical sciences (such as in hot plasma theory), there is an obvious advantage in obtaining solutions on a closed surface. Of course, enthusiasm for this approach must be tempered by the fact that neocortex is not a spherical surface and, in any case, neocortical eigenfunctions are altered by inhomogeneity and anisotropy of the corticocortical fiber systems.

One-dimensional solutions to the brain wave equations for a finite loop of cortex

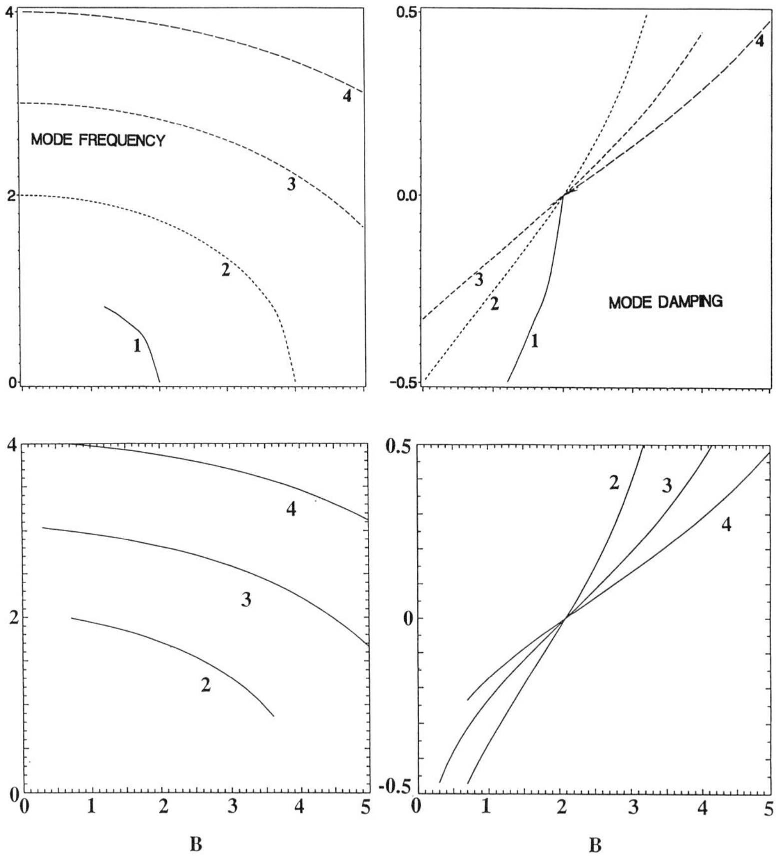

Figure 11-30. Normalized frequency ($\omega_R/\lambda_E v_E$) and damping (γ/ω_R) for "brain waves" in a closed loop of cortex. The modes m = 1 through 4 are shown. The plots in the upper row were obtained from the solutions for an infinite loop (11.14) and (11.15) with boundary conditions applied post hoc. The plots in the lower row were obtained for a finite neocortex using (A.15) of the Appendix. Both solutions were obtained for $\lambda_E L = 2\pi$, where L is the circumference of the loop or $\lambda_E R = 1$, where R is the radius of the loop that forms a circle. The two solutions mostly agree, except mode m = 1 does not occur in the finite loop solution.

by Srinivasan (1994) are outlined in the Appendix and compared with solutions obtained in an infinite loop in Figure 11-30. As expected, predicted normal mode frequencies generally correlate with solutions for an infinite medium if wave lengths are short compared with the circumference of the loop. Thus the main difference is the absence of the mode m = 1 in the finite loop solution. Here we concentrate on solutions on the surface of a homogeneous sphere, as developed independently by Katznelson (1981, 1982). Differences in the presentation are due mainly to more realistic choice of parameter ranges and closer connection to the one-dimensional theory. The assumptions of peaked velocity of action potential propagation, a single long-range excitatory fiber system ($n \rightarrow E$), exponential decrease of inhibitory connection number density, and linearization about a fixed state g_0 are also made in Katznelson's two-dimensional solution of (11.1) and (11.2). Modulation of excitatory synaptic action $H_E(\theta, \phi, t)$ is expanded in a series of spherical harmonics $Y_{\ell m}(\theta, \phi)$ where θ and ϕ are the usual spherical coordinates of a system originating at the center of a "spherical cortex" of radius R, as indicated in Figure 2-5. That is

$$H_E(\theta, \phi, t) = \sum_{\ell=0}^{\infty} \sum_{m=-\ell}^{+\ell} H_{E\ell m} Y_{\ell m}(\theta, \phi) \tag{11.42}$$

The input-output relation for the cortex is then expressed by

$$H_{E\ell m}(\omega) = \frac{U_{\ell m}(\omega)}{D_\ell(\omega)} \tag{11.43}$$

where the indices (ℓ, m) denoting different eigenfunctions on the cortical surface replace the wave numbers k_m for waves in a closed strip of cortex, in a manner analogous to the examples of waves on a spherical surface discussed in Chapter 9. The dispersion functions $D_\ell(\omega)$ are associated with each of the spherical harmonics $Y_{\ell m}(\theta, \phi)$.

The assumption of a spherical, homogeneous, isotropic cortical surface leads to a degeneracy in the temporal behavior of normal modes; that is, the transfer function $D_\ell^{-1}(\omega)$ is independent of the m index so that the dispersion relation

$$D_\ell(\omega) = 0 \tag{11.44}$$

yields roots ω_ℓ, which do not change as the index m varies from $-\ell$ to $+\ell$. A genuine cortex–corticocortical system would, of course, be nonspherical, anisotropic, and inhomogeneous so that splitting of the modes would be expected, as discussed in Chapter 9. Realistic parameter ranges yield a dispersion relation

$$1 - B_{2D} S_{E\ell}(Z) = 0 \tag{11.45}$$

where the functions S_ℓ are defined recursively in the Appendix and the variable Z is defined by

$$Z \equiv j \frac{\omega R}{v_E} + \lambda_E R \tag{11.46}$$

Because the complex frequency is $\omega = \omega_R - j\gamma$, wave damping is denoted by

$$\frac{\gamma R}{v_E} = \text{Real}(Z) - \lambda_E R \tag{11.47}$$

The two-dimensional cortical control parameter

$$B_{2D} \approx \frac{Q_E \rho_E}{Q_I \rho_I} \left(\frac{1 + \lambda_E^2 R^2}{1 + e^{-\pi \lambda_E R}} \right) \tag{11.48}$$

has the same order of magnitude as the equivalent one-dimensional parameter (B

$= Q_E\rho_E/Q_I\rho_I$) obtained in the basic one-dimensional solution of the section Basic Global Theory (assuming that all excitatory fibers are long range) for realistic values of the nondimensional parameter $\lambda_E R \sim 1$.

Numerical solutions to (11.45) were obtained for modes $\ell = 0, 10$. In particular, we searched for weakly damped or unstable oscillatory modes

$$\begin{aligned} |\omega_R R/v_E| &\leq 10 \\ |\gamma/\omega_R| &> -0.5 \end{aligned} \tag{11.49}$$

Reported cortical surface areas range from about 1,600 to 4,000 cm^2 corresponding to effective sphere radii of $R \sim 11$ to 18 cm. A reasonable guess for the decrease in number of synaptic connections in the longest corticocortical fiber system is perhaps $\lambda_E \sim 0.05$ to 0.2 cm^{-1} as discussed in the section Alternate Functional Forces for Corticocortical Fiber Distribution. We considered numerical solutions for the apparently realistic parameter range $\lambda_E R \sim 0.7$ to 1.5.

Frequencies and damping for modes $\ell = 1, 6$ with $\lambda_E R = 0.7$ are plotted versus the one-dimensional cortical control parameter B in Figure 11-31 (the mode $\ell = 0$ has no oscillatory solutions). As the cortical control parameter increases from zero, the $\ell = 3$ mode with frequency $|\omega_R R/v_E| \sim 2$ and the $\ell = 2$ mode with $|\omega_R R/v_E| \sim 1$ appear first near $B = 0.5$. The $\ell = 2$ mode with frequency ≤ 1 becomes more weakly damped for $B \sim 1.5$ and unstable for $B \sim 1.7$. As B is increased further, higher modes first become weakly damped and then unstable.

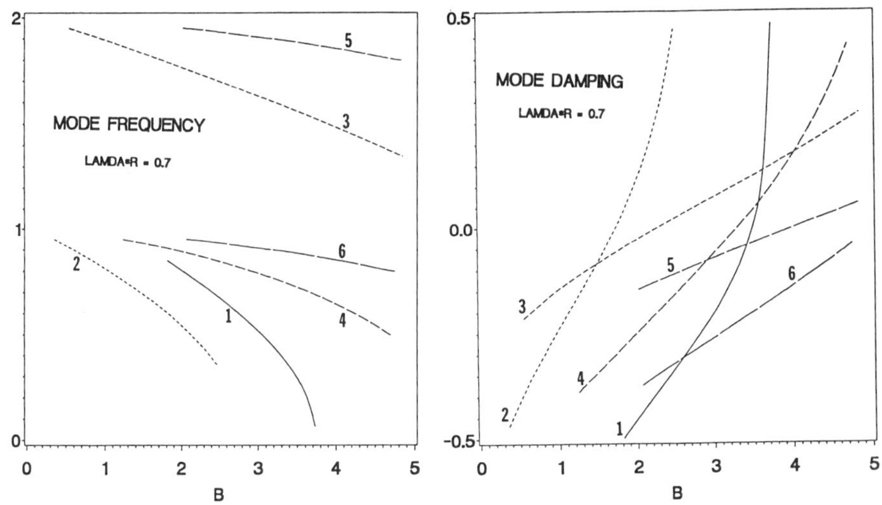

Figure 11-31. Normalized frequency ($\omega_R R/v_E$) and damping (γ/ω_R) for "brain waves" on a spherical surface as obtained from a numerical solution of (11.45) with $\lambda_E R = 0.7$. The modes $\ell = 1, 6$ are shown. In contrast to the one-dimensional theory of the section Basic Global Theory, higher modes ($\ell > 2$) yield weakly damped or unstable solutions for $\omega_R R/v_E \leq 2$. Frequency plots (*left*) are shown only if oscillatory solutions were obtained with $\gamma/\omega_R > -0.5$. The horizontal axis is the one-dimensional control parameter B.

Furthermore, the frequency of each mode decreases with increasing B. We can speculate that unstable modes in the linear theory may actually undergo limit cycle oscillations, as discussed in relation to the quasi-linear approach. The case $\lambda_E R = 1.5$ is shown in Figure 11-32. The results are similar to the case $\lambda_E R = 0.7$ except that weakly damped and unstable oscillations are less abundant. The $\ell = 3$ and 5 modes become unstable at $B \sim 3.7$ and 4.8, respectively. No other weakly damped or unstable modes were found over the range of control parameter $0 \leq B \leq 5$ for $\lambda_E R = 1.5$.

An important finding in the theory for waves on a sphere is that for this range of B, nearly all the weakly damped or unstable solutions to (11.45) with $\ell = 1$, 10 occur at low frequency, that is in the approximate range

$$0.3 < \left| \frac{\omega_R R}{v_E} \right| < 2.0 \tag{11.50}$$

With the exception of the mode $\ell = 1$, odd modes occur near frequencies $\omega_R R/v_E \sim 2$, whereas even modes occur near frequencies $\omega_R R/v_E \sim 1$ for smaller B values. This result is in sharp contrast to the behavior of nearly all known linear wave phenomena, for which higher spatial modes correspond to progressively higher frequencies. A few moderately damped oscillations at frequencies greater than 2.0 were found from (11.45) over narrow B ranges, but none were weakly damped or unstable. With $R = 11$ to 18 cm and $v_E = 600$ to 900 cm/second,

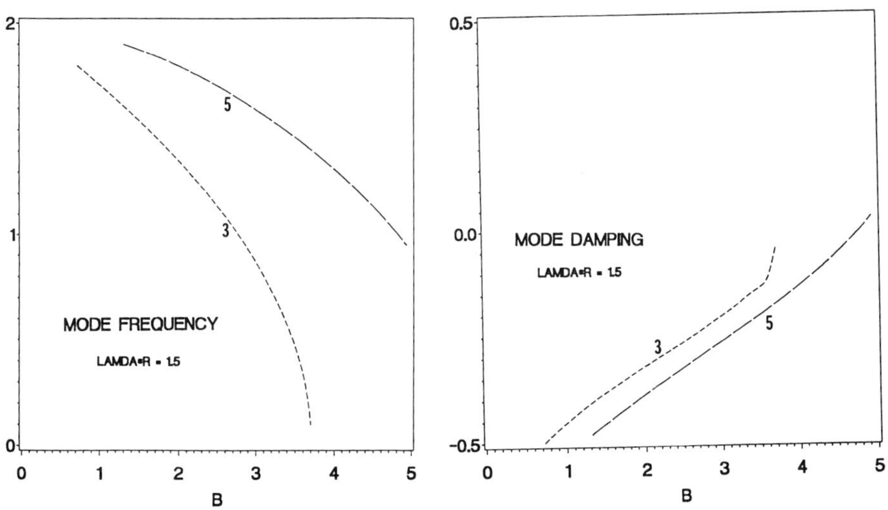

Figure 11-32. Normalized frequency and damping as a function of cortical control parameter B. This is identical to Figure 11-31 except $\lambda_E R = 1.5$, that is corticocortical fibers are shorter with respect to sphere radius. Weakly damped or unstable oscillations are less common in this case. Plots were obtained by solving (11.45).

(11.50) yields a predicted range for human spontaneous EEG of

$$f \sim 2 \text{ to } 26 \text{ Hz} \tag{11.51}$$

This result is relatively independent of uncertainties in physiologic parmeters and is consistent with experimental observations.

Comparison of One- and Two-Dimensional Theories

We can compare the predictions of the one-dimensional and two-dimensional versions of the global theory if the one-dimensional waves are assumed to occur in a closed strip forming a circumference of the same sphere used in the two-dimensional version. In this case, the allowed wave numbers are those of (9.35) with L equal to the sphere circumference, that is,

$$k_\ell = \frac{\ell}{R} \qquad \ell = 1, 2, 3 \ldots \tag{11.52}$$

With this interpretation of the modes k_ℓ, the expression for wave frequency obtained for one-dimensional waves (11.14) is

$$\frac{\omega_R R}{v_E} = (\lambda_E R)\left[\left(\frac{\ell}{\lambda_E R}\right)^2 - \frac{B^2}{4}\right]^{1/2} \qquad \ell = 1, 2, 3 \ldots \tag{11.53}$$

Mode-independent damping is obtained from (11.15), that is

$$\frac{\gamma R}{v_E} = -(\lambda_E R)\left(1 - \frac{B}{2}\right) \tag{11.54}$$

The control parameter for waves on a sphere B_{2D} is related simply to the one-dimensional control parameter B by comparison of (11.48) and (11.19) if all excitatory fibers are long range. More realistically, the definition (11.48) may be modified in the two-dimensional theory to include short excitatory fibers, as in (11.19). Thus, with these modifications, the parameters and nondimensionalization of the one-dimensional version are equal to those of the two-dimensional version of the global theory. Frequencies and relative damping for modes $\ell = 1, 4$ based on (11.53) and (11.54) are plotted versus the cortical control parameter B in Figure 11-30 for $\lambda_E R = 1$. Analogous plots obtained from the two-dimensional version are shown in Figure 11-33. A comparison of the two sets of predictions shows similarities and a few important differences, as listed below.

Mode Frequency Dependence on the Cortical Control Parameter

In both versions of the theory, the frequency of each mode ℓ decreases with increasing values of the control parameter B until a critical value $B_{\ell c}$ is achieved. At larger values of B, these modes disappear from the EEG signal. In contrast to the infinite one-dimensional predictions, no weakly damped $\ell = 1$ mode is pre-

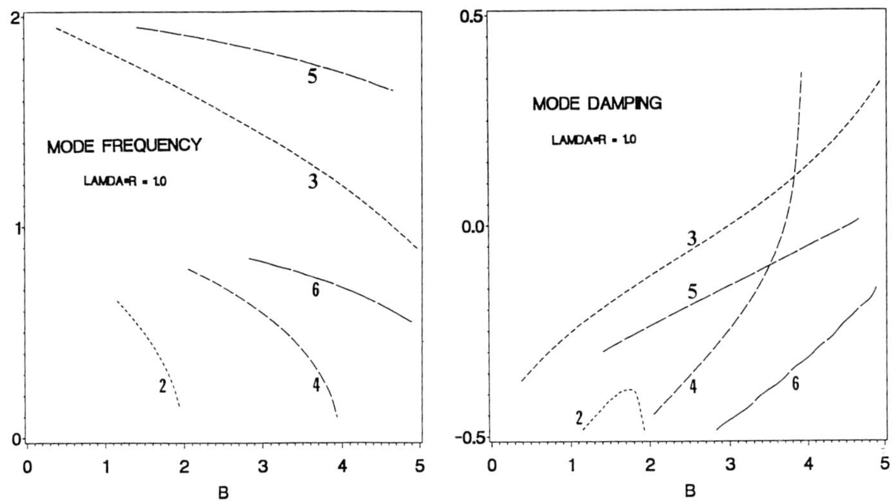

Figure 11-33. Normalized frequency and damping as a function of cortical parameter B for $\lambda_E R = 1.0$ for "brain waves" on a spherical surface. Plots were obtained by solving (11.45) with B calculated from B_{2D} in (11.48) so that direct comparison was obtained between Figures 11-30 and 11-33.

dicted by either of the finite versions for $\lambda_E R = 1$. This descrepancy is not surprising because an infinite medium was assumed in the infinite one-dimensional version with boundary conditions applied post hoc. This approximation was thought valid only for waves of wavelength substantially shorter than the system size $L = 2\pi R$. The solutions for waves in a finite loop or on the surface of sphere are consistent with this idea.

Mode Number Dependence on Frequency

In the one-dimensional versions, higher modes yield higher frequencies, as indicated by (11.53) and Figure 11-30. The fundamental mode ($\ell = 1$) frequency is $|\omega_R R/v_E| \leq 1$. In the two-dimensional version, the $\ell = 1$ mode does not occur when $\lambda_E R = 1$; however, all modes contribute low-frequency oscillations with $|\omega_R R/v_E| \leq 1$ for $\ell = 2, 4, 6 \ldots$ or $|\omega_R R/v_E| \leq 2$ for $\ell = 3, 5, 7 \ldots$. The highest frequencies of each mode occur at smaller B values as indicated in Figure 11-33. With the finite, one-dimensional solution, some higher spatial modes may also contribute to the low-frequency range.

Mode Damping and Instability

As B increases, all modes first become less damped and then go unstable ($\gamma_\ell > 0$) at some value $B_{\ell u}$. This general result applies to all versions of the theory. In the infinite one-dimensional version with $f(v) = \delta(v - v_E)$, all modes become unstable at B = 2.0. In contrast, instability of waves on a sphere is mode dependent. For example, Figure 11-33 indicates no instability for $\ell = 1$ or 2, but higher mode instabilities at the following values of the control parameter $B_{3u} \sim 3.0$, $B_{4u} \sim 3.7$, $B_{5u} \sim 4.3$, and $B_{6u} \sim 5.4$ (not shown). The one-dimensional quasi-linear theory suggests that unstable oscillatory modes actually may become limit cycle oscillations for each mode. This is predicted because the cortical control parameter becomes weakly dependent on mode amplitude. An analogous argument can be applied to the two-dimensional theory, which has the same presumed physiologic bases and control parameter B.

Effect of Fiber Length on Damping and Instability

As the parameter $\lambda_E R$ increases (corresponding to shorter corticocortical fibers relative to effective cortical radius), the critical value $B_{\ell c}$ (at which the frequency of the ℓ mode becomes zero) becomes smaller in all versions of the theory. That is, larger values of $\lambda_E R$ (shorter corticocortical fibers in relation to sphere radius) make oscillatory solutions less likely at any fixed value of the control parameter B.

In summary, one- and two-dimensional versions of the theory agree qualitatively and, in most important cases, semi-qualitatively, except for low pass properties of the two-dimensional theory not predicted by the infinite one-dimensional theory (with $f_E(v)$ equal to a delta function). The low pass behavior predicted by the two-dimensional theory occurs because higher modes mainly contribute low frequency oscillations. Low pass behavior predicted by the infinite one-dimensional theory (and, by implication, also in the two-dimensional theory) occurs in the presence of a spread in the corticocortical velocity distribution $f_E(v)$. This is due to the elimination of weakly damped higher modes at any fixed value of the cortical control parameter B. Because of the anisotropy of long corticocortical fibers (such as the long front-back connections), it is not clear whether the finite one-dimensional or two-dimensional version of the theory represents real brains most accurately. In any case, the general predictions of the two versions are similar. Several EEG experiments described in Chapter 12 appear to agree qualitatively and, in several cases, quantitatively with the global wave theory outlined in this chapter.

Symbols for Chapters 11 and 12

The following definitions apply to symbols used in Chapters 11 and 12. The physical dimensions are shown in parentheses. Nondimensional quantities have no parentheses.

a, b Inverse of rise times of EPSPs and IPSPs, respectively (second^{-1})

B_{2D}, B, B(k)	Cortical control parameter (believed to be only weakly k dependent), which partly determines physiologic state
$B_{\ell c}$	Value of control parameter for which oscillatory mode ℓ disappears from one-dimensional or two-dimensional solutions
$B_{\ell u}$	Value of control parameter for which oscillatory mode ℓ becomes unstable in any version of the linear theory
c, d	Inverse of characteristic lengths for the decrease in number of intracortical excitatory and inhibitory synapses from a single cell (cm^{-1})
E	Index indicating excitatory synaptic action; specific fiber system $n \rightarrow E$
$D_G(k, \omega)$	Global dispersion function (11.10), (11.11) or (11.33) that is, inverse of global transfer function
$D_L(k, \omega)$	Local dispersion function (5.1)
$D(k, \omega)$	Combined local and global dispersion function (11.27)
f	Frequency measured in Hertz
$f_n(v)$, $f_E(v)$	Velocity distribution functions for action potential propagation in nth (or specific, E) corticocortical fiber system (second/cm)
$F(k, \omega)$	Function defined by (11.26)
$g(\mathbf{r}, t)$	Number density of action potential firings in a cortical column (cm^{-3})
$G(\mathbf{k}, \omega)$	Fourier transform of modulation of $g(\mathbf{r},t)$ (second/cm, two-dimensional theory)
$h_E(\mathbf{r}, t)$, $h_I(\mathbf{r}, t)$	Number densities of excitatory and inhibitory synaptic action in a cortical column (cm^{-3})
$H_E(\mathbf{r}, t)$, $H_I(\mathbf{r}, t)$	Modulation of $h_E(\mathbf{r},t)$ or $h_I(\mathbf{r}, t)$ around some fixed level associated with fixed physiologic state (cm^{-3})
i	Index indicating ith pair of complex roots to a polynomial dispersion relation
j	Square root of minus one
k, **k**	Wave number or "spatial frequency" in one or two surface directions (cm^{-1})
L	Characteristic length representing "circumference" of fissured cortical surface, as estimated from circumference of a sphere having the same surface area as that of neocortex (cm)
ℓ, *m*	Indices indicating mode or eigenfunction for standing waves, m used in one-dimensional theory; (ℓ, *m*) used for waves on a sphere
n	Index indicating excitatory fiber system; see (11.7) and Figure 11-6
Q	Strength of intracortical coupling in local theory, that is, local control parameter; proportional to numbers of excitatory and inhibitory synaptic feedback connections and to transmembrane potentials caused by a single synaptic activation

Q_E Increase in number density of action potentials δg in a cortical column caused by increase in number density of excitatory synaptic input δh_E in a fixed physiologic state; see (11.4) and Figures 11-5 and 11-26

Q_I Decrease in number of action potentials ($-\delta g$) in a cortical column caused by increase in number density of inhibitory synaptic input δh_I in a fixed physiologic state; see (11.4) and Figures 11-5 and 11-26

r Vector locating point on "inflated" cortical surface, which smooths fissures and sulci (cm); see Figure 11-4

$R_E(\mathbf{r}, \mathbf{r}_1, v)$ Distribution function indicating the number of excitatory fibers connecting locations **r** and $\mathbf{r}_1$ and having action potential velocity v (second/cm^3 in two-dimensional theory; second/cm^2 in one-dimensional theory)

$R_I(\mathbf{r}, \mathbf{r}_1)$ Distribution function indicating the number of inhibitory fibers connecting locations **r** and $\mathbf{r}_1$ (cm^{-2} in two-dimensional theory; cm^{-1} in one-dimensional theory)

R Radius of equivalent spherical cortex, defined in terms of cortical surface area (cm)

s Length of corticocortical fibers when all are the same length; see (11.34) (cm)

$S_{E\ell}$, $S_{n\ell}$ Functions defined by (A.39) in the Appendix, $n \rightarrow E$ is specific fiber system

$T(k,\omega)$ Transfer function; inverse of dispersion function $D(k,\omega)$

$u(\mathbf{r}, t)$ Number density of excitatory (afferent) synaptic input from the midbrain (cm^{-3})

u_0 Number density of inhibitory (afferent) synaptic input from the midbrain (cm^{-3})

$U(\mathbf{r}, t)$, $U(\mathbf{k}, \omega)$ Modulation of $u(\mathbf{r}, t)$ and its spatial–temporal Fourier transform (cm^{-3} and second/cm, respectively, for two-dimensional theory)

v, v_E Action potential velocity in corticocortical fibers (cm/second); v_E refers to peak in velocity distribution (cm/second)

v_{min} Minimum action potential velocity in corticocortical fibers (cm/second)

v_p Phase velocity (cm/second)

v_G Group velocity (cm/second)

$V(k, \omega)$ Total synaptic output from a neocortical mass due to midbrain and nonlocal cortical input (second/cm in two-dimensional theory)

x, x_1 Coordinate along the cortical surface, in and out of fissures sulci (cm)

Z Variable defined by (11.46)

γ, γ_i Imaginary part of complex frequency for ith branch of dispersion relation; defined such that negative values indicate damping ($second^{-1}$)

ω_{Ri} Real part of complex frequency for ith branch of dispersion relation; when only one branch occurs, ω_R is used ($second^{-1}$), $f_{Ri}(Hz) = \omega_{Ri}/2\pi$

λ_n, λ_E Inverse of characteristic length for decrease of number of corticocortical synapses in nth fiber system (or specific excitatory system E) (cm^{-1}); also λ is used for alternate distribution of corticocortical fibers R_E in (11.32) (cm^{-1})

$\lambda_I = d$ Inverse of characteristic length for decrease of number of intracortical inhibitory synapses (cm^{-1})

$\omega_i = \omega_{Ri} - j\gamma_i$ Complex frequency or ith pair ($\pm$ values) of complex roots of dispersion relation ($second^{-1}$); index i refers to the different branches of the dispersion relation

ρ_n, ρ_E Number of excitatory synapses from fiber system *n* (or specific long-range excitatory system E) per cortical neuron

ρ_I Number of inhibitory synapses per cortical neuron

Δv Spread in the velocity for action potential propagation in one of the corticocortical fiber systems (cm/second)

Λ Spatial wavelength of wave (cm)

References

Abeles, M. *Local Cortical Circuits.* New York: Springer-Verlag, 1982.

Biedenbach, M.A., DeVito, J.L., and Brown, A.C. Pyramidal tract of the cat: Axon size morphology. *Exp. Brain Res.* 61:303–310, 1986.

Bishop, G.H. and Smith, J.M. The size of nerve fibers supplying cerebral cortex. *Exp. Neurol.* 9:483–501, 1964.

Braitenberg, V. *On the Texture of Brains.* New York: Springer-Verlag, 1977.

Braitenberg, V. and Schuz, A. *Anatomy of the Cortex, Statistics and Geometry.* New York: Springer-Verlag, 1991.

Creutzfeldt, O.D. The neuronal generation of EEG. In: *Handbook of Electroencephalography and Clinical Neurophysiology. Vol. 2. Part C: The Neuronal Generation of EEG.* (O.D. Creutzfeldt, Ed.) Amsterdam: Elsevier, 1974.

Creutzfeldt, O.D. The neocortical link: Thoughts on the generality of structure and function of the neocortex. In: *Architectronics of the Cerebral Cortex.* (M.A.B. Brazier and Petsche, H., Eds.) New York: Raven Press, 1978.

DeMeyer, W. Number of axons and myelin sheaths in adult human medullary pyramids. *Neurology* 9:42–47, 1959.

Freeman, W.J. *Mass Action in the Nervous System.* New York: Academic Press, 1975.

Freeman, W.J. Analytic techniques used in the search for the physiological basis of the EEG. In: *Handbook of Electroencephalography and Clinical Neurophysiology.* Vol. 1 (Revised series). (A.S. Gevins and Remond, A., Eds.) New York: Elsevier, pp. 583–664, 1987.

Garey, L.J. Mammalian neocortical commissures. In: *Structure and Function of Cerebral*

Commissures. (I.S. Russel, Van Hof, M.W., and Berlucchi, G., Eds.) Baltimore: University Park Press, 1979.

Gasser, H.S. and Grundfest, H. Axon diameters in relation to spike dimensions and the conduction velocity in mammalian A fibers. *Am. J. Physiol.* 127:393–414, 1939.

Katznelson, R.D. Deterministic and stochastic field theoretic models in the neurophysics of EEG. Ph.D. Dissertation. San Diego, CA: University of California at San Diego, 1982.

Katznelson, R.D. Normal modes of the brain: Neuroanatomical basis and a physiological theoretical model. In: *Electric Fields of the Brain: The Neurophysics of EEG* (P.L. Nunez), New York: Oxford University Press, 1981.

Kowalski, K. and Nunez, P.L. A mathematical study of a dispersion relation for brain waves using MACSYMA. *Brain Physics Group Report.* January 15, 1991.

Krieg, W.J.S. *Connections of the Cerebral Cortex.* Evanston, IL: Brain Books, 1963.

Krieg, W.J.S. *Architectronics of the Human Cerebral Fiber System.* Evanston, IL: Brain Books, 1973.

Kunzle, J. Cortico-cortical efferents of primary motor and somatosensory regions of the cerebral cortex in Macaca fascicularis. *Neuroscience* 3:25–39, 1978.

Lee, K.H., Chung, K., Chung, J.M., and Coggeshall, R.E. Correlation of cell body size, axon size, and signal conduction velocity for individually labelled dorsal root ganglion cells in the cat. *J. Comp. Neurol.* 243:335–346, 1986.

Montgomery, D.C. and Tidman, D.A. *Plasma Kinetic Theory.* New York: McGraw-Hill, pp. 51–65, 1964.

Nunez, P.L. Longitudinal wave propagation in a plasma containing an external time-dependent electric field. *Physics of Fluids* 14:633–638, 1971.

Nunez, P.L. The brain wave equation: A model for the EEG. Presented at the American EEG Society Meeting, Houston, 1972.

Nunez, P.L. The brain wave equation: A Model for the EEG. *Mathematical Biosciences* 21:279–297, 1974a.

Nunez, P.L. Wave-like properties of the alpha rhythm. *IEEE Trans. Biomed. Eng.* 21:473–482, 1974b.

Nunez, P.L. *Electric Fields of the Brain: The Neurophysics of EEG.* New York: Oxford University Press, 1981a.

Nunez, P.L. A study of origins of the time dependencies of scalp EEG: I. Theoretical basis. *IEEE Trans. Biomed. Eng.* 28:271–280, 1981b.

Nunez, P.L. A study of the origins of the time dependencies of scalp EEG: II. Experimental support of theory. *IEEE Trans. Biomed. Eng.* 28:281–288, 1981c.

Nunez, P.L. Global contribution to cortical dynamics: Theoretical and experimental evidence for standing wave phenomena. In: *Dynamics of Sensory and Cognitive Processing by the Brain.* (E. Baser, Ed.) New York: Springer-Verlag, 1988.

Nunez, P.L. Generation of human EEG by a combination of long and short range neocortical interactions. *Brain Topography* 1:199–215, 1989a.

Nunez, P.L. Towards a physics of neocortex. In: *Advanced Methods of Physiological Systems Modeling.* Vol. 2 (V.Z. Marmareliz, Ed.) New York: Plenum Press, pp. 241–259, 1989b.

Nunez, P.L. and Srinivasan, R. Implications of recording strategy for estimates of neocortical dynamics with EEG. *Chaos: An Interdisciplinary Journal of Nonlinear Science* 3:257–266, 1993.

Purpura, D.P. Intracellular stûdies of synaptic organizations in the mammalian brain. In:

Structure and Function of the Synapses. (G.D. Pappas and Purpura, D.P., Eds.) New York: Raven Press, pp. 257–302, 1972.

Rall, W. Core conductor theory and cable properties of neurons. In: *Handbook of Physiology. Vol. 1. The Nervous System*. (E.T. Kandel, Ed.) Bethesda: American Physiological Society, 1977.

Rall, W.A. A statistical theory of monosynaptic input-output relations. *J. Cell. Comp. Physiol*. 46:373–411, 1955a.

Rall, W.A. Experimental monsynaptic input-output relations in mammalian spinal cord. *J. Cell. Comp. Physiol*., 46:413–437, 1955b.

Scheibel, M.E. and Scheibel, A.B. Elementary processes in selected thalamic and cortical subsystems—the structural substrates. In: *The Neurosciences: 2nd Study Program*. (F.O. Schmitt, Ed.) New York: Rockefeller University Press, pp. 443–457, 1970.

Sholl, D.A. *The Organization of the Cerebral Cortex*. New York: Wiley, 1956.

Srinivasan, R. An experimental and theoretical study of neocortical dynamics. Ph.D. Dissertation. New Orleans, LA: Tulane University, 1994.

Swadlow, H.A., Rosene, D.L, and Waxman, S.G. Characteristics of interhemispheric impulse conduction between prelunate gyri of the rhesus monkey. *Exp. Brain Res*. 33:455–467, 1978.

Swadlow, H.A., Waxman, S.G., and Geshwind, N. Small-diameter nonmyelinated axons in the primate corpus callosum. *Arch. Neurol*. 37:114–115, 1980.

Swadlow, H.A. and Waxman, S.G. Variations in conduction velocity and excitability following single and multiple impulses of visual callosal axons in the rabbit. *Exp. Neurol*. 53:128–150, 1976.

Szentagothai, J. Local neuron circuits of the neocortex. In: *The Neurosciences 4th Study Program*. (F.O. Schmitt and Worden, F.G., Eds.) Cambridge, MA: MIT Press, pp. 399–415, 1979.

Tomasch, J. Size, distribution and number of fibers in the human corpus callosum. *Anat. Rec*. 119:119–135, 1954.

van Rotterdam, A., Lopes da Silva, F.H., van der Ende, J., Viergever, M.A., and Hermans, A.J. A model of the spatial-temporal characteristics of the alpha rhythm. *Bull. Math. Biol*. 44:283–305, 1982.

Waxman, S.G. and Bennett, M.V.L. Relative conduction velocities of small myelinated and non-myelinated fibers in the central nervous system. *Nature New. Biol*. 238:217–219, 1972.

Wilson, H.R. and Cowan, J.D. A mathematical theory of the functional dynamics of cortical and thalmic nervous tissue. *Kybernetik*. 13:55–80, 1973.

Wright, J.J. and Lilley, D.T.J.: Personal communication, 1994.

12

Experimental Connections Between EEG Data and the Global Wave Theory

PAUL L. NUNEZ

Overview of the Global Theory

A global theory of electroencephalographic (EEG) generation in a cortex-like model medium was developed in Chapter 11. This theory contains no free parameters; that is, all physiologic and anatomic parameters can be, in principle, measured. The theory has been purposely formulated so that the most uncertain parameters are combined in a single, nondimensional cortical control parameter B, which is thought to change as a result of alterations in diffuse cortical input from the midbrain. In this manner, EEG waveforms are predicted to change with physiologic state. Of course, any theory purporting to describe, even very approximately, the complex dynamics of neocortex must involve assumptions so mathematical development may be accomplished and the number of parameters may be limited to manageable ranges. Then there is the question of the dependence of the theory's predictions on these assumptions. With bad theories, conclusions are simply the summation of assumptions.

The critical assumption issue was addressed in Chapter 11 in several ways. The assumed parameter ranges were justified as much as possible with anatomic and physiologic data. Furthermore, separate sections of Chapter 11 examined separate effects of the various assumptions. Overall, the predictions of weakly damped or limit cycle standing waves appear to be relatively insensitive to these assumptions. That is, details of the wave behavior change with different asumptions, as expected. However, qualitative and several semiquantitative predictions of the theory seem robust.

We can also judge a theory by its ability to make predictions of experiments that have not been conducted. In fact, several of the experiments discussed in this chapter were performed specifically to test the theory. Many apparent agreements between theory and experiment are found; however, the theory is proposed only as a tentative step toward quantitative description of neocortical dynamics. For example, many important issues regarding nonlinear effects and spatial-temporal scale are not addressed by the global theory. Some of these issues are considered in Chapter 14 in relation to the statistical mechanical approach to neocortical dynamics. Experimental connections to the global theory (mainly without considering possible contributions from the local circuit delays) are outlined in the following sections. The manner in which neocortical dynamics may change between global and local states is discussed in Chapter 13.

We can describe the global EEG theory in general, qualitative terms with still another metaphor that is aimed partly at readers who avoid (perhaps because of the mathematics) the physiologically based theoretical study of Chapter 11. Both spinal cord and brain develop from the neural tube of the embryo. The spinal cord contains an outer layer of white matter, consisting of axons carrying ascending and descending action potentials, and central gray matter in which synaptic action occurs. In the following thought experiment, we imagine the construction of a crude, one-dimensional model of neocortex and its corticocortical connections by joining ends of a spinal cord to form a closed loop of neural tissue.

We also imagine that ends of axons form gray matter excitatory synapses, but that axons have different lengths that vary from about 1 to 20 cm, thereby mimicking corticocortical fibers. The circumference of our synthetic spinal cord is the anterior-posterior circumference of the neocortex, that is, about 50 to 100 cm, with the former distance measured along the free surface and the latter more applicable to axons following the folded surface (Nunez, 1981a).

Our synthetic spinal cord is similar to the closed loop of transmisson line discussed in Chapters 2 and 9, except propagation velocities in the cord are distributed because of varying (myelinated) axon diameters. Stimulation of the cord at any location causes dispersive wave fronts of compound action potential to propagate in both directions away from the origin. If gray matter neurons are in the appropriate background state (as determined by external control systems that provide chemical and electrical input to the cord), sufficient excitatory synaptic inputs (which occur within short time intervals) to gray matter regions cause secondary neurons to fire action potentials. In this case, wave fronts can be relayed around the entire circumference of the cord. Alternately, inhibitory synaptic action may be dominant in other states, in which serial activation is inhibited and compound action potential wavefronts are strongly attenuated over distances longer than the average axon length.

We imagine EEG experiments involving electrodes placed in gray matter. Electric potential oscillations occur as a result of local synaptic action modulation, which is determined by external control mechanisms and by relays from other spinal cord regions through spinal cord axons. Random input (in time and location) to our synthetic cord creates complex wave fields of compound action potentials and causes modulation of synaptic action, the later superimposed on background synaptic activity.

The synthetic spinal cord acts as a spatial-temporal filter. That is, any spatial pattern of modulation of synaptic action can be represented as a superposition of spatial Fourier components, representing standing waves with different integer numbers of wavelengths over the circumference of the loop of cord. Integer wavelengths are required so dependent variables and their spatial derivatives (such as modulation of synaptic action) are single-valued functions of position along the cord (as required if these variables represent actual physiological quantities). Thus cord system geometry partly determines the manner in which variables are spatially filtered. Other possible contributions to spatial filtering may occur because of inhibitory damping mechanisms that depend on wavelength. Temporal filtering occurs as a result of spatial filtering and the detailed dynamic behavior of the cord system, which may dictate a wave dispersion relation relating spatial and temporal frequencies of the resulting oscillations.

The resonant modes (normal mode frequencies) of this kind of system generally depend on distribution of propagation velocities, local synaptic delays, circumference of the closed loop, and magnitudes of control parameters, as described in Chapter 11 for one- and two-dimensional versions of the synthetic spinal cord or neocortical system. In either case, standing waves are predicted for a variety of parameter choices.

In What Sense Is the Theory Right or Wrong?

We make no claim that the global wave theory of EEG is "right" in any absolute sense. Rather it may be viewed as a succession of concepts starting from plausible notions of general wave motion and progressing to more speculative ideas that are less likely to be valid. This chain of concepts may be outlined in qualitative terms as follows.

Perturbations of neocortical state variables defined at macroscopic scales (such as synaptic action density) may propagate through the neocortical medium like traveling waves as the result of progressive synaptic activation. These general types of phenomenon are predicted by nearly all serious EEG theories regardless of whether corticocortical fibers are included in the analyses. The putative traveling waves are generally nonlinear, although plausible linear approximations often appear to be consistent with small perturbations of background activity. Weakly damped traveling waves on the closed neocortical surface interfere to form spatial patterns that are partly determined by global boundary conditions. With linear or quasilinear waves, such patterns are accurately described as standing waves. The medium then acts as a multiple band pass spatial filter, which implies bandpass temporal filtering in the case of linear wave phenomena. Interference phenomena also occur for nonlinear traveling waves, but additional effects may complicate the simple linear picture, as discussed in more detail in Chapters 10 and 14.

Interference of traveling waves on a spherical surface is illustrated in Figure 12-1. In this example, perturbations of the wave medium originate at eight "epicenters" on the surface of the sphere. Whether we observe traveling or standing waves in experimental data depends partly on the period of observation and spatial

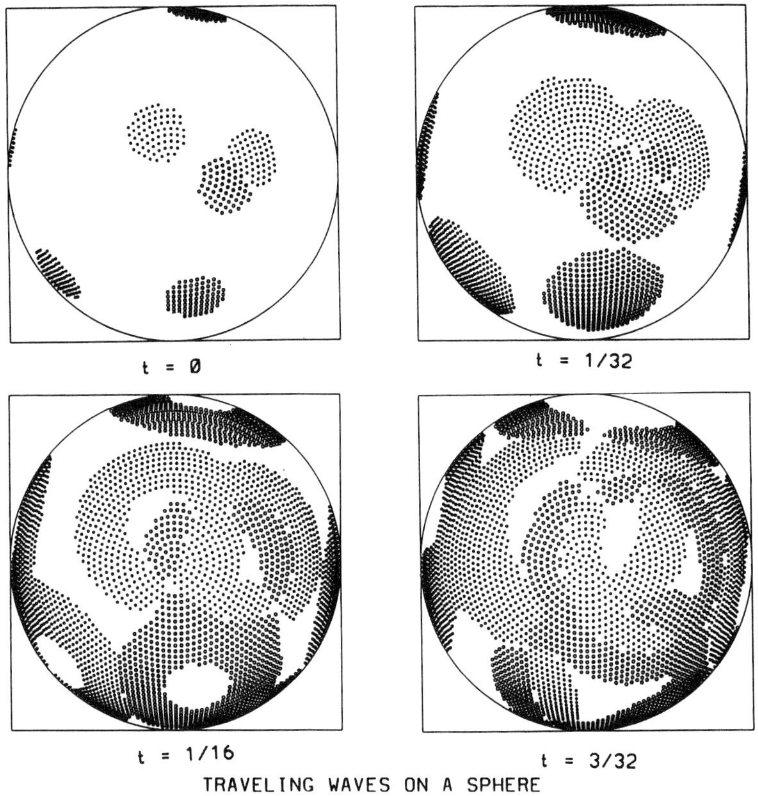

Figure 12-1. Nondispersive traveling waves (theoretical) on the surface of a sphere are simulated. This figure illustrates a transient solution; Figures 12-2 and 12-13 through 12-15 illustrate a steady-state solution for the same phenomenon, that is, standing waves. These waves are similar to the Schumann waves of electromagnetic field caused by lightning strikes in the earth's atmosphere described in Chapters 2 and 9. Wave fronts originate at eight discrete locations at t = 0. Seven in the northern hemisphere are shown in the t = 0 plot and one in the southern hemisphere first appears in the right side of the t = 1/32 plot. Dots indicate positive and open circles indicate negative perturbations of some field variable. Empty spaces are regions where the field is close to equilibrium. Constructive and destructive interference are first seen in the center of the t = 1/32 plot. Holes in the patterns (two at the bottom and one at the top of the t = 1/16 plot, for example) occur after each wave front has moved a distance that is about equal to the width of the wave packet. The time t = 1/2 is the time for a single packet to move to the opposite pole of the sphere.

extent over which recordings are obtained. For example, local electrode arrays (such as on the cortex) used near one of the epicenters illustrated in Figure 12-1 measure traveling waves for early times, that is, before substantial interference from other wave fronts obscures this interpretation. Alternately, the same phenomenon observed over large regions and longer periods (such as the time

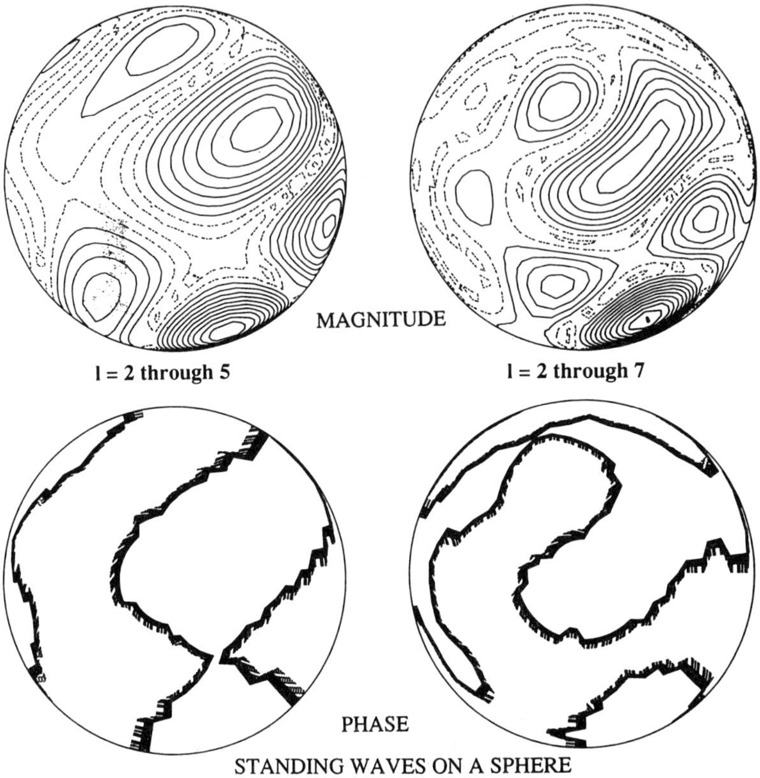

Figure 12-2. Nondispersive standing waves (theoretical) on the surface of a sphere are simulated. The surface waves are driven by point sources at 100 locations similar to those shown in Figure 12-1, except these occur randomly in time. The resulting spatial patterns are very complicated and change continuously with time; such plots are not very illuminating. Here we show magnitude and cosine (phase) plots corresponding to broad frequency bands. Above-average magnitudes are indicated by solid lines, below-average magnitudes by dashed lines. Cosine (phase) intervals are fixed at 0.15. The first column is a linear combination of modes $\ell = 2$ through 5 and the second column involves modes $\ell = 2$ through 7, where mode frequency is proportional to $[\ell(\ell + 1)]^{1/2}$, as in (9.40). That is, if we were to Fourier transform a multichannel record of data based on this physical process and obtained sufficient spatial resolution, we would expect magnitude and phase plots over the two broad frequency ranges to be similar to the plots in columns 1 or 2. Magnitude and phase patterns for individual ℓ modes are shown in Figures 12-13 through 12-15.

required for a wave to travel around the surface) reveal standing waves, provided the waves are weakly damped.

To demonstrate the general patterns of magnitude and phase plots produced by standing waves on a surface, consider nondispersive weakly damped waves on a sphere. That is we present forced solutions of (9.1) with α and $\omega_0 \simeq 0$. The driving term in these examples is

$$v(\theta, \phi, t) = \sum \delta(t - t_i) \sum_{n=1}^{N} D_{ni}\, \delta(\cos\theta - \cos\theta_n)\, \delta(\phi - \phi_n) \tag{12.1}$$

In this manner, wave motion over the surface of a sphere is stimulated by point sources that occur randomly at times t_i and at random locations over the surface, as determined by latitude and longitude coordinates (θ_n, ϕ_n). This might correspond physically to random lightning strikes in the atmosphere that disturb the electromagnetic field in the resonant cavity formed by the earth's surface and the bottom of the ionosphere. Figure 12-2 depicts the case of N = 100 activated source regions. We first chose the example of simple (that is linear, nondispersive) wave motion, rather than our putative brain waves, to emphasize that qualitative features of these results are applicable to nearly any linear surface waves. The solution (a scalar electric or magnetic field component, for example) is given by (9.39), with coefficients $A_{\ell m}$ determined by parameters in (12.1) except that ω_ℓ replaces $\omega_{\ell m}$ in (9.39) as a result of spherical symmetry. To match procedures applied to spontaneous EEG data (Chapter 3), we take the Fourier transform of (9.39) and evaluate the solution at fixed frequency ω_ℓ, that is,

$$\Psi(\theta, \phi, \omega_\ell) \sim \sum_{m=-\ell}^{+\ell} A_{\ell m} Y_{\ell m}(\theta, \phi) \tag{12.2}$$

Magnitude and phase plots of the function $\Psi(\theta, \phi, \omega_\ell)$ are shown for linear combinations (ℓ = 2 to 7) of the modes in Figure 12-2. Specific values of the complex coefficients $A_{\ell m}$ in (12.2) depend on the details of the input function (12.1), such as on the locations of input (θ_n, ϕ_n), times t_i at which they occur, and the magnitudes and signs of the input coefficients D_{ni}. However, we can make some remarks about the general kinds of magnitude and phase plots to be expected in this type of system when viewed over periods long compared with times required for waves to travel over the entire surface, that is, after substantial interference of traveling waves has produced standing waves.

1. The phase of Ψ exhibits nodal lines separating regions of the surface that oscillate 180° out of phase. These spatial patterns are linear combinations of the eigenfunctions $Y_{\ell m}(\theta, \phi)$ obtained from (12.2).
2. The magnitude of Ψ is largest in regions between nodal lines, which have zero magnitude at all times if spatial patterns are fixed. This feature is illustrated in Figure 12-2.
3. With the simple waves considered in this section, the number of nodal lines in the phase plot, as determined by the index ℓ, corresponds with the frequency ω_ℓ given by (9.40). That is, higher temporal frequencies occur with higher spatial frequencies. This particular feature of simple wave phenomena may not, however, apply to the putative standing brain waves described in Chapter 11. That is, low-frequency oscillations on a spherical brain-like surface can occur with higher eigenfunctions (large ℓ).

The idea of traveling waves on a closed surface that interfere to form standing waves can apply to local circuit models (discussed in Chapters 5 and 8) or to global theories. In either case, wave damping is generally a function of wave number. Thus waves in certain wave number ranges are weakly damped and are predicted to propagate over long distances (such as the entire cortical surface). When a wave packet of inhibition coalesces with a wave packet of excitation, partial cancellation occurs (interference). The main difference between local and global theories discussed in this book is that, in strictly local theories, wave propagation is provided exclusively by intracortical fibers, and wave propagation velocity is determined by local synaptic delays and intracortical fiber lengths. In contrast, in the purely global theory, wave propagation is due to delays in corticocortical axon propagation. We have argued here that the two processes are complementary and follow naturally from apparently realistic features of physiology and anatomy. However, several EEG phenomena are predicted with the purely global theory, without needing to consider local circuit effects.

Multiple branches of dispersion relations are proposed for waves in the neocortical medium. Some branches are associated with local delays (such as postsynaptic potential [PSP] rise and decay times), whereas other branches are associated with global delays due to finite velocity of action potential propagation in corticocortical fibers. Thus different types of "brain waves" are predicted to coexist in an (assumed) homogeneous neocortex. These wave branches generally produce different resonant frequency ranges; however, several branches may produce similar resonant frequencies that are in the general range of spontaneous EEG.

Instability of some spatial modes predicted with linear approximations may undergo limit cycle oscillations. Although the specific quasi-linear solution outlined in Chapter 11 cannot be regarded too seriously due to the mathematical approximations and requirement of additional unknown parameters, this general type of behavior is common in complex physical systems that share important properties with neocortex. Limit cycles at the local circuit level may also occur, such as the general type described by Wilson and Cowan (1974). In this view, the epilepsies are phenomena for which control parameters assume values that cause neocortical dynamics to change from linear or quasi-linear ranges to more strongly nonlinear ranges. Chaotic dynamics may or may not characterize such states. In any case, chaos in EEG depends in part on the spatial scale of measurement (Nunez and Srinivasan, 1993).

Whereas the "brain wave equations" (11.1) and (11.2) have not been studied in detail for inhomogeneous neocortex, we can anticipate some general characteristics of such solutions based on experience with similar physical phenomena. For example, suppose that local and global control parameters (Q and B, respectively, of Chapter 11) vary over the cortical surface such that local and global effects are dominant in different regions, as depicted symbolically in Figure 12-3. Traveling waves may be heavily damped as they cross boundaries of the local regions but weakly damped in the global region B. Or local circuit oscillations

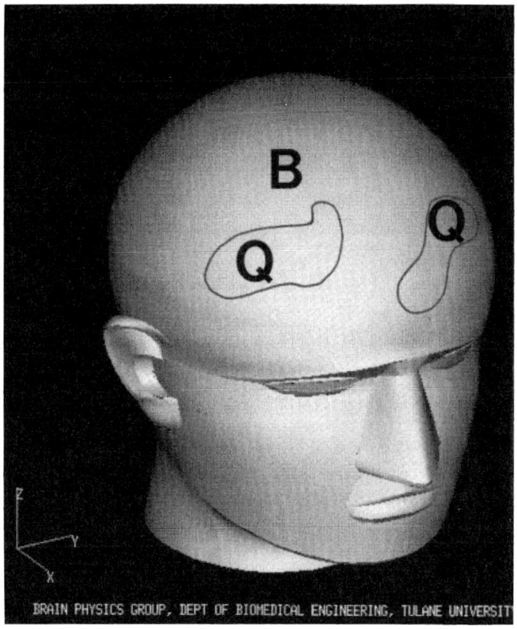

Figure 12-3. Symbolic representation of different regions of a theoretical neocortex in which local or regional (Q) and global (B) processes are dominant. Q and B may have different magnitudes in different regions (see Chapters 11 and 13). Standing waves might occur as a result of interference of waves traveling in region B; such waves might be damped in Q regions. Oscillations due mainly to intracortical circuits are imagined to be dominant in Q regions, with coherence between remote Q regions facilitated by specific corticocortical axons. Evidence for this qualitative idea is provided by Thatcher and colleagues (1986) and by data presented in Chapters 3 to 7 and 13.

may coexist with standing waves of the same frequency. If traveling waves find continuous paths in the global region and interfere on the closed neocorticl surface, standing waves can occur in region B simultaneously with local or distributed circuits in multiple local regons Q. If the total area occupied by regions Q is small compared with region B, global normal mode frequencies can be expected to approximately equal frequencies obtained for a homogeneous neocortex, which occurs when all Q regions shrink to zero size. In contrast, if the Q regions become so large and numerous that they block global wave interference, spatial patterns associated with global resonance may disappear altogether.

In addition to these general, qualitative ideas, the global theory provides specific quantitative predictions: EEG resonant frequencies, wave propagation velocities, magnitudes of the global control parameter at which specific modes are most likely to appear in the EEG, and so on. Quantitative connections between theory and experiment are often difficult to obtain, partly because the theory is approximate and because of problems in interpreting experimental results. However, in the following sections, we outline several of these quantitative connections and also more general associations.

One of the strongest motivations for the more tentative, preliminary experimental connections described in the folowing sections is to guide new experimental studies. That is, some of these data can be compared with theory only qualitatively rather than quantitatively because the investigators did not know the theoretical basis for EEG proposed here, and thus missed relatively easy opportunities to check theoretical predictions.

Prediction of the Approximate Frequency Range of Spontaneous EEG from the Underlying Physiologic and Anatomic Parameters

The theory suggests weakly damped (or perhaps limit cycle) oscillations of lower modes of approximate normalized frequency $\omega_R R/v_E \sim 1$ or 2 for relatively small values of the cortical control parameter B. Using realistic ranges for effective cortical radius R and corticocortical propagation velocity v_E and (11.53), this prediction corresponds to a frequency range of about $f \sim 2$ to 26 Hz. As the control parameter increases (due perhaps to removal of inhibitory influence from the midbrain), the frequency of each mode tends to decrease, but at a different rate for each mode. That is, there is a critical value of B for each mode ($B_{\ell c}$) such that an abrupt decrease in the ℓth mode frequency occurs as B approaches $B_{\ell c}$. Further increases in B may cause the ℓth mode to disappear from the EEG, cause an abrupt decrease in the frequency of a higher mode $>\ell c$, or both.

This predicted behavior is superficially similar to that observed in EEG during the transition from the awake to sleeping state and during some sleep stages. That is, an abrupt decrease occurs in the dominant EEG frequency components at sleep onset to the 1-Hz range. In addition, some higher frequency components can be observed during different sleep stages. In the context of the global theory, these may be viewed as higher modes that are overdamped at lower B values, that is modes only observed over the range of B values for which they are "efficient." This *mode scanning* feature of the theory is considered further in the context of EEG during anesthesia in the next section.

Higher EEG frequencies tend to be limited by several aspects of the theory. In addition to the mode scanning response of cortex predicted by theory, a spread in the distribution of corticocortical velocities acts as a low pass filter of neocortical waves for any fixed control parameter B. Furthermore, the theory for waves on a sphere predicts that both high and low spatial modes produce standing wave frequencies in the low range of $\omega_R R/v_E \sim 1$ or 2. The predicted low pass behavior of neocortex agrees with the general character of human EEG, as discussed in Chapter 3. Because the basic theory was first presented (Nunez, 1972, 1974a) before comprehensive data on corticocortical propagation velocity were fully available (or at least known to the author), we can perhaps claim that the theory makes an approximate prediction of average corticocortical propagation velocity based on known EEG frequency ranges.

Mode Scanning with Halothane Anesthesia

Several sections of Chapter 11 describe different theoretical bases for mode scanning effects. In the greatly oversimplified case of waves in an infinite "loop" of neocortex, (11.15) suggests that all values of the control parameter B > 2 result in unstable waves in the linear theory (such as limit cycles). However, the more accurate solutions for one-dimensional waves in a finite loop (see the Appendix), waves in a medium with distributed corticocortical propagation velocities (Chapter 11, Effects of Spreads in Action Potential Velocity Distribution), and brain waves on a spherical surface (Chapter 11, Brain Waves on a Spherical Surface) suggest more complex selection of modes. That is, certain ranges of the neocortical control parameter B are more "efficient" for specific global modes. In this section, we summarize some experimental results that provide qualitative support for global mode scanning. These halothane EEG data were recorded in an operating room; mode scanning properties were first discussed in connection with the solution for brain waves on a sphere, originally obtained from (11.1), (11.2) and (11.3), by Katznelson (1981, 1982).

Several hours of seven-channel EEG recordings were obtained from each of eight subjects who were placed under varying levels of halothane anesthesia as part of an unrelated cardiovascular study (Nunez et al, 1976; Stockard and Bickford, 1975). These data had the following general characteristics in all eight subjects:

1. Large-amplitude (100 to 250 μv) oscillations were recorded over all scalp locations. The dominant frequencies of these rhythms depend strongly on inspired halothane concentration. Dominant frequencies vary between 4 and 16 Hz as inspired concentration varies between 4% and 0.5%. The exact range of frequencies is somewhat subject-dependent; however, lower frequencies are associated with deeper anesthesia states in all subjects. Thus the general EEG effect of halothane is to "tune" neocortex to certain preferred frequency ranges in a manner similar to that predicted by theoretical mode-scanning mechanisms.
2. Multiple global modes are observed in all subjects. This effect is demonstrated for one of them in Figure 2-13 and for three others in Figure 12-4. We are apparently justified in calling these modes "global" because they appear and disappear simultaneously at all scalp locations as halothane concentration is varied. The relative amplitudes of different modes may vary with recording location, orientation of bipolar electrodes, or both, as illustrated in Figure 12-4. This effect can be explained by noting that recorded magnitudes of standing wave phenomena depend on the relative locations of nodal lines and recording points (see Chapter 9). Of course, we cannot rule out local circuit contributions to the dominant frequencies shown in Figure 12-4, but such contributions apparently are not needed to explain these data. In fact, EEG measured under anesthesia is less variable among participants than is EEG in waking states (Stockard and Bickford, 1975). This finding is consistent with the idea that anesthetics produce standing waves that are determined primarily by a few global parameters, with minimal influence from specific distributed circuits that may have different characteristics in different persons and different cognitive states.
3. Low-frequency modes emerge in the data in an orderly manner as halothane concentration is increased; a propitious concentration range appears to exist for each mode. Three separate dominant modes are evident in Figure 12-4, together with many closely spaced weak modes in the 15- to 25-Hz range. All modes show decreased frequency with increased halothane concentration. Also the relative frequency shift appears to be about the same in a given participant. That

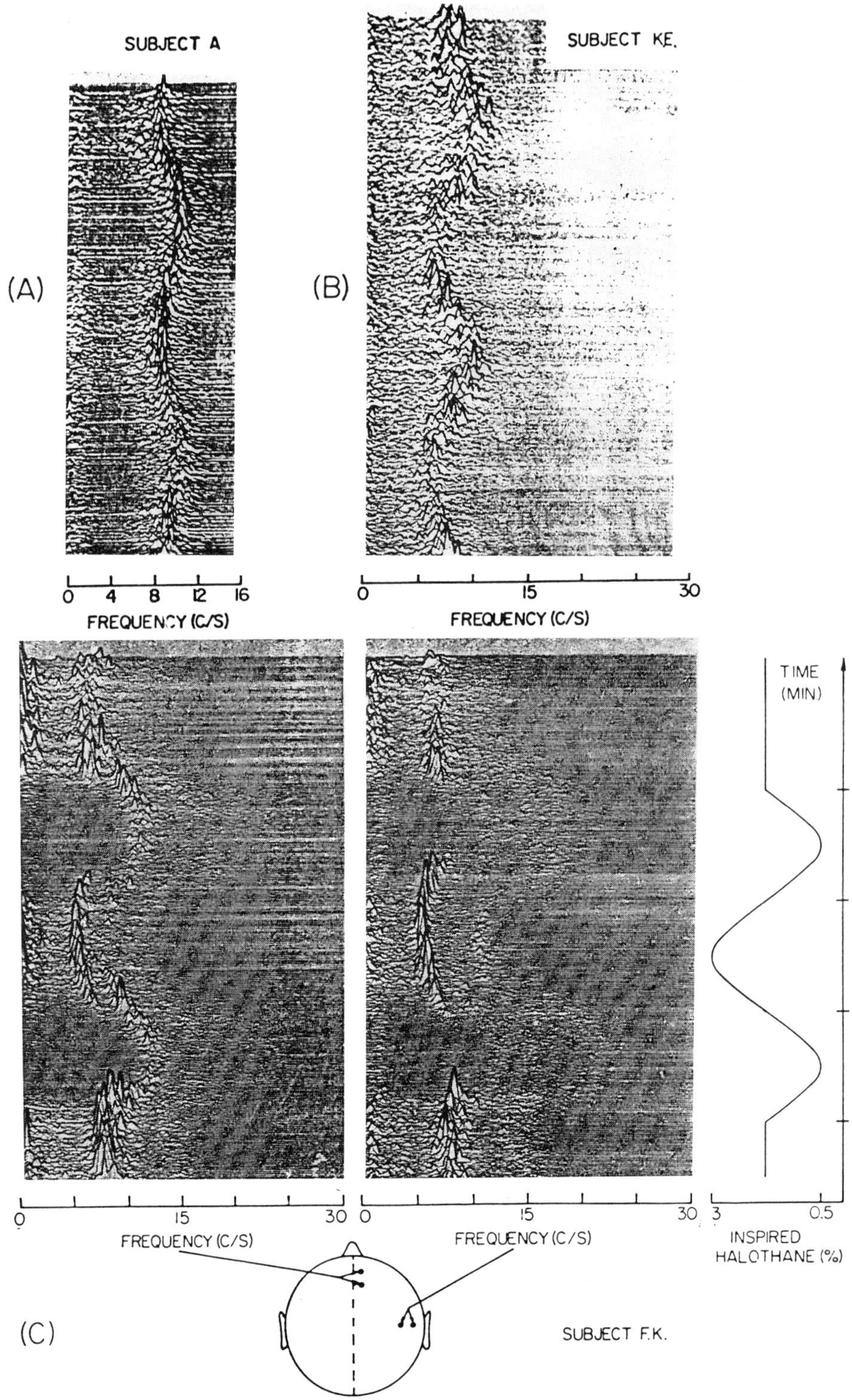
SUBJECT A
(A)
0 4 8 12 16
FREQUENCY (C/S)
SUBJECT K.E.
(B)
0 15 30
FREQUENCY (C/S)
TIME (MIN.)
45
30
15
0
0 15 30
FREQUENCY (C/S)
0 15 30
FREQUENCY (C/S)
3 0.5
INSPIRED HALOTHANE (%)
(C)
SUBJECT F.K.

is, higher frequencies have larger frequency changes for a given concentration change.

These data have several qualitative and semiquantitative features in common with the theoretical mode scanning mechanisms illustrated in Figures 11-30 through 11-33. How the neocortical control parameter B may be expected to change with anesthetic depth is a complex but important question. Halothane causes decreases in action potential firing rate in some subcortical neural populations, and increases in others (Shimoji and Bickford, 1971). Furthermore, depression of brainstem systems evidently can result in either net excitatory or inhibitory influences on neocortex because of a complex collection of chemical and electrical input mechanisms (see Chapters 4, 5 and 13). Studies of the effects of some anesthetic agents show that they may produce depression or excitation of various neural structures in brainstem, limbic system, and neocortex, either simultaneously or in sequence (Stockard and Bickford, 1975).

For our purposes, the primary issue is the net effect of all halothane influences on the background excitability of neocortex, that is, the relative magnitudes of the control parameter B at different concentrations. We note that most general anesthetics can produce electrocerebral seizure activity, which suggests an overall excitatory influence on neocortex (Stockard and Bickford, 1975). This observation is reasonably consistent with a general amplitude property of most anesthetics. That is, when anesthetic depths at moderate concentrations are increased, amplitudes of sinusoidal EEG typically increase, although very high concentrations may produce nonsinusoidal EEG (such as "burst suppression") of lower amplitude and finally a flat EEG trace at maximal concentrations (Stockard and Bickford, 1975). From these data, we conclude that at moderate halothane concentrations (as used clinically and in these experiments), increases in concentration should have a net excitatory influence on neocortex, that is increase the control parameter B.

For illustrative purposes, consider the following scenario based on theoretical mode frequencies and damping shown in Figure 11-33. Although nondimensional mode frequencies ($\omega_R R/v_E$) are plotted, it is more convenient to assume that $v_E/2\pi R = 10$ Hz to make arguments easier to follow. This value of the parameter is apparently accurate within a factor of two, so specific frequency estimates have the same potential error. From Figure 11-33, a control parameter $B = 2$ results in theoretical prediction of a weakly damped mode ($\ell = 3$) of about 17 Hz and a moderately damped mode ($\ell = 5$) of about 19 Hz. This is approximately consistent with experimental observations that halothane produces 12- to 18-Hz sinusoidal EEG at very light (subanesthetic) concentrations (Stockard and Bickford, 1975).

Figure 12-4. Compressed spectral arrays for three subjects (A, B, C) anesthesized to varying depths with halothane. Inspired concentration of halothane for subject C is the function of time, shown at the lower right. Higher concentrations reduce the frequencies of all modes, possibly as a result of increasing the global control parameter B. (Reproduced with permission from Katznelson, 1981).

As B is increased to values between 2 and 4, both frequencies and damping of the $\ell = 3$ and 5 modes gradually decrease. Based partly on the quasi-linear solution of the section Quasi-linear Effects of Chapter 11, we expect corresponding increases in amplitudes of these modes for values of B where the linear theory predicts instability. When B is less than about 3, the mode $\ell = 4$ is heavily damped and not expected to be observable. However, as B increases to values greater than 3, frequency and damping of the $\ell = 4$ mode rapidly decrease. The frequency of the $\ell = 4$ mode is about 7 Hz for B = 3 and near 1 Hz for B = 4, a result that agrees semiquantitatively with Figure 12-4. Further increases in the control parameter B result in the introduction of a succession of new odd modes that first appear with small amplitudes and frequencies in the 10- to 20-Hz range. As B increases, the frequencies of these modes decrease and amplitudes increase. New even modes also appear with initial frequencies typically in the 5- to 10-Hz range; these frequencies also decrease and amplitudes increase as B increases. Very large B values may lead to nonsinusoidal or flat EEGs, depending on both nonlinear and low pass effects discussed in Chapter 11, although too many confounding variables may make reasonable theoretical predictions for large B values more difficult.

This scenario is based on a characteristic length for corticocortical fibers (compared with sphere radius R) of $\lambda_E R = 1$. However, qualitatively similar results are predicted for $\lambda_E R = 0.7$ (Figure 11-31) and $\lambda_E R = 1.5$ (Figure 11-32). The main difference is that the number of weakly damped modes possible in the model neocortex is reduced substantially for larger values of $\lambda_E R$, that is as corticocortical fiber lengths become shorter in relation to sphere radius.

A compressed spectral array of EEG in a dog anesthetized with halothane is shown in Figure 12-5 (Rampil et al, 1980). The dog EEG shows characteristics qualitatively similar to those observed in humans as inspired concentration changes. The main difference is evidently that canine frequency peaks occur at roughly twice the human peak frequencies observed at the same halothane concentrations. This effect is expected if canine brains are scaled down by a linear factor of two, with all other physiology and anatomy features fixed (including axon diameter; that is, characteristic axon propagation velocity v_E). This prediction follows simply from fixed application of the global theory based on the nondimensional frequency $(\omega_R R/v_E)$. As indicated in Table 2-1, the canine linear scale factor is about 0.36, indicating a "naive" frequency ratio of 2.8. Canine axon diameters may be a little smaller than human axon diameters so that the effective v_E is lower, but of course many important physiologic and anatomic differences other than scale probably contribute to frequency differences. In any case, the dog EEG data are qualitatively consistent with the global theory.

Finally, many of these general ideas about mode scanning in the EEG may be applicable to other states. For example, the appearance of multiple modes that occur in some sleep stages but not in others also may be due to changes in the neocortical control parameter B. Spectral analysis of various sleep stages may be found in Johnson and coworkers (1969), Nunez (1981a), and in Chapter 4. In later sections, we consider additional experimental methods to study mode scanning,

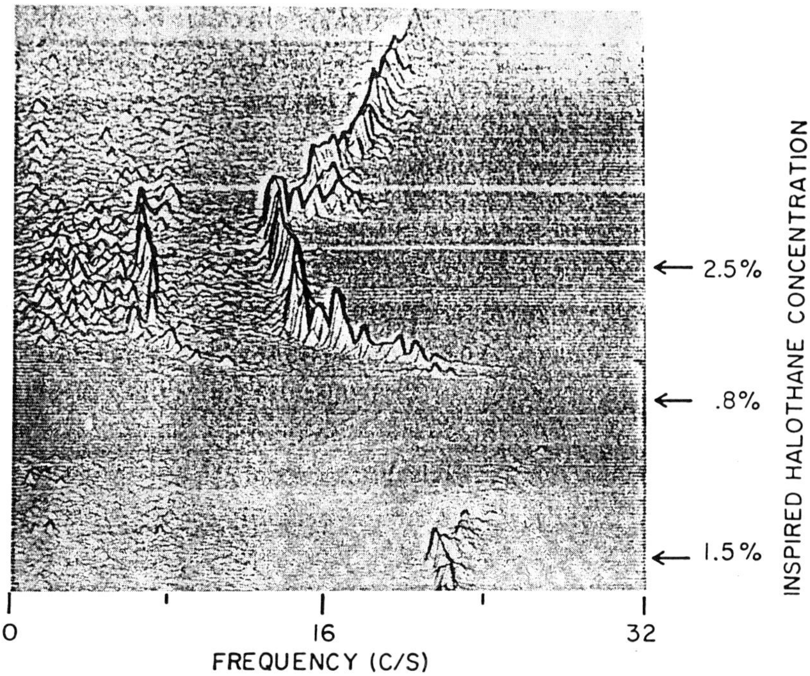

Figure 12-5. Compressed spectral array showing different mode frequencies as a function of inspired concentration of halothane in a dog. (Reproduced with permission from Rampil et al, 1980.)

including methods that may allow independent estimation of magnitudes of the control parameter B.

Quasi-stable Spatial Structure of EEG with Apparent Nodal Lines

Spontaneous EEG data presented in Chapter 3 and steady-state visual evoked potential data presented in Chapter 6 suggest quasi-stable, partly coherent spatial structures. A short period of alpha rhythm which is free of obvious artifact is shown in Figure 12-6. Potential maps for the extrema of the P4 potential labeled 1 through 4 are shown in Figure 3-13. Corresponding Laplacian maps are shown in Figure 3-14. Extrema potential plots 5 through 12 are shown in Figures 12-7 and 12-8. Corresponding Laplacian maps are shown in Figures 12-9 and 12-10. Corresponding cortical image maps are shown in Figures 12-11 and 12-12. The potential maps suggest a large scale anterior-posterior oscillation which persists for the five alpha rhythm cycles shown. The Laplacian and cortical image maps show more detail, for example spatial patterns appear relatively stable over the period 1 through 7 (300 milliseconds) with change to a new state at time 8. The relation of such

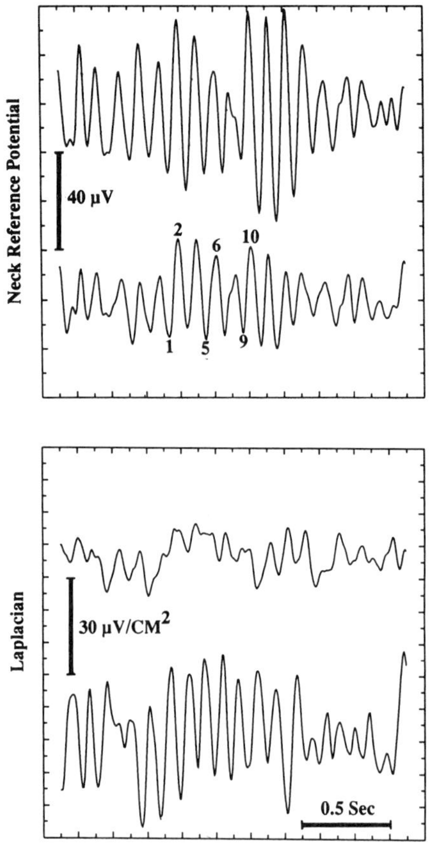

Figure 12-6. Alpha rhythm waveforms. Same data shown in Figure 3-12 over a shorter time. Upper plots in each box are P3 potential or Laplacian; lower curves are P4 potential or Laplacian. Extrema 1 through 12 are the times at which contour maps were obtained.

patterns (called "microstates") to cognitive processing has been studied by Lehmann and colleagues (Wackermann et al., 1993). There is nothing special about these data other than all 64 channels are free of artifact over the period shown. Locating periods of data which is free of obvious artifact can be the most time-consuming part of EEG data analysis.

Spatial properties of EEG can also be considered on longer time scales. The 10-Hz magnitude and phase plots of alpha rhythm described in Chapter 3 show similar structure when viewed over successive 1-second periods. When viewed over successive 1-minute periods, spatial structure at these large scales is constant if the brain's physiologic and cognitive state is relatively fixed.

Ideally, we would like to study the detailed spatial properties (requiring 64 or more electrodes) of EEG under halothane anesthesia because these rhythms appear to exhibit multiple global modes. However, because such data are not available now, we consider magnitude and phase plots for the alpha rhythm data discussed in Chapter 3. The following issues tend to obscure comparisons between experimental data and theoretical predictions of spatial-temporal properties:

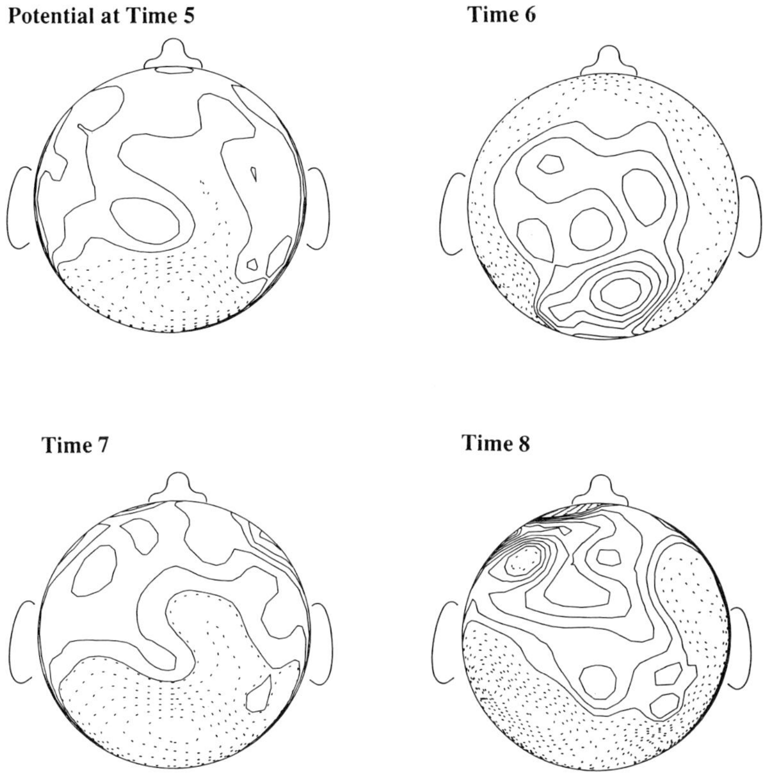

Figure 12-7. Potential maps at times 5 through 8 shown in Figure 12-6. Potential maps for times 1 through 4 are shown in Figure 3-13.

1. Detailed spatial maps of EEG recorded from human neocortex are not available. Unprocessed scalp potential measurements represent a low pass spatially filtered estimate of cortical potential, most sensitive to the lower modes, as shown in Figure 1-28. In contrast, the surface Laplacian is relatively insensitive to lower modes. The sampled Laplacian sensitivity (such as estimated with our spline algorithm) depends on the relative locations of sources and electrodes, but provides a sensitivity that approximates that of the analytic Laplacian if 64 or more electrodes are used. EEG experiments are now planned by the Melbourne group using 131 electrodes so that the accuracies of the spatial maps can be further verified (see Chapter 6).

2. With nondispersive standing waves on a sphere, as illustrated by the theoretical examples in Figure 12-2 and Figures 12-13 through 12-15, choosing a narrow frequency band with the Fourier transform results in spatial patterns that correspond to fixed ℓ modes. The spatial patterns (magnitude and phase) at fixed frequency can, however, change because they generally involve different sums over the m index, that is different $A_{\ell m}$ values in (12.2). But we generally expect to observe more nodal lines in phase plots corresponding to higher frequencies because frequency is proportional to $[\ell(\ell + 1)]^{1/2}$ for linear, nondis-

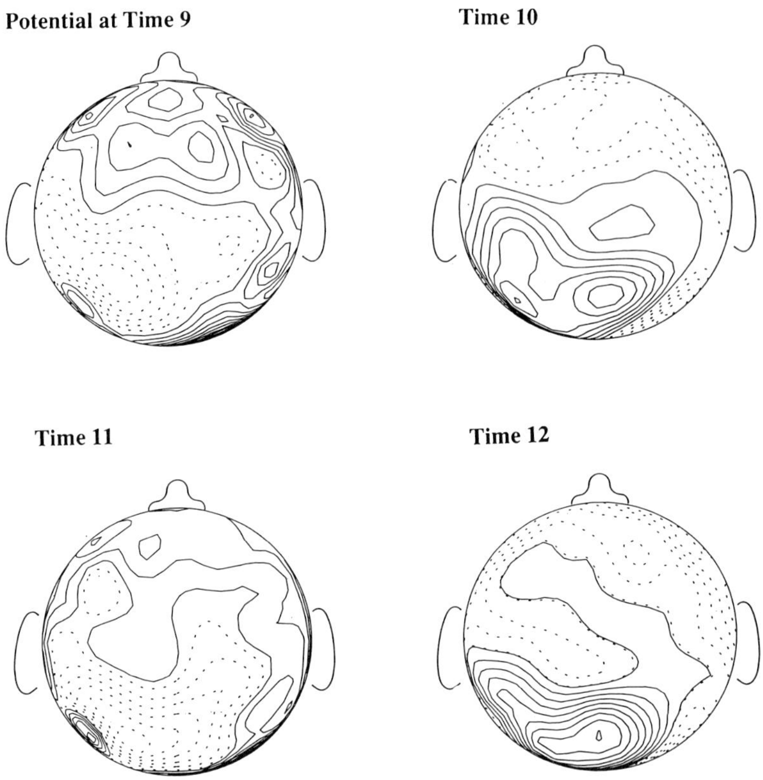

Figure 12-8. Potential maps at times 9 through 12 shown in Figure 12-6.

persive waves on a spherical surface. Thus, if brain waves were this simple, magnitude and phase plots of EEG at different frequencies could be used as a direct check for the presence of standing wave phenomena.

3. The putative brain waves predicted by the methods described in Chapter 11 are, however, more complicated than the simple waves considered above. The geometry clearly is not spherical and the medium is inhomogeneous so that splitting of ℓ modes is expected, that is a single ℓ index may correspond to several normal mode frequencies. With waves on a prolate spheroid (Chapters 2 and 9), different frequencies occur with different m indices, for example. If the modes are closely spaced, we may not be able to display a single mode from EEG data with our Fourier transform. Although we can improve frequency resolution by increasing Fourier transform epoch lengths, a small drift in mode frequencies (due, for example, to small changes in control parameters) may cause overlapping modes.

4. Our putative brain waves are generally dispersive and have multiple branches of the dispersion relation. Higher ℓ modes can oscillate at frequencies near the fundamental, that is $\omega_R R/v_E \sim 1$ or 2, as outlined previously. Thus a Fourier transform of this type of field evaluated at some fixed frequency may pick out a combination of ℓ modes, even for waves on a homogeneous, isotropic spherical

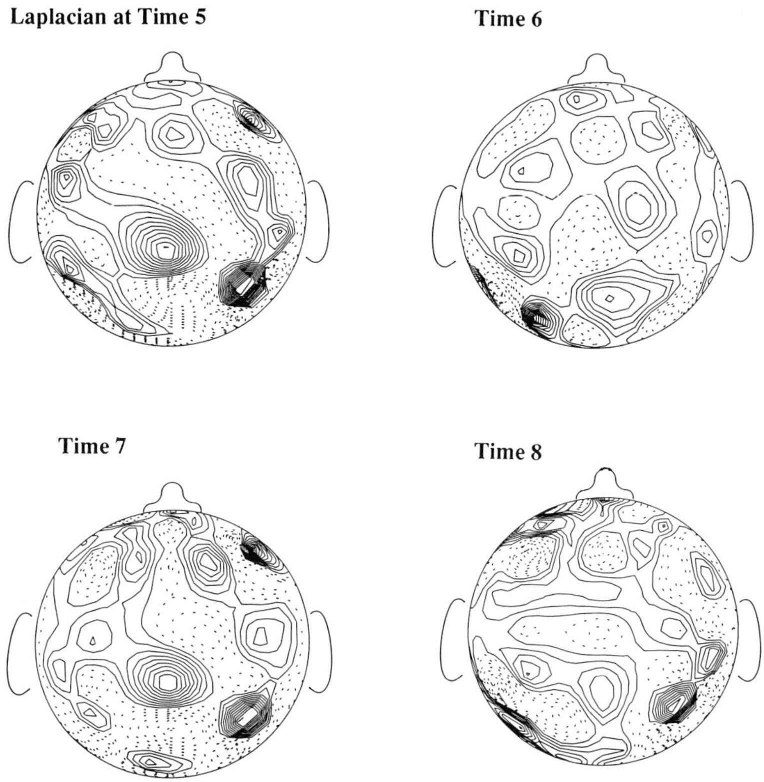

Figure 12-9. Laplacian maps at times 5 through 8. Laplacian maps for times 1 through 4 are shown in Figure 3-14.

surface. In theory, we can control the relative contributions of different ℓ modes by varying the global control parameter B, by varying anesthetic depth, for example. A few example magnitude and phase plots (theoretical) for nondispersive standing waves on a sphere that involve linear combinations of m modes are shown in Figures 12-13 through 12-15. These may be compared with similar plots of alpha rhythm potential and Laplacian maps shown in Figures 12-16 through 12-18. We expect our spline-Laplacian (64 electrodes) to be sensitive to a broader and higher range of spatial frequencies than is unprocessed scalp potential. This theoretical prediction is consistent with differences observed in the potential and Laplacian maps of alpha rhythm shown in Figures 12-16 and 12-17.

Despite problems of interpretation, the magnitude and phase plots shown here and in Chapter 3 are highly suggestive of standing waves at large scales. Apparent nodal lines occur in nearly all of the Laplacian and cortical image phase plots. Furthermore, a correspondence often occurs between large magnitude and regions between apparent nodal lines in phase plots, as would be expected of standing

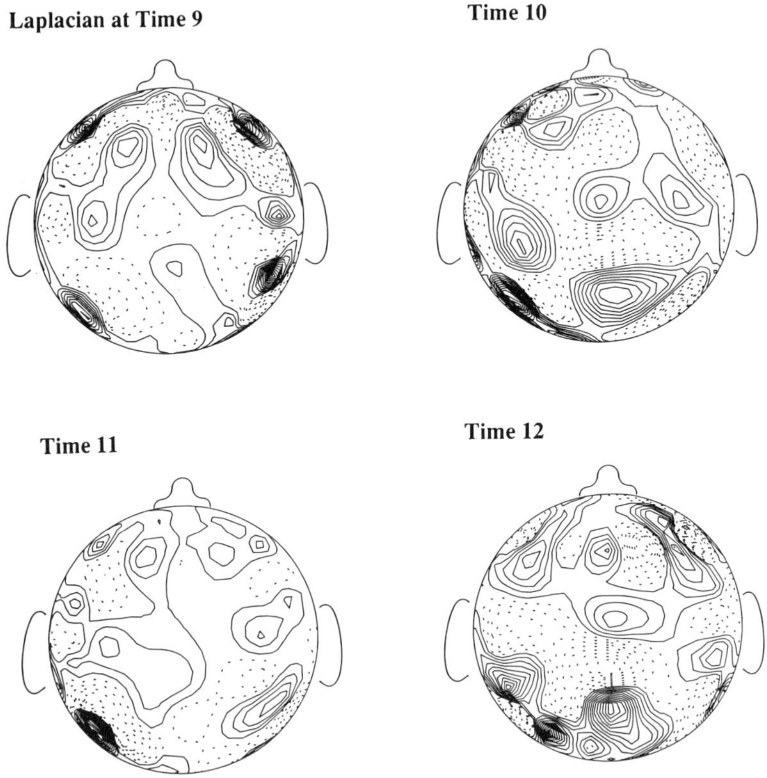

Figure 12-10. Laplacian maps at times 9 through 12.

waves, which is illustrated by the simple theoretical waves of Figures 12-2 and 12-13 through 12-15. Furthermore, the spatial patterns evoked by sine wave-modulated light change as a function of driving frequency, as discussed in Chapter 6 and a later section. Thus it does not appear that nodal lines are fixed by brain anatomy such as fissures and sulci.

Frequency Dependence on Size of the Neural System

If the general idea of standing brain waves is correct, we expect that larger brains will, on the average, produce lower EEG frequencies. With a spherical cortex, this prediction follows directly from the relation $(\omega_R R/v_E) \sim 1$ to 2 obtained in Chapter 11; however, the general idea that mode frequencies decrease with surface area is expected regardless of the nature of the wave (as described by the dispersion relation) or shape of the cortical surface, especially for linear or quasi-linear waves. With elementary physical waves, dispersion relations ensure that higher temporal frequencies tend to occur with higher spatial frequencies, in the usual manner of

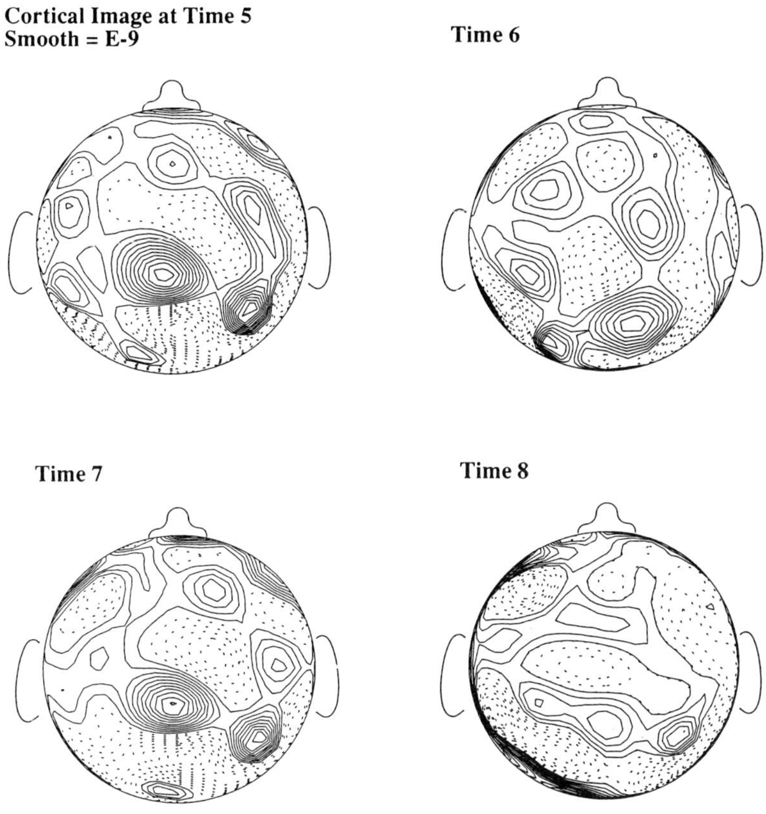

Figure 12-11. Cortical image maps at times 5 through 8.

"waves" (as discussed in Chapter 9). Lower spatial frequencies are allowed, by the boundary conditions, to persist on larger cortical surfaces because of interference of waves traveling in different directions. Thus larger surfaces allow for lower fundamental mode frequencies, and higher frequency overtones also occur. With putative standing neocortical waves on a spherical surface, predicted in Chapter 11, many higher spatial modes contribute to the low temporal frequency range, and thus this issue is somewhat more complicated than that of waves with simple dispersion relations. However, a size-frequency dependence is still predicted, that is, $f \sim (1 \text{ to } 2)\,(v_E/2\pi R)$.

Several difficulties with this idea tend to obscure the postulated correlation between cortical surface area and EEG frequency, as listed below.

1. Brain size is highly correlated to the volume of the skull (correlation coefficient ~ 0.83), but the correlation between brain size and more convenient linear measures of head size is somewhat smaller (Blinkov and Glezer, 1968). Accurate estimation of cortical surface area apparently would require magnetic resonance images (MRI) for every participant.
2. In one study (Blinkov and Glezer, 1968), the average volume of the brain

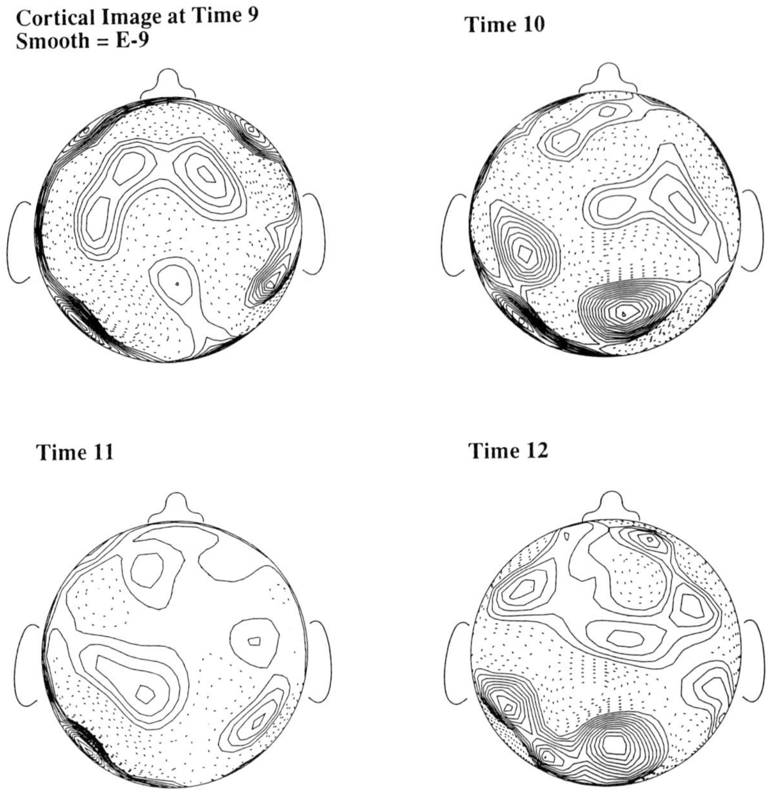

Figure 12-12. Cortical image maps at times 9 through 12.

in a group of 228 was 1260 cm^3, with a minimum volume of 984 cm^3 and a maximum volume of 1610 cm^3. This variation in volume corresponds to a change of only $\pm 8\%$ in effective cortical radius (that is, linear scale factor as in Table 2-1) from the average. Because mode frequencies vary inversely with sphere radius, we expect a change in the frequency spectrum due only to brain size differences of this same magnitude. Many brains would then be needed to obtain significant correlations.

3. In even the most simplified version of the global theory, the frequency of the fundamental mode of alpha rhythm is thought to depend on at least two parameters other than brain size, such as the average propagation velocity of the action potential in association fibers and the cortical control parameter B. If local effects make important contributions to EEG frequency, at least one additional control parameter must occur in addition to several other parameters associated with local time delays. However, if cortical state is fixed, as may be the approximate case during "resting" alpha rhythm, we can conjecture that control parameter influences on EEG frequency would be minimized.

4. If all neural structures, including corticocortical axon diameter, were to scale equally, no size–frequency relation would be predicted by the theory.

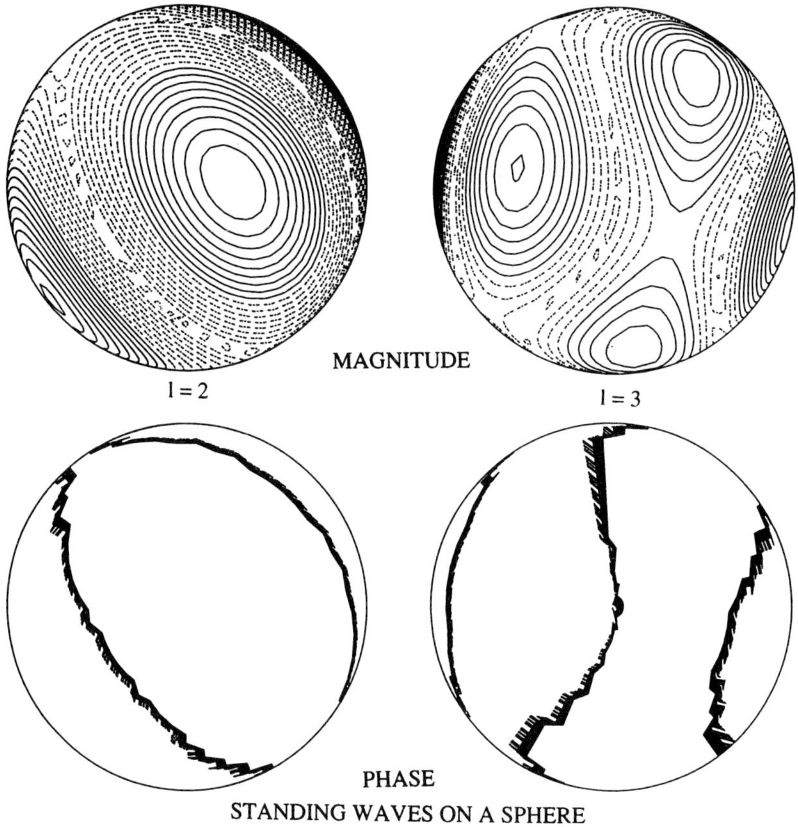

Figure 12-13. Standing nondispersive waves on a spherical surface (theoretical) due to continuous random input are simulated using (12.1). The surface potential distribution is viewed over a long period and Fourier transformed in time so that individual mode frequencies can be viewed. Here the modes $\ell = 2$ and 3 (ω_2 and ω_3) are shown. Degeneracy of the m modes causes these plots to be linear combinations of different m modes, as given by (12.2).

That is, corticocortical propagation velocity in myelinated fibers is proportional to axon diameter, so that both v_E and R in (11.58) would change in the same proportion. The available data on variations of axon diameter between individual persons is insufficient to address this question; however, a reasonable guess (based on animal data) is that axon diameter variations do not vary systematically with human brain size. Comparisons of EEG frequencies with other mammals are partly inconclusive for this reason. In addition, there may be substantial problems associated with cross-species comparisons of EEG, which must be recorded in equivalent physiologic states, as discussed in Chapters 2 and 5.

5. The alpha rhythm spectrum may contain several closely spaced modes, as a result of lack of symmetry of cortical geometry and possible inhomogeneity of the connection parameters. We can only hope to measure the average frequency of closely spaced modes.

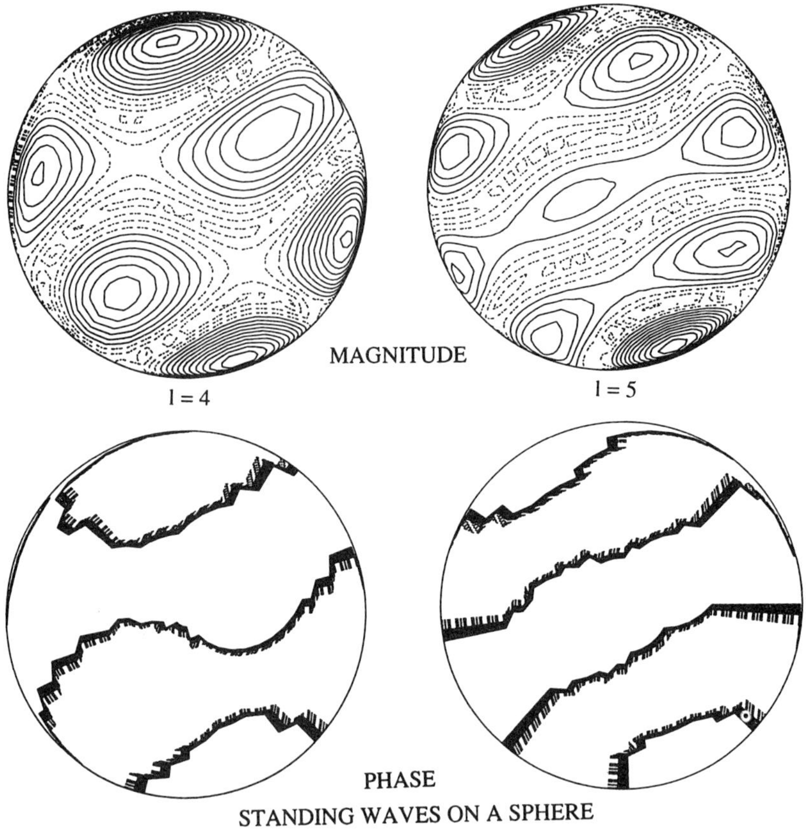

Figure 12-14. This figure is identical to Figure 12-13, except that modes $\ell = 4$ and 5 (ω_4 and ω_5) are shown. With simple, nondispersive waves, larger ℓ indices correspond to higher frequencies ω_ℓ. However, the putative "brain waves" on a spherical surface described in Chapter 11 do not necessarily follow this rule. See, for example, Figures 11-30, 11-31, and 11-33.

6. With nonlinear waves, the size–frequency relation is even less clear. However, as suggested by the quasi-linear solution for brain waves and in several examples of nonlinear physical phenomena (Chapter 10), it is not unreasonable to expect more dominance of lower frequency activity in larger cortices, even with nonlinear brain waves and in the presence of temporal chaos. Consider, for example, the famous Lorenz equations (10.22) that exhibit chaotic behavior in certain parameter ranges. The nondimensional time in these equations is proportional to (fluid depth)$^{-2}$. Thus, if we consider fluids in tanks of different sizes, but with the parameters A, B, C of (10.22) held fixed (including the ratio of depth to width), dynamic behavior in the different tanks based on the Lorenz equations is identical except that all oscillation frequencies (peaks in the temperature perturbation spectra, for example) are inversely proportional to tank size squared. This observation is, however, complicated by the fact that the

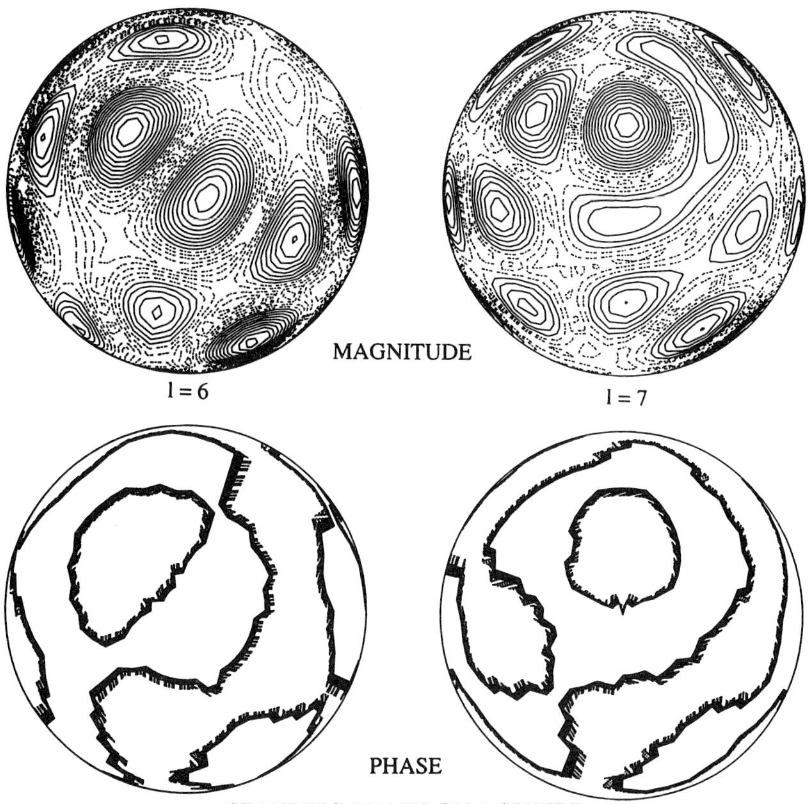

Figure 12-15. This is identical to Figures 12-13 and 12-14 except that modes $\ell = 6$ and 7 (ω_6 and ω_7) are shown.

normalized Rayleigh number B depends on the width and depth of the tank and on other parameters associated with the fluid. Thus these fluid parameters must change between tanks of different sizes to keep parameter B fixed. However, if we observe many such systems in which parameters are allowed assume wide ranges of values, higher frequency oscillations generally would be expected in smaller systems, but with many individual exceptions to this general trend.

These considerations suggest that, even if the global wave theory is correct, the correlations between head size and EEG frequency might be too small to observe in an experiment involving a reasonable number of participants. Nevertheless, we performed such a study of human alpha rhythm (Nunez et al, 1978; Nunez, 1981a). Participants were chosen through newspaper ads seeking volunteers with either very large or very small heads. Head size was defined as the cube root of the product of three standard linear measures (ear to ear, nasion to inion, and circumference). Although many of the respondents had nearly normal head size, a maximum variation in linear head size of −14% and +15% from the mean was obtained in a subject population of 123 having a peaked alpha rhythm

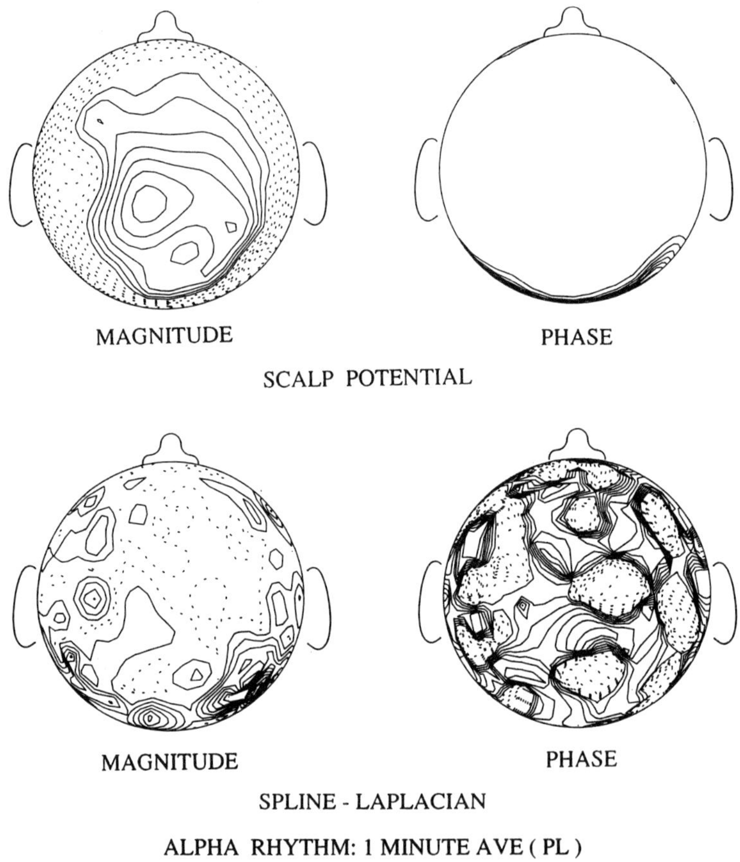

Figure 12-16. Magnitude and phase plots at 10 Hz for 1 minute of alpha rhythm (eyes closed) in subject PL. Raw scalp potential obtained from a 64-channel recording is shown in the upper row. Corresponding spline-Laplacian estimate of cortical surface potential is shown in the lower row. Raw scalp potential tends to pick up mainly the lower modes, whereas the spline-Laplacian is more sensitive to higher modes. See Figure 1-28.

frequency. The scatter diagram, shown in Figure 12-19, indicates a small ($r = -0.206$) but significant ($p = 0.02$) negative correlation between head size and peak alpha frequency, as anticipated by the global wave theory. Furthermore, the average frequency of the five size groups, shown by the solid circles, decreased progressively with increasing head size. A similar correlation also occurred between "maximum frequency" (as defined by the peak power histogram) and head size ($r = -0.233$, $p = 0.01$).

We considered whether this study measured only sex differences in alpha frequency. The negative correlation between head size and alpha frequency was also observed when applied to men and women separately, although, in this case, the small variation in head size within each subgroup caused the significance to be

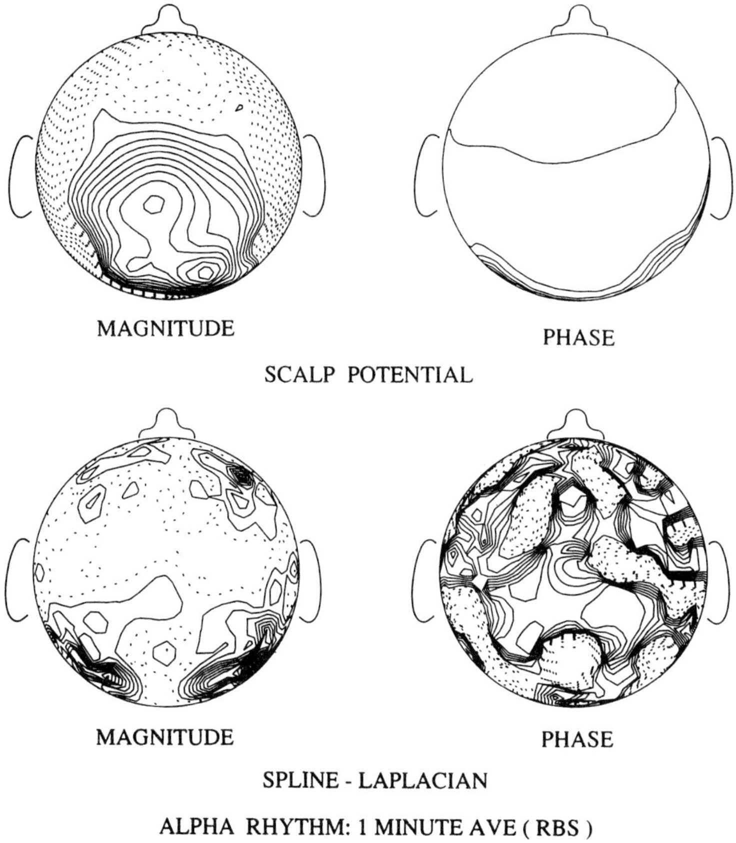

Figure 12-17. Potential and Laplacian magnitude and phase plots at 10 Hz for 1 minute of alpha rhythm (eyes closed) in subject RBS.

somewhat inconclusive ($r = -0.186$ for men; $r = -0.139$ for women). Also these same data were later analyzed in a separate study (Hayes and Katznelson, 1979). The corresponding linear regression coefficients for the two scatter diagrams (with men and women analyzed separately) were not significantly different, suggesting that the observed frequency differences between small and large heads were not due to smaller head sizes in the women.

Another question to address is the possible effect of age on alpha frequency. Earlier data suggest that no systematic change in alpha frequency occurs with age, except in persons older than 60 years, in whom frequency decreases substantially (Nunez, 1981a). To study this question further, the data were separated into six age groups (17–23, 24–29, 30–39, 40–49, 50–59, and 60–78) and linear regression analyses were performed for each group (Hayes and Katznelson, 1979). All six regression equations had a negative slope (negative correlation coefficient), thereby further supporting the hypothesis that brain size is negatively correlated with alpha frequency.

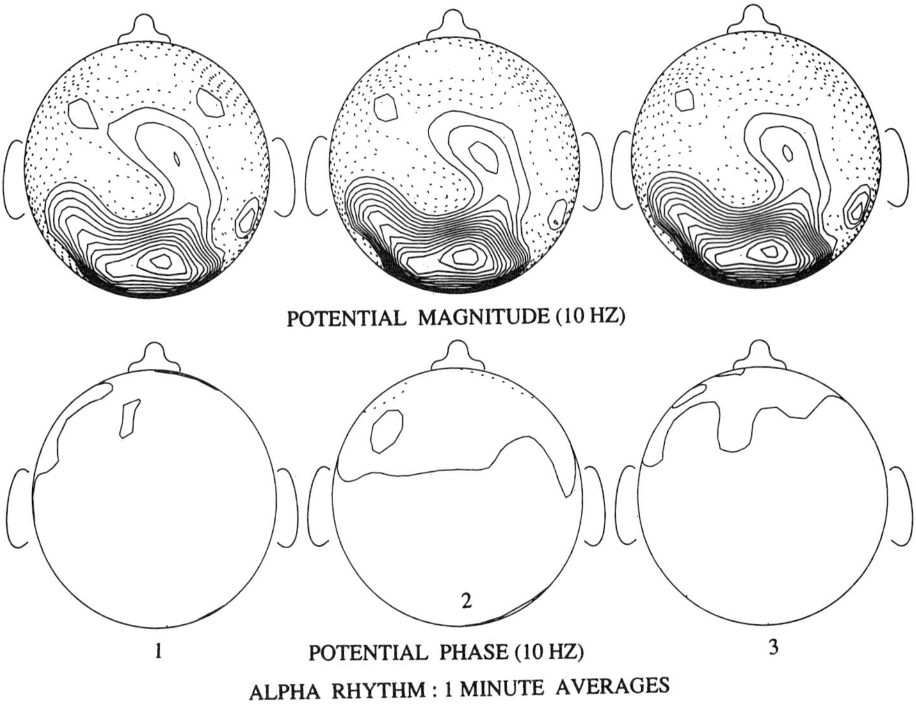

Figure 12-18. Magnitude and phase plots at 10 Hz for three successive 1 minute periods of alpha rhythm (eyes closed) in subject PLN. Laplacian magnitude and phase plots for the entire 3 minute period are shown in the left column of Figure 3-23.

Maturation of the Alpha Rhythm

The study of the correlation between head size and alpha frequency excluded children, mainly because substantial myelination of corticocortical axons occurs in humans during maturation, apparently even through age 30 years (Yakovlev and Lecours, 1967; Courchesne, 1990). Myelination of axons increases propagation velocity by a factor of about 5 or 10 for small fibers of the same diameter, as discussed in Chapter 11. Furthermore, brain size undergoes relatively small changes after about age 2 years. For example, brain weights of 2 and 5 year olds have been reported to be 74% and 93%, respectively, of their adult values (Blinkov and Glezer, 1968). These values correspond to effective brain radii R of 90% and 98%, respectively, of adult values. Because our predicted fundamental mode frequency is expressed approximately by $f \sim v_E/2\pi R$, we would expect large increases in EEG frequency during childhood because of relatively large average propagation velocity increases, with negligible effects due to size changes.

The maturation of EEG rhythms for a group of children between ages 1 and 10 years is shown in Figure 12-20 (Bickford, 1973). The expected progressive shift in the spectrum from lower to higher frequencies is evident. Of course, it is

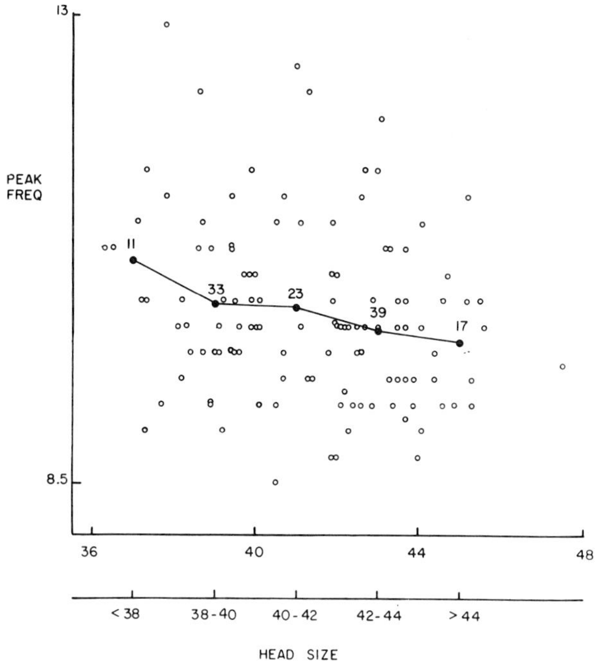

Figure 12-19. Head size is plotted versus alpha rhythm peak frequency in 123 subjects. Same data shown in Figure 2-9. (Reproduced with permission from Nunez, 1981.)

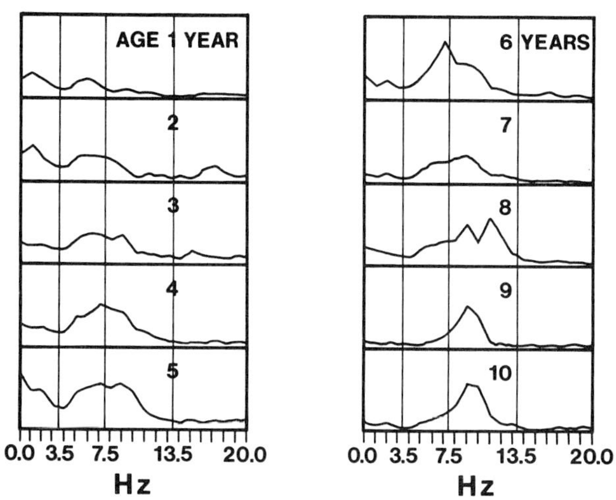

Figure 12-20. Series of amplitude spectra showing changes in the alpha rhythm in children ages 1 to 10 years. (Reproduced with permission from Bickford, 1973.)

difficult to make a quantitative comparison with theory because of the many confounding variables. For example, we do not know the percentage of myelinated fibers as a function of age, so we cannot estimate changes in the velocity distribution function $f_E(v)$. Nor do we have any information on how the cortical control parameter B might change with age. In addition, local circuit changes may occur with age that change the local cortical control parameter Q as discussed in Chapter 11.

Methods To Estimate EEG Phase and Group Velocities

The predicted and observed spatial-temporal properties of EEG are complicated. Cortical potentials are perhaps composed of many waves simultaneously traveling in different directions (by analogy to waves caused by rain drops on a pond), which partly combine also to form standing waves forced by global boundary conditions. That is, we should evidently view EEG as a combination of forced and free oscillations because noecortex receives continual input from various midbrain regions. This is consistent with local and global theories. However, a one or two order of magnitude difference exists between the velocities predicted by local and global theories because the former predict propagation due solely to intracortical interactions, whereas the latter emphasizes propagation along corticocortical fibers (see Chapters 5 and 8).

Two basic types of wave propagation velocity characterize wave phenomena, phase velocity, and group velocity. An elementary discussion of these concepts is given in Chapters 1 and 9 and by Pain (1978) and Nunez (1981a). Sinusoidal waves of different temporal frequencies have different wave numbers k, as expressed by the wave dispersion ralation $\omega = \omega(k)$. The phase velocity is defined by

$$v_p = \frac{\omega(k)}{k} \tag{12.3}$$

Often waves are composed of short pulses (that is, regions of disturbance) that propagate through the wave medium, as illustrated in Figure 12.1. Such pulses can be considered to be composed of many sinusoidal (in both space and time) components of different spatial frequencies (that is wave numbers, k) and corresponding temporal frequencies $\omega(k)$. If the medium is nondispersive, that is if $\omega = vk$, all wave components travel with the same velocity v. All components travel together and the pulse retains its shape as it travels along, which explains the label "nondispersive."

With dispersive wave media, some sinusoidal components lag behind or run ahead of others so that the pulse is broadened or dispersed as it travels. The compound action potential of a nerve fiber behaves like this because it is composed of many axons with different diameters, that is different propagation velocity. Each axon carries a pulse of constant shape, but the composite wave form due to all axons forms a dispersive wave pulse. The group velocity is the velocity with which an amplitude function impressed on a carrier wave travels (somewhat like the velocity of the "center of mass" of the pulse). Often the group velocity has a simple physical interpretation, that is, it is the velocity with which the energy of the pulse travels. Exceptions are cases of anomalous dispersion, in which group velocity has no easy physical interpretation. For example, group velocity sometimes may become greater than the velocity of light or negative over narrow wave number ranges. In the usual case of nonanomalous dispersion, group velocity may be larger or smaller than the phase velocity. With nondispersive waves, phase and group velocities are equal. Group velocity generally is expressed by

$$v_G = \frac{d\omega(k)}{dk} \tag{12.4}$$

With waves traveling on a surface, the wave number **k** is a vector representing propagation in two directions. However, the global theory suggests a possible predominance of waves traveling parallel to the longest corticocortical fibers (that is, in the anterior/posterior direction) because the nondimensional parameter $\lambda_E R$ is smaller in this direction. Furthermore, we can more easily resolve spatial resolution problems in EEG experiments in this longitudinal direction due to the longer space available to place electrodes over a single hemisphere. For this reason, we first take a simplistic view that cortical waves of potential travel front to back and back to front (x direction) according to the usual expression for waves traveling in two directions

$$\Psi(x, t) \cong \sum_{n=1}^{N} [A_n \cos(\omega_n t + k_n x) + B_n \cos(\omega_n t - k_n x)] \tag{12.5}$$

In writing (12.5), we included the possibility of both free and forced oscillations so that there may be many more n waves than ℓ modes of standing waves.

Another way to view the proposed EEG process is to allow the traveling waves to combine due to interference. That is, by using common trigonometric identities, (12.5) yields

$$\Psi(x, t) \cong \sum_{n=1}^{N} [2A_n \cos(\omega_n t)\cos(k_n x) + (B_n - A_n)\cos(\omega_n t - k_n x)] \tag{12.6}$$

This form emphasizes that, in general, $\Psi(x, t)$ is composed of both standing (first half of sum) and traveling waves (second half of sum). Generally, we would expect to observe traveling wave phenomena in short time segments of spontaneous EEG records. In contrast, records over longer time intervals (such as more than 1 second) may reveal standing waves due to the interference of many waves traveling in different directions.

The special case $A_n = B_n$ corresponds to a pure standing wave n, as shown most readily in (12.6). In contrast, the cases A_n or $B_n = 0$ denote pure traveling waves in the positive or negative x directions, respectively, as shown by either (12.5) or (12.6). In addition, each wave n can be expected to satisfy a dispersion relation $\omega_n = \omega(k_n)$, otherwise it would not normally be classified as wave. The phase difference θ_n and corresponding time lags Δt_n associated with waves traveling between two locations separated by distance x are related to the phase velocity v_{pn} of the nth mode by

$$\Delta t_n = \frac{\theta_n}{\omega_n} = \frac{x}{v_{pn}} \tag{12.7}$$

Given these considerations, several questions concerning phase and group velocities can be posed about EEG data. The situation just described is greatly oversimplified, even with respect to the global theory (which is a vast oversimplification of real neocortical dynamics). However, it may be close enough to the true picture so that some approximate estimates of phase and group velocity can be obtained. There are also considerable difficulties from the experimental side. Data obtained from the scalp suffers from poor spatial resolution due to space averaging by tissue (which limits information at high spatial frequencies) and the limited region over which electrodes can be placed (which limits information at low spatial frequencies). Despite such difficulties, substantial experimental connections are possible, as discussed in the following sections.

We want to consider one type of experiment in which estimates of phase velocity are obtained as a function of frequency. This is most easily accomplished using EEG or MEG evoked by sinusoidally modulated light because wave propagation is expected in the posterior-anterior direction. Also we may be able to obtain some crude estimates from short segments of spontaneous EEG that show continuous phase shifts in a particular direction, that is, cases in which the A_n in (12.6) are small. Several reports of apparent traveling waves of spontaneous EEG are found in the literature, as discussed in later sections.

We can write phase velocity (12.3) as

$$v_p(\omega) = \frac{\omega}{k(\omega)} \tag{12.8}$$

and differentiate both sides with respect to ω to obtain

$$\omega \frac{dv_p}{d\omega} = v_p \left[1 - v_p \frac{dk(\omega)}{d\omega}\right] \tag{12.9}$$

If derivatives are estimated experimentally by finite differences, the following relation is obtained

$$v_p/v_G \sim 1 - \frac{\omega}{\Delta\omega}\frac{\Delta v_p}{v_p} \tag{12.10}$$

That is, a certain fractional change in driving frequency $\Delta\omega/\omega$ results in a corresponding fractional change in phase velocity $\Delta v_p/v_p$, thereby yielding an estimate of the ratio of phase to group velocity as a function of frequency for evoked waves traveling through neocortex. Actually, (12.10) is highly idealized because the global EEG theory for waves in finite media predicts multiple branches of the dispersion relation; that is, several modes (with different effective k) can contribute to the same narrow frequency band. This implies a range of phase and group velocities within narrow frequency bands.

Despite these problems in interpretation, we can obtain a direct comparison of (12.10) with the one-dimensional theory for the infinite loop of neocortex, in which only one branch of the dispersion relation is predicted. In this manner, we can search for very approximate comparisons with experiment. With an infinite loop of cortex, theoretical phase velocity is given by (11.14), that is

$$v_p = \frac{\omega}{k} = v_E \left[1 - \left(\frac{\lambda_E B}{2k}\right)^2\right]^{1/2} \quad (12.11)$$

This approximate solution can only be valid for waves having wavelengths that are short compared with brain circumference. Theoretical group velocity is obtained by differentiating (12.11) with respect to k to obtain

$$v_G \equiv \frac{d\omega}{dk} = \frac{v_E^2}{v_p} \quad (12.12)$$

Here v_E is the characteristic velocity for action potential propagation in corticocortical fibers. Because (12.11) shows that $v_p \leq v_E$, (12.12) indicates that theoretical group velocity v_G is greater than or equal to theoretical phase velocity v_p. This prediction correlates qualitatively with experiment if a positive change in phase velocity Δv_p is measured when sinusoidal driving frequency $\Delta\omega$ in (12.10) is increased. By combining (12.11) and (12.12), we find

$$\frac{v_p}{v_G} = 1 - \left(\frac{\lambda_E B}{2k}\right)^2 \quad (12.13)$$

Comparison of (12.10) and (12.13) yields a potential method to estimate the effective neural parameter $\lambda_E B$ directly from EEG data. That is, comparison of the theoretical relations (12.13) with the corresponding experimental relation (12.10) yields the estimate

$$\frac{\lambda_E B}{k(\omega)} \sim 2\left(\frac{\omega}{\Delta\omega}\frac{\Delta v_p}{v_p}\right)^{1/2} \quad (12.14)$$

The approximation (12.14) applies only to wavelengths that are short compared with brain circumference. The combined brain hemispheres are approximately shaped as a single prolate spheroid with a free anterior-posterior circumference of about 45 cm (Nunez, 1981a), or about 100 cm along the folded surface. Thus, (12.14) can be valid only for waves in the anterior-posterior direction along the cortical surface with wave numbers k that are large compared with 0.06 cm^{-1}.

If the quantity under the square root in (12.14) is positive (the data presented in the following sections suggest this is the case), (12.14) provides a method to estimate the effective product $\lambda_E B$, if estimates of wave numbers $k(\omega)$ for each driving frequency are obtained independently. The parameter for decrease in corticocortical axon connection density λ_E is fixed by the anatomy. In contrast, the control parameter B is thought to vary with physiologic state.

Preliminary data presented in the next section suggest that if average phase velocities for steady-state evoked potentials with driving frequency in the range $f \sim 10$ Hz are used in (12.14),

$$\frac{f}{\Delta f} \cdot \frac{\Delta v_p}{v_p} \sim 1 \tag{12.15}$$

This follows from the observation that the average wave number changes little with driving frequency over the narrow range studied. Averaged wave numbers k for these same data are about $0.18\ \text{cm}^{-1}$ on the scalp, or about $0.09\ \text{cm}^{-1}$ along the cortical surface. Because the approximate dispersion relation (12.11) is limited to short wavelengths, these estimates are crude approximations. The anatomic data reviewed in Chapter 11 suggest a reasonable guess for decrease in corticocortical fiber density along the cortical surface of $\lambda_E \sim 0.05$ to $0.2\ \text{cm}^{-1}$. Thus the following crude estimate for the range of cortical control parameter B is obtained from (12.14) and (12.15)

$$B \sim 2k/\lambda_E \sim 0.9 \text{ to } 3.6 \tag{12.16}$$

This estimated range of control parameter B obtained from experimental EEG combined with anatomic data on corticocortical fiber lengths correlates fairly well with the crude estimate of B obtained in Chapter 11. The later estimate, based on independent physiologic and anatomic data, is

$$B \sim 0.4 \text{ to } 9.0 \tag{12.17}$$

Equations (12.16) and (12.17) correlate approximately within the apparent limits of theoretical and experimental uncertainty. We can imagine more accurate experiments in which sinusoidal visual evoked potentials are obtained during awake states, during some sleep stages, or for various depths of anesthesia. In this manner, we can try to fit the individual λ_E and B to experimental data. If this is accomplished, additional checks for self-consistency of parameters may be developed using independent experiments.

Phase Velocities Forced by Visual Evoked Potentials

Estimates of phase velocity obtained from progressive phase shifts of sinusoidal visually evoked potentials recorded by the Melbourne group are described in Chapter 6. We briefly outline these results here to help complete this chapter. The phase velocity v_{pn} associated with a particular driving frequency ω_n may be estimated from the phase difference between recording sites separated by distance x from (12.7). Here we interpret separation distance x as measured along the neocortical surface, that is, x is interpreted as 2.1x (distance measured along the scalp surface). There is some uncertainty in these estimates because multiple corticocortical fiber systems may have different geometrical relations to the cortical surface (see Chapter 11); however, these phase velocity estimates should incur error due to uncertain geometry on axon paths by no more than a factor of about two.

An unstructured sinusoidal stimulus (10 Hz) was chosen to provide input of relatively low spatial frequency. Approximately 40% of subjects showed a smooth variation of phase of the visual evoked potential in the posterior-anterior direction, as expected for waves traveling away from visual cortex. Phase velocities were estimated using (12.7) in these subjects with reference EEG, bipolar EEG, and magnetoencephalography (MEG). The reference EEG data are thought to be in error because of the confounding effects of volume conduction. Phase velocity (v_p) estimates after correcting for the folded neocortical surface (presented in Chapter 6) are reference EEG, 10 to 18 m/second; bipolar EEG, 6 to 13 m/second; MEG, 5 to 8 m/second.

The MEG and bipolar EEG experimental estimates correlate closely with the general idea of waves traveling away from visual cortex in which progressive delays Δt_n in (12.7) are due to propagation velocity ($v_E \sim 6$ to 9 m/second) in corticocortical fibers. Other studies also support estimates of traveling waves with phase velocities in this range, such as Hughes and colleagues (1992), who reported transient event-related potentials that are consistent with cortical traveling waves that have phase velocities of about 4 to 7 m/second.

In the steady-state studies, phase velocity could be estimated only from (12.7) in 40% of participants who showed continuous phase changes along the midline. Approximately 30% showed a sharp 180° phase shift between electrodes placed in the parietal and midline positions. These sharp boundaries may be nodal lines of standing waves. That is, the separation of scalp potential into standing and traveling waves (12.6) is consistent with these data, if the two major terms on the right side of (12.6) have different magnitudes in different subjects. For example, if waves traveling away from visual cortex are heavily damped in mesial cortex (due perhaps to inhomogeneous damping mechanisms), only traveling waves might be observed on the upper scalp surface; that is, the A_n in (12.6) might be very small. Alternatively, weakly damped waves may combine to form standing waves with $A_n \sim B_n$, so the second term on the right side of (12.6) is small. In other subjects, the two major terms of (12.6) might have approximately equal magnitudes, so neither pure traveling nor pure standing waves are evident.

The phase velocity estimates cited above are based on several minutes of data. Another way to estimate average phase velocities of traveling waves is to identify short segments of EEG that exhibit a continuous phase shift in a particular scalp direction, such as along the midline. This procedure was applied by the New Orleans group to steady-state evoked potentials recorded by the Melbourne group in five subjects. Frequencies of the visual stimulus were varied over the range of 9 to 13 Hz. Data were digitized at exactly 16 samples per stimulus cycle to obtain accurate estimates of single-cycle Fourier coefficients, which were used to determine phases for each short segment (77 to 142 milliseconds) of data. Neck reference data were recorded from nine midline channels, and eight bipolar records were formed from adjacent electrodes. The total length of the array in the posterior-anterior direction was 24 cm (electrode spacing was about 3 cm).

Electroencephalographic records based on 1760 or 2336 cycles of the visual stimulus were obtained for each stimulus frequency. Correlation coefficients were obtained for each short data segment (single cycle of the stimulus) to flag linear relations between phase and electrode separation distance, as would be expected of simple waves traveling along the midline. The criteria for possible single-cycle traveling waves are based on linear regression studies of positive phase shifts in the posterior-anterior direction. If the significance level for phase versus distance plots based on bipolar recordings for the eight scalp locations was less than 1%, the short data segment was identified as a putative traveling wave. The correlation coefficient corresponding to the 1% significance level is 0.8343.

Phase velocity estimates for single cycles of steady state evoked potentials in

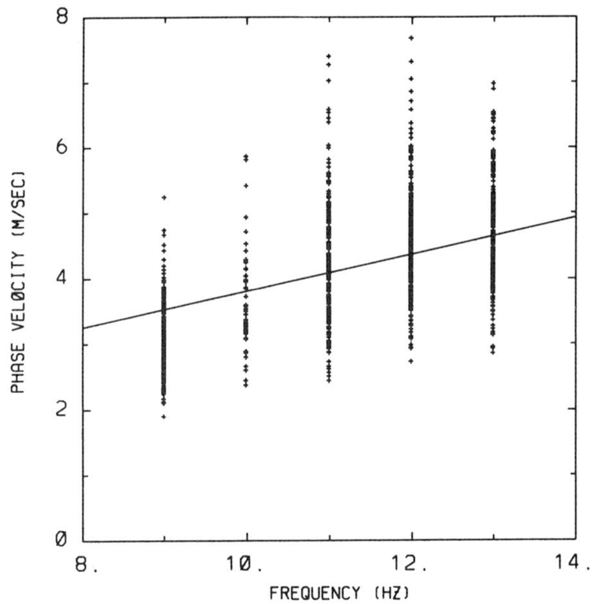

Figure 12-21. Phase velocity estimates (at the scalp) based on single-cycle Fourier coefficients obtained from steady-state visual evoked potentials. Velocities along the cortical surface are about twice as large. Horizontal axis is driving frequency. "Phase velocity" is defined based on linear shifts in phase along the posterior-anterior direction with statistical significance at the 1% level. About 8% of the cycles passed this test. The linear regression line is also plotted. Data were recorded at the Swinburne Centre for Applied Neuroscience in Melbourne and studied by the Brain Physics Group at Tulane University in New Orleans, Louisiana. Subject RBS.

one subject are plotted versus driving frequency in Figure 12-21. These results are typical for the five subjects studied. The first point concerns the many cycles that satisfied the criterion of a linear phase shift along the midline, that is 966 of a possible (5 × 2336 = 11,680) cycles or about 8%. In contrast, the number of cycles passing this same test using fields of random phases or the same phases at random locations was less than 0.1%. Thus we conclude that evidence exists for propagating EEG activity. Furthermore, the bulk of phase velocity estimates shown in Figure 12-21 (and for the other four subjects) are in the range 3 to 5 m/second along the scalp or about 6 to 10 m/second along the cortical surface.

Individual cycles with lower apparent phase velocities (that is larger wave numbers) were searched for separately by looking for progressive phase shifts involving either 7, 6, 5, or 4 contiguous scalp positions along the midline. The correlation coefficients corresponding to 1% significance levels for these different points in linear regression calculations are 0.8745, 0.9172, 0.9587, and 0.9900, respectively. With this approach we should be able to identify traveling waves with wavelengths as short as about 12 cm, that is, with phase velocities as low as 1 m/second. A total of 3192 phase velocity estimates were obtained in this manner, and all such phase velocity estimates were greater than 1.9 m/second. Average phase velocity estimates at each driving frequency were about 3 to 5 m/second, that is, the results were not much different from those based on 8 scalp positions, as illustrated in Figure 12-21. Thus no evidence for traveling waves with wavelengths shorter than 20 cm or phase velocities less than 1.9 m/second was found in these scalp potential data. Only 14 (0.4%) of the phase velocity estimates were greater than 10 m/second; these may be due only to chance.

These are very crude arguments that, at best, provide a greatly oversimplified explanation of the steady-state evoked potential data (see Chapter 6 for more details). However, the main results of this section are clear. First evidence suggests the existence of waves traveling away from visual cortex. Second, estimated phase velocities along the neocortical surface of human scalp evoked potentials are typically about 6 to 10 m/second. In contrast, estimates of phase velocities of 10-Hz activity obtained with electrodes on the cortical surfaces of dogs and cats are about 0.1 to 0.5 m/second, that is 10 to 100 times slower (see Chapters 5 and 6). The animal experiments apparently apply to much smaller spatial scales of EEG activity that cannot be observed with scalp recordings, and animal phase velocities appear to be due only to delays in intracortical circuits. We also note the progressive increase in average phase velocity with driving frequency shown in Figure 12-21. This result is expected if group velocity is greater than phase velocity, as predicted previously.

Phase Velocity Estimates for Spontaneous EEG

The direct method of estimating phase velocity is to search EEG records for segments of data in which progressive phase shifts occur along a particular scalp direction, as discussed previously for evoked potentials. Several of these experiments have involved searches for traveling waves in spontaneous EEG data, with estimates of phase velocity along the scalp for alpha rhythm of about 3 to 10 m/second. These estimates translate to a range 6 to 20 m/second for waves traveling along the cortical surface. Higher estimates are obtained using reference recording methods; they may be about 50% to 100% too high because of volume conduction-induced errors, as shown in Chapter 6.

We consider here a study of posterior-anterior phase differences of EEG recorded in 200 children ranging in age from 5 to 18 years (average age, 10 years) (Thatcher et al, 1986). These data present several interpretation problems in obtaining comparisons with theory. In particular, reference data are presented, and the wide age range of the children suggests a possible wide range in characteristic corticocortical propagation velocity v_E. Nevertheless, the data averaged over the 200 children show a progressive phase shift over about 21 cm in the posterior-anterior direction for alpha rhythm (that is, the broad band of 7 to 13 Hz). This phase shift corresponds to a phase velocity of about 6 m/second along the scalp or about 12 m/second along folded neocortex. Again, we expect this estimate to be too high by 50% to 100% because of unprocessed reference electrode data were used. Of course, it would be interesting to obtain phase velocity as a function of age in these data, but this information was not published.

Other frequency bands also indicated some evidence of progressive midline phase shifts, but phase-versus-distance plots deviate more from a linear relation than did the alpha data. However, crude estimates of apparent midline phase velocity v_p from these data are delta (0.5 to 3.5 Hz), 1.5 m/second; theta (3.5 to 7.0 Hz), 3 m/second; alpha (7.0 to 13.0 Hz), 6 m/second; and beta (13.0 to 22.0 Hz), 11 m/second. These values are uncorrected for either folded neocortical surface or volume conduction (two effects that tend to cancel). Although these estimates are very rough, (1) alpha phase velocities are fairly consistent (within a factor to about two) with similar experimental estimates and with the theoretical predictions of Chapter 11; and (2) phase velocity estimates progressively increase with EEG frequency, suggesting that group velocity is greater than phase velocity, as suggested by the previous theoretical arguments.

In another study of data recorded by the Melbourne group (Nunez et al, 1994) the method of searching for short data segments of linear phase shifts along the midline (discussed previously) was applied to adult human alpha rhythm. Estimated phase velocities at 10 Hz are plotted versus cycle number for one subject in Figure 12-22. Scalp phase velocity estimates for single 100-millisecond segments of data are nearly all about 3 to 7 m/second (6 to 14 m/second along the cortex).

Group Velocity Estimates for Spontaneous EEG

In an experimental study designed to estimate group velocities (Nunez, 1974b), electrodes were placed in a linear array along the right side of the midline, as indicated by Figure 2-7. Bipolar recordings from closely spaced pairs of electrodes were obtained, thereby gaining improvement in spatial resolution over reference

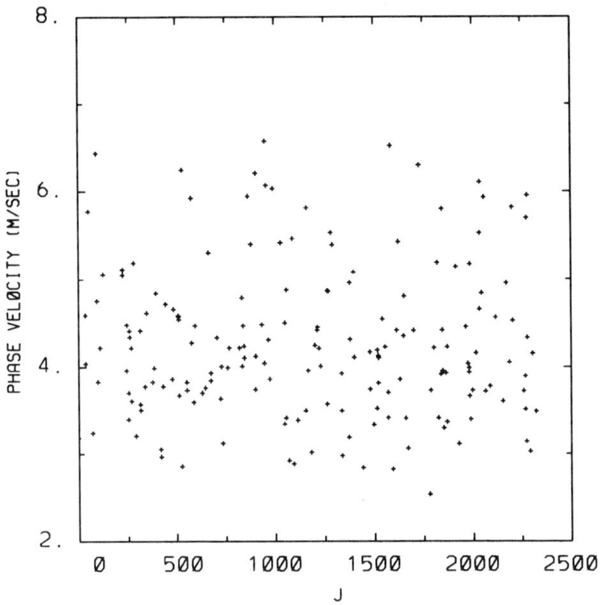

Figure 12-22. Phase velocity estimates (at the scalp) based on single-cycle Fourier coefficients obtained from 10-Hz alpha rhythm (eyes closed). Phase velocity is defined in the same manner as in Figure 12-20. Phase velocity estimates for alpha rhythm are here plotted versus cycle number (J). The plot contains 180 estimates of 2336 possible cycles (8%) that satisfied the 1% significance criterion. Subject RBS.

recordings, as discussed in Chapters 1 and 6. Each bipolar record provided an estimate of the time history of the local, tangential electric field in the scalp. Frequency-wave number spectra were obtained using standard fast-Fourier transform computer methods. If we assume waves traveling only in one direction (anterior-to-posterior, for example), the tangential scalp electric field associated with the nth wave is obtained from (12.5) with the $B_n = 0$

$$\varepsilon_n(x, t) = A_n k_n \cos(\omega_n t + k_n x) \qquad (12.18)$$

An estimate of the spatial-temporal Fourier transform of (12.18) for frequencies ω near ω_n is (Bendat and Piersol, 1986)

$$\varepsilon_n(k, \omega) \sim \left[\frac{\sin(k - k_n)\frac{a}{2}}{(k - k_n)\frac{a}{2}} \right] \left[\frac{\sin(\omega - \omega_n)\frac{T}{2}}{(\omega - \omega_n)\frac{T}{2}} \right] \qquad (12.19)$$

where $T = 2$ seconds is the epoch length and $a \sim 20$ cm is the length of the electrode array. There are about 20 cycles in the time epoch, but approximately only one cycle in the spatial domain, so we can approximate (12.19) by

$$\varepsilon_n(k, \omega) \sim \left[\frac{\sin(k - k_n)\frac{a}{2}}{(k - k_n)\frac{a}{2}}\right] \delta(\omega - \omega_n) \tag{12.20}$$

We cannot make the analogous approximation for the factor involving wave number because of the short electrode array length compared with the dominant spatial wavelengths in the signal. In the experiment described here, fast-Fourier transforms yield estimates of the spectral density function at discrete frequencies and wave numbers expressed by

$$\begin{aligned} \omega &= \omega_i = \frac{2\pi i}{T} \qquad i = 0, I \\ k &= k_j = \frac{2\pi j}{a} \qquad j = 0, 1, 2, 3 \end{aligned} \tag{12.21}$$

where the maximum frequency $\omega_I \sim \pi\Delta t$ and wave number $k_3 \sim \pi\Delta x$ in the estimate are determined by the temporal sampling interval $\Delta t = 128$ second^{-1} and center-to center electrode spacing $\Delta x \sim 2$ to 3 cm, respectively.

The results of this experimental study are summarized in Table 12-1. Thirteen experiments involved eight subjects (indicated by the letter in the first column), with some persons tested on several different days. The frequency peak in the spectral density function was determined from artifact-edited records of several minutes duration. It was also postulated that the "alpha rhythm" might be composed of several different waves n with nearly identical frequencies, as indicated, for example, by (12.5). Frequency-wave number spectra were obtained from the data for frequencies just below and just above the peak frequency. By comparison of these spectra with (12.20) it was determined that the experimental spectra in the alpha band are consistent with dominant waves of spatial wavelength somewhat longer than one half the electrode array length plus additional acivity at shorter wavelengths. Crude estimates of dominant wavelengths (and corresponding phase velocities) were obtained by matching either the ratio of $j = 0$ to $j = 1$ power (estimate 1) or just the $j = 0$ power (estimate 2) to (12.20). (Spectral power is expressed as a percentage of total power in the $j = 0, 1, 2,$ and 3 wave number bands obtained from the fast-Fourier transform.)

All experiments of this study showed apparent shifts of power in the wave number spectrum from $j = 0$ to $j = 1$ as the frequency increased across the alpha band. That is, higher alpha frequencies corresponded to higher wave numbers (shorter wavelengths) as expected if a dispersion relation $\omega = \omega(k)$ across part of the alpha band exists. This result is not anticipated by nonwave theories of EEG, for example, by models consisting of multiple, independent sources. This shift in the spectrum did not occur with jaw muscle artifact or when electrode arrays were

Table 12-1.

	Experimental EEG Data							Theoretical Estimates			
				% Power in the Wave, j =				"Long" Wave Length (cm)		Phase Velocity (cm/sec)	
Record	Array Length (cm)	Peak Alpha Frequency	Frequency Range (Hz)	0	1	2	3	1	2	1	2
K1	21.0	10.5	09.0–10.0	24	42	21	13	13.40	12.90	140	134
			11.0–12.0	19	44	23	14	13.10	12.60		
K2	21.0	11.0	09.5–10.5	28	38	21	13	13.65	13.10	149	143
			11.5–12.5	24	39	23	15	13.45	12.90		
K3	17.5	11.0	09.5–10.5	34	37	16	13	11.60	11.15	126	121
			11.5–12.5	26	41	17	15	11.25	10.80		
M1	17.5	11.5	10.0–11.0	24	40	23	13	11.20	10.75	127	122
			12.0–13.0	20	41	23	16	11.00	10.55		
M2	17.5	10.5	09.0–10.0	23	39	22	14	11.20	10.70	117	112
			11.0–12.0	20	44	21	13	10.95	10.55		
M3	21.0	10.5	09.0–10.0	27	40	22	10	13.55	13.05	140	135
			11.0–12.0	20	50	21	9	13.00	12.65		
J	17.5	09.8	08.0–09.0	40	30	17	13	11.95	11.40	114	109
			10.0–11.0	27	38	22	13	11.35	10.85		
V	17.5	09.5	08.0–09.0	43	33	16	10	11.95	11.55	114	109
			10.5–11.5	41	31	18	9	11.90	11.45		
G	21.0	09.3	07.5–08.5	33	33	20	14	14.00	13.35	129	123
			10.0–11.0	30	35	21	14	13.80	13.20		
H	19.3	11.5	10.0–11.0	41	33	14	12	13.05	12.60	146	141
			12.0–13.0	28	44	14	14	12.35	12.00		
F1	19.3	09.8	08.0–09.0	32	41	18	9	12.55	12.20	120	117
			10.5–11.5	24	47	21	8	12.15	11.80		
P1	17.5	10.5	09.0–10.0	33	35	21	12	11.60	11.10	118	114
			11.0–12.0	20	49	20	11	10.85	10.55		
P2	07.0	11.0	09.5–10.5	61	17	11	11	No estimate due to short array length			
			11.5–12.5	49	24	15	12				
Average		10.5		32	37	19	12	12.10	11.85	126	122
P2 excluded				25	42	20	13	11.75	11.45		

Estimate 1: Match ratio of j = 0 to j = 1 power to Equation (12.20).
Estimate 2: Match j = 0 power.

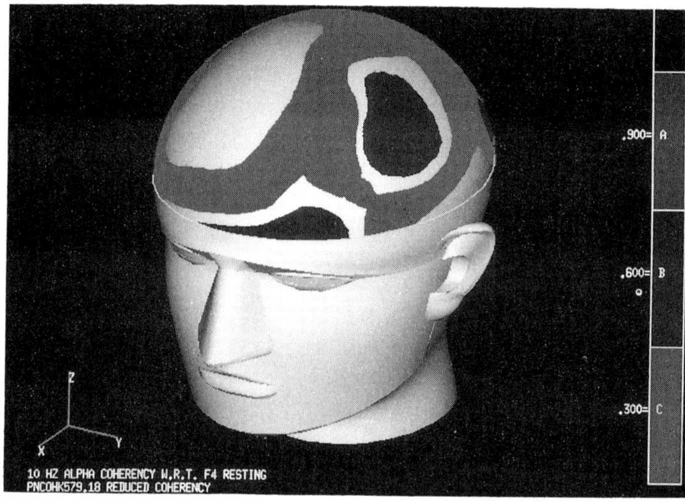
.900= A
.600= B
.300= C
Z
X
Y
10 HZ ALPHA COHERENCY W.R.T. F4 RESTING
PNCOHK579,18 REDUCED COHERENCY

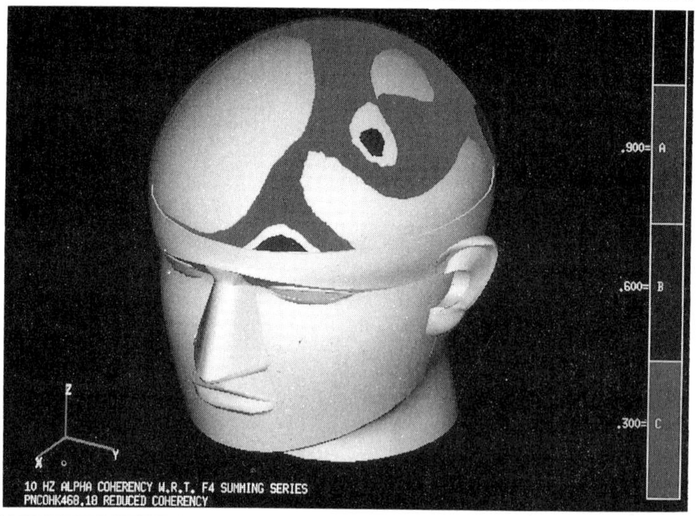
.900= A
.600= B
.300= C
Z
X
Y
10 HZ ALPHA COHERENCY W.R.T. F4 SUMMING SERIES
PNCOHK468,18 REDUCED COHERENCY

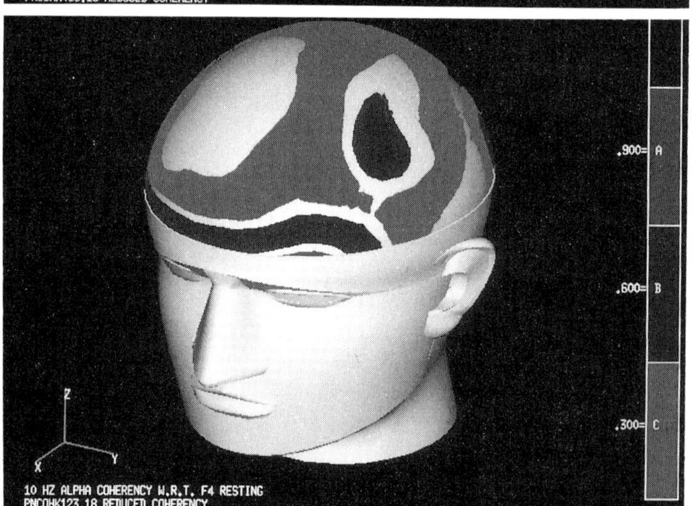
.900= A
.600= B
.300= C
Z
X
Y
10 HZ ALPHA COHERENCY W.R.T. F4 RESTING
PNCOHK123,18 REDUCED COHERENCY

placed laterally across the midline, possibly because such arrays cover waves traveling in opposing directions in separate hemispheres.

One way to estimate group velocity from the data is based on the fractional changes in phase velocity with corresponding frequency changes (12.10). From Table 12-1, we obtain the following crude estimates based on data averaged over 12 experiments: $(\Delta v_p/v_p) \sim 22/128 \sim 0.17$ (independent of correction for surface folding) and $(\omega/\Delta\omega) \sim 10/2 = 5$. Phase velocity estimates apply to a broad range of wave numbers and cannot be regarded too seriously. Also, (12.10) is sensitive to small errors in these estimates in this range. In any case, (12.10) yields

$$v_G \sim 7v_p \qquad (12.22)$$

The exact values of these estimates are not reliable. However, we note the following. (1) All 13 experiments resulted in a negative shift of wavelength with a positive frequency change Δf. That is, all individual group velocity estimates are positive, suggesting the possible existence of a nonanomalous dispersion relation for alpha rhythm in the narrow 2-Hz band width centered at the peak frequency. Data presented in Chapter 2 suggests the existence of a dispersion relation over a broad band (>10 Hz) above the alpha peak frequency. (2) Group velocities are apparently larger than phase velocities as predicted by the theory of Chapter 11, as indicated previously in this chapter.

Coherent Spatial Structures of EEG

Data presented in this book suggest that patterns of coherency in spontaneous EEG (Chapter 3), patterns of covariance in transient evoked potentials (Chapter 7), and patterns of magnitude and phase in steady-state visual evoked potentials (Chapter 6) change in regular and reproducible ways when specific cognitive tasks are performed. Distinct, coherent spatial structures are associated with different mental states because of the involvement of changing functional "networks" of neural tissue distributed throughout the brain.

An example of EEG coherency as a function of scalp location and cognitive state is illustrated in Figures 12-23 and 12-24. Because of the confounding effects of volume conduction on coherency estimates (discussed in Chapter 3), we define "reduced coherency" as the portion of coherency that cannot be accounted for by volume conduction. That is, Figure 3-10 provides an estimate of coherency versus

←

Figure 12-23. Reduced coherency (at 10 Hz) of the right frontal region (F4) with respect to other scalp locations for 3 minutes of resting (upper), 3 minutes of mental task (summing a series, middle), and 3 minutes of resting (lower). Similar to data presented in Figure 3-24, with 1-minute states combined (that is 1, 2, 3; 4, 6, 8, and 5, 7, 9), except for the use of "reduced coherency" (that which cannot be explained by volume conduction). No estimates are obtained near F4 because reduced coherency cannot be obtained between close locations. Frontal-to-frontal coherencies consistently decrease during the mental task. Subject PLN.

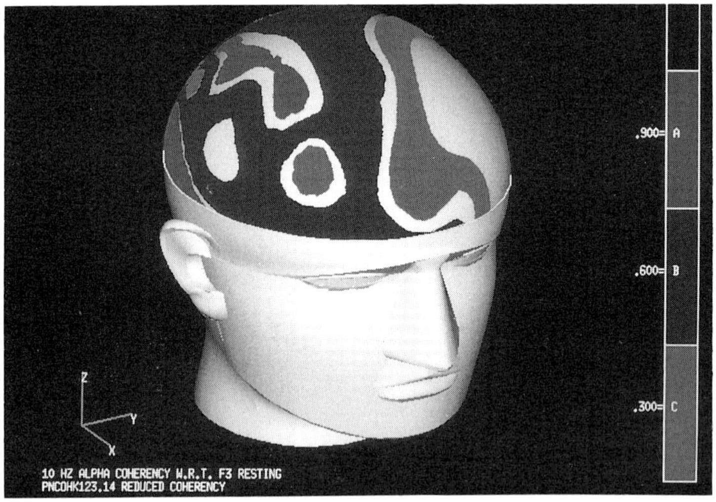
.900= A
.600= B
.300= C
Z
Y
X
10 HZ ALPHA COHERENCY W.R.T. F3 RESTING
PNCOHK123.14 REDUCED COHERENCY

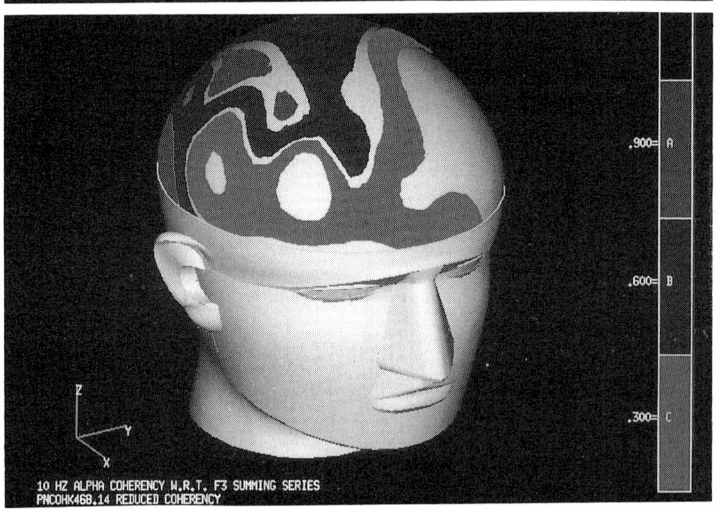
.900= A
.600= B
.300= C
Z
Y
X
10 HZ ALPHA COHERENCY W.R.T. F3 SUMMING SERIES
PNCOHK468.14 REDUCED COHERENCY

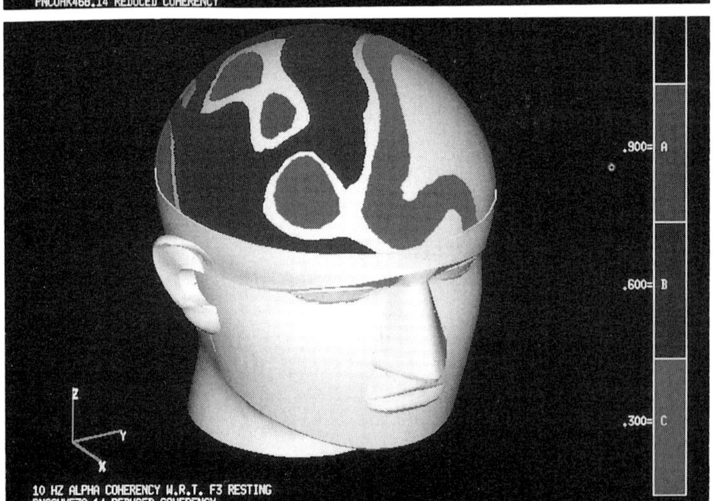
.900= A
.600= B
.300= C
Z
Y
X
10 HZ ALPHA COHERENCY W.R.T. F3 RESTING
PNCOHK579.14 REDUCED COHERENCY

scalp electrode separation distance when the underlying neocortical sources are entirely incoherent (the "random coherency"). We define reduced coherency as the measured coherency (neck reference) less the random coherency obtained from Figure 3-10 (upper left), with the constraint that negative reduced coherency values are set to zero. With this definition, we can only estimate reduced coherency at distances greater than about 5 to 7 cm because volume conduction and source coherency cannot be distinguished at short distances with scalp recordings.

Reduced coherency (10-Hz alpha rhythm) between right frontal cortex (F4) and the other 63 scalp locations is plotted in Figure 12-23. Three states are shown (3 minutes each): resting, summing a series, resting (see Chapter 3 for task and recording details). Reduced coherency between left frontal cortex (F3) and the other 63 scalp locations is shown in Figure 12-24. These data suggest the following. (1) Coherency between distant cortical source regions (such as those greater than 10 cm) in the eyes-closed resting alpha rhythm can often be 0.5 or higher. Although the (neck) reference electrode may contribute erroneously, the bipolar and Laplacian data presented in Chapter 3 suggest that this general conclusion is justified. (2) Many frontal-to-frontal coherencies decrease substantially during the cognitive task. However, other coherencies may remain fixed or increase.

Another indication of the standing wave nature of EEG is that of coherency patterns as a function of interelectrode distance for the steady-state visual evoked potential shown in Figure 12-25. The plot in the upper left is obtained for spontaneous EEG with eyes open for comparative purposes. This coherency distribution is somewhat similar to that obtained in simulated data for random neocortical sources, shown in the upper left of Figure 3-10. In contrast, the ($64 \times 63/2 = 2016$) coherency estimates for driving frequencies of 9, 10, and 13 Hz are much higher. Coherency estimates for driving at 11 and 12 Hz are generally low. This is strong evidence for global dynamic behavior that is sensitive to driving frequency, consistent with resonant global modes.

Potential and Laplacian magnitude and phase maps produced by steady-state visual evoked potentials at driving frequencies 9 through 12 Hz are shown in Figures 12-26 through 12-29. These are the same data shown at these frequencies in the coherency plots of Figure 12-25. Phase patterns are seen to change for small changes in the driving frequency, suggesting that phases are not fixed by cortical anatomy such as fissures and sulci. These are preliminary data, but similar pattern changes were observed in several subjects. Additional work to quantify pattern changes with frequency and changes over time in different frequency bandwidths is planned by the Melbourne and New Orleans groups.

←

Figure 12-24. Reduced coherency (at 10 Hz) of the left frontal region (F3) with respect to other scalp locations. Same data and methods shown in Figure 12-23. These data were recorded at the Swinburne Centre for Applied Neuroscience in Melbourne and analyzed at Tulane University in New Orleans, Louisiana.

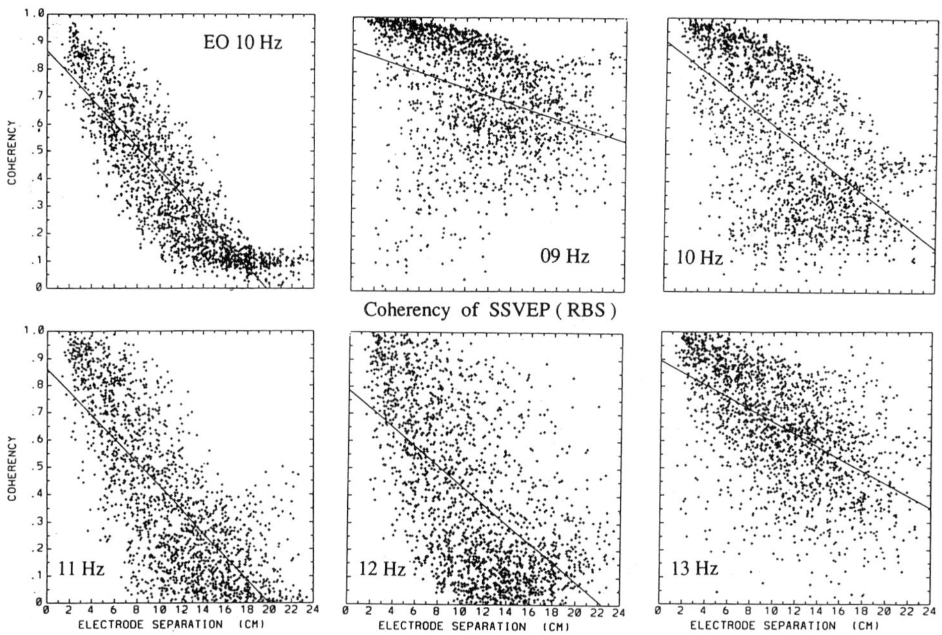

Figure 12-25. Coherency is plotted as a function of distance between 2016 electrode pairs in 64-channel recordings. All coherency estimates are based on 2336 cycles of either the 10-Hz spontaneous EEG (eyes open, upper left) or 2336 cycles of the steady-state visual evoked potential (see Chapters 3 and 6 for details). By contrast to eyes open data, eyes closed spontaneous EEG (alpha rhythm) yields high coherencies (similar to the 13 Hz plot), not shown. Subject RBS.

Spatial Principal Components of EEG

Another way to represent spatial properties is to calculate empirical orthogonal functions from the data. This approach is typically called the Karhunen-Loéve expansion by physical scientists and principal components analysis (PCA) by biological scientists. Since we have been interested in evidence for standing waves in EEG, a temporal frequency approach to spatial PCA was adopted in earlier studies of EEG (Nunez, 1981a, 1981b). That is, the EEG was assumed to be distributed over a sphere that approximates a subject's head. The EEG was represented by the following series of orthogonal functions.

$$\mathrm{EEG}(\theta, \phi, t) = \sum_{n=0}^{N} \sum_{j=1}^{J} A_{nj} Z_{nj}(\theta, \phi) e^{j\omega_n t} \qquad (12.23)$$

Here the $Z_{nj}(\theta, \phi)$ are the empirical orthogonal functions on a sphere (spatial principal components) corresponding to the nth temporal frequency component of the EEG. That is, each frequency component in an EEG record has its own spatial properties, given by $Z_{nj}(\theta, \phi)$. The subscript j refers to a particular or-

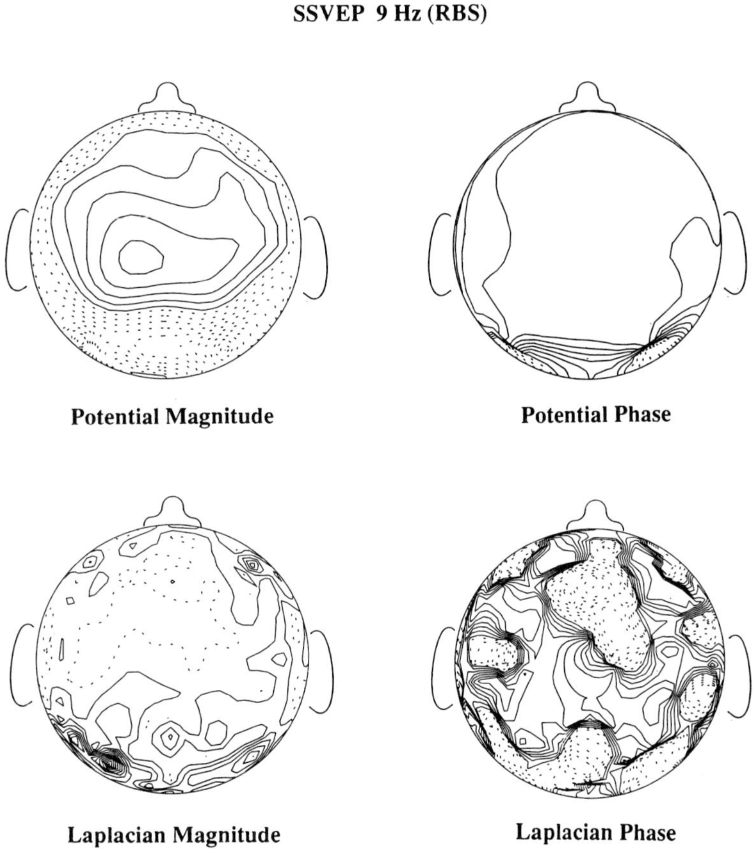

Figure 12-26. Magnitude and phase maps for the steady-state visual evoked potential (SSVEP, 9 Hz). Frequency resolution is 0.004 Hz. Above average magnitudes are solid lines, below average magnitudes are dashed lines. Contour intervals are 0.1 microvolts for the potential magitude and 0.67 microvolts per square centimeter for the Laplacian magnitude. Cosine phase contours are 0.15 for both potential and Laplacian plots. Local maxima in the potential magnitude near visual cortex cannot be seen in this plot since these peaks are too low on the surface displayed. Data recorded in Melbourne. Subject RBS.

thogonal function in a set of J functions, where J is also the number of EEG channels. The orthogonal functions may be placed in decreasing order of significance as determined by the series coefficients (or weighting constants) A_{nj}. This approach will be most useful when most of the orthogonal functions are negligible, that is, when most of the coefficients A_{nj} for $j > 1$ are much smaller than A_{n1}. The orthogonal functions Z_{nj} are analogous to the orthogonal functions $\sin(k_{xn}x)\sin(k_{ym}y)$, where the single subscript j takes the place of the subscripts n and m, denoting different wave numbers. However, the functions Z_{nj} are defined only at the discrete scalp locations of the electrodes (θ_j, ϕ_j), $j = 1, J$. The functions Z_{nj} are the eigenvectors of the complex covariance matrix formed by a multichannel

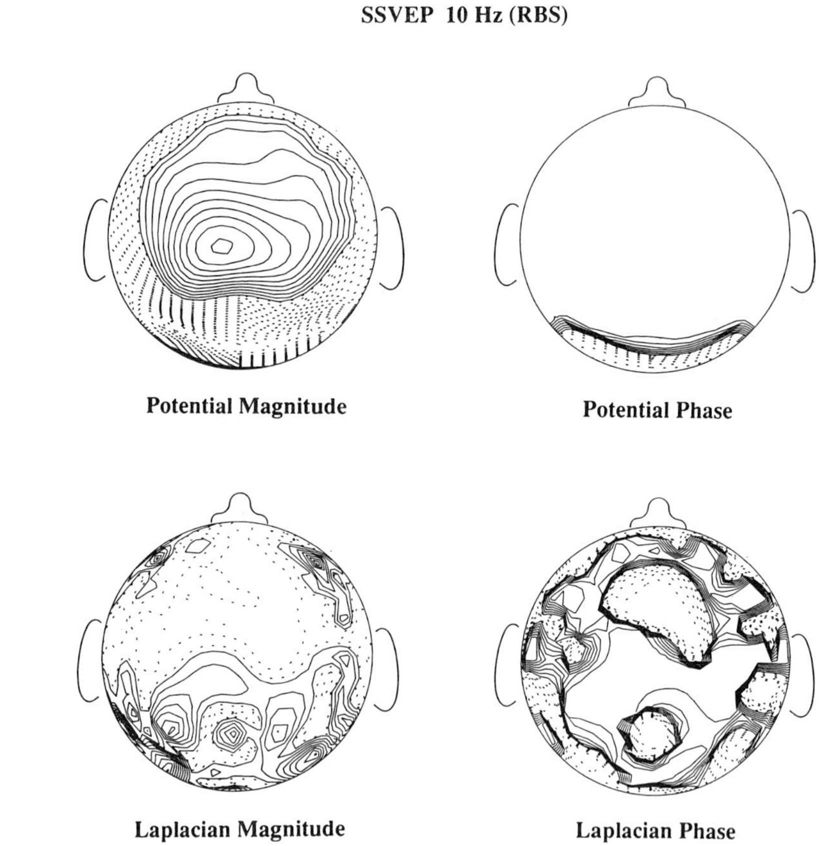

Figure 12-27. Contour intervals are identical to plots in Figure 12-26. SSVEP frequency is 10 Hz.

data set and the squared coefficients A^2_{nj} are the corresponding eigenvalues. The principal components Z_{nj} and the corresponding coefficients A_{nj} have the following properties:

1. The Z_{nj} provide the most efficient method of compressing the spatial data. These orthogonal functions are complex since they contain phase information.
2. The Z_{nj} may be regarded as uncorrelated modes of variability of the potential.
3. The A^2_{nj} are the portions of the overall variance associated with the corresponding eigenvector (or orthogonal function), Z_{nj}. The A_{nj} are real.

The spatial principal components for a 71 second period of alpha rhythm are plotted in Figures 12-30 through 12-34, corresponding to frequencies 8 Hz through 12 Hz. These data were selected from a 180 second period in order to eliminate all artifact. Suspected artifact occurred over short periods in 2 channels of the 64 channel data. These channels were eliminated so that all plots are based on the

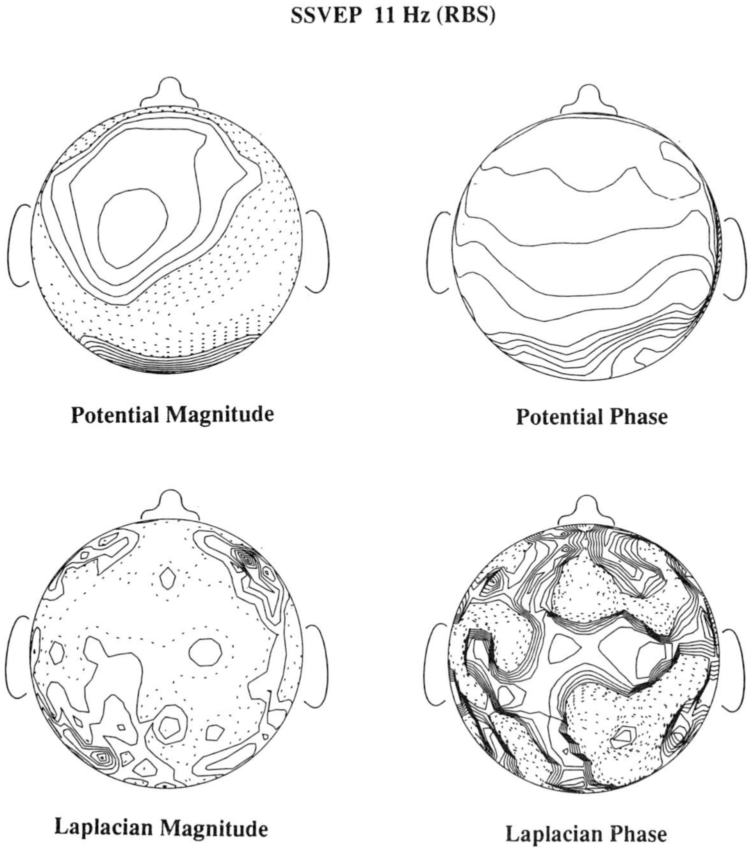

Figure 12-28. Identical to Figure 12-26 except SSVEP frequency is 11 Hz. Magnitude and phase changes as SSVEP changes from 10 Hz to 11 Hz parallel coherency changes between these frequencies as shown in Figure 12-25.

remaining 62 channels. Fourier transforms of 1-second epochs from each data channel were obtained and complex covariance matrices for each frequency calculated as described in Nunez (1981a, 1981b). This procedure was applied to the unprocessed potential data which is spatially low-pass filtered by the head volume conductor. The potential-based principal components are shown in the first columns of Figures 12-30 through 12-34. The same procedure was applied to data passed first through the spline-Laplacian algorithm which provides a spatial band-pass filter of the data which complements the unprocessed potential data. The Laplacian-based principal components are shown in the second columns of Figures 12-30 through 12-34.

Some results of this preliminary PCA study are:

1. A substantial portion of the overall variances are associated with the first few eigenvectors (Z_{nj} or principal components). For example, the eigenvalue

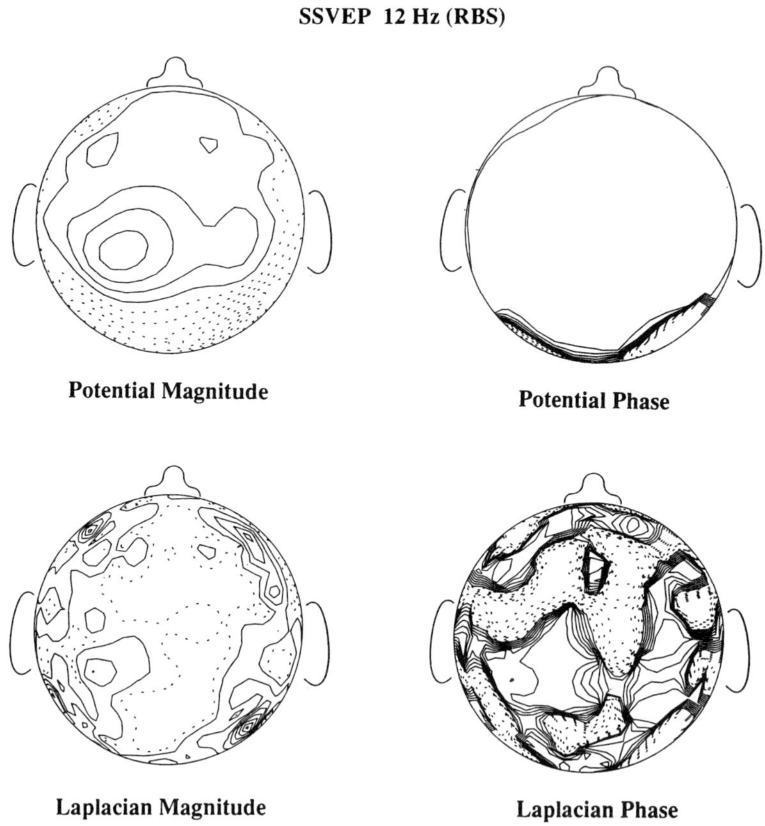

Figure 12-29. Identical to Figure 12-26 except SSVEP frequency is 12 Hz.

A^2_{n1} based on spatially incoherent noise averaged over more than 30 epochs is approximately 1/62 or 1.6% (Nunez 1981a). By contrast, the A^2_{n1} obtained from the alpha potential and Laplacian data range from 19% to 59%.

2. The neck reference potential data (which was spatially low-pass filtered by the head volume conductor) shows large changes in the spatial structure of the first principal component Z_{n1} through the alpha band ($n = 8$ through 12). By contrast, the spline-Laplacian maps of Z_{n1} (for which the lowest spatial frequencies make minimal contribution) are relatively constant over the alpha band. These data are consistent with Table 12-1 which suggests that the alpha band is composed of more than one mode.

3. The first principal component of the 9 Hz potential data (Figure 12-31) looks like the mode $\ell = 2$ of a standing wave (see Figure 12-13). This is the closest component to the peak power in the spectrum which is a little higher than 9 Hz (Peak frequencies typically drift over ± 0.25 Hz).

4. The Laplacian Z_{n1} maps are more like the $\ell = 4$ through 7 modes shown in Figures 12-14 and 12-15. One may conjecture that they represent standing waves with higher modes, local circuits, regional circuits (discussed in Chapter 13), or some combination.

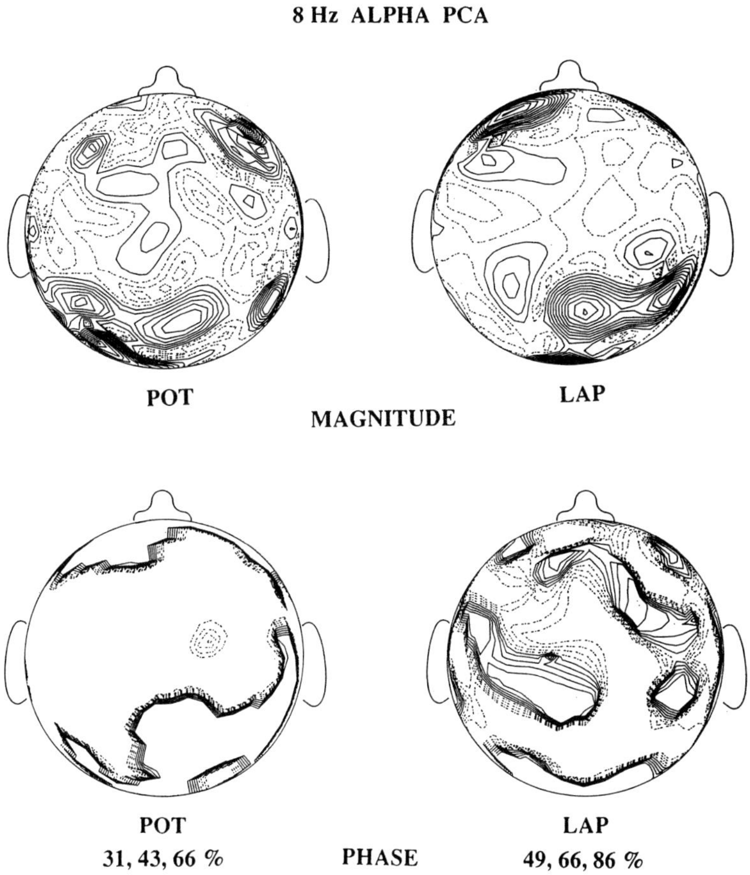

Figure 12-30. First spatial principal component $Z_{8,1}$ (empirical orthogonal function) of the 8 Hz frequency component for 71 seconds of resting alpha rhythm. The first column contains magnitude and phase plots of the first component associated with unprocessed scalp potential. The second column is the first component associated with the spline-Laplacian. The three numbers at the bottom of each column indicate the percentage of variance accounted for by the first spatial principal component, the first 2 principal components, and the first 5 principal components. Subject PLN.

These PCA data do not provide definitive answers to the underlying dynamics of EEG. Rather they suggest new approaches to further study, discussed in the next section.

Synergetic Studies of EEG Data

A theory of neocortical dynamic function was derived from known anatomic and physiologic data in Chapter 11. Synaptic action modulation $H(\mathbf{r}, t)$ (and EEG by

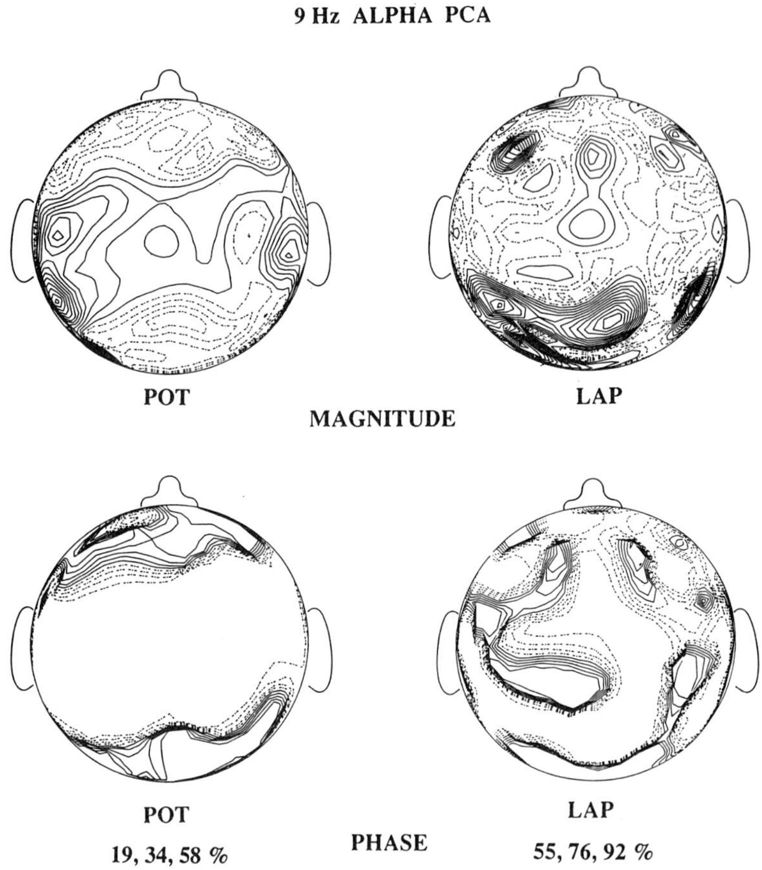

Figure 12-31. Identical to Figure 12-30 except that principal components $Z_{9,1}$ are the 9 Hz Fourier components.

implication) was represented in series of coherent spatial modes of the general form

$$H(\mathbf{r}, t) = \sum_k H_k(t) Z_k(\mathbf{r}) \tag{12.24}$$

The spatial functions Z_k of the surface coordinate **r** might be sinusoidal functions (one-dimensional global theory), spherical harmonics (two-dimensional global theory as in [11.42]), or empirical orthogonal functions. The functions $H_k(t)$, called order parameters in the parlance of dynamical systems theory, are the solutions of ordinary differential equations (generally nonlinear) such as (11.39). Chapter 12 has outlined connections between this physiologically based theory and EEG data.

A separate but complementary approach was recently initiated by the Institute for Theoretical Physics and Synergetics in Stuttgart, Germany. These studies used

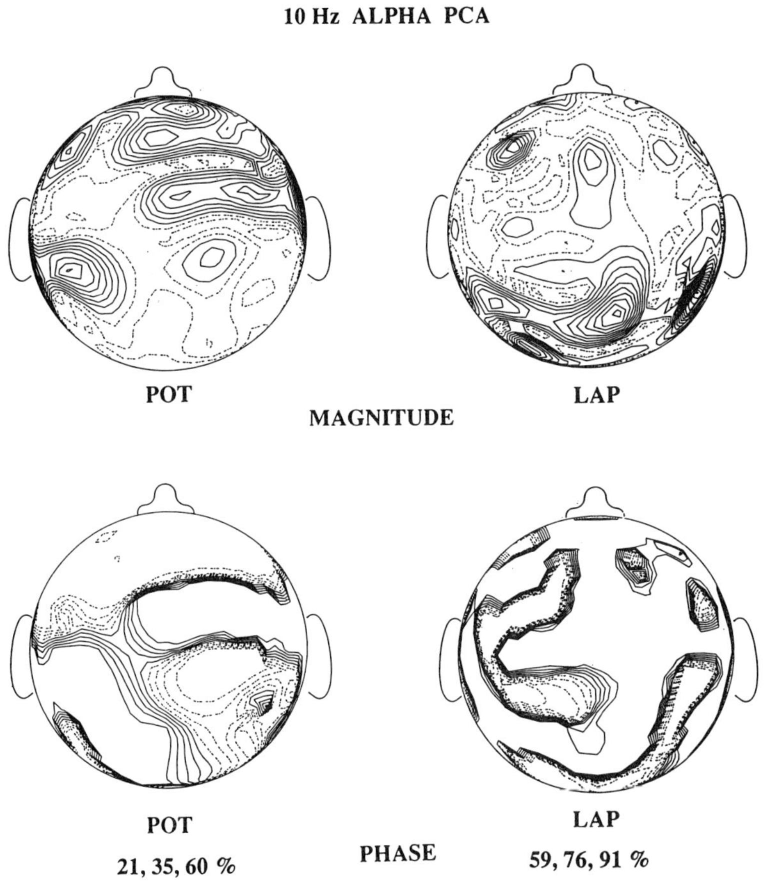

Figure 12-32. Identical to Figure 12-30 except $Z_{10,1}$ are the 10 Hz components.

EEG data recorded by D. Lehmann at University Hospital, Zurich, Switzerland (Friedrich et al, 1991; Friedrich and Uhl, 1992) and MEG data recorded at the Center for Complex Systems at Florida Atlantic University in Boca Raton (Fuchs et al, 1992; Jirsa et al, 1994). Data were described by a few spatially coherent modes as in (12.24). The dynamic behavior was determined by the order parameters $H_k(t)$. Changes of physiologic state (phase changes in the parlance of dynamical system theory) were quantified by order parameter changes.

Preliminary results of these studies are apparently consistent with the theoretical predictions of Chapter 11. For example, both alpha rhythm and seizure data exhibited coherent spatial structures in the EEG that showed complex temporal evolution (Friedrich et al, 1991). The basis functions $Z_k(\mathbf{r})$ for alpha rhythm were interpreted as the spherical harmonics $Y_{\ell m}(\theta, \phi)$ with $\ell = 2$ and different m values. A mixture of standing and "rotating" waves described the scalp recorded data. A covergence of physiologically based theory with such experimentally based

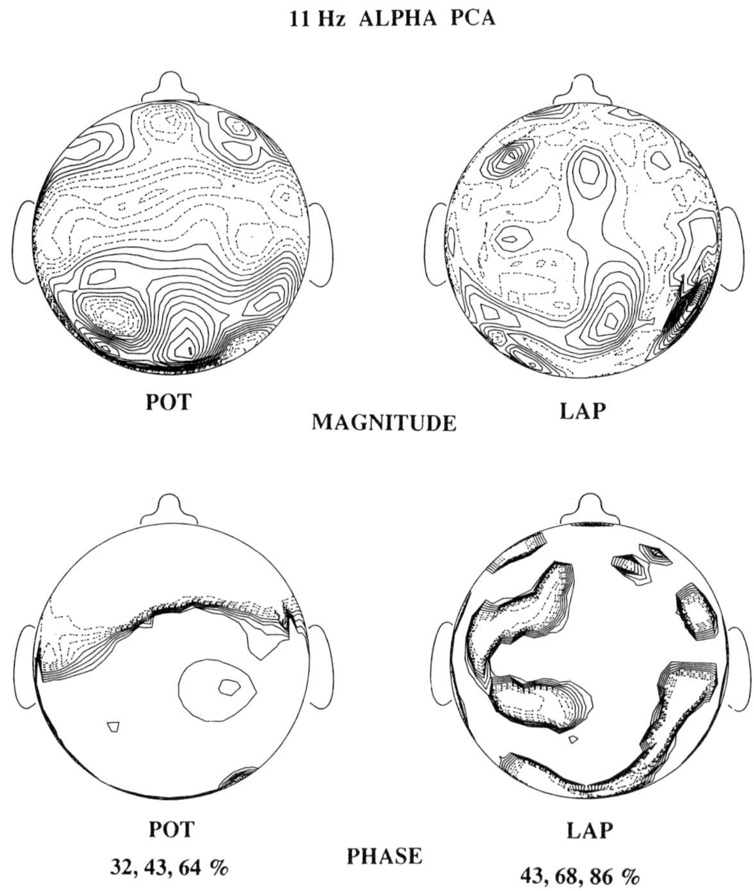

Figure 12-33. Identical to Figure 12-30 except $Z_{11,1}$ are the 11 Hz components.

synergetic studies is now required. Additional studies in the field of nonlinear neocortical dynamics are described in Chapter 14.

EEG Recorded from the Cortical Surface

We conclude this chapter with a discussion of the classic studies of epilepsy patients by Penfield (a neurosurgeon) and Jasper (an electroencephalographer) in the context of EEG standing waves. Penfield is famous for his studies of patient response to electrical stimulation of the cortical surface, a procedure required prior to surgery. During these procedures, EEG was recorded from different locations in many patients so that recordings from the entire upper surface of the cortex were apparently obtained in the patient population. These results are summarized in Figure 12-35 which shows that alpha rhythm was recorded from almost the entire

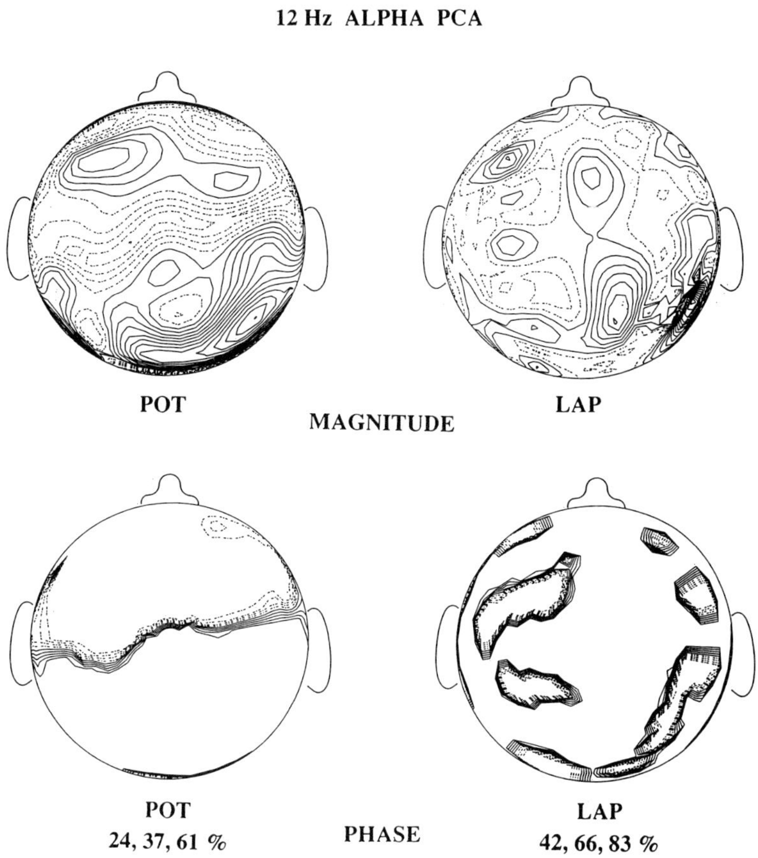

Figure 12-34. Identical to Figure 12-30 except $Z_{12,1}$ are the 12 Hz components.

ventral surface. The regions for which no alpha rhythm was reported are mainly along the central motor strip where beta rhythms were recorded. In order to evaluate these data in a modern theoretical context, we note the following:

1. These studies were performed before spectral analysis became an EEG tool. Thus the categories "alpha" and "beta" were assigned by counting zero crossings of the waveforms, a procedure still commonly used in EEG. This approach often results in broad band EEG or EEG composed of narrow band alpha and broad band beta (as determined by spectral analysis) being classified as "beta rhythm."
2. Production of widely distributed alpha rhythm in the awake state normally requires a healthy relaxed experimental subject. Penfield's patients had their EEG's recorded while on the operating table with portions of their skulls removed prior to brain surgery. Such conditions are not well-suited for alpha rhythm production.

If synaptic action in the neocortex is modulated in the 10 Hz range and a nodal

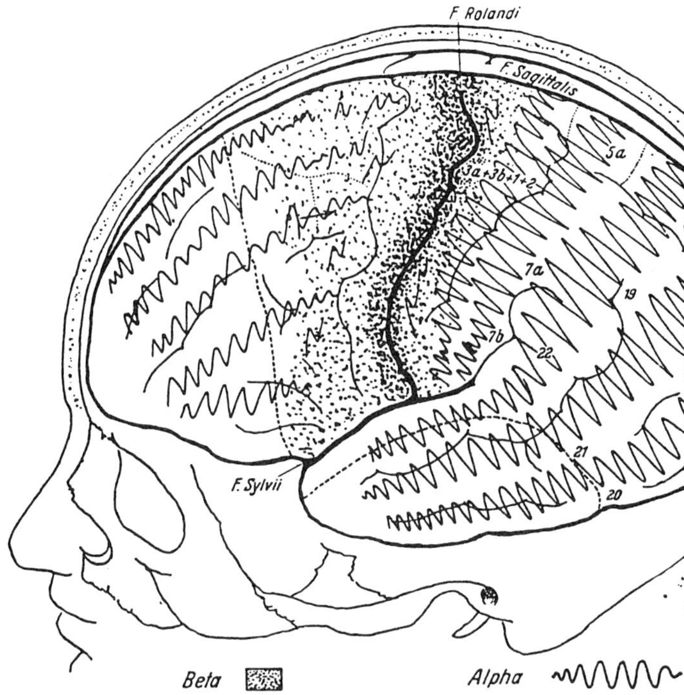

Figure 12-35. Diagram of areas in which alpha rhythm was recorded from the cortical surface in epilepsy surgery patients (wavy lines). Dotted area indicates locations of beta recording. Alpha and beta were defined by zero crossings of time records; that is, these data were not Fourier transformed. (Reproduced with permission from Jasper and Penfield, 1949.)

line lies along the motor strip, the amplitude distribution of a pure standing wave would be similar to that shown in Figure 12-35. (Possible facilitation of this nodal line by neuromodulators is discussed in Chapter 13.) However, we might expect anterior and posterior magnitudes to be more equal than shown in this figure. This apparent discrepancy can perhaps be explained by a cortex with inhomogeneous damping, a cortex in which both local and global processes contribute to alpha rhythm, or both. For example, a global 10 Hz modulation of synaptic action may exist, but for this standing wave of synaptic action to be recorded as EEG, perhaps local (Q) and global (B) control parameters must be in ranges that produce synaptic modulation of sufficient magnitude. A similar argument may apply to other frequency bands which have different nodal lines and different responses to Q and B, as suggested in Chapter 11.

Chapter 11 outlined a theoretical framework for the spatial-temporal structures of EEG that may consist of different mixtures of standing waves, local circuits, and regional circuits which vary in location and relative importance with brain state. In this chapter we presented a variety of EEG data which appear to fit this framework naturally. Chapter 13 presents data from neuropharmacology and neuroanatomy which is also consistent with this theoretical framework.

References

Bendat, J.S. and Piersol, A.G. *Random Data: Analysis and Measurement Procedures.* Second ed. New York: Wiley, 1986.

Bickford, R.G. *Clinical Electroencephalography.* New York: Medcom, 1973.

Blinkov, S.M. and Glezer I.I. *The Human Brain in Figures and Tables.* New York: Plenum Press, 1968.

Courchesne, E. Chronology of postnatal human brain development: Event-related potential, positron emission tomography, myelinogenesis, and synaptogenesis studies. In: *Event-Related Potentials of the Brain.* (J. W. Rohrbaugh, Parasuraman, R., and Johnson, R., Eds.) New York: Oxford University Press, pp. 210–241, 1990.

Friedrich, R., Fuchs, A., and Haken, H. Spatio-temporal EEG patterns. In: *Rhythms in Physiological Systems.* (H. Haken and Koepchen H.P., Eds.) Berlin, Springer-Verlag, pp. 315–338, 1991.

Friedrich, R. and Uhl, C. Synergetic analysis of human electroencephalograms: petit-mal epilepsy. In: *Evolution of Dynamical Structures in Complex Systems.* (R. Friedrich and Wunderlin, A., Eds.) Berlin, Springer-Verlag, pp. 249–265, 1992.

Fuchs, A., Kelso, J.A.S., and Haken, H. Phase transitions in the human brain: spatial mode dynamics. *International Journal of Bifurcation and Chaos.* 2:917–939, 1992.

Hayes, R. and Katznelson, R.D. Unpublished data, 1979.

Hughes, J.R., Kuruvilla, A., and Fino, J.J. Topographic analysis of visually evoked potentials from flash and pattern reversal stimuli: Evidence for "travelling waves," *Brain Topography.* 4:215–228, 1992.

Jasper, H.D. and Penfield, W. Electrocorticograms in man: Effect of voluntary movement upon the electrical activity of the precentral gyrus. *Archiv. Für Psychiatrie und Zeitschrift Neurologie* 183:163–174, 1949.

Jirsa, V.K., Friedrich, R., Haken, H., and Kelso, J.A.S. A theoretical model of phase transitions in the human brain. *Biological Cybernetics.* 71:27–35, 1994.

Johnson, L., Lubin, A., Naitoh, P., Nute, C., and Austin, A. Spectral analysis of the EEG of dominant and non-dominant alpha subjects during waking and sleeping. *Electroencephalogr. Clin. Neurophysiol.* 26:361–370, 1969.

Katznelson, R.D. Deterministic and stochastic field theoretic models in the neurophysics of EEG. Ph.D. Dissertation, San Diego, CA: University of California at San Diego, 1982.

Katznelson, R.D. Normal modes of the brain: neuroanatomical basis and a physiological theoretical model. In: *Electric Fields of the Brain: The Neurophysics of EEG.* (P. L. Nunez, Author) New York: Oxford University Press, 1981.

Nunez, P.L. The brain wave equation: A model for the EEG, American EEG Society Meeting, Houston, Texas, 1972.

Nunez, P.L. The brain wave equation: A model for the EEG. *Mathematical Biosciences* 21:279–297, 1974a.

Nunez, P.L. Wave-like properties of the alpha rhythm, *IEEE Trans. Biomed. Eng.* 21:473–482, 1974b.

Nunez, P.L. *Electric Fields of the Brain: The Neurophysics of EEG*. New York: Oxford University Press, 1981a.

Nunez, P.L. A study of the origins of the time dependencies of scalp EEG. II Experimental support of theory. *IEEE Trans. Biomed. Eng.* 28:281–288, 1981b.

Nunez, P.L., Stockard, J.J, and Smith, N.T., unpublished data, 1976.

Nunez, P.L., Reid, L., and Bickford, R.G. The relationship of head size to alpha frequency with implications to a brain wave model. *Electroencephalogr. Clin. Neurophysiol.* 44:344–352, 1978.

Nunez, P.L., Silberstein, R.B., Cadusch, P.J., Wijesinghe, R., Westdorp, A.F., and Srinivasan, R. A theoretical and experimental study of high resolution EEG based on surface Laplacians and cortical imaging. *Electroencephalogr. Clin. Neurophysiol.* 90:40–57, 1994.

Nunez, P.L. and Srinivasan, R.A. Implications of recording strategy for estimates of neocortical dynamics with EEG. *Chaos: An Interdisciplinary Journal of Nonlinear Science* 3:257–266, 1993.

Pain, H.J. *The Physics of Vibrations and Waves*. New York: Wiley, 1978.

Penfield, W. and Jasper, H.D. *Epilepsy and the Functional Anatomy of the Human Brain*. London: Little, Brown, and Co., 1954.

Rampil, I.J., Sasse, F.J., Smith, N.T., Hoff, B.H., and Fleming, D.C. Spectral edge frequency—A new correlate of anesthetic depth. *Anesthesiology*. 53:3S12, 1980.

Shimoji, K. and Bickford, R. Differential effects of anesthetics on mesencephalic reticular neurons: I. Spontaneous firing patterns. *Anesthesiology*. 35:68–88, 1971.

Stockard, J.J. and Bickford, R.G. The neurophysiology of anaesthesia. In: *A Basis and Practice of Neuroanaesthesia II*. (E. Gordon, Ed.) Amsterdam: Excerpta Medica, pp. 3–46, 1975.

Thatcher, R.W., Krouse, P.J., and Hrybyk, M. Cortico-cortical associations and EEG coherence: A compartmental model. *Electroencephalogr. Clin. Neurophysiol.* 64:123–143, 1986.

Wilson, H. R. and Cowan, J. D. A mathematical theory of the functional dynamics of cortical and thalmic nervous tissue. *Kybernetik*. 13:55–80, 1973.

Yakovlev, P.I. and Lecours, A.R. The myelogenetic cycles of regional maturation of the brain. In: *Regional Development of the Brain in Early Life*. (A. Minkowski, Ed.) Philadelphia, F.A. Davis, pp. 3–70, 1967.

13

Neuromodulation of Neocortical Dynamics

RICHARD B. SILBERSTEIN

The relation between the electroencephalographic (EEG) and cognitive processes suggests an association between the different EEG-generating mechanisms and higher cortical functions as discussed in Chapter 4. This chapter explores these links in the context of a model that relates brain stem neurotransmitters to local and global EEG-generating mechanisms, reviewing briefly features of neocortical physiology, architecture, and brain stem neurotransmitter systems. Neocortical dynamic states are profoundly influenced by brain stem neurotransmitters that may change the level of corticocortical coupling. Changes in the level of corticocortical and intracortical coupling are a central feature of this "coupling model." In the light of this proposed coupling model, some cognitive and neuropsychiatric implications are considered.

Our understanding of the role and function of brain stem neurotransmitters is still evolving and this model cannot yet incorporate all the reported effects of brain stem neurotransmitters on neocortical dynamics. However, substantial consistencies in some of these experimental data suggests certain speculations about the interrelation of neocortical architecture, neuromodulation, and the genesis of neocortical rhythmic activity. As such, this proposed coupling model should be considered primarily a speculative conceptual framework that stimulates further, theoretically based experimentation.

Neocortical Structures Mediating Global Resonances

A distinctive feature of global EEG theories is the central role of the corticocortical fibers (see Chapters 2 and 11). This fiber system rapidly distributes neural activity and permits the development of traveling and standing waves in the neocortex, as shown in Chapters 6 and 12. In addition to the corticocortical fibers, an extensive network of intracortical fibers comprises the unmyelinated axon collaterals of the pyramidal cells. These collaterals rarely extend beyond 7 mm and conduct at speeds of 0.1 to 0.5 m/second. The role of such intracortical fibers in the generation of local resonances is considered subsequently.

Traveling waves on the closed neocortical surface permit the development of standing waves with particular spatial distribution (eigenstates). Such eigenstates are associated with specific "resonant" frequencies (see Chapters 2, 3, 11, and 12). Thus neocortex may behave like an electrical or mechanical linear filter with a high "gain" at certain resonant frequencies. In this context, the scalp-recorded EEG is a manifestation of neocortical filtering of input originating in the thalamus. Evoked potentials elicited by transient sensory stimuli can be considered the impulse response of such a neocortical resonant system. Such a view is consistent with observations that transient evoked potentials have the same frequency composition as the background EEG (Sayers, 1974; Basar, 1980; Basar et al, 1992).

Before considering the nature of local and global mechanisms, we review some of the neuroanatomy and neurophysiologic features of the neocortex. Although subject to some variability, the neocortex is generally considered a six-layered structure, as shown in Figure 13-1. This is already an oversimplification because the number of layers varies considerably and each of the original six layers have been subdivided into sublayers (Barbas, 1986; Jones, 1985, Pandya and Yeterian, 1985). Layer 1 (the most superficial layer) is frequently described as the most "primitive" layer in the cortex (Vogt, 1991). In primates it is almost completely cell free and consists of the dendrites of cells located in layers 2, 3, and 5; collateral axons from deeper cells; axon terminations originating from layer 6, 3, and 2; axons from other cortical regions of the ipsilateral and contralateral hemispheres; and nonspecific thalamic nuclei (Jones, 1984). The outer part of the primate layer 1 has a high concentration of gamma-aminobutyric acid (GABA) receptors and the GABA synthetic enzyme glutamic acid decarboxylase (GAD), suggesting strong inhibitory modulation of inputs (Houser et al, 1984; Vogt, 1991).

Layers 2 and 3 comprise pyramidal and various classes of nonpyramidal cells. These layers are the "association" layers of the cortex, because the pyramidal cell axons constitute the corticocortical fibers that project exclusively to other cortical regions. Fibers from these layers tend to terminate in layer 4 of the receiving cortex, although there is considerable variability, with some fibers terminating in more superficial layers (Barbas, 1986; Fellerman and Van Essen, 1991; Jones, 1984; Maunsell and Van Essen, 1983). The two major inputs to the pyramidal cells in layers 2 and 3 arise from axonal terminations in layer 1, thalamic inputs to layer 3, and excitatory stellate cells in layer 4 (Mitzdorf, 1985). Inputs from layers 1 and 2 to pyramidal cells are processed by the apical dendritic structures, whereas inputs from layer 4 are processed more by basal dendritic structures. The apical shaft dendrites traversing layers 2 and 3 are often free of dendritic spines, which suggests that two functional dendritic compartments, a basal one conveying information from layers 4 and 3 and a superficial apical one, convey information from layer 1, as shown in Figure 13-2 (Vogt, 1991). The idea that these two dendritic compartments may be functionally independent is strengthened by recent investigations showing the existence of dendritic action potentials

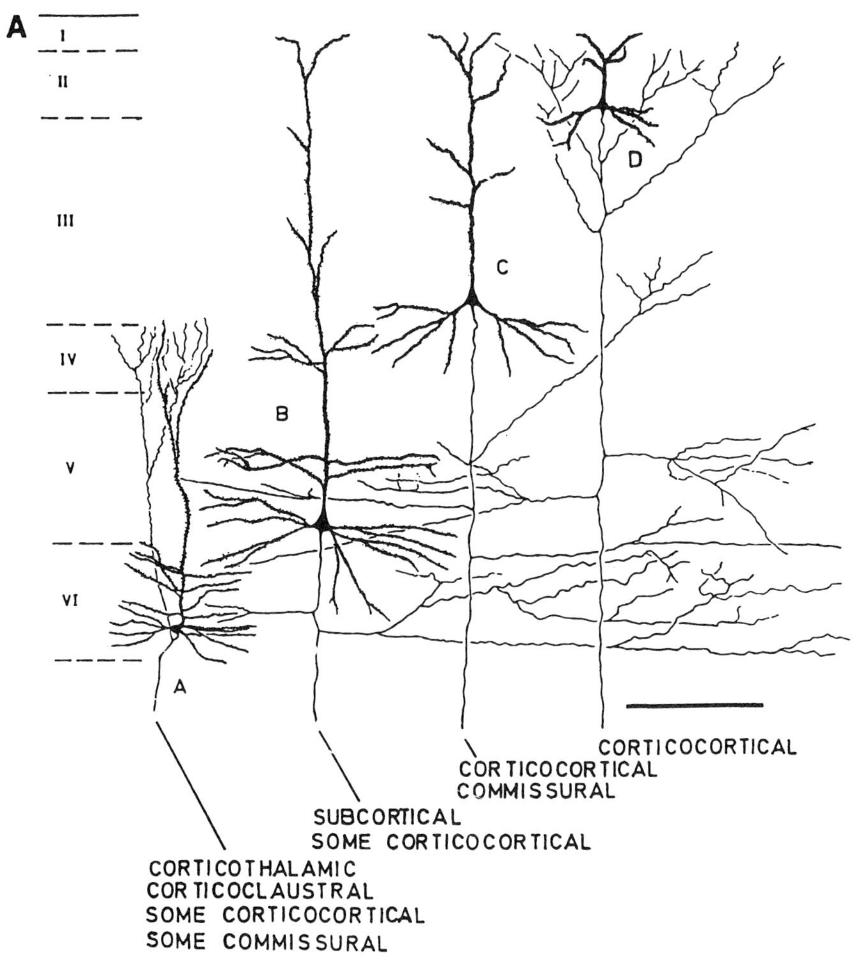

Figure 13-1. Schematic drawing of major targets of pyramidal cells in different layers in monkey motor cortex. Also see Figure 4-2. (From Jones, 1986.)

(Wang et al, 1979; Mitgaard, 1994). This contrasts with the traditional view that regards dendrites as purely passive structures that integrate postsynaptic dendritic potentials by electronic conduction.

Layer 4 is sometimes called the "sensory" or input layer. This layer is most prominent in the primary sensory regions and is composed of various stellate cells. It is relatively free of pyramidal cells and thus is frequently called the agranular layer. This region receives inputs from specific thalamic relay nuclei and corticocortico fibers from neocortical pyramidal cells in layers 2 and 3. The input fibers tend to synapse on excitatory spiny stellate cells that supply a strong excitatory synaptic drive to cells in layers 2 and 3 and to those in layers 5 and 6. Pyramidal cells in layer 5 tend to project to various subcortical nuclei, to layers 1, 2, and 5;

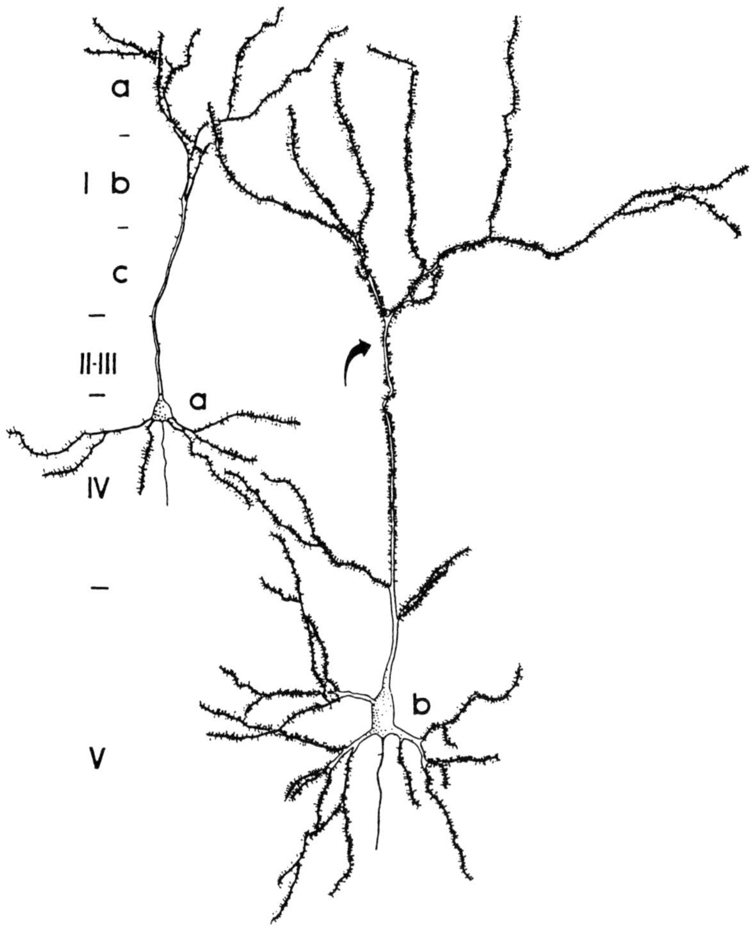

Figure 13-2. Pyramidal cells from layers 2 to 3 and layer 5 in rat posterior cingulate cortex. The dendritic spines, or synaptic contacts, are organized in two regions, an apical dendritic and a basal dendritic region. These two regions are separated by a relatively spine-free apical shaft. The capacity for dendrites to support action potentials suggests that these two zones could act as separate integrative compartments for inputs from layer 1 for the apical dendritic compartment and layer 4 for the basal dendritic region. (From Vogt, 1991.)

and to cells of other neocortical regions. In contrast, pyramidal cells in layer 6 project to the nonspecific thalamus (Jones, 1985). Layers 5 and 6 are sometimes called the "output" layers of the cortex.

The relation between various neocortical areas involved in the processing of sensory or motor information, although complex, obeys certain principles. First, almost all relations between regions are reciprocal, with both regions receiving and projecting fibers to and from each other. Many regions appear to be hierarchically related such that information is processed by a particular cortical region before being passed onto another region higher in the hierarchy. The relation between the visual primary or striate cortex and the visual association cortex is an example of such a reciprocal hierarchic relation. The fiber system that conveys information from the primary to the association cortex is the "feed-forward" system, and the reverse flow is mediated by the "feed-back" system.

The laminar features of these projections differ in that feed-forward projections generally originate in layers 2 and 3 and project principally to layer 4 and, to a lesser but still important extent to layers 2 and 3 of the region receiving the projection. The feed-back projections originate principally in layers 5 and 6 and, to a lesser extent, to layers 2 and 3 and project primarily to layer 1 and, to a lesser extent, to layers 5 and 6 as indicated in Figure 13-3 (Barbas, 1986; Fellerman and Van Essen, 1991). The most consistent difference is that feed-back projections tend to avoid layer 4 whereas feed-forward projections terminate principally in layer 4 with a smaller projection to layers 2 and 3. This description is an oversimplification, however. Evidence shows a range of other possibilities already identified in the primate neocortex. Readers interested in a more detailed account of these interconnections should consult the review by Fellerman and Van Essen (1991).

Feed-back loops with substantial (if not predominantly) inhibitory feed-back mediated by the superficial component of layer 1 (Vogt, 1991) suggests the possibility of resonance processes based on such regional feed-back structures. The frequency of such proposed resonance structures would be a function of both synaptic time constants and propagation delays (dendritic and axonal). Typically, two reciprocally connected regions separated by 5 cm and 4 to 7 synapses yielding

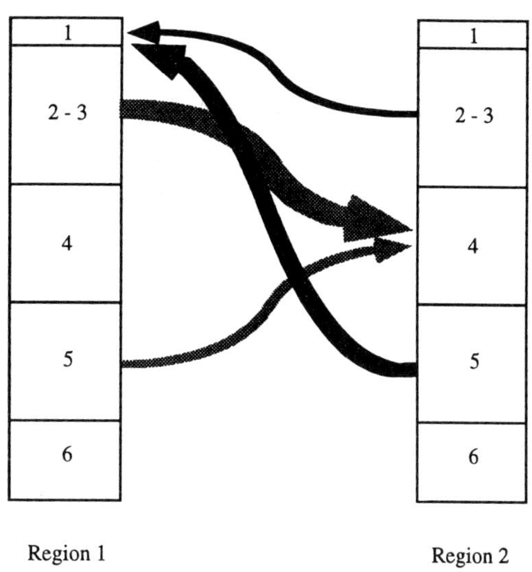

Figure 13-3. Linkage between two related neocortical areas, R1 and R2. In this diagram, R1 is situated below R2 in the information processing hierarchy. In this situation, cells in layers 2, 3, and, to a lesser extent, layer 5 of a R1 project to layer 4 of the R2. The feed-back fibers originate primarily in layer 5 and, to a lesser extent, layers 2 and 3 of the R2 region and project back to layer 1 of R1. The high GABAergic levels in the superficial components of layer 1 suggests negative feed-back from R2 to R1.

axonal delays of 10 to 20 milliseconds with synaptic delays of 2 to 35 milliseconds may be expected to produce resonant frequencies corresponding to approximately twice the loop time or 9 to 17 Hz. Such resonances are here called "regional resonances" and clearly may exist across a range of spatial scales and coexist with higher-order global resonances. The issue of interactions at multiple spatial scales is considered in more detail in Chapters 2 and 14. Both regional and global resonances depend on the flow of activity through layer 1 to the pyramidal cells in layers 2 and 3. Layer 1 thus appears to play a central functional role in mediating regional and global resonances. Global and regional resonances may be the origin of various EEG rhythms with frequencies less than 20 Hz. Any pathologic disruption or damage to the fiber systems mediating the regional resonances will reduce the corresponding regional resonant frequency. Axonal delays will increase due to local demyelination, whereas disruptions of synaptic contacts effectively increases the synaptic delay. This may partly account for the localized EEG slowing that is a feature of regional brain damage. Another possible contribution to local slowing is interruption of local pathways for neuromodulators, thereby altering control parameters.

The Thalamus

The thalamus plays an important role in generating brain rhythmic activity and is frequently considered the principal pacemaker for cortical activity (Buzsaki 1991; Steriade et al, 1991a, 1991b). Thalamic anatomy is discussed in Chapter 4. The delta rhythm, sleep spindles, and possibly some high frequency beta activity have been attributed exclusively to the thalamus. Buzsaki (1991) stated this most unambiguously when he wrote ". . . a general consensus today is that neocortical rhythmicity is due to the oscillatory behavior of the intrathalamic or thalamocortical circuits." In contrast, the view presented in this book is that neocortex and the thalamus play complementary roles in generating brain rhythmic activity. The violin metaphor illustrates the proposed relation between the thalamus and neocortex in Chapter 3. The sounds produced by a violin are determined by the resonant modes of its cavity. The role of violin strings is thus to activate selectively the desired resonant modes of the cavity. It is proposed that neocortex determines the resonant modes of the brain and the thalamus selectively activates different modes, thereby yielding the EEG resonances.

Extensive evidence shows that the thalamus can generate a range of rhythmic activities in the low-frequency range (1 to 4 Hz), an intermediate-frequency range (12 to 17 Hz), and a high-frequency range (approximately 20 to 60 Hz) (Steriade, 1991; Steriade et al, 1990). The reticularis nucleus of the thalamus (NRT) is thought to play a central role in thalamic rhythmogenesis. It forms a thin layer around the dorsolateral border of the thalamus and receives inputs from thalamocortical and corticothalamic axons. The NRT cells project exclusively back into the thalamus through GABAergic synapses, where they act on relay and inhibitory interneurons as shown in Figure 4-4B. (Jones, 1985; Steriade and Deschenes, 1984). The behavior of NRT cells appears to depend strongly on the state of membrane polarization. When the resting membrane potential is between −60 mv and −65 mv, a low-threshold calcium current is activated that produces bursts of action potentials associated with spindlelike oscillations in the 7 to 14 Hz range (Steriade and Deschenes 1984; Steriade et al, 1991a). Hyperpolarization of NRT and thalamic relay cells between −65 mv and −90 mv yield rhythmic spike bursts in the 1 to 4 Hz range (Steriade et al, 1991b). In contrast, when NRT cells are depolarized to a transmembrane voltage greater than −60 mv, they are more likely to respond at high rates of approximately 40 Hz (McCormick, 1992; Pinault and Deschenes, 1992b). These three rhythmic modes therefore can be impressed on the specific and nonspecific thalamic relay nuclei and then onto the cortex. The specific thalamocortical fibers terminate primarily in layer 4, whereas the nonspecific fibers terminate mainly in layer 1 (Herkenhamm, 1986).

The nonspecific thalamic activation of neocortical lamina 2 and 3 cells through lamina 1 at specific frequencies should preferentially activate global and regional resonances. This suggestion is supported by features of the recruiting response. This response consists of electrocortical responses of progressively increasing amplitude, elicited by repetitive electrical stimulation of nonspecific thalamic nuclei at certain frequencies (Foster, 1980; Steriade, 1991). In the context of global and regional resonances, the recruiting response can be interpreted as the response of a highly tuned system (the cortex) to a series of impulses occurring at a neocortical resonant frequency. The slow increase and decrease in recruiting response amplitude after the start and finish of electrical stimulation are typical of the behavior of highly tuned systems. Figure 13-4 illustrates the feline recruiting response and the response of a mechanical or electrical filter showing damped simple harmonic motion. In both cases, the effect of the stimulus pulses delivered at the resonant frequency is a response at the stimulus frequency with an amplitude that slowly increases with time.

A neocortical origin for the recruiting response is suggested by observations of a preserved recruiting response in the absence of the thalamic nuclei (Mitzdorf, 1985). Laminar analysis of neocortical current flows during the recruiting response suggests that thalamic activation excites cells in layers 2 and 3 through layer 1 while simultaneously inhibiting cells in layer 5 (Foster, 1980). A neocortical contribution to rhythmogenesis was demonstrated in a study of the canine alpha rhythm by Lopes da Silva et al. (1980). In this study, simultaneous recordings were obtained from neighbouring occipital neocortical sites and the lateral geniculate nucleus and pulvinar nucleus of the thalamus. The method of partial coherence was used to estimate the intracortical contribution to the coherence between various neocortical recording sites after the thalamic contribution had been mathematically removed. The paper concluded that ". . . there are thalamocortical and cortico-cortical components which interact in the generation of cortical alpha rhythms" (Lopes da Silva, 1980).

The idea that neocortical resonances determine the dominant EEG rhythms elicited by thalamic activity requires reconciliation with two features of thalamic

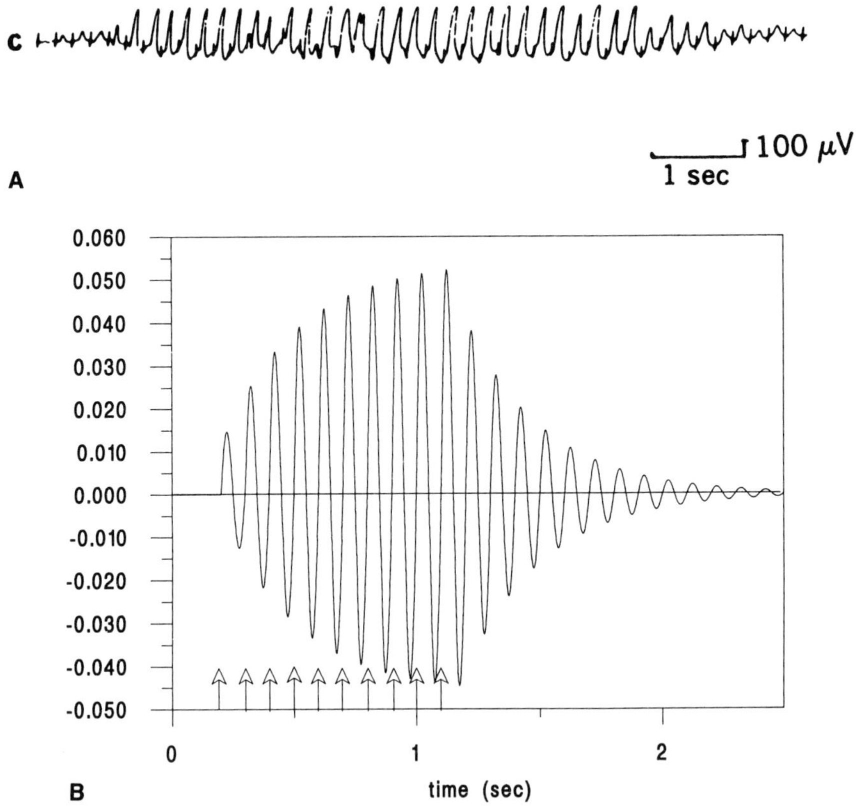

Figure 13-4. **A** illustrates the recruiting response elicited by regular electrical stimulation of the cat nucleus centralis medialis, a nonspecific nucleus projecting to layer 1. **B** illustrates the response of damped second-order system stimulated by impulses occurring at the resonant frequency. The arrows on the time axis indicate the timing of the impulses. Note the slow increase in amplitude and the corresponding slow decay of the oscillations. The recruiting response is a neocortical resonance phenomenon similar to the simulated system. (Figure 4A from Jasper, 1960.)

behavior. First, the thalamus can generate several specific rhythms that seem to coincide with the proposed neocortical resonant frequencies. Second, the thalamic sleep spindles of 11 to 17 Hz are preserved in cats that had their entire neocortex removed (Morrison and Bassett, 1945). Both of these features have been proposed to favor a thalamic pacemaker model, with the neocortex assigned a passive role in determining the EEG rhythms. Thalamic sleep spindles are especially intriguing because they occur at the frequencies thought to be mediated by neocortical regional resonances.

A mechanism that could reconcile the proposed role of the neocortex as the prime factor determining the EEG resonant frequencies with the thalamus' ability to generate such rhythms independently, involves the thalamus' ability to adjust

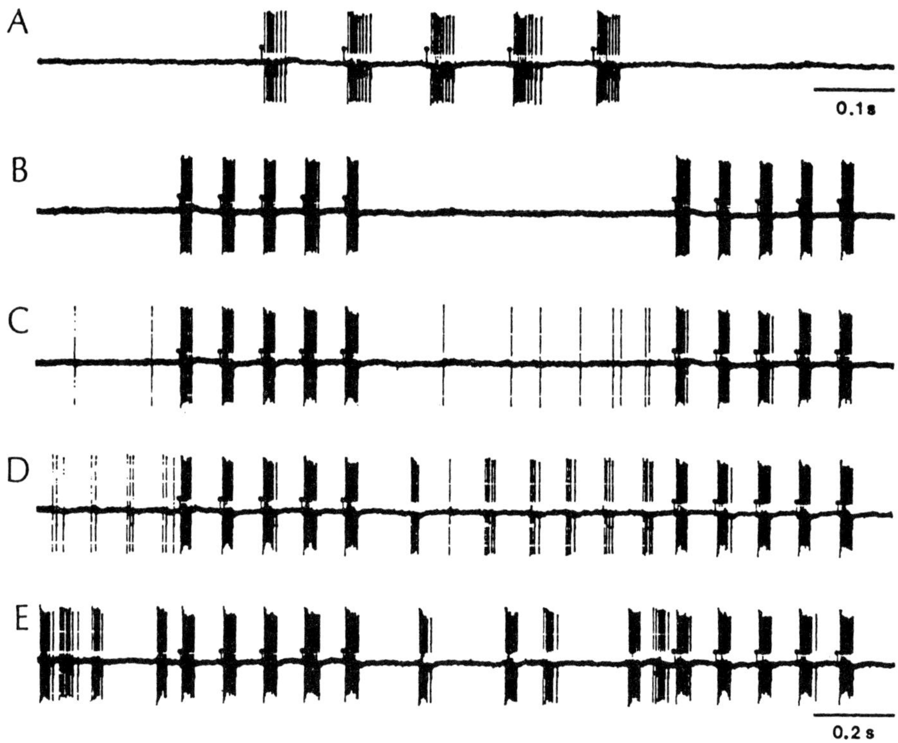

Figure 13-5. Single unit activity recorded in ventrolateral thalamic neurons in a cat in response to motor cortex stimulation with five shocks at 10/second delivered every 1.3 seconds. Top row (**A**) illustrates the activity with higher temporal resolution. Row **B** illustrates the response at the beginning of the stimulation sequence, whereas row **E** shows the response after 28 seconds. The appearance of spontaneous bursts of activity with similar time course to the stimulated response suggests a "frequency plasticity" effect. This effect could be the mechanism whereby the thalamus adjusts the frequency of various spontaneous rhythms to match those of the neocortical resonant frequencies. (From Steriade 1991.)

its resonant frequencies. The possibility that the thalamus adjusts its modal frequencies to coincide with neocortical resonant frequencies was introduced in Chapter 3. Evidence for such "frequency plasticity" was reported by Steriade and colleagues (Steriade et al, 1976). In that study, the motor cortex was stimulated by a sequence of five pulses delivered at a rate of 10 pulses per second every 2 seconds. At first each stimulus elicited a brief (fewer than 50 milliseconds) bursting response from the thalamic ventrolateral cell. After only 28 shock trains, the thalamic neuron spontaneously produced a rhythmic burst response near the original driving frequency, this process is illustrated in Figure 13-5.

Thalamic frequency plasticity and the reciprocal relation between the nonspecific thalamic nuclei and neocortex could comprise a mechanism that may account for production of rhythmic activity at neocortical resonant frequencies by thalamic nuclei. A thalamic rhythm occurring at a neocortical global or regional resonant frequency will yield a larger neocortical response than one elicited by a thalamic rhythm unrelated to the neocortical resonances. The larger neocortical resonant response, coupled with the frequency plasticity effect, in turn modifies the thalamic spontaneous frequency to approximate the neocortical resonant frequency. Reports of thalamic sleep spindles in the absence of neocortex therefore could be an indication of thalamic frequency plasticity operating during the animal's lifetime. This mechanism is consistent with reports that human sleep spindles comprise two independent components, each having a specific frequency and topography. One component with a frontal focus has a frequency of 12 Hz whereas the other has a central parietal focus and a frequency of 14 Hz (Jobert et al, 1992). Such findings are consistent with the idea that the frequency and topography of the frontal and parietal sleep spindles are determined by frontal and parietal regional resonances, respectively.

In summary, thalamic frequency plasticity suggests a mechanism that reconciles the EEG primacy of neocortical resonances with observations of independent thalamic rhythms at neocortical resonant frequencies. The thalamus may be tuned by the neocortex to the neocortical resonant frequencies, a process which is similar to the violin analogy introduced in Chapter 3. In this case, the violin cavity (cortex) adjusts the tension in the violin strings (thalamus) so that their resonant frequencies match.

Local Resonances

In the context of this chapter, local resonances are those rhythmic processes in the 30 to 80 Hz range due to tissue with spatial extent in the millimetric range (see Figure 13-6). Such local resonances might comprise cortical macrocolumns or thalamic pacemakers. An important feature of such local resonant processes is that their frequencies are independent of the spatial extent of the neural region involved (in a manner similar to typical electric circuits). Furthermore, these resonant frequencies are determined almost exclusively by the synaptic delays, that is the rise and fall times of postsynaptic potentials and, in some cases, the dynamics of membrane conductances (Llinas, 1992; Nunez, 1989). Many local theories of neocortical rhythmic activity highlight the role of the inhibitory stellate cells in an inhibitory feed-back loop (Wilson and Cowan, 1973; Freeman, 1975, 1992; Lopes da Silva, 1991). Such negative feed-back circuits have resonance properties with frequencies determined by the loop times of the circuits. Freeman (1992) noted that the loop times involving neocortical pyramidal and inhibitory stellate cells are consistent with resonances at approximately 40 Hz. In a recent study based on quantitative estimations of intracortical coupling, Wright and Liley (1994) proposed a model of neocortical rhythmic activity that, under specific circumstances, can generate 40-Hz activity. In all such models, 40-Hz activity appears spontaneously if the loop gain is great enough. The loop gain associated with high-frequency local resonances is related to the local resonance control parameter Q

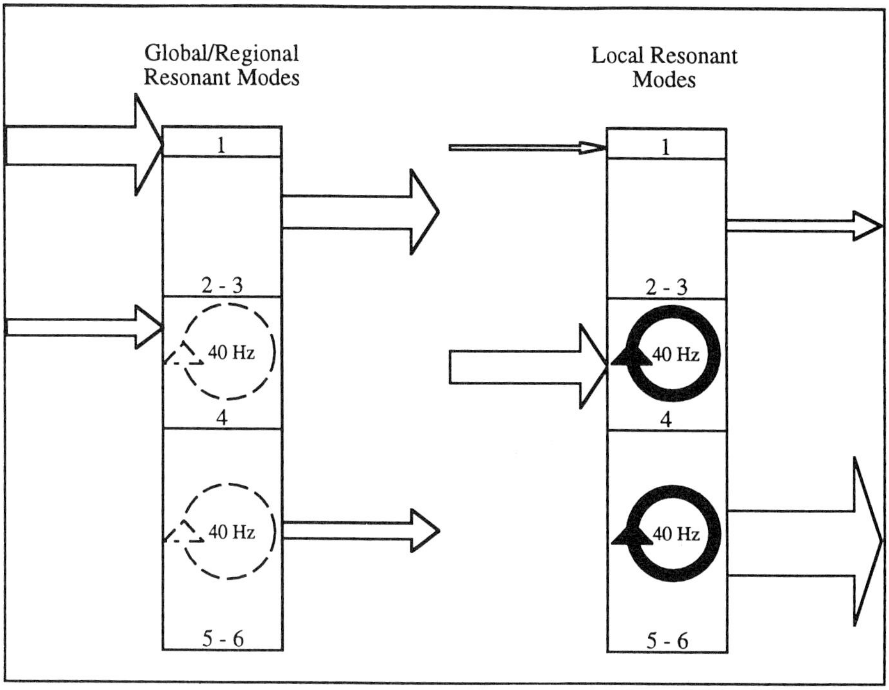

Figure 13-6. Symbolic representation of global–regional and local neocortical resonant modes. In global and regional resonant modes, layer 1 is a major input zone to cells in the microcolumn with the response of cells in layers 2 and 3 facilitated. At the same time, cells in layers 5 and 6 are inhibited by pre- and postsynaptic inhibitory processes. This inhibition reduces the gain of the feed-back loops generating 40-Hz activity in the deeper layers leading to suppression of such activity. In the local resonant mode, inputs from layer 1 are inhibited and layer 4 is the major input zone to the neocortical column. Excitation of deeper cells increases gain of the deeper 40-Hz, feed-back loops.

discussed in Chapters 3, 5, 8, and 11. In addition to the high-frequency activity generated by neural networks with negative feed-back, evidence shows some inhibitory stellate cells with intrinsic high-frequency (40 Hz) rhythmicity (Llinas, 1992).

Probably the thalamus is also an important factor in determining the appearance of local 40-Hz activity. High-frequency activity in the NRT affects specific thalamic nuclei than in turn project to layer 4, where they elicit a 40-Hz cortical response (Llinas and Ribary, 1992, 1993).

An important distinction between local and global–regional resonant modes is that the local resonant modes need not be coherent over distances of more than a few millimeters. In contrast, human regional and global resonant modes are coherent over distances of many centimeters. Cognitive, behavioral, or perceptual states requiring a high degree of spatiotemporal specificity in neocortical activation may be consistent only with local states as suggested in Chapter 12. A skilled

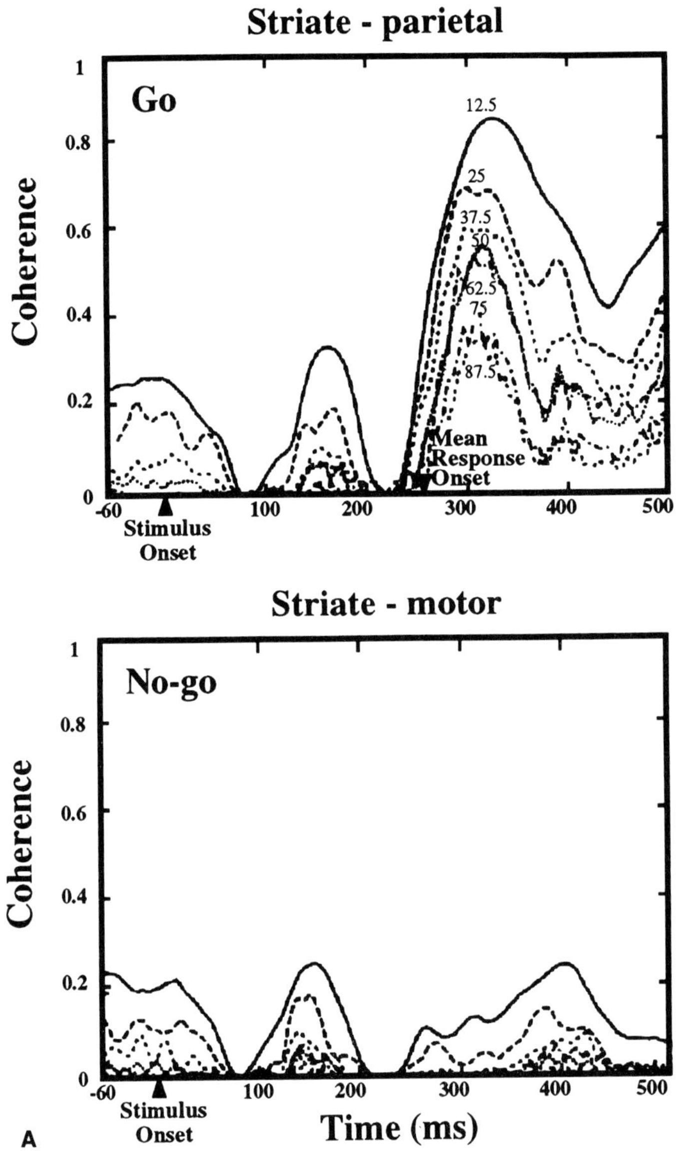

A

Figure 13-7. Changes in coherence between striate and motor cortex (**A**) and between striate and parietal cortex (**B**). The coherence is illustrated for seven frequencies, 12.5 Hz, 25 Hz, 37.5 Hz, 50 Hz, 62.5 Hz, 75 Hz, and 87.5 Hz. The left panel shows the coherences when a motor response was required (that is, Go), whereas the right panels show the situation for no motor response (No-Go). The striate-motor coherencies showed a substantial increase in the Go but not the No-Go situation. In contrast, the striate-parietal coherencies showed an increase in coherencies regardless of whether a motor response was required. (From Bressler et al, 1993.)

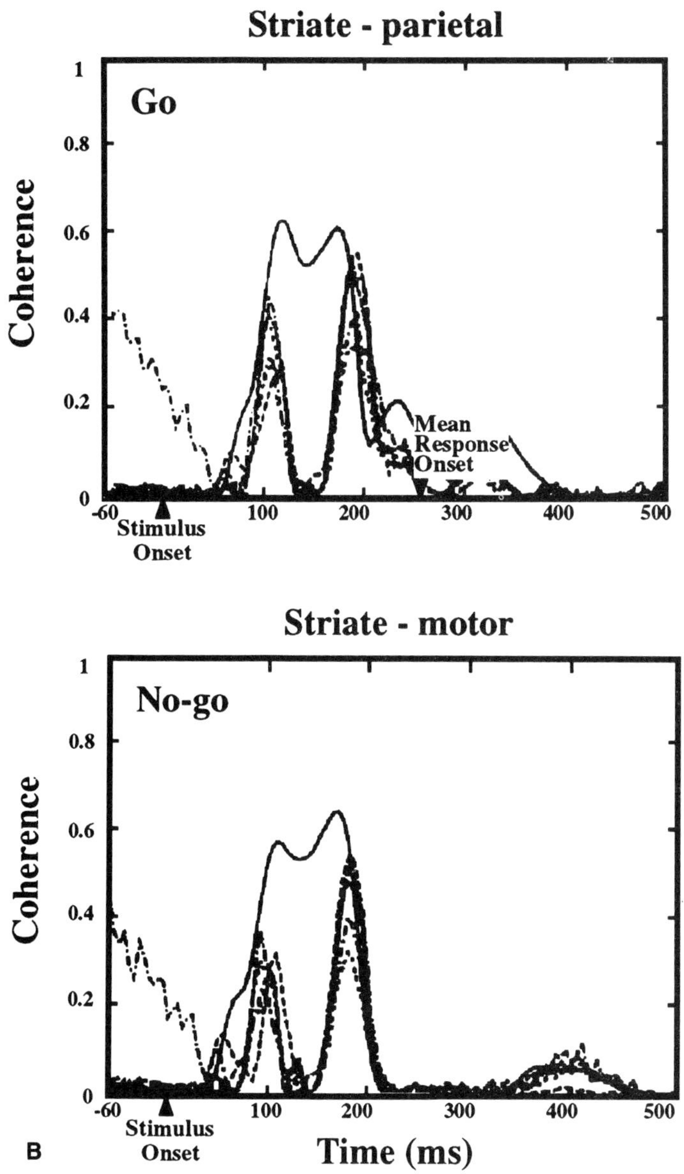

B

Figure 13-7. *(Continued)*

movement, for example, is associated with a very precise sequence of cortical activation. Under some circumstances, we can observe evidence of widely distributed yet coherent local modes in the scalp EEG and single cell recordings. Rougeul-Buser (1984) reported prominent 40-Hz electrocortical activity in cats when in a state of focused arousal whereas Sheer (1976, 1984, 1989) found 40-Hz human EEG activity while subjects were in a state of focused arousal and engaged in problem solving. Neurodegenerative diseases such as Alzheimer dementia greatly reduce this activity (Loring et al, 1985). The distribution of high frequency activity is widespread at the outset of a novel task but decreases in extent as tasks become familiar. Pfurtscheller and Neuper (1992) reported transient increases in 40-Hz activity over the motor cortex when participants perform unimanual finger movements, and Tiitinen and associates (1993) showed that selective attention enhanced the 40-Hz auditory response.

Evidence for widespread synchronization of high-frequency, single cell activity in the visual system was also reported (Engel et al, 1990). This synchronization is thought to play a central role in integrating neural activity over widely separate areas of the cortex. Bressler and coworkers (1993) reported widespread and task-related transient increases in high-frequency coherence in the monkey neocortex (see Figure 13-7). While monkeys performed a pattern-discrimination task, high-frequency activity in the motor and striate cortexes were briefly correlated when a motor response occurred and were uncorrelated when no response was required. In contrast, the high-frequency activity in the striate and parietal cortex was briefly correlated after the presentation of the stimulus, regardless of whether a motor response was required. These findings suggest that the increases in coherence are functionally related to the cognitive and motor aspects of the task. The appearance of widely separated spatially coherent local processes also suggests that the synchronization is mediated by the fast corticocortical fiber system. The time course of high-frequency coherence between the striate–parietal and striate–motor areas lasts 50 to 200 milliseconds and is illustrated in Figure 13-7. These authors noted that activity at 12.5-Hz showed increases in coherence at the same times that the higher harmonics of 12.5 Hz showed such increases (that is, 25 Hz, 37.5 Hz, 50 Hz, 62.5 Hz, and so on). They commented that this appears to be at variance with the reports of Pfurtscheller and Neuper (1992), who showed reductions in alpha activity with increases in 40-Hz activity. Several factors may account for this. First, Bressler and associates (1993) analyzed intracortical field potentials that were recorded from closely spaced electrode pairs. This would attenuate field potentials generated by more remote sources and bias the response to higher spatial frequencies. In contrast, the scalp-recorded potentials reported by Pfurtscheller and Neuper (1992) spatially average the activity over a larger scale and therefore are biased to lower spatial frequencies. Global and regional resonances, by virtue of their spatial extent, occur over low spatial frequencies (Nunez et al, 1994; Chapters 2 and 3) and may have been attenuated by the high common-mode rejection bipolar recording system used by Bressler and associates (1993).

Another factor that may contribute to the difference between this and Pfurtscheller and Neuper's (1992) findings concerns the nature of the 12.5-Hz activity. The rapid changes in high-frequency activity in the 30 to 80 Hz range can be modeled as amplitude modulation of a broadband signal. In this case, the broadband carrier is modulated by a signal with a bandwidth as large as 20 Hz. This follows from the fact that the minimum duration of the transient increase in high-frequency power is approximately 50 milliseconds. Amplitude modulation of a sinusoidal signal yields additional signals at the sums and differences of the carrier and modulating signal. Thus a 20-Hz signal amplitude modulating a 30 to 80 Hz broadband carrier will generate activity in the 10 to 60 Hz range and the 50 to 100 Hz range. The 12.5-Hz activity reported by Bressler and associates (1993) therefore may be a manifestation of the local resonances and be distinct from the regional and global resonances that also yield activity in this frequency range.

The scalp-recorded, 40-Hz activity may constitute a special case in which several prolonged, 40-Hz sources are spatially coherent. The more general situation may comprise widely distributed high frequency sources that are only briefly spatially coherent. In this situation, the EEG would simply appear as "fast desynchronized" activity.

Modulation of Global/Regional Resonances

The neocortex utilizes a variety of neorotransmitters which mediate rapid information processing and transmission (see Chapters 4 and 5). The major excitatory neurotransmitters comprise glutamate and aspartate while the principal inhibitory neurotransmitter is gamma-aminobutyric acid (GABA). Complementing the intrinsic neurotransmitters are a diverse range of slow acting neurotransmitters which include acetylcholine (ACh), noradrenaline (NA), dopamine (DA) and 5-hydroxytryptamine or serotonin (5-HT). These neurotransmitters are thought to modulate the response of neocortical cells to the intrinsic neurotransmitters GABA, glutamate and aspartate and have been termed neuromodulators. A number of features distinguish neuromodulators from the intrinsic neurotransmitters, these include the relatively slow time course of their action and the diffuse nature of their distribution. Such features enable neuromodulators to play a central role in the control of the excitability and patterns of activity in the thalamocortical system, in a state dependent manner (McCormick 1992).

The list of recognized neuromodulators has increased drastically in the last two decades. In addition to ACh, NA, DA, and 5-HT, histamine and a range of neuropeptides appear to play a crucial role in modifying the response to the neuromodulators. The action of this vast array of active compounds has not been characterized adequately. Each compound appears to act on several receptor types (see Table 4-2). Thus ACh can have a rapid depolarizing effect when acting on nicotinic receptors and have a very slow depolarizing effect when acting on muscarinic receptors. The situation is made more complex by the fact that different receptors for the same neuromodulator can have opposing effects. Thus the alpha NA receptor may have a depolarizing effect when the beta NA receptor simultaneously induces a hyperpolarizing state (McCormick, 1992). Given the limitations imposed by space and the state of current knowledge, this chapter focuses primarily on the roles of NA, DA, 5-HT, and ACh, neuromodulators whose roles have been studied most extensively.

The primary source of neocortical NA is a brain stem nucleus called the "locus coeruleus" (LC) (see Figure 4-7). The LC is remarkable in that only 26,000 neurons innervate the entire cortex, subcortical regions, and the spinal cord (Foote et al, 1983; Foote and Morrison, 1987; Aston-Jones, 1985). Although all regions of the cortex receive an NA innervation from the LC, the density and laminar distribution of this innervation varies greatly among regions. The somatosensory and motor regions are heavily innervated in all six layers, whereas the temporal cortex receives a weak innervation restricted to layer 1 (Vogt, 1991). The activity of the LC is strongly influenced by the behavioral or cognitive state of the subject; heightened arousal, environmental novelty, and anxiety are some of the factors that increase LC activity (Aston-Jones, 1985). On the other hand, a resting or inattentive state decreases the levels of LC activity with evidence of spontaneous bursts of activity occurring every 2 to 5 seconds (Foote et al, 1983).

The reported effects of NA on neocortical pyramidal cells have been mixed. Iontophoretic application of NA is generally associated with hyperpolarization and thus inhibition (McCormick, 1992), although other studies report that electrical stimulation of the LC strongly inhibits spontaneous activity in pyramidal cells and only weakly inhibits stimulus-related activity (Foote and Morrison, 1987). This led to the "signal to noise" enhancement theory of the role of the LC. The dual excitatory and inhibitory effects of NA have been illustrated most clearly by Sato and coworkers (1989); electrical stimulation of the feline LC was found to predominantly inhibit stimulus-related activity in pyramidal cells in layers 2 and 3 while simultaneously facilitating stimulus-related activity in layers 5 and 6 pyramidal cells. The inhibitory effect is mediated by beta receptors and excitation is mediated by alpha receptors (McCormick, 1992). Sato and coworkers (1989) found no evidence of an enhanced signal-to-noise ratio after LC stimulation. Cells with background activity that was suppressed by LC stimulation also showed inhibition of sensory-evoked activity and vice versa.

The effects of NA on neocortical dynamics can be appreciated when we note that the major synaptic inputs to the cells in layers 2 and to a lesser extent layer 3 of the neocortex originate in layer 1. In contrast, the cells in layers 5 and 6 receive their strongest synaptic input from deeper layers, which include layers 3, 4, and 5 (Vogt, 1991). Noradrenaline-mediated inhibition of cells in layers 2 and 3 thus would selectively inhibit layer 1 activation to these cells. Because the regional and global resonances described earlier depend crucially on inputs to layer 1, NA may weaken or decouple the corticocortico interactions that depend on layer 1. This decoupling would suppress or eliminate the regional and global resonances mediated by the corticocortico systems. Excitation of pyramidal cells in the deeper layers could simultaneously facilitate high-frequency local resonances in layers 5 and 6. The reduction in occipitoparietal alpha activity and central mu rhythm may be specific examples of such corticocortico decoupling. Such reductions in alpha and mu activity and corresponding increases in high-frequency beta activity are a recognized effect of drugs that increase brain NA levels (Herning et al, 1985; Mock and Kunkel, 1982; Rougeul-Buser, 1984). In terms of the mechanisms described in Chapters 11 and 12, this NA-mediated decoupling of corticocortical communication would be equivalent to reducing the control parameter (B) describing the strength of corticocortical interactions. This can also be illustrated in terms of the nonlinear spring and linear string analogy introduced in Chapter 2. The effects of increasing NA would be to weaken the string tension (corticocortical coupling) and increase the stiffness of the springs (local loop gain), whereas reduced NA levels would have the opposite effect. These effects can also be shown by a simple analogy consisting of two inhibitory feed-back systems linked by long-range fibers with an inhibitory feed-back component (see Figure 13-8). When the effect of the long-range coupling q_l is larger than the effect of the short-range coupling q_s, low- frequency responses emerge (Figure 13-B). When the opposite occurs, high-frequency activity is observed (Figure 13-C). In the context of Figure 13-8, NA would increase q_s and reduce q_l. The linked oscillators in Figure 13-8 represent only an analogy, and the short- and long-range delays were selected specifically to yield frequencies of 8 Hz and 43 Hz.

The dopaminergic fibers have their primary origin in the substantia nigra and the ventral tegmental area. The projections of the substantia nigra show considerable regional and laminar variations. Layer 1 receives a strong DA innervation throughout the neocortex whereas layers 5 and 6 also receive a less pronounced innervation that extends throughout the neocortex (Smiley et al, 1992). The DA synapses in layers 2 and 3 are less pronounced with some areas, such as the visual cortex, devoid of DA terminals. Throughout the neocortex, layer 4 has the lowest DA terminal levels (Berger et al, 1991).

The effects of DA on pyramidal cells are similar to those of NA; that is, a predominantly inhibitory effect on cells in layers 2 and 3 and a predominantly excitatory effect on cells in layer 5 (Sawaguchi et al, 1986). The inhibitory mechanism in layers 2 and 3 involves specialized synaptic contacts known as "triadic complexes." These consist of a dendritic spine in contact with a DA terminal or varicosity and a synaptic excitatory fiber. These triadic complexes are frequently found most in association with nonspecific thalamic projections to layer 1 and feedback corticocortico fibers from layers 5 and 6 (Berger et al, 1991; Smiley et al, 1992). The triadic complexes are thus well placed to suppress inputs from these sources. The high DA levels in layer 1 coupled with specific ultrastructural features, such as triadic complexes, suggest that DA, like NA, is ideally situated to shift the operating point of the neocortex from low-frequency global–regional resonance modes to high-frequency local resonance modes.

Dopamine may play an analogous role in the vertebrate retina. In the retina, specialized horizontal cells link several rods and cones to convey their summed generator potentials to the ganglion cells. This mechanism increases light sensitivity and operates in low light or scotopic conditions (Brown, 1980). This increase in sensitivity is associated with larger ganglion cell receptive fields and thus a reduction in spatial resolution. At higher light levels, where photopic vision operates, this horizontal cell-mediated coupling is inhibited when specialized retinal cells secrete DA. The reduced size of the receptive fields and the operation of lateral inhibition increases the spatial resolution associated with photopic vision (Brown, 1980). The effect of DA is thus to decouple the relatively long-range interactions mediated by the horizontal cells and facilitate localized retinal pro-

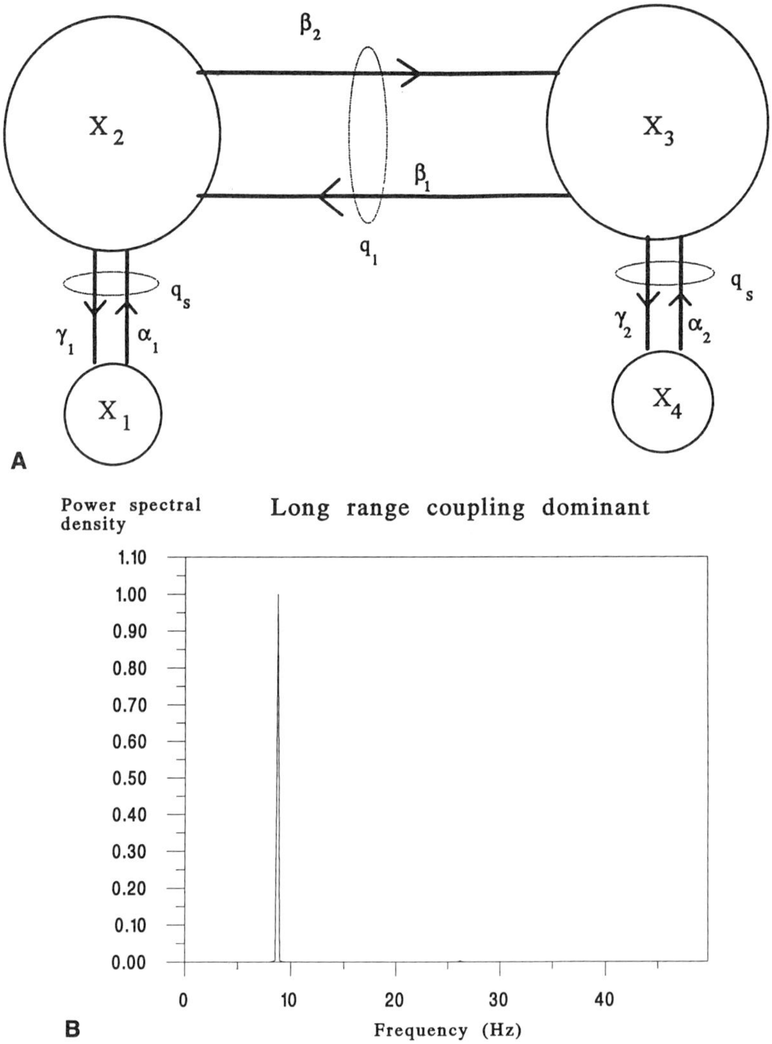

Figure 13-8. (**A**) illustrates a simple oscillatory system consisting of two local inhibitory feed-back systems X_1/X_2 and X_3/X_4. The X_1/X_2 and X_3/X_4 connections are considered local and are characterized by feed-forward and feed-back dispersive delays of 5 milliseconds. The feed-forward components (γ) are excitatory, whereas the feed-back components (α) are always inhibitory, with a strength 10% of the feed-forward component. The X_2/X_3 connections are meant to represent the corticocortical connections with feed-forward and feed-back dispersive delays of 25 milliseconds, representing a regional resonance. The feed-forward component (β_2) is excitatory and the feed-back component (β_1) is inhibitory, with a strength 10% of the feed-forward component. The local delays yield a resonance at approximately 43 Hz, whereas the corticocortical delays yield a resonant frequency of approximately 8 Hz. The strength of the corticocortical system is given by q_1 and the strength of the local system is q_s. Noradrenaline reduces the strength of corticocortical coupling or q1 and increases the strength of the local feed-back loop (q_s). (**B**) illustrates the

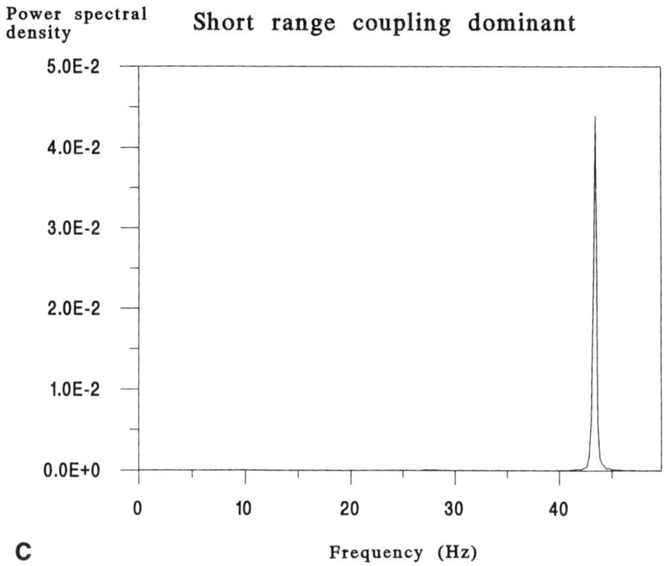

response of the system when X_2 and X_3 are driven by two independent white noise sources and the corticocortical coupling (q_1) dominates. In this case, the response is a resonance peak at 8 Hz. (C) illustrates the complementary situation in which local coupling qs dominates. The local resonance peak is situated at 43 Hz. (The model illustrated in Figure 13-8 is only meant to be considered an analogy of the actual details of corticocortico and intracortical connectivity.)

cessing (Rogawski, 1987; Wassle and Boycott, 1991). The central role of DA in decoupling retinal receptive fields is confirmed by findings that DA cell loss in Parkinson disease is associated with reduced visual contrast sensitivity at high spatial frequencies (Bodis-Wollner, 1990). It must be emphasized that these retinal effects of DA are only presented as an analogy and do not in themselves constitute strong evidence for the decoupling role of DA in the neocortex.

The proposed role of DA in shifting neocortical operating points from regional–global to local states is consistent with a range of neuropharmacologic and electrophysiologic findings. High-frequency, 40-Hz EEG activity requires an intact dopaminergic system (Lopes da Silva, 1991; Montaron et al, 1982). Furthermore, drugs that increase DA activity such as dihydroxyphenylalanine, apomorphine, and amphetamine, also enhance 40-Hz activity in cats (Rougeul-Buser, 1984). Like NA, DA is a neuromodulator that reduces the global control parameter B while increasing the local control parameter.

Acetylcholine is often considered a complementary neurotransmitter to NA and DA. In primates, the major source of ACh is the nucleus basalis of Meynert (NBM) in the basal forebrain (McCormick and Prince, 1988, Mesulam 1988). The cholinergic fibers innervating the neocortex do not collateralize to the same extent as the LC fibers and there is a capacity to vary selectively cholinergic drive to particular neocortical and subcortical regions (Foote, 1987). The activity of the

NBM is strongly influenced by behavioral state, with the highest NBM activity levels found in conditions of focused arousal (Celesia and Jasper, 1966; Rougeul-Buser, 1984; Mesulam, 1988). Levels of ACh vary greatly with cortical region and lamina, but the highest levels are found in the limbic region, especially the hippocampus and amygdala (Mesulam, 1988). Within the neocortex, the highest ACh levels are observed in the primary sensory–motor cortex (Mesulam, 1988, 1992). Acetylcholine has a direct excitatory effect on pyramidal cells, with nicotinic receptors generating rapid, short-lived excitation and muscarinic receptors responsible for slower, long-lasting excitation (McCormick, 1988). The pyramidal cell effects of ACh vary with neocortical layer. Cells in layers 5 and 6 are strongly excited and tend to respond with a high-frequency burst of activity (Steriade et al, 1991). In contrast, cells in layers 2 and 3 are inhibited as a consequence of cholinergic excitation of muscarinic receptors on GABAergic inhibitory stellate cells (McCormick, 1990; McCormick and Prince, 1988). These inhibitory stellate cells in layers 2 and 3 are enveloped in cholinergic fibers (Mesulam et al, 1992), suggesting that the cholinergic input is especially powerful. Acetylcholine could act to decouple corticocortical interactions through the strong inhibition of pyramidal cells in layers 2 and 3 while simultaneously facilitating high-frequency local resonance modes in layers 5 and 6. Therefore, acetylcholine would reduce the global control parameter B while simultaneously increasing the local control parameter Q. This idea is supported by EEG findings that a loss of cholinergic input to the cortex invariably leads to reduced high-frequency EEG activity and the appearance of pathologic low-frequency EEG activity (Lopes da Silva, 1991; Loring et al, 1985; McCormick, 1992; McCormick and Prince, 1988; Mesulam, 1988; Riekkinen et al, 1991; Sheer, 1984, 1989).

The final monoamine to be considered, 5-HT, is synthesized in the mesencephalic raphe nuclei (MRN) situated within the brain stem reticular formation (Foote and Morrison, 1987) as indicated in Figure 4-7. "Serotonergic neurons comprise the most expansive neurochemical network in the vertebrate [central nervous system]. These midline brain stem neurons innervate virtually all portions of the neuraxis" (Jacobs and Azmitia, 1992). The raphe nuclei are most active during rhythmic "vegetative" states such as feeding, licking, and grooming, whereas the activity is decreased at times of heightened arousal and orientation (Jacobs and Fornal, 1993). This behavioral specificity complements that of NA, where the LC activity is highest during arousal. The activity of the serotonergic MRN neuron is characterized by low frequency (3 to 5 Hz) and regularity (Jacobs and Azmitia, 1992). Like other monoamines, 5-HT has a distinctive regional and laminar distribution. Serotonergic fibers appear to comprise at least two types in the cerebral cortex. The classification is based on the size and distribution of the 5-HT presynaptic terminals or varicosities. The large varicosities are prominent in layers 1 to 3, whereas the fine varicosities are distributed more uniformly, with tendency to peak in layer 4 (Mamounas et al, 1992; McCormick, 1992; Jacobs and Azmatia, 1992). Neocortical areas with the highest levels of 5-HT terminals include the striate, parietal, and temporal cortex and the lowest levels are found in the motor cortex (Azmitia and Gannon, 1986).

The pyramidal cell effects of 5-HT are determined by the type of receptor activated, and more than six distinct subtypes of 5-HT receptors have been identified. Although 5-HT_{1A} receptors are found in all neocortical layers, their levels tend to be higher in layers 1 to 3 (Jacobs and Azmitia, 1992). The direct effect of 5-HT_{1A} receptors on pyramidal cells is a hyperpolarization, an effect seen most clearly in layers 5 and 6 (McCormick, 1992). In neocortical layers 1, 2, and 3, the 5-HT_{1A} receptors are associated with GABAergic cell bodies and dendrites (Mamounas et al, 1992). Specialized networks of 5-HT synapses surround the GABAergic cells in "baskets or pericellular arrays" (Mulligan and Tork, 1988). The hyperpolarization of these inhibitory cells produces disinhibition of the pyramidal cells in the superficial layers (Joyce, 1993). The net effect of 5-HT_{1A} receptors therefore is to suppress local resonant modes by inhibiting cells in layers 4, 5, and 6 while enhancing the appearance of global–regional modes by exciting cells in layers 1 to 3. These effects mirror those associated with ACh. Acetylcholine excites cells in layers 5 and 6 by direct depolarization and inhibits cells in layers 2 and 3 by excitation of GABAergic cells and dendrites in layers 1, 2, and 3. The idea that 5-HT and ACh have complementary roles in layers 2 and 3 is reinforced by the fact that 5-HT pericellular arrays are remarkably similar to the network of ACh fibers that envelope superficial GABAergic cells.

The 5-HT_{1B} receptors operate primarily by activating presynaptic inhibitory processes in pyramidal and stellate cells in layers 4, 5, and 6 (Tanaka and North, 1993). Such inhibition would decrease the flow of information processed by these cells and would also decrease the gain of the excitatory and inhibitory feed-back loops described earlier. The effect of the 5-HT_{1B} receptor is synergistic with the 5-HT_{1A} receptor because it suppresses the appearance of local resonant modes through presynaptic inhibition, whereas the 5-HT_{1A} receptor yields a similar effect through postsynaptic inhibition.

The concentration of 5-HT_2 receptor is highest in layer 4 of the sensory cortex, especially the striate cortex. The direct effect of 5-HT_2 receptor activation is membrane depolarization, which can subsequently yield several effects. Depolarization and hyperpolarization of pyramidal cells in layers 5 and 6 have been reported, possibly as a consequence of depolarization of GABAergic interneurons (Ashby and Wang, 1990; McCormick, 1992). The fact that drugs which block 5-HT_2 receptors, prevent the excessive drowsiness or catalepsy associated with neuroleptic drug treatment of schizophrenia (Seeman 1990) suggests 5-HT_2 receptors may suppress local resonant modes. In the context of the current model, suppression of local modes implies that the 5-HT_2 receptors may have a predominantly inhibitory effect on pyramidal cells in layers 5 and 6. The effects of 5-HT_{1a}, 5-HT_{1B}, and 5-HT_2 receptors shift the neocortical operating point toward global–regional resonance and away from local resonance modes. The effects of 5-HT also can be described as increasing the global control parameter B and reducing the local control parameter Q. This is consistent with the finding that L-tryptophan, the precursor of 5-HT, increases EEG alpha theta activity in humans (Spinweber et al, 1983). These 5-HT effects complement the effects of DA, NA, and ACh that move the neocortical operating point toward local resonance states. Table 13.1 summarizes the laminar effects of these neuromodulators.

Previously we noted that the retinal effects of DA were to decouple the relatively long-range interaction mediated by the retinal horizontal cells. Serotonin, and melatonin, one of its derivatives, have retinal effects that complement those of DA. In conditions of dim light, melatonin is synthesized and secreted in the retina. This inhibits DA release and enhances horizontal cell linkage of the rod photoreceptors (Krause and Dubocovich, 1990). It is tempting to speculate that melatonin may have analogous effects in the neocortex. Apart from the retina, the sole source of melatonin is the pineal gland, where its secretion follows a circadian rhythm, with a maximum occurring between midnight and 2 A.M. local time (Cassone, 1990). Melatonin receptors were identified in the neocortex, and administration of melatonin promotes sleep and increases slow-wave activity (Brailowsky, 1976; Miles and Philbrick, 1988; Stankov et al, 1991). Melatonin may be another compound that enhances global and regional resonant modes, although it could operate on a longer time scale (days to weeks) to regulate the levels of ACh and DA receptors. Like the retinal effects of DA, the retinal effects of 5-HT and melatonin are introduced only as a suggestive analogy.

In summary, it is suggested that NA, DA, and ACh are well positioned to reduce corticocortical coupling (B) and increase the local loop gain (Q). In contrast, 5-HT could reduce the local loop gain and increase corticocortical coupling. Neocortical states characterized by reduced corticocortical coupling are here called "hypocoupled states," whereas those characterized by increased corticocortical coupling subsequently are called "hypercoupled states." Hypocoupled states are associated with high-frequency EEG, whereas hypercoupled states are associated with lower frequency EEG activity that is spatially coherent over distances of at least several centimeters. The effects of NA, DA, and ACh could be to move the neocortical operating point in the hypocoupled direction while 5-HT moves the operating point in the hypercoupled direction. The resulting EEG rhythms thus may depend on the current balance between these control processes as illustrated in Figure 13-9.

A range of experimental findings may be considered in the context of this coupling model. It accounts for task-related changes in the 13-Hz, steady-state,

Table 13.1. Summary table outlining the effects of various neuromodulators on superficial (layers II and III) and deep (layers V and VI) pyramidal cells.

Neuromodulator	NA		DA	ACh		5-HT	
Receptor type	α	β		muscarinic	5-HT^{1A}	5-HT^{1B}	5-HT_2
Effects on layers II & III		−	−	−	+		
Effects on layers V & VI	+		+	+	−	−	?−

The receptors mentioned in the text and thought to mediate either excitation (+) or inhibition (−) are listed under their respective neuromodulators. The question mark associated with the 5-HT_2 receptor indicates that these effects are partly inferred from EEG and behavioural observations.

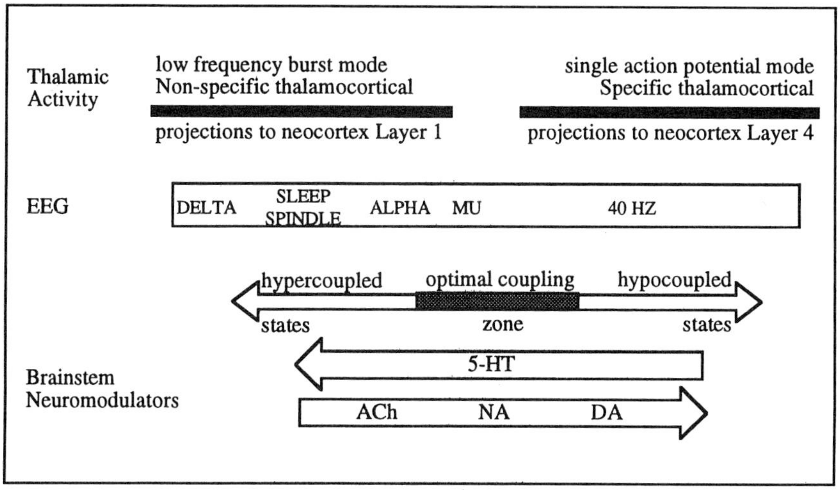

Figure 13-9. Summary of the relation between the various neocortical resonant modes, the brain stem neuromodulators, and the EEG rhythms. One parameter used to characterize the resonant state is the strength of long-range corticocortical coupling. Neocortical states associated with strong corticocortical coupling are called hypercoupled and are associated with global or regional resonant modes. Neocortical states associated with weak corticocortico coupling are called hypocoupled and are associated with local resonances.

visually evoked potential (SSVEP) elicited by a uniform visual flicker. A range of cognitive tasks yields site-specific SSVEP amplitude reductions. These reductions were interpreted as increases in cortical activity (see Chapter 6 and Silberstein et al, 1990, 1994). Such an interpretation is consistent with the idea that the 13-Hz SSVEP amplitude indexes the amplitude of regional resonances in the alpha frequency range. The reductions in SSVEP amplitude are a consequence of neuromodulator-mediated corticocortical decoupling that leads to decreased regional resonances.

A related phenomenon is event-related desynchronization (Pfurtscheller and Aranibar, 1977; Pfurtscheller and Klimesch, 1990), which consists of transient decreases in alpha activity associated with specific cognitive and motor tasks. These reductions have differing task-dependent topographies that are consistent with neuropsychologic data. Thus a unimanual motor task shows alpha attenuation over the contralateral motor cortex, whereas a reading task shows comparable attenuation in the temporal cortex. The decreases in alpha activity could be considered a consequence of increased monoaminergic and possibly cholinergic activation of the neocortical regions participating in the cognitive–motor task. These increased neuromodulatory levels decouple the corticocortical fibers that sustain the alpha frequency regional resonances. The decreases in alpha activity are also associated with corresponding increases in 40-Hz activity (Pfurtscheller and Neuper, 1992).

Both the alpha attenuation and the 40-Hz activity increase are consistent with the idea of neuromodulatory-mediated decreases in regional resonant modes and increases in local resonant modes.

In a relaxed, low-vigilance state, the locus coeruleus shows slow, irregular changes in activity (Foote et al, 1983; Marshal and Finlayson, 1988). Fluctuations in LC and neocortical NA levels could dynamically alter the level of corticocortical coupling. This would suggest increases in alpha activity during intervals of low LC activity and decreases in alpha activity during transient increases in LC activity. This mechanism may also account for reported stable alpha topographies or "alpha spindles" (Lehmann et al, 1987, 1989; Williamson et al, 1990). Such alpha spindles last 0.2 to 1 second and have a stable topography during this interval. When an alpha spindle is terminated, the new spindle frequently possesses a different topography (Lehmann, 1989; Lehmann et al, 1987).

These observations can be interpreted in terms of the following mechanisms. A transient decrease in LC activity results in an associated strengthening of the corticocortical system underpinning the regional and global resonances; that is, a shift in the neocortical operating point in the hypercoupled direction. This permits the emergence of sharply tuned regional and possibly global resonances. A feature of sharply tuned linear systems is an inverse relation between sharpness of the resonance peak and the rate at which the system characteristics change (Papoulis, 1977). The temporal stability of the alpha spindle is thus a consequence of the sharpness of the regional–global resonances that yield the alpha spindle. A subsequent transient surge of LC activity will decouple the system and thus eliminate the regional–global resonance condition and its associated alpha spindle. After the transient LC burst of activity, the decrease in neocortical NA levels permits the reestablishment of corticocortical coupling through layer 1, and the global–regional modes are reestablished. The new stable structure or eigenstate is determined by the spatial distribution of the B and Q parameters. Specifically, low B and high Q regions will form the boundary conditions for the new alpha spindle eigenstate. In conditions of low arousal, the onset of transient LC activity and the collapse of an alpha spindle correlate. Although I am not aware of published findings that address this issue directly, sleep spindles and LC activity appear synchronized in the rat. In a study reported by Aston-Jones and Bloom (1981), sleep spindles were synchronized with LC activity, with the onset of a burst of LC activity occurring before the termination of a sleep spindle. This finding is consistent with the idea that the sleep spindle is terminated by an increase in LC activity. The mechanisms responsible for the termination of a sleep spindle and an alpha spindle thus may be the same; that is, a transient surge of LC activity. Increases in LC activity also effect the thalamus by inhibiting the burst firing modes seen during sleep spindles and alpha activity (McCormick, 1992).

The slow scalp potentials associated with a range of cognitive and motor tasks (Birbaumer et al, 1990) also may be a manifestation of the effects of brain stem neuromodulators such as ACh. The possibility of cholinergic involvement in the genesis of slow potentials is supported by the findings of Pirch and associates

(1986), who noted that subdural applications of atropine, an ACh muscarinic blocker, powerfully reduce slow cortical potentials in the rat.

Some Cognitive and Clinical Speculations

Purposive behavior, cognition, and learning are three states that depend on the selective engagement of particular spatiotemporal patterns of neural activity (Engel et al, 1990; Gray et al, 1990). Examples of the spatiotemporal specificity of neural activation have been reported for sensory and motor tasks (Georgopoulos et al, 1993; Richmond and Optican, 1990; Richmond et al, 1990). Such spatiotemporal specificity is only consistent with the high-frequency local resonant modes, because only these modes can change their activity levels in the brief intervals in which information processing occurs. Furthermore, only high-frequency, local resonant modes have the spatial specificity consistent with the need to activate particular neocortical populations. Regional and global resonances do not have the required spatial specificity or capacity for rapid change that underlies the neural correlates of cognitive processes. Such modes are more consistent with low demand states such as the mu rhythm in conditions of muscle relaxation and the alpha rhythm in conditions of visual inattentiveness.

Why should the global–regional resonant modes appear during low arousal states? Why not electrical silence? Spontaneously active systems may have low-frequency oscillatory limit cycles as their lowest energy state (see Chapters 11 and 12). A complementary biological explanation suggests that the optimum operation of the brain depends on a continuous exchange of trophic substances between nerve cells. Neurotransmitters frequently serve multiple functions, such as a medium for information transmission and a trophic substance. Global–regional states thus may be an efficient way to prevent the emergence of local states and maintain the necessary interaction between nerve cells.

According to the proposed coupling model, the level of corticocortical coupling that determines the balance between local and global–regional states is a function of the activity of brain stem neuromodulators, which in turn depend on the behavioral state of the subject. The operating point, on the hypo- to hypercoupled continuum, of any part of the neocortex is then determined by the spatial distribution and activation of brain stem neuromodulators and their receptors. The motor cortex, supplementary motor cortex, and prefrontal cortex have the heaviest neocortical DA innervation (Foote and Morrison, 1987). This suggests that the operating point of these regions may be biased in the hypocoupled direction. Such biasing would be consistent with the need to rapidly elicit specific patterns of neural activity associated with motor behavior. The important role of DA, in biasing the motor and prefrontal cortex, is illustrated in an eye-movement study by Sawaguchi and Goldman-Rakic (1994). In that study, an oculomotor delayed-response task performed by a monkey deteriorated with the localized application of a DA_1 receptor blocker. In the context of this coupling model, this effect may be interpreted as the DA_1 blocker preventing the required corticocortical decoupling and associated activation of local resonances.

Low DA levels, found in such conditions as Parkinson disease, compromise rapid initiation of thoughts and actions. Consequently, symptoms of Parkinson disease are, in the context of our model, the manifestation of excessive hypercoupled states in those regions that depend heavily on DA to bias the operating modes. The EEG of Parkinsonian patients is characterized by increased slow-wave activity (Fungeld, 1989; Helkala et al, 1991; Soikkeli et al, 1991), which is also consistent with increased global–regional modes. The converse situation, of excess DA activity in the motor and supplementary motor cortex, could lead to the disorganized emergence of local states associated with specific motor manifestations. Tourette syndrome may be an example of such a situation, which manifests as tics or sudden unintended movements such as excessive blinking, grimacing, and vocalization (Corbett and Turpin, 1990). The tic frequency typically increases in association with elevated brain monoamine levels, leading to anxiety or arousal (Robertson, 1989; Handley and Dursun, 1992). The involvement of DA in Tourette syndrome is also suggested by the effectiveness of DA blocking to treat this condition (Cohen et al, 1980).

Neocortical regions operating in states of pathologic hypocoupling results in disorganized emergence of local resonant modes. The specific symptoms elicited by such aberrant local resonant modes would depend on the neocortical regions involved. Aberrant local resonant modes in the temporal and prefrontal cortex may manifest as psychotic states or disordered thought processes. The possibility that such disorders are a manifestation of hypocoupled states is supported by the findings that drugs that increase brain NA and DA levels may produce psychotic states (Jaffe, 1992). Drugs that block 5-HT could also permit the emergence of aberrant local resonances because this neuromodulator enhances global–regional resonant modes and suppresses local resonant modes. The specific manifestations of these aberrant modes would be determined by the neocortical regions most strongly affected by the 5-HT blockers. Drugs that block 5-HT release, such as LSD-25, tend to produce vivid visual hallucinations, a feature consistent with the high levels of 5-HT_2 receptors in the visual cortex.

Speculations on Schizophrenia and Aberrant Local Resonant Modes

In this section, the possibility that schizophrenia may be a manifestation of aberrant local resonant modes is discussed. As a preface to these discussions, it must be emphasized that this section constitutes the most speculative portion of a speculative chapter. It's inclusion is made on the grounds that it may yield a range of testable hypotheses in the disciplines of biological psychiatry and neuropsychiatry. Symptoms of schizophrenia are frequently classified into positive and negative categories. Negative symptoms are characterized by apathy, withdrawal, and emotional flattening, whereas positive symptoms are characterized by severe hallucinations, delusions, illogical thinking, and bizarre behavior (Andreasen et al,

1991; Mackert et al, 1991; Crow, 1985; Marneros and Andreasen, 1991). Negative symptoms may be associated with gross neuroanatomic changes such as cortical shrinkage and increases in ventricular size (Andreasen et al, 1991). The EEG associated with negative symptoms tends to be characterized by excessive theta and delta activity, with a reduction in alpha frequency (Guenther et al, 1988; Itil, 1980; Kemali et al, 1988). Persons with schizophrenia with predominantly negative symptoms tend to respond poorly to antipsychotic medication based on DA receptor blockers (Crow, 1985; Lieberman et al, 1991).

Persons with schizophrenia having positive symptoms, on the other hand, tend not to have such gross neuroanatomic changes, and they respond better to DA blocking agents (Carlson, 1987; Crow, 1980, 1985; Huber et al, 1980). When symptoms are positive, the EEG is more likely to be characterized by prominent high-frequency beta activity that is suggestive of excessive local modes (Itil, 1980; Karson et al, 1988; Kemali et al, 1988; Scarone et al, 1987). This high-frequency activity in persons with schizophrenia with positive symptoms is consistent with neocortical hypocoupled states and aberrant local resonant modes. Excess high-frequency activity also has been reported in asymptomatic children at risk from developing schizophrenia (Itil et al, 1974). The association of positive schizophrenic symptoms with hypocoupled states and aberrant local resonances is supported by findings of reduced responsiveness of patients with schizophrenia to photic drive or a steady-state visual flicker in the alpha frequency range (Jin et al, 1990; Ciorciari, 1994). In a study of five patients with schizophrenia with predominantly positive symptoms, Ciorciari (1994) reported that the occipital response to a 13-Hz visual flicker was normal or elevated, whereas the frontal response was severely attenuated. These findings are consistent with the idea that positive schizophrenia is associated with reduced global–regional resonance modes and increased local resonant modes, especially in the frontal cortex (low B, high Q). Dopamine receptor blockers are the most common drugs used to treat schizophrenia. A favorable response to these drugs is associated with decreased high-frequency activity and correspondingly increased in alpha activity (Itil, 1980). These electrophysiologic changes are consistent with the idea that DA blockers move the neocortical operating point in the hypercoupled direction.

Positive symptoms such as those found in schizophrenia have been reported when drugs such as amphetamines increase neocortical NA or DA levels (Jaffe, 1992; Leach, 1991), in temporal lobe epilepsy (Reynolds and Trimble, 1981; Trimble and Robertson, 1987), and in certain forms of narcolepsy (Douglass et al, 1991). Positive symptoms therefore may be a diagnostic categorization that covers a range of underlying causes. The neurophysiologic counterpart of this diagnostic categorization are aberrant local resonant modes. Such aberrant local resonant modes in the prefrontal cortex, temporal cortex, and the limbic system may yield positive symptoms of schizophrenia. Furthermore, the emergence of aberrant local resonant modes can be a direct or indirect consequence of disturbances to several neuromodulatory systems.

Although the role of DA has traditionally been considered central in schizophrenia with positive symptoms (Carlson, 1987; Crow, 1980, 1985; Joyce, 1993;

Mackay et al, 1982; Van Kammen et al, 1991), evidence also implicates excess NA activity with positive symptoms (Bird et al, 1979; Breier et al, 1990; Gomes et al, 1980; Kemali et al, 1988; Lake et al, 1980; Van Kammen et al, 1991; Horcnykiewicz, 1982). Kemali et al (1988) reported that cerebrospinal fluid levels of NA were higher in persons with schizophrenia and positive symptoms and that these levels were positively correlated with the amplitude of frontal beta EEG activity and negatively correlated with frontal alpha activity. More recently, Van Kammen and colleagues (1994) reported that brain NA levels were positively correlated with the rate of psychotic relapse after the withdrawal of DA blocking drugs. There has been renewed interest recently in the role of 5-HT disturbances in schizophrenia. The development of effective antipsychotic drugs that preferentially effect 5-HT rather than DA receptors suggests an important role for this neuromodulator (Meltzer, 1991).

Reports suggest a possible role for ACh in some forms of schizophrenia. Douglass and associates (1991) described five patients with a variant of narcolepsy with hallucinatory and other psychotic symptoms indistinguishable from positive schizophrenic symptoms. They suggest that these symptoms are a manifestations of "dream intrusions" into the waking state. The central role of ACh in rapid eye movement (REM) or dreaming sleep (Hobson, 1990), together with the findings of Douglass and associates (1991), suggests that disturbances in the cholinergic system may, infrequently, precipitate positive schizophrenic symptoms. This possibility is consistent the proposed model, because ACh facilitates the emergence of local resonant modes. The possible role of ACh in schizophrenia is also supported by findings of

- reduced REM latency in schizophrenia (Caldwell and Domino, 1967; Zarcone et al, 1975);
- statistically significant negative correlation between REM latency and plasma cholinesterase levels in persons with schizophrenia (Keshavan et al, 1992); and
- increased cholinergic cells in the NBM of patients with schizophrenia compared with age-matched psychiatric controls (Karson et al, 1991).

Compared with DA, the role of ACh in schizophrenia is controversial. A factor that may contribute to the uncertainty of the role of ACh in schizophrenia is that ACh overactivity may cause depression (Janowsky and Davis, 1979; Mesulam, 1988). Such depressive states yield symptoms that are common to negative schizophrenia and include affective flattening, loss of drive, and poverty of speech. That ACh overactivity may precipitate depressive psychotic states and negative-symptom schizophrenia was noted by Kanson and colleagues (1991) and is supported by some electrophysiologic observations. The contingent negative variation, a slow brain potential, is larger in depressed patients and those with negative symptoms of schizophrenia (Thier et al, 1986; Oke et al, 1994). Because cholinergic processes appear to play a central role in the genesis of slow cortical potentials (Pirch et al, 1986), enhanced slow potentials in depression and negative-symptom schizophrenia suggest ACh overactivity in these conditions. The possibility of ACh involvement in negative symptomatology schizophrenia is also suggested by the actions of Clozapine, a relatively new "atypical" antipsychotic drug which appears more effective in the treatment of negative symptoms (Meltzer 1991). In addition to blocking 5-HT_2 receptors, Clozapine is a powerful blocker of ACh muscarinic receptors (Seeman 1990).

That positive-symptomatology schizophrenia is the behavioral manifestation of aberrant local resonant modes suggests that any pathophysiologic mechanisms that can generate aberrant local resonant modes could cause such symptoms. Given the central roles of DA, NA, 5-HT, and ACh in setting the neocortical operating point, disturbances to any one or more of these neuromodulators could result in aberrant local modes that manifest as positive- (and sometimes negative-) symptom schizophrenia. We do not suggest that the neurochemical disturbances that may lead to schizophrenia are necessarily limited to abnormalities of these neuromodulatory systems (see Lieberman and Koreen, 1993). Any neurochemical disturbance that yields aberrant local resonant modes in the appropriate neocortical and subcortical structures may manifest as symptoms of schizophrenia.

Concluding Remarks

Researchers recognized the EEG effects of brain stem neuromodulators shortly after the EEG was discovered. Such effects are now generally interpreted in terms of membrane current mechanisms thought to underpin the rhythmic activity of neocortical and thalamic neurons. This chapter presents a conceptual framework that has emergent neocortical rhythmic properties at its focus. Central to this framework are the notions of global, regional, and local neocortical resonances whose properties are determined by a few control parameters. These control parameters describe both the level of corticocortical coupling (B) and local loop gain (Q). We suggest that these control parameters are determined by the balance of neuromodulator activity. Acetylcholine, NA, and DA may reduce corticocortical coupling and increase local loop gain, thereby facilitating local resonances. 5-Hydroxytryptamine may also play a complementary role in increasing corticocortical coupling and reducing local loop gain, thereby facilitating global and regional resonances. The possible relation between various neocortical resonance processes and cognitive–affective states suggests the feasibility of an explicit link between these control parameters, the EEG, and some disturbances of higher cortical function. The conceptual framework presented in this chapter, while admittedly speculative, should facilitate a growing dialogue between the often disparate fields of brain physics, neurochemistry, neuroanatomy, and neuropsychiatry. This dialogue will suggest new experiments which focus on measures of neocortical dynamic function.

Acknowledgments

The author would like to acknowledge the advice, encouragement and critical comments on earlier drafts of these chapters offered by Alex Sergejew, Ben

Ramsden, Fernando Lopes da Silva, Joseph Ciorciari and Pierre Etevenon. Peter Cadusch was especially helpful in frequent discussions and also derived the feedback model illustrated in Figure 13.8. Some components of chapter 13 were presented at the 2nd Pan Pacific Conference on Brain Electric and Magnetic Topography in Sydney Australia, in February 1994.

References

Andreasen, N.C., Flaum, M., Arndt, S., Alliger, R., and Swayzw, V.W. Positive and negative symptoms: Assessment and validity. In: *Negative Versus Positive Schizoprenia* (A. Marneros, Andreasen, N.C., and Tsuang, M.T., Eds.) New York: Springer-Verlag, pp. 28–51, 1991.

Ashby, C.R., Jr. and Wang, R.Y. Effects of antipsychotic drugs on 5-HT_2 receptors in the medial prefrontal cortex: Microiontophoretic studies. *Brain Res.* 506:346–348, 1990.

Aston-Jones, G. Behavioral functions of locus coeruleus derived from cellular attributes. *Physiological Psychology* 13:118–126, 1985.

Aston-Jones, G. and Bloom, F.E. Activity of norepinephrine-containing locus coeruleus neurons in behaving rats anticipates fluctuations in the sleep waking cycle. *J. Neurosci.* 1:876–886, 1981.

Azmittia, E.C. and Gannon, P.J. Anatomy of the serotonergic system in the primate and sub-primate brain. *Adv. Neurol.* 43:407–468, 1986.

Barbas, H. Pattern in the laminar origin of corticocortical connections. *J. Comp. Neurol.* 252:415–422, 1986.

Basar, E. *EEG Brain Dynamics: Relation Between EEG and Brain Evoked Potentials.* Amsterdam: Elsevier, 1980.

Basar, E., Basar-Eroglu, C., Parnefjord, R., Rahn, E., and Schurmann, M. Evoked potentials: Ensembles of brain induced rhythmicities in the alpha, theta and gamma ranges. In: *Induced Rhythms in the Brain* (E. Basar and Bullock, T.H., Eds.) Boston: Birkhauser, pp. 155–181, 1992.

Berger, B., Gaspar, P., and Verney, C. Dopaminergic innervation of the cerebral cortex: Unexpected differences between rodents and primates. *Trends in Neurosciences* 14:21–27, 1991.

Berger, B., Trottier, S., Verney, C., Gaspar, P., and Alvarez, C. Regional and laminar distribution of the dopamine and serotonin innervation in the macaque cerebral cortex: a radioautographic study. *J. Comp. Neurol.* 273:99–119, 1988.

Birbaumer, N., Elbert, T., Canavan, A.G.M., and Rockstroh, B. Slow potentials of the cerebral cortex and behavior. *Physiol. Rev.* 70:1–41, 1990.

Bird, E.D., Spokes, E.G., and Iversen, L.L. Brain norepinephrine and dopamine in schizophrenia. *Science* 204:93–94, 1979.

Bodis-Wollner, I. Visual deficits related to dopamine deficiency in experimental animals and Parkinson's disease patients. *Trends in Neurosciences* 13:296–302, 1990.

Brailowsky, S. Effects of melatonin on the photosensitive epilepsy of the baboon, Papio Papio. *EEG and Clin. Neurophysiol.* 41:314–319, 1976.

Breier, A., Wolkowitz, O.M., Roy, A., Potter, W.Z., and Pickar, D. Plasma norepinephrine in chronic schizophrenia. *Am. J. Psychiatry* 147:1467–1470, 1990.

Bressler, S.L., Coppola, R., and Nakamura, R. Episodic multiregional cortical coherence at multiple frequencies during visual task performance. *Nature* 366:153–156, 1993.

Brown, K.T. Physiology of the retina. In: *Medical Physiology* (V. B. Mountcastle, Ed.) Chicago: Mosby, pp. 504–543, 1980.

Buzsaki, G. The thalamic clock: Emergent network properties. *Neuroscience* 41:351–364, 1991.

Caldwell, D.F. and Domino, E.F. Electroencephalographic and eye movement patterns during sleep in chronic schizophrenic patients. *Electroencephalogr. Clin. Neurophysiol.* 22:414–420, 1967.

Carlson, A. The dopamine hypothesis of schizophrenia 20 years later. In: *Search for the Causes of Schizophrenia* (H. Hafner, Gattaz, W.H., and Janzarik, W., Eds.) Berlin: Springer-Verlag, pp. 223–235, 1987.

Cassone, V.M. Effects of melatonin on vertebrate circadian systems. *Trends in Neurosciences* 11:457–464, 1990.

Celesia, G.C. and Jasper, H.H. Acetylcholine released from cerebral cortex in relation to state of activation. *Neurology* 16:1053–1083, 1966.

Ciorciari, J. Brain electrical activity topography in schizophrenia. Unpublished PhD thesis. Swinburne University of Technology, 1994.

Cohen, D.J., Detlor, J., Young, J.B., and Shaywitz, B.A. Clonidine ameliorates Gilles de la Tourette syndrome. *Arch. Gen. Psychiatry* 37:1350–1357, 1980.

Corbett, J.A. and Turpin, G. Tics and Tourette's syndrome. In: *Children and Adolescent Psychiatry, Modern Approaches, 2nd Ed.* (M. Rutter and Hersov, L., Eds.) Oxford: Blackwell Scientific Publications, pp. 516–525, 1990.

Crow, T.J. Positive and negative symptoms and the role of dopamine. *Br. J. Psychiatry.* 137:383–386, 1980.

Crow, T.J. Two syndromes in schizophrenia? In: *Transmitters in Action.* (D. Bousfield, Ed.) New York: Elsevier, pp. 279–285, 1985.

Douglass, A.B., Hays, P., Pazderka, F., and Russell, J.M. Florid refractory schizophrenias that turn out to be treatable variants of HLA-associated narcolepsy. *J. Nerv. Ment. Dis.* 179:12–17, 1991.

Engel, A.K., Konig, P., Gray, C.M., and Singer, W. Stimulus dependent neuronal oscillations in cat visual cortex: Intercolumnar interactions as determined by cross-correlation analysis. *Eur. J. Neurosci.* 2:586–606, 1990.

Fellerman, D.J. and Van Essen, D.C. Distributed hierarchical processing in the primate cerebral cortex. *Cerebral Cortex* 1:1–47, 1991.

Foote, S.L., Bloom, F.E., and Aston-Jones, G. Nucleus locus ceruleus: New evidence of anatomical and physiological specificity. *Physiol. Rev.* 63:844–914, 1983.

Foote, S.L. and Morrison, J.H. Extrathalamic modulation of cortical function. *Ann. Rev. Neurosci.* 10:67–95, 1987.

Foster, J.A. Intracortical origin of recruiting responses in the cat cortex. *Electroencephalogr. Clin. Neurophysiol.* 48:639–653, 1980.

Freeman, W.J. *Mass Action in the Nervous System.* New York: Academic Press, 1975.

Freeman, W.J. Predictions on neocortical dynamics derived from studies in palepcortex. In: *Induced Rhythms in the Brain* (E. Basar and Bullock, T.H., Eds.) Boston: Birkhauser, pp. 183–199, 1992.

Fungeld, E.W. Spectral and frequency analysis of the central EEG activity in Parkinson's disease patients with Alzheimer's disease: The development during nootropic therapy. In: *Topographic Brain Mapping of EEG and Evoked Potentials.* (K. Maurer, Ed.) Berlin: Springer-Verlag, pp. 233–240, 1989.

Georgopoulos, A.P., Taira, M., and Lukashin, A. Cognitive neurophysiology of the motor cortex. *Science* 260:47–52, 1993.

Gomes, U.C.R., Shanley, B.C., Potgieter, L., et al. Noradrenergic overactivity in chronic schizophrenia: Evidence based on cerebrospinal fluid noradrenaline and cyclic nucleotide concentrations. *Br. J. Psychiatry* 137:346–351, 1980.

Gray, C.M., Engel, A.K., Konig, P., and Singer, W. Stimulus-dependent neuronal oscillations in cat visual cortex: Receptive field properties and feature dependence. *Eur. J. Neurosci.* 2:607–619, 1990.

Guenther, W., Davous, P., Godet, J.L., Guillibert, F., Brietling, D., and Rondot, P. Bilateral brain dysfunction during motor activation in type II schizophrenia measured by EEG mapping. *Biol. Psychiatry* 23:295–311, 1988.

Handley, S.L. and Dursun, S.M. Serotonin and Tourette's syndrome: Movements such as head-shakes and wet-dog shakes may model human Tics. In: *Serotonin, CNS Receptors and Brain Function* (P.B. Bradley, Handley, S.L., Cooper, S.J., Key, B.J., Barnes, N.M., and Coote, J.H., Eds.) New York: Pergamon Press, pp. 235–253, 1992.

Helkala, E.-L., Laulumaa, V., Soikkeli, R., Partanen, J., Soininen, H., and Riekkinen, P.J. Slow-wave activity in the spectral analysis of the electroencephalogram is associated with cortical dysfunctions in patients with Alzheimer's disease. *Behav. Neurosci.* 105:409–415, 1991.

Herkenhamm, M. New perspectives on the organization and evolution of nonspecific thalamocortical projections. In: *Cerebral Cortex, Volume 5* (E.G. Jones and Peters, A., Eds.) New York: Plenum Publishing, pp. 403–445, 1986.

Herning, R.I., Jones, R.T., Hooker, W.D., Mendelson, J., and Blackwell, L. Cocain increases EEG beta: A replication and extension of Hans Berger's historic experiments. *Electroencephalogr. Clin. Neurophysiol.* 60:470–477, 1985.

Hobson, J.A. Sleep and dreaming. *J. Neurosci.* 10:371–382, 1990.

Hornykiewicz, O. Brain catecholamines in schizophrenia—a good case for noradrenaline. *Nature* 299:484–485, 1982.

Houser, C.R., Vaughn, J.E., Hendry, S.H.C., Jones, E.G., and Peters, A. GABA neurons in the cerebral cortex. In: *Cerebral Cortex, Volume 2.* (A. Peters and Jones, E.G., Eds.) pp. 63–89, 1984.

Itil, T.M. Computer-analyzed electroencephalogram to predict the therapeutic outcome in schizophrenia. In: *Perspectives in Schizophrenia Research* (C. Baxter and Melnechuk, T., Eds.) New York: Raven Press, pp. 61–80, 1980.

Itil, T.M., Hsu, W., Saletu, B., and Mednick, S. Computer EEG and auditory evoked potential investigations in children at high risk for schizophrenia. *Am. J. Psychiatry* 131:892–900, 1974.

Jacobs, B.L. and Azmitia, E. Structure and function of the brain serotonin system. *Physiol. Rev.* 72:165–229, 1992.

Jacobs, B.L. and Fornal, C.A. 5-HT and motor control: A hypothesis. *Trends in Neurosciences* 16:346–352, 1993.

Jaffe, J.H. Drug addiction and drug abuse. In: *The Pharmacological Basis of Therapeutics.* (A.G. Gilman, Rall, T.W., Nies, A.S., and Taylor, P., Eds.) New York: McGraw-Hill, pp. 522–573, 1992.

Janowsky, D.S. and Davis, J.M. Psychological effects of cholinomimetic agents. In: *Brain Acetylcholine and Neuropsychiatric Disease* (K.L. Davis and Berger, P.A., Eds.) New York: Plenum Press, pp. 3–14, 1979.

Jasper, H.H. Unspecified thalamocortical relations. In: *Handbook of Psychology, Neurophysiology Section* (H.W. Magoun, Ed.) Baltimore: Williams & Wilkins, 1960.

Jin, Y., Potkin, S.G., Rice, D., Sramek, J., Costa, J., Isenhart, R., Heh, C., and Sandman,

C.A. Abnormal EEG responses to photic stimulation in schizophrenic patients. *Schizophr. Bull.* 16:627–634, 1990.

Jobert, M., Poiseau, E., Jahnig, P., Schultz, H., and Kubicki, S. Topographical analysis of sleep spindle activity. *Neuropsychobiology* 26:210–217, 1992.

Jones, E.G. Connectivity of the primate sensory-motor area. In: *Cerebral Cortex, Volume* 5. (E.G. Jones and Peters, A., Eds.) New York: Plenum Publishing, pp. 113–183, 1986.

Jones, E.G. Identification and classification of intrinsic circuit elements in the neocortex. In: *Dynamic Aspects of Neocortical Function.* (G.M. Edelman, Gall, W.E., and Cowan, W.M., Eds.) Chicago: Wiley, pp. 7–40, 1984.

Jones, E.G. *The Thalamus.* New York: Plenum Press, 1985.

Joyce, J.N. The dopamine hypothesis of schizophrenia: Limbic interactions with serotonin and norepinephrine. *Psychopharmacology* 112:S16–S34, 1993.

Karson, C.N., Coppola, R., Daniel, D.G., and Weinberger, D.R. Computerized EEG in schizophrenia. *Schizophr. Bull.* 14:193–197, 1988.

Karson, C.N., Garcia-Rill, E., Biedermann, J., Mrak, R.E., Husain, M.M., and Skinner, R.D. The brain stem reticular formation in schizophrenia. *Psychiatry Res.* 40:31–48, 1991.

Kemali, D., Galderisi, S., and Maj, M. EEG correlates of clinical heterogeneity of schizophrenia. In: *The EEG of Mental Activities.* (D. Giannitrapani and Murri, L., Eds.) Basel: Karger, pp. 169–181, 1988.

Keshavan, M.S., Mahadik, S.P., Reynolds, C.F., Mukerjee, S., Korenovsky, A., Houck, P., and Jarrett, D.B. Plasma cholinesterase isozymes and REM latency in schizophrenia. *Psychiatry Res.* 43:23–29, 1992.

Krause, D.N., and Dubocovich, M.L. Regulatory sites in the melatonin system of mammals. *Trends in Neurosciences* 13:464–470, 1990.

Lake, C.R., Sternberg, D., van Kammen, D.P., Ballenger, F.C., Zielger, M.G., Post, R.M., Kopin, J.F., and Bunney, W.E. Schizophrenia: Elevated cerebrospinal fluid norepinephrine. *Science* 207:331–333, 1980.

Leach, A.M. Stimulants and psychosis. *Current Opinion in Psychiatry* 4:47–50, 1991.

Lehmann, D. Microstates of the brain in EEG and ERP mapping studies. In: *Springer Series in Brain Dynamics* 2. (E. Basar and Bullock, T.H., Eds.) Berlin: Springer-Verlag, pp. 72–83, 1989.

Lehmann, D., Ozaki, H., and Pal, I. EEG Alpha map series: Brain microstates by space-oriented adaptive segmentation. *Electroencephalogr. Clin. Neurophysiol.* 67:271–288, 1987.

Lieberman, J.A., Jody, D., Alvir, J.M.J., Borenstein, M., Mayerhoff, D.I., Geisler, S., Szymanski, S., Gonzales, A., Bogerts, B., and Ashtari, M. Negative symptoms in schizophrenia: Relationship to positive symptoms and outcome. In: *Negative Versus Positive Schizoprenia* (A. Marneros, Andreasen, N.C., and Tsuang, M.T., Eds.) New York: Springer-Verlag, pp. 109–125, 1991.

Lieberman, J.A. and Koreen, A.R. Neurochemistry and neuroendocrinology of schizophrenia: A selective review. *Schizophr. Bull.* 19:371–429, 1993.

Llinas, R.R. Oscillations in CNS neurons: A possible role for cortical interneurons in the generation of 40-Hz oscillations. In: *Induced Rhythms in the Brain* (E. Basar and Bullock, T.H., Eds.) Boston: Birkhauser, pp. 269–283, 1992.

Llinas, R.R. and Ribary, U. Coherent 40-Hz oscillation characterizes dream state in humans. *Proc. Natl. Acad. Sci. USA.* 90:2078–2081, 1993.

Llinas, R.R. and Ribary, U. Rostrocaudal scan in human brain: A global characteristic of the 40-Hz response during sensory input. In: *Induced Rhythms in the Brain* (E. Basar and Bullock, T.H., Eds.) Boston: Birkhauser, pp. 147–154, 1992.

Lopes da Silva, F.H. Neural mechanisms underlying brain waves: From neural membranes to networks. *Electroencephalogr. Clin. Neurophysiol.* 79:81–93, 1991.

Lopes da Silva, F.H., Vos, F. E., Mooibroek, F., and Van Rotterdam, A. Relative contribution of intracortical and thalamo-cortical processes in the generation of alpha rhythms, revealed by partial coherence analysis. *Electroencephalogr. Clin. Neurophysiol.* 50:449–456, 1980.

Loring, D., Sheer, D.E., and Largen, J. Forty Hertz EEG activity in dementia of Alzheimer type and multi-infarct dementia. *Psychophysiology* 22:121–166, 1985.

Mackay, A.V.P., Iversoen, L.L., Rossor, M., Spokes, E., Bird, E., Arregui, A., Creese, I., and Snyder, S.H. Increased brain dopamine and dopamine receptors in schizophrenia. *Arch. Gen. Psychiatry* 39:991–997, 1982.

Mackert, A., Fletchtner, K.-M., Woyth, C., and Frick, K. Increased blink rates in schizophrenia: Influence of neuroleptics and psychopathology. *Schizophrenia Research* 4:41–47, 1991.

Mamounas, L.A., Wilson, M.A., Axt, K.J., and Molliver, M.E. Morphological aspects of serotonergic innervation. In: *Serotonin, CNS Receptors and Brain Function* (P.B. Bradley, Handley, S.L., Cooper, S.J., Key, B.J., Barnes, N.M., and Coote, J.H., Eds.) New York: Pergamon Press, pp. 97–118, 1992.

Marneros, A. and Andreasen, N.C. Positive and negative symptomatology: The state of affairs. In: *Negative Versus Positive Schizoprenia* (A. Marneros, Andreasen, N.C., and Tsuang, M.T., Eds.) New York: Springer-Verlag, pp. 441–460, 1991.

Marshall, K.C. and Finlayson, P.G. Synaptic regulation of locus coeruleus neuronal activity. In: *Neurotransmitters and Cortical Function* (M. Avoli, Reader, T.A., Dykes, R.E., and Gloo, P., Eds.) New York: Plenum Press, pp. 373–390, 1988.

Maunsell, J.H.R. and Van Essen, D.C. The connections of the middle temporal visual area (MT) and their relationship to a cortical hierarchy in the macaque monkey. *J. Neurosci.* 3:2563–2586, 1983.

McCormick, D.A. Cellular mechanisms of cholinergic control of neocortical and thalamic neuronal excitability. In: *Brain Cholinergic Systems* (M. Steriade and Biesold, D., Eds.) New York: Oxford University Press, pp. 236–264, 1990.

McCormick, D.A. Neurotransmitter actions in the thalamus and cerebral cortex and their role in neuromodulation of thalamocortical activity. *Prog. Neurobiol.* 39:337–388, 1992.

McCormick, D.A. and Prince, D.A. Postsynaptic actions of acetylcholine in the mammalian brain in vitro. In: *Neurotransmitters and Cortical Function* (M. Avoli, Reader, T.A., Dykes, R.E., and Gloo, P., Eds.) New York: Plenum Press, pp. 287–302, 1988.

Meltzer, H.Y. The mechanism of action of novel antipsychotic drugs. *Schizophr. Bull.* 17:263–287, 1991.

Mesulam, M.-M. Central cholinergic pathways: Neuroanatomy and some behavioral implications. In: *Neurotransmitters and Cortical Function* (M. Avoli, Reader, T.A., Dykes, R.E., and Gloo, P., Eds.) New York: Plenum Press, pp. 237–260, 1988.

Mesulam, M.-M., Hersh, L.B., Mash, D.C., and Geula, C. Differential cholinergic innervation within functional subdivisions of the human cerebral cortex: A choline acetyltransferase study. *J. Comp. Neurol.* 318:316–328, 1992.

Midtgaard, J. Processing of information from different sources: Spatial synaptic integration in the dendrites of vertebrate CNS neurons. *Trends in Neurosciences* 17:166–173, 1994.

Miles, A. and Philbrick, D.R.S. Melatonin and psychiatry. *Biol. Psychiatry* 23:405–425, 1988.

Mitzdorf, U. Current source-density method and application in cat cerebral cortex: Investigation of evoked potentials and EEG phenomena. *Physiol. Rev.* 65:37–100, 1985.

Mock, H. and Kunkel, H. EEG-profile of mepindolol as compared to diazepam and placebo. In: *Electroencephalography in Drug Research* (W.M. Herrmann, Ed.) London: Gustav Fischer-Butterworths, pp. 509–521, 1982.

Montaron, M.F., Bouyer, J.J., Rougeul, A., and Buser, P. Ventral mesencephalic tegmentum (VMT) controls electrocortical beta rhythms and associated attentive behaviour in the cat. *Behav. Brain Res.* 59:978–996, 1982.

Morrison, R.S. and Bassett, D.L. Electrical activity of the thalamus and basal ganglia in decorticate cats. *J. Neurophysiol.* 8:309–314, 1945.

Mulligan, K.A. and Tork, I. Serotonergic innervation of the cat cerebral cortex. *J. Comp. Neurol.* 270:86–110, 1988.

Nunez, P.L. Generation of human EEG by a combination of long and short range neocortical interactions. *Brain Topography* 1:199–215, 1989.

Oke, S., Saatchi, R., Allen, E., Hudson, N.R., and Jervis, B.W. The contingent negative variation in positive and negative types of schizophrenia. *Am. J. Psychiatry* 151:432–433, 1994.

Pandya, D.N. and Yeterian, E.H. Architecture and connections of cortical association areas. In: *Cerebral Cortex, Volume 4.* (A. Peters and Jones, E.G., Eds.) New York: Plenum Publishing, pp. 3–61, 1985.

Papoulis, A. *Signal Analysis.* New York: McGraw-Hill, 1977.

Pfurtscheller, G. and Aranibar, A. Event-related cortical desynchronization detected by power measurements of scalp EEG. *Electroencephalogr. Clin. Neurophysiol.* 42:817–826, 1977.

Pfurtscheller, G. and Klimesch, W. Topographic display and interpretation of event-related desynchronization during a visual-verbal task. *Brain Topography* 3:85–93, 1990.

Pfurtscheller, G. and Neuper, C. Simultaneous EEG 10Hz desynchronization and 40Hz synchronization during finger movements. *Neurology Report* 3:1057–1060, 1992.

Pinault, D. and Deschenes, M. Control of 40-Hz firing of reticular thalamic cells by neurotransmitters. *Neuroscience* 51:259–268, 1992A.

Pinault, D. and Deschenes, M. Voltage-dependent 40-Hz oscillations in rat reticular thalamic neurons in vivo. *Neuroscience* 51:245–258, 1992B.

Pirch, J.H., Corbus, M.J., Rigdon, G.C., and Lyness, W.H. Generation of cortical event-related slow potentials in the rat involves nucleus basalis cholinergic innervation. *Electroencephalogr. Clin. Neurophysiol.* 63:464–475, 1986.

Reynolds, E.H. and Trimble, M.R. *Epilepsy and Psychiatry.* London: Churchill Livingstone, 1981.

Richmond, B.J. and Optican, L.M. Temporal encoding of two-dimensional patterns by single units in primary visual cortex II. Information transmission. *J. Neurophysiol.* 64:370–380, 1990.

Richmond, B.J., Optican, L.M., and Spitzer, H. Temporal encoding of two-dimensional patterns by single units in primary visual cortex. I. Stimulus-response relations. *J. Neurophysiol.* 64:351–369, 1990.

Riekkinen, P., Buzsaki, G., Riekkinen, P., Soininen, H., and Partanen, J. The cholinergic system and EEG slow waves. *Electroencephalogr. Clin. Neurophysiol.* 78:89–96, 1991.

Robertson, M.M. The Gilles de la Tourette syndrome: The current status. *Br. J. Psychiatry*. 154:147–169, 1989.

Rogawski, M.A. New directions in neurotransmitter action: Dopamine provides some important clues. *Trends in Neurosciences*. 10:200–205, 1987.

Rougeul-Buser, A. Monoamines, cortical rhythms and attentive behaviour in cat. In: *Modulation of Sensorimotor Activity During Alterations in Behavioral States* (R. Bandler, Ed.) New York: Alan R. Liss, pp. 139–149, 1984.

Sato, H., Fox, K., and Daw, N.W. Effect of electrical stimulation of locus coeruleus on the activity of neurons in the cat visual cortex. *J. Neurophysiol*. 62:946–958, 1989.

Sawaguchi, T. and Goldman-Rakic, P.S. The role of D1-dopamine receptor in working memory: Local injections of dopamine antagonists into the prefrontal cortex of rhesus monkeys performing an oculomotor delayed-response task. *J. Neurophysiol*. 71:515–528, 1994.

Sawaguchi, T., Matsumura, M., and Kubota, K. Catecholamine sensitivities of motor cortical neurons of the monkey. *Neurosci. Lett*. 66:135–140, 1986.

Sayers, B. The mechanism of auditory evoked EEG responses. *Nature* 247:481–483, 1974.

Scarone, S., Gambini, O., Colombo, C., Cattaneo, R., Bellodi, L., and Pugnetti, L. Electrophysiological characteristics of hemispheric functioning in schizophrenic disorders: Diagnostic and pathophysiological correlates. In: *Cerebral Dynamics, Laterality and Psychopathology* (R. Takahashi, Flor-Henry, P., Gruzelier, J., and Niwa, S., Eds.) New York: Elsevier, pp. 115–124, 1987.

Seeman, P. Atypical neuroleptics: role of multiple receptors, endogenous dopamine, and receptor linkage. *Acta. Psychiatr. Scand*. 82(Suppl.358):14–20, 1990.

Sheer, D.E. Biofeedback training of 40Hz EEG and behavior. In: *Biofeedback and Self-Control* (J. Kamiya, Barber, T.X., Miller, N.E., Shapiro, D., and Styva, J., Eds.) Chicago: Aldine, pp. 435–472, 1976.

Sheer, D.E. Focussed arousal, 40Hz EEG and dysfunction. In: *Self-Regulation of the Brain and Behavior* (T. Elbert, Rockstroh, B., Lutzenberger, W., and Birbaumer, N., Eds.) New York: Springer, pp. 63–84, 1984.

Sheer, D.E. Sensory and cognitive 40Hz event-related potential: Behavioral correlates, brain function and clinical application. In: *Springer Series in Brain Dynamics* (E. Basar and Bullock, T.H., Eds.) New York: Springer, pp. 339–374, 1989.

Silberstein, R.B., Ciorciari, J., and Pipingas, A. Steady state visually evoked potential topography during the Wisconsin card sorting test. *Electroencephalogr. Clin. Neurophysiol*. (In press), 1994.

Silberstein, R.B., Schier, M.A., Pipingas, A., Ciorciari, J., Wood, S.R., and Simpson, D.G. Steady state visually evoked potential topography associated with a visual vigilance task. *Brain Topography* 3:337–347, 1990.

Smiley, J.F., Williams, S.M., Szigeti, K., and Goldman-Rakic, P.S. Light and electron microscopic characterization of dopamine-immunoreactive axons in human cerebral cortex. *J. Comp. Neurol*. 321:325–335, 1992.

Soikkeli, R., Partanen, J., Soininen, H., Paakkonen, A., and Riekkinen P. Sr. Slowing of EEG in Parkinson's disease. *Electroencephalogr. Clin. Neurophysiol*. 79:159–165, 1991.

Spinweber, C.L., Ursin, R., Hilbert, R.P., and Hilderbrand, R.L. L-Tryptophan: Effects on daytime sleep latency and the waking EEG. *Electroencephalogr. Clin. Neurophysiol*. 55:652–661, 1983.

Stankov, B., Fraschini, F., and Reiter, R.J. Melatonin binding sites in the central nervous system. *Brain Research Reviews* 16:245–256, 1991.

Steriade, M. Alertness, quiet sleep, dreaming. In: *Cerebral Cortex, Volume* 9 (A. Peters, Ed.) New York: Plenum Publishing, pp. 279–357, 1991.

Steriade, M. Spindling, incremental thalamocortical responses, and spike-wave epilepsy. In: *Generalized Epilepsy* (M. Avoli, Gloo, P., Kostopoulos, G., and Naquet, R., Eds.) Boston: Birkhauser, pp. 161–180, 1990.

Steriade, M. and Deschenes, M. The thalamus as a neuronal oscillator. *Brain Research Reviews* 8:1–63, 1984.

Steriade, M., Dossi, R.C., and Nunez, A. Network modulation of a slow intrinsic oscillation of cat thalamocortical neurons implicated in sleep delta waves: Cortically induced synchronization and brainstem cholinergic suppression. *J. Neurosci.* 11:3200–3217, 1991A.

Steriade, M., Dossi, R.C., Pare, D., and Oaken, G. Fast oscillations (20–40 Hz) in thalamocortical systems and their potentiation by mesopontine cholinergic nuclei in the cat. *Proc. Natl. Acad. Sci. USA.* 88:4396–4400, 1991B.

Steriade, M., Gloor, P., Llinas, R.R., Lopes da Silva, F.H., and Mesulam, M.-M. Basic mechanisms of cerebral rhythmic activities. *Electroencephalogr. Clin. Neurophysiol.* 76:481–508, 1990.

Steriade, M., Oakson, G., and Diallo, A. Cortically elicited spike-wave discharge in thalamic neurons. *Electroencephalogr. Clin. Neurophysiol.* 41:641–644, 1976.

Tanaka, E. and North, R.A. Actions of 5-hydroxytryptamine on neurons of the rat cingulate cortex. *J. Neurophysiol.* 69:1749–1757, 1993.

Thier, P., Axmann, D., and Giedke, H. Slow brain potentials and psychomotor retardation in depression. *Electroencephalogr. Clin. Neurophysiol.* 63:570–581, 1986.

Tiitinen, H., Sinkkonen, J., Reinikainen, K., Alho, K., Lavikainen, J., and Naatanen, R. Selective attention enhances the auditory 40-Hz transient responses in humans. *Nature* 364:59–60, 1993.

Trimble, M.R. and Roberston, M.R. Laterality and psychopathology: Recent findings in epilepsy. In: *Cerebral Dynamics, Laterality and Psychopathology* (R. Takahashi, Flor-Henry, P., Gruzelier, J., and Niwa, S., Eds.) New York: Elsevier, pp. 359–369, 1987.

Van Kammen, D.P., Agren, H., Yao, J.K., O'Connor, D.T., Gurklis, J., and Peters, J.L. Noradrenergic activity and prediction of psychotic relapse following haloperidol withdrawal in schizophrenia. *Am. J. Psychiatry* 151:379–384, 1994.

Van Kammen, D.P., Mouton, A., Kelley, M., Breeding, W., and Peters, J.L. Explorations of dopamine and noradrenaline activity and negative symptoms in schizophrenia: Concepts and controversies. In: *Negative Versus Positive Schizoprenia* (A. Marneros, Andreasen, N.C., and Tsuang, M.T., Eds.) New York: Springer-Verlag, pp. 317–340, 1991.

Vogt, B.A. The role of layer I in cortical function. In: *Cerebral Cortex, Volume 9.* (A. Peters and Jones, E.G., Eds.) New York: Plenum Publishing, pp. 49–80, 1991.

Wassle, H. and Boycott, B.B. Functional architecture of the mammalian retina. *Physiol. Rev.* 71:447–480, 1991.

Williamson, S.J., Wang, J.Z., and Ilmoniemi, R.J. Method for locating sources of alpha activity. In: *Advances in Biomagnetism* (S.J. Williamson, Hoke, M., Stroink, G., and Kotani, M., Eds.) New York: Plenum Press, pp. 257–260, 1990.

Wilson, H.R. and Cowan, J.D. A mathematical theory of the functional dynamics of cortical and thalamic nervous tissue. *Kybernetik* 13:55–80, 1973.

Wong, R.K.S., Prince, D.A., and Basbaum, A.J. Intradendritic recordings from hippocampal neurons. *Proc. Natl. Acad. Sci. U.S.A.* 76:986–990, 1979.

Wright, J.J. and Liley, D.T.J. A millimetric scale simulation of electrocortical wave dynamics based on anatomical estimates of cortical synaptic density. *Network: computation in neural systems.* 5:191–202, 1994.

14

Statistical Mechanics of Multiple Scales of Neocortical Interactions

LESTER INGBER

General Philosophy

In many complex systems, as spatial-temporal scales of observation increase, new phenomena arise through synergistic interactions among smaller-scale entities (perhaps more properly called "quasi-entities") that explain much observed data in a parsimonious, usually mathematically esthetic, manner (Haken, 1983; Nicolis and Prigogine, 1973). For example, in classical thermodynamics of equilibrium systems, we can move from microscopic molecular scales to macroscopic scales, using the macroscopic concept of temperature to describe the average kinetic energy of microscopic molecular activity or the macroscopic concept of pressure to describe the average rate of change of momentum per unit area of microscopic molecules bombarding a cavity wall.

However, many complex systems are not in equilibrium, being driven by nonlinear and stochastic interactions of many external and internal degrees of freedom. For these systems, classical thermodynamic concepts typically do not apply (Ma, 1985). For example, descriptions of weather and ocean patterns, which try to include important features such as turbulence, rely on semiphenomenologic mesoscopic models that correlate with molecular theories but cannot be derived rigorously from them. Phase transitions in magnetic systems, and many systems similarly modeled (Ma, 1976; Wilson, 1979; Wilson and Kogurt, 1974), require careful treatment of a continuum of scales near critical points. Generally, rather than having a general theory of nonequilibrium nonlinear process, several approaches overlap that are typically geared to classes of systems, usually expanding on nonlinear treatments of stochastic systems (Gardiner, 1983; Haken, 1983; Kubo et al, 1973; Nicolis and Prigogine, 1973; van Kampen, 1981). Many biological systems yield phenomena at overlapping spatial-temporal scales. For example, the coiling of DNA is reasonably approached by blending microscopic molecular-dynamic calculations with mesoscopic diffusion equations to study angular winding

(Cartling, 1989). These approaches have been directed to study electroencephalography (EEG) (Basar, 1980) and other biological systems (Goel and Richter-Dyn, 1974).

Therefore, it is not surprising that the complex human brain supports many phenomena arising at different spatial-temporal scales. What is perhaps surprising is that we are apparently able to study truly macroscopic neocortical phenomena such as EEG using a chain of arguments dealing with overlapping microscopic and mesoscopic scales. A series of papers has developed this statistical mechanics of neocortical interactions (SMNI) (Ingber, 1981a, 1982, 1983a, 1984a, 1985a, 1985b, 1985c, 1986a, 1988a, 1988b, 1988c, 1991a, 1992, 1993a; Ingber and Nunez, 1990). This approach allows us to identify models of EEG whose variables and parameters are reasonably identified with ensembles of synaptic and neuronal interactions. This approach was made possible by developments in mathematical physics since the late 1970s in the field of nonlinear nonequilibrium statistical mechanics. This theory originates in quantum and gravitational field theory.

As discussed in Chapter 10, many physical systems have different degrees of theoretical support leading to Fokker-Planck partial differential equation descriptions. Here new problems arise in nonlinear nonequilibrium systems, often requiring modeling with a nonconstant coefficient of the second-derivative "diffusion" term. The spatial second-derivative term usually represents the kinetic energy when the first derivative represents the momentum in the differential equation description of a system. It was noticed early that similar treatment of the gravitational equation (DeWitt, 1957) required a modification of the potential term of the corresponding Lagrangian. We now better understand the mathematical and physical similarities between classical stochastic processes described by Fokker-Planck equations and quantum processes described by the Schrödinger equation (Langouche et al, 1982). The Lagrangian, essentially equal to the kinetic energy minus the potential energy, to first order in an expansion about the most probable state of a quantum or stochastic system, provides a global formulation and generalization of the relation force equals mass times acceleration (Feynman et al, 1963). In the neocortex, the velocity corresponds to the rate of firing of a column of neurons, and a potential is derived that includes nearest-neighbor interactions between columns. The Lagrangian formulation also accounts for the influence of fluctuations about such most probable paths of the evolution of a system, by using a variational principle associated with its development. Therefore the Lagrangian is often more useful than the Hamiltonian, which is equal to the kinetic energy plus the potential energy. As we will demonstrate, this is especially useful to obtain information about the system without solving the time-dependent Fokker-Planck equation; however, we will also describe neocortical phenomena that require the full solution.

In its differential form, the momentum is proportional to the derivative operator. For classical systems, the coefficient of the square of the momentum is twice the diffusion, such as the second moment of a probability distribution that describes some systems. The introduction of a nonconstant coefficient of even the first-derivative term requires careful treatment. Such a problem arises for a charged particle in an electromagnetic field (Schulman, 1981), which was first treated by physical arguments to enforce "minimal coupling," whereby the momentum p is simply replaced by p − Ae/c, where A is the electromagnetic potential, e is the electric charge, and c is the speed of light. Minimal coupling excludes other A^2 terms from appearing in the equation of evolution, such as Schrödinger's equation. Such problems are related to the operator-ordering of the derivative operators with respect to their nonconstant coefficients. For classical systems, the analogous expression to Ae/c is the drift—the first moment of a probability distribution describing some systems. In neocortex, we derive nonlinear expressions for both the drift and diffusion, for example. The detailed mathematical relation to the physical content of these issues was only clarified in the late 1970s and early 1980s, and is relevant to the mathematics of the neocortex. The first real breakthrough was achieved by noting how these issues should be treated in the context of classical nonlinear nonequilibrium statistical mechanics (Graham, 1977a; Graham, 1977b).

Although these new mathematical physics techniques have been applied in quantum and classical statistical mechanics (Ingber, 1983b, 1984b, 1986b), we are not merely bringing techniques to neuroscience from other disciplines for the sake of curiosity. Indeed, the contention appears to be well supported that a mathematical investigation of the neocortex demands these mathematical techniques to such an extent that it can be argued that, if the neocortex had been studied and sufficient data collected before the mathematical development of quantum or gravitational theory, then these mathematical techniques might have been developed in neuroscience first. The brain is sufficiently complex that it requires the same tools that are used for similarly complex physical systems. In many ways, we may consider the brain as the prototypical information-processing system, and the mathematical techniques used here may be viewed rigorously as filters to describe the processing of this information.

This statistical-mechanics approach, at many junctions in its development, may be intuitively compared with the approach used in simple magnetic systems, a comparison made early in neuronal modeling (Cragg and Temperley, 1954). Although we must be cautious to respect the integrity of the neocortical system, such comparisons can be useful pedagogically. The mathematical approach presented here also has been useful to describe phenomena in social systems, ranging from military command, control, and communications (Ingber 1991b, 1993b; Ingber et al, 1991; Ingber and Sworder, 1991), to political systems (Weidlich and Haag, 1983), to pricing bonds on financial markets (Ingber, 1984c, 1990; Ingber et al, 1991). In this context, the activity of neurons may resemble the activity of a throng of people, in which interactions occur at multiple hierarchical levels (Bullock, 1980). The numeric algorithms used in SMNI were developed, in part, in the process of investigating these other systems.

Top-down Versus Bottom-up

This admittedly complex technical approach can be presented in at least two ways. First, summarizing material presented in Chapters 2 and 11, we take the top-down approach, essentially examining some macroscopic issues in EEG measurement. This motivates us to look to a bottom-up approach, starting with microscopic synaptic activity and neuronal interactions, then scaling up through mesocolumnar activity of columns of neurons, to finally achieve a reasonable macroscopic description of EEG activity. The confluence of these approaches is expected to yield a tractable approach to EEG analyses (Ingber, 1985a, 1991a; Ingber and Nunez, 1990; Nunez, 1989).

This chapter's organization closely follows a more technical format (Ingber, 1991a), in which more details and references can be found. We tried to convey the foundation, general description, and verification of SMNI. Typically each section first gives an "executive summary" of the main concepts being developed and fortifies this with some sampling of more mathematical arguments. The references provide more details.

Top-down String Model

Modeling of Observables

As discussed in Chapter 2, a stretched string displacement Φ (potential within the cortex) is expressed by the wave equation

$$\frac{\partial^2\Phi}{\partial t^2} - c^2\frac{\partial^2\Phi}{\partial x^2} + [\omega_0^2 + f(\Phi)]\Phi = 0 \tag{14.1}$$

in terms of the string displacement Φ, represented by a Fourier series

$$\Phi(x, t) = \sum_{n=1}^{\infty} G_n(t)\sin k_n x \tag{14.2}$$

where we have assumed zero boundary conditions at the ends of the string for simplicity of presentation, but our observed $\hat{\Phi}$ (referenced as $\Phi^\dagger$ in the SMNI literature) is expressed by

$$\hat{\Phi}(x, t) = \sum_{n=1}^{M} G_n(t)\sin k_n x \tag{14.3}$$

With respect to the cortical medium, we address the question, What can we say about $\hat{\Phi}(x, t)$, the macroscopic observable displacement potential on the scalp or cortical surface? Based on previous studies of EEG dispersion relations (Ingber, 1982; Nunez, 1981a), we should be able to describe $\hat{\Phi}$ as a linear or quasi-linear variable influenced by the local nonlinear behavior that crosses the hierarchical level from mesoscopic to macroscopic columnar dipoles. How do we mathematically articulate this intuition to consistently describe and lay the foundation for future detailed numeric calculations? The "bottom-up" approach part of this chapter suggests some answers to these questions.

We examine these issues by using reasonable synaptic parameters, developing the statistical mechanics of neocortical interactions, and then determining whether they are consistent with observed EEG data. In fact, we fit multichannel human scalp EEG data to these algebraic forms. We are currently investigating the response of the cortical system to given initial driving forces that match or mismatch firing patterns of columnar firings possessed by a given set of synaptic parameters, and under conditions that plastically change synaptic parameters and reflect changes of these patterns. This should help clinicians to make diagnoses using EEG.

Outline of Derivation of the Nonlinear String Model

We use a mechanical analog model, the string model, derived explicitly for neocortical interactions using SMNI (Ingber and Nunez, 1990). This defines a probability distribution of firing activity, which can be used to investigate further the existence of other nonlinear phenomena, such as bifurcations or chaotic behavior, in brain states (Rapp et al, 1989).

Previous studies have suggested that the predominant physics of short-term memory and of short-fiber contribution to EEG phenomena occurs in a narrow "parabolic trough" in M^G space, approximately along a diagonal line (Ingber, 1984a). G represents E or I, M^E represents contributions to columnar firing from excitatory neurons, and M^I represents contributions to columnar firing from inhibitory neurons. The object of interest within a short refractory time, τ, approximately 5 to 10 milliseconds, is the Lagrangian $\underline{L}$ for a mesocolumn, described in more detail below. $\tau\underline{L}$ can vary by as much as a factor of 10^5 from the highest peak to the lowest valley in M^G space. Therefore, we can assume that a single independent firing variable might offer a crude description of the physics. Furthermore, the scalp potential Φ can be considered a function of this firing variable. ("Potential" refers to the electric potential, not the potential term in the Lagrangian derived below.) In an abbreviated notation subscripting the time dependence

$$\Phi_t - \langle\langle\Phi\rangle\rangle = \Phi(M_t^E, M_t^I) \approx a(M_t^E - \langle\langle M^E\rangle\rangle) + b(M_t^I - \langle\langle M^I\rangle\rangle) \quad (14.4)$$

where a and b are constants, and $\langle\langle\Phi\rangle\rangle$ and $\langle\langle M^G\rangle\rangle$ represent typical minima in the trough. In the context of fitting data to the dynamic variables, there are three effective constants, $\{a, b, \phi\}$

$$\Phi_t - \phi = aM_t^E + bM_t^I \quad (14.5)$$

We scale and aggregate the mesoscopic probability distributions P over this columnar firing space to obtain the macroscopic conditional probability distribution over the scalp-potential space

$$P_\Phi[\Phi] = \int dM^E dM^I P[M^E, M^I]\delta[\Phi - \Phi'(M^E, M^I)], \quad (14.6)$$

in an abbreviated notation expanded below. The parabolic trough described above justifies a form

$$P_\Phi = (2\pi\sigma^2)^{-1/2} \exp\left(-\Delta t \int dx\, L_\Phi\right),$$

$$L_\Phi = \frac{\alpha}{2}|\partial\Phi/\partial t|^2 + \frac{\beta}{2}|\partial\Phi/\partial x|^2 + \frac{\gamma}{2}|\Phi|^2 + F(\Phi), \tag{14.7}$$

$$\sigma^2 = 2\Delta t/\alpha$$

where $F(\Phi)$ contains nonlinear qualities away from the trough, σ^2 is about $1/N$ given the derivation of $\underline{L}$ above, and the integral over x is taken over the spatial region of interest. In general, there also will be terms linear in $\partial\Phi/\partial t$ and in $\partial\Phi/\partial x$.

Previous calculations of EEG phenomena, described below (Ingber, 1985a), show that the short-fiber contribution to the alpha frequency and the movement of attention across the visual field are consistent with the assumption that the EEG physics is derived from an average over the fluctuations of the system, represented by σ in the above equation, for example. This is described by the Euler-Lagrange equations derived from the variational principle possessed by L_Φ (essentially the counterpart to force equals mass times acceleration), but more properly by the "midpoint-discretized" Feynman L_Φ, with its Riemannian terms, as discussed below (Ingber, 1982, 1983a, 1988c). Thus we can use the variational principle

$$0 = \frac{\partial}{\partial t}\frac{\partial L_\Phi}{\partial(\partial\Phi/\partial t)} + \frac{\partial}{\partial x}\frac{\partial L_\Phi}{\partial(\partial\Phi/\partial x)} - \frac{\partial L_\Phi}{\partial\Phi} \tag{14.8}$$

The result is

$$\alpha\frac{\partial^2\Phi}{\partial t^2} + \beta\frac{\partial^2\Phi}{\partial x^2} + \gamma\Phi - \frac{\partial F}{\partial\Phi} = 0 \tag{14.9}$$

If regions in neocortical parameter space exist such that we can identify $\beta/\alpha = -c^2$, $\gamma/\alpha = \omega_0^2$ (such as explicitly calculated below)

$$\frac{1}{\alpha}\frac{\partial F}{\partial\Phi} = -\Phi f(\Phi) \tag{14.10}$$

and *x* is one dimensional, we can recover our nonlinear string, described by (14.1). Terms linear in $\partial\Phi/\partial t$ and in $\partial\Phi/\partial x$ in L_Φ in Eq. (14.7) can make other contributions, such as giving rise to damping terms, as discussed in Chapter 10.

The path–integral formulation of the long-time evolution of the distribution P_Φ has a utility beyond its deterministic Euler-Lagrange limit. We have used this to examine the long-time evolution of systems explicitly, to compare models to long-time correlations in simulation data (Ingber, 1993b; Ingber et al, 1991), to approach similar problems in finance (Ingber, 1990; Ingber et al, 1991) and in EEG modeling as described here. Similar advantages of this approach are available for EEG analyses.

Macroscopic Coarse Graining and Renormalization

We can address how to justify the intuitive coarse graining of Φ to get $\hat{\Phi}$. In L_Φ above, consider terms of the form

$$\begin{aligned}\int \Phi^2\, dx &= \int dx \sum_n^\infty \sum_m^\infty G_n G_m \sin k_n x \sin k_m x \\ &= \sum_n \sum_m G_n G_m \int dx \sin k_n x \sin k_m x \\ &= (2\pi/R) \sum_n G_n^2\end{aligned} \tag{14.11}$$

By similarly considering all terms in L_Φ, we effectively define a short-time probability distribution for the change in node n, defined by

$$p_n[G_n(t + \Delta t) | G_m(t)] \tag{14.12}$$

where, in general, the $F(\Phi)$ term in L_Φ requires coupling between $G_n(t + \Delta t)$ and $G_m(t)$, $n \neq m$, probably including more than one m. Therefore, we can define

$$P_\Phi = p_1 p_2 \cdots p_\infty \tag{14.13}$$

Now we can physically and mathematically define a coarse graining

$$P_{\hat{\Phi}} = \int dk_{M+1}\, dk_{M+2} \cdots dk_\infty p_1 p_2 \cdots p_M p_{M+1} p_{M+2} \cdots p_\infty . \tag{14.14}$$

Because we have a bona fide probability distribution P_Φ, we can integrate over those fine-grained variables, which are not observed. This procedure is one contribution to algorithms used in "renormalization group" theory (Ma, 1976) to account for multiple intermediate scales of interactions. Although other criteria in that specific theory are not present here, we should recognize that this is a reasonable phenomenologic approach to integrating over many scales of neocortical interactions.

The integration over the fine-grained wave numbers tends to smooth the influence of the k_n values for $n > M$, effectively "renormalizing"

$$\begin{aligned} G_n &\rightarrow G_n^\dagger \\ \Phi &\rightarrow \hat{\Phi} \\ L_\Phi &\rightarrow L_{\hat{\Phi}}^\dagger \end{aligned} \tag{14.15}$$

Eventually, laminar circuitry should be included in the local and global models. Previous articles have described how this can be realized, but more numeric-based study is needed to determine the degree to which this can be accomplished. As reported here, the solutions are being tested by their goodness of fit to existing EEG data using methods of very fast simulated reannealing (Ingber, 1989, 1993c), the precursor to a more powerful code, adaptive simulated annealing (ASA) (Ingber, 1993a).

Bottom-up SMNI Model

Rationale

We begin our "bottom-up" approach by taking the view that because much progress has been made in mathematically describing the physics at finer spatial-temporal scales, we should use these descriptions to derive a development of the coarser EEG macroscopic scale described previously. Statistical mechanics of neocortical interactions reasonably detail a consistent physics that at least parallels, with striking numeric specificity, short-term memory (STM) and EEG phenomena at the mesocolumnar scale of hundreds of neurons to the macrocolumnar scale of hundreds of thousands of neurons, in terms of aggregated physics occurring at the single-neuronal level. Details of this SMNI development of STM and EEG support the "top-down" development described previously.

An important contribution of SMNI is its analytic treatment of minicolumns (Mountcastle, 1978). Minicolumns span approximately 7×10^2 μm^2, as discussed in Chapter 2. Mesocolumnar domains are defined as physiologic (functional) units, with input converging from an anatomic (structural) macrocolumn extent of approximately 1000 minicolumns, and output diverging from an anatomic minicolumn to a macrocolumnar extent. Calculations support observations of periodically alternating firings of columnar structures (Fitzpatrick and Imig, 1980; Goldman and Nauta, 1977; Hubel and Wiesel, 1962; Hubel and Wiesel, 1977; Jones et al, 1978). As pictured in Figure 14-1, this microscopic scale is larger (by several orders of magnitude) than the moleculear scale of membrane biophysics. "Macrocolumns" spanning about 7×10^5 μm^2 have been defined as another physiologic entity observed in the neocortex (Mountcastle, 1978), but the macroscopic regions considered here are larger than these by several orders of magnitude. Mesocolumnar domains are sufficiently close to the scale of microscopic neurons to allow direct dependence of this theory on neuronal chemical and electrical properties. The proper stochastic treatment of their interaction permits their development into macroscopic regions responsible for global neocortical information processing. Thermodynamic entities corresponding to the "free-energy" potential, "temperature," and order parameters of these macroscopic regions are derived from a statistical-mechanics paradigm but with no recourse to quasi-equilibrium limits (Landau et al, 1980).

Relative to other biological entities, the intrinsic synaptic activity of the most highly evolved mammalian human neocortex functions through the most degenerate and the shortest-range neuronal interactions (measured in micrometers). "Degenerate" reflects the mesoscopic state of approximate redundancy of connectivity among microscopic neurons to describe this coarser scale. This suggests that many collective aspects of this system can be fruitfully studied similarly to other collective systems, such as magnetic systems, lasers, and more general information-theoretic systems (Haken, 1988; van Kampen, 1981). Collective effects, from clustering (Szentágothai, 1975; Szentágothai and Arbib, 1974) or from statistical interactions (Katchalsky et al, 1974), are proposed as mechanisms of

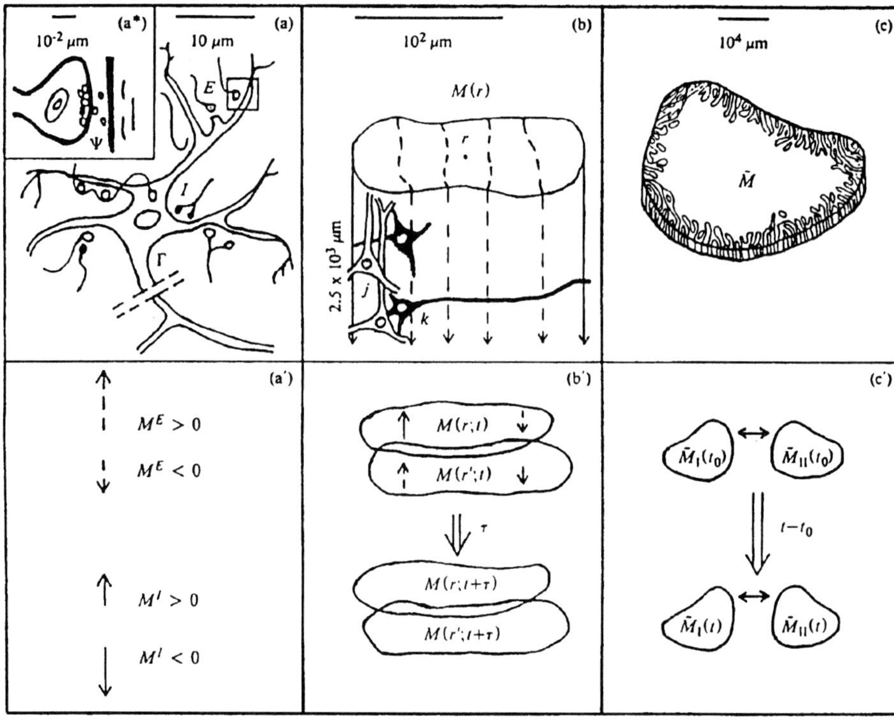

Figure 14-1. Three biophysics scales of neocortical interactions: (**a**), (a*), (a′) microscopic neurons; (**b**) and (b′) mesocolumnar domains; (**c**) and (c′) macroscopic regions. In (a*) synaptic interneuronal interactions, averaged by mesocolumns, are phenomenologically described by the mean and variance of a distribution Ψ. Similarly in (a), intraneuronal transmissions are phenomenologically described by the mean and variance of Γ. Mesocolumnar averaged excitatory (E) and inhibitory (I) neuronal firings are represented in (a′). In (b), the vertical organization of minicolumns in sketched together with their horizontal stratification, yielding a physiologic entity, the mesocolumn. In (b′), the overlap of interacting mesocolumns is sketched. In (c), macroscopic regions of the neocortex are depicted as arising from many mesocolumnar domains. These are the regions designated for study here. (c′) shows how regions may be coupled by long-range interactions.

information processing, in addition to the "hard-wiring" mechanisms also possessed by other more ordered cortical entities (Afifi and Bergman, 1978; Sommerhoff, 1974).

Reasonable criteria for any physical approach to the neocortex should include three basic features that illustrate the appropriate analogies between the neocortex and other collective physical systems.

1. Interactions. Short-range neuronal interactions over periods of several milliseconds should be derived from even more microscopic synaptic activities (Shepherd, 1979) (Figure 14-1a). Long-range spatial interactions from specific neuronal pathways, primarily composed of long excitatory fibers from ipsilateral

association, contralateral commissural, and thalamocortical processes, must be treated consistently. These long-range interactions are also important for collective activity in the mammalian cortex (Braitenberg, 1978), and they are included in this study. Longer time, weaker, and modulatory nonsynaptic influences arising from humoral and electronic interactions (Dismukes, 1979; McGeer et al, 1978; Schmitt et al, 1976) are included, but only as their averaged properties affect synaptic parameters.

2. Statistics. Neurons separated by large distances, across 10^3 to 10^8 neurons, can be coupled statistically through their short-range interactions (Figure 14-1c). Order parameters, the underlying independent variables at the appropriate scale of the theory, must be identified, and intrinsic fluctuations from the microscopic synaptic and neuronal systems (diffusion effects) must be included. There also are fluctuations of the mesoscopic system because of their aggregated neuronal interactions, derived here as gradient couplings between neighboring mesoscopic cells. These spatially ordered mesoscopic domains respect the observed anatomic and physiologic character of the neocortex (Szentágothai, 1975; Szentágothai and Arbib, 1974), and complement earlier theories hypothesizing random neural networks (Griffith, 1971; McCulloch and Pitts, 1943).

3. Dynamics. A viable formalism must be adopted to describe the statistical time evolution of the macroscopic nonequilibrium system over scales of 10^2 to 10^4 milliseconds.

Although cooperativity between distant neurons is typically low (Adey, 1978), except perhaps in homologous regions of separate hemispheres, macroscopic regions reflect cooperative behavior, which can be best understood as initiated at the mesoscopic level of interaction. Collective spatial-temporal activity, embedded in a spontaneous noisy background, is supported by statistical analyses of EEG and MEG recordings (John, 1972; Williamson et al, 1979). As long as collective mechanisms that arise in a physical system characterized by these three features are viable sources of collective neocortical phenomena, then these features are correctly formulated by SMNI.

A large body of literature addresses neuronal mechanisms and intuits phenomenologic differential equations from rates of change of average excitatory and inhibitory neuronal firings, and searches for collective behavior, limit cycles, and oscillatory behavior (Babloyantz and Kaczmarek, 1979; Freeman, 1975; Kaczmarek and Babloyantz, 1977; Wilson, 1977; Wilson and Cowan, 1972; Wilson and Cowan, 1973). Mechanisms are sought to explain varied phenomena such as hysteresis in perception (Wilson, 1977), perception and learning (Hebb, 1949; Takeuchi and Amari, 1979), and ontogenesis of columnar formation (Takeuchi and Amari, 1979; von der Marlsburg, 1979). Comparisons with applications of these techniques to those used in other physical systems (Haken, 1983) show that the pioneering application of these appropriate formalisms to the neocortical system is still valuable. Much inspiration for these applications has come from work in nonequilibrium thermodynamics, which has been applied to specific systems, such as chemical reactions, lasers, magnetic systems, fluids, spin glasses, and so forth, and to the general formulation of complex nonlinear systems (Haken, 1983; Katchalsky et al, 1974; Kubo et al, 1973; Nicolis and Prigogine, 1973; van Kampen, 1976).

This study also distinguishes neuronal mechanisms the neocortex uses to process information from the structures of information processed by the neocortex. A Lagrangian is derived that operates on firings of the system. When integrated over a time period, it yields the nonequilibrium equivalent of a "thermodynamic potential." This Lagrangian is derived, not conveniently defined or hypothesized, from the short-time evolution of the probability distribution of columnar firing states. The exponential of minus the Lagrangian, essentially this short-time distribution up to an important normalization factor, operates as a weighting factor on all possible states, filtering or transforming (patterns of) input firings into output firings. "Information" is a concept defined in terms of the probability eigenfunctions of electrical–chemical activity of this Lagrangian. The path–integral formulation presents an accurate intuitive description of an initial probability distribution of patterns of firings that are filtered by the (exponential of the) Lagrangian, resulting in a final probability distribution of firing patterns.

At the end of this chapter is a brief summary of the advantages of the SMNI model in the context of its practical application to enhancing the extraction from EEG data of signal from noise.

Microscopic Neurons

General Description

Figure 14-1a illustrates the microscopic neuronal interaction scale, which is several micrometers. Neocortical neurons typically have many dendrites that receive quanta of chemical postsynaptic stimulation from many other neurons. The distribution of quanta transmitted across synapses occurs on the scale of 10^{-2} μm, as illustrated in the inset of Figure 14-1a. Each quantum has thousands of molecules of chemical neurotransmitters that affect the chemically gated postsynaptic membrane. Chemical transmissions in the neocortex are thought to be either excitatory (E), such as glutamic acid, or inhibitory (I), such as gamma aminobutyric acid. Many transmitters and other chemicals that modulate their effects exist, but after millions of synapses between hundreds of neurons are averaged over, we can ascribe a distribution function Ψ with a mean and variance for E and I interneuronal interactions.

Some neuroscientists do not accept the assumption that simple algebraic summation of excitatory depolarizations and inhibitory hyperpolarizations at the base of the inner axonal membrane determines the firing depolarization response of a neuron within its absolute and relative refractory periods (Shepherd, 1979), that is, including the absolute refractory time after a firing during which no new spikes can be generated, and the relative refractory period during which spikes can be produced only at a decreased sensitivity (Sommerhoff, 1974). However, many other neuroscientists agree that this assumption is reasonable when describing the activity of large ensembles of neocortical neurons, each one typically having many thousands of synaptic interactions.

This same averaging procedure allows us to ascribe a distribution function Γ with a mean and variance for E and I intraneuronal interactions. A Gaussian Γ describes the distribution of electrical polarizations caused by chemical quanta impinging on the postsynaptic membrane. These polarizations yield a resultant polarization at the base of the neuron, the axon (extension in Figure 14-1a cut by the double broken line). The base of the axon of a large fiber may be myelinated. However, smaller neurons typically lack these distinguishing features. Experimental techniques are not sufficiently advanced to attempt the explicit averaging procedure necessary to establish in vivo the means and variances of Ψ and Γ and their parameters (Vu and Krasne, 1992). Differential attenuations of polarizations from synapses to the base of an axon are only phenomenologically accounted for by including these geometric and physiologic effects into Γ.

With a sufficient depolarization of approximately 10 to 20 mV at the soma, within an absolute and relative refractory period of approximately 5 milliseconds, an action potential is pulsed down the axon and its many collaterals, affecting voltage-gated presynaptic membranes to release quanta of neurotransmitters. Not detailed here is the biophysics of membranes, of thickness $\approx 5 \times 10^{-3}$ μm, composed of biomolecular leaflets of phospholipid molecules (Caillé et al, 1980; Scott, 1975; von der Heydt et al, 1981). Ψ and Γ approximate this biophysics for macroscopic studies. We can apply the formalism adopted in this study to use new microscopic functional dependences, gleaned from other experimental or theoretical investigations, and extend them to obtain similar macroscopic descriptions. Chemical independence of excitatory depolarizations and inhibitory hyperpolarizations are well established in the neocortex, and this independence is retained throughout this study.

Experimental studies initially used to infer Ψ and Γ (such as at neuromuscular junctions) were made posible by deliberately reducing the number of quanta by decreasing external calcium concentrations (Boyd and Martin, 1956; Katz, 1966). Ψ was Poissonian, but in that system, where hundreds of quanta are transmitted in vivo, Ψ may be otherwise, such as Gaussian with independent mean and variance. Current research suggests a binomial distribution, having a Poisson limit (Ingber, 1982; Korn et al, 1981; Perkel and Feldman, 1979). Some investigators have shown that a Bernoulli distribution is more accurate in some cases (Ingber, 1982; Korn and Mallet, 1984; Perkel and Feldman, 1979), and that the concept of quantal transmission is under review, despite the fact that good fits to experimental data are achieved with this concept. In the neocortex, probably few quanta are transmitted at synapses, but other effects, such as nonuniformity and nonstationarity of presynaptic release sites and nonlinear summation of postsynaptic potentials, may detract from a simple phenomenologic Poisson description (Shepherd, 1979). This short description highlights possible differences in Ψ resulting from many sources. However, the derivation of synaptic interactions given here makes it plausible that for reasonable neuronal parameters, the statistical folding of Ψ and Γ is independent of the functional form assumed for Ψ, just requiring specification of its numeric mean and variance.

From this analysis, we can calculate the transition probability of the firing of neuron j, p_{σ_j}, given its interaction with its neighbors that also may or may not fire. The result is the tabulated error function. Within the range in which the total influences of excitatory and inhibitory firings match and exceed the average threshold potential of a given neuron, the probability of that neuron firing receives its major contribution to increase from 0 toward 1. A step function derived as $\tanh F^G$ is defined by the threshold factor F_j. That is, for $F^G >> 1$, $\tanh F^G \rightarrow 1$, whereas for $F^G << 1$, $\tanh F^G \rightarrow -1$; so the threshold region of $-1 < F^G < 1$ sensitively controls this important $\tanh F^G$ contribution to the drifts (the driving terms) in the Lagrangian. The mesoscopic development discussed below retains this sensitivity.

This is similar to the mathematical result obtained by others (Little, 1974; Little and Shaw, 1978; Shaw and Vasudevan, 1974) who modeled the neocortex using magnetic systems (Cragg and Temperley, 1954). However, the following is derived more generally and has the neural parameters more specifically denoted with different statistical significances given to Ψ and Γ, as described previously.

Conditional Probability

Consider $10^2 < N < 10^3$ neurons, labeled k, interacting with a given neuron j. Each neuron may contribute many synaptic interactions to many other neurons. A neuron may have as many as 10^4 to 10^5 synaptic interactions. Within time $\tau_n \approx 5$ milliseconds, Ψ is the distribution of q quanta of chemical transmitter released from neuron k to neuron j ($k \neq j$), with mean a_{jk}, where

$$a_{jk} = A_{jk}(\sigma_k + 1)/2 + B_{jk} \qquad (14.16)$$

A_{jk} is the conductivity weighting transmission of polarization, dependent on k firing

$$\sigma_k = \begin{cases} 1, & \text{k fires,} \\ -1, & \text{k does not fire} \end{cases} \qquad (14.17)$$

and B_{jk} is a background including some nonsynaptic and long-range activity. Of course, A and B are complicated functions of kj. This definition of σ_k permits a decomposition of a_{jk} into two physical contributions. At this point we can make a reasonable analogy with magnetic systems, in which σ_k might represent a unit spin. However, the details of the interactions between neurons differ from those between magnetic spins, and this greatly affects such comparisons.

Further SMNI development yields the conditional probability, p_{σ_j}, of neuron j firing given previous firings within τ of other neurons k

$$p_{\sigma_j} = \pi^{-1/2} \int_{(\sigma_j F_j \sqrt{\pi}/2)}^{\infty} dz \exp(-z^2)$$

$$= \frac{1}{2} [1 - \mathrm{erf}(\sigma_j F_j \sqrt{\pi}/2)], \tag{14.18}$$

$$F_j = \frac{V_j - \sum_k a_{jk} v_{jk}}{\left(\pi \sum_{k'} a_{jk'} (v_{jk}^2 + \phi_{jk'}^2)\right)^{1/2}} .$$

"erf" is the tabulated error function, simply related to the normal probability function (Mathews and Walker, 1970). F_j^G is a threshold factor, as p_{σ_j} increases from 0 to 1 between $\infty > \sigma_j F_j > -\infty$ sharply within the range of $F_j \approx 0$.

If

$$|\sigma_j F_j| < 1 \tag{14.19}$$

then an asymptotic expression for p_{σ_j} is

$$p_{\sigma_j} \approx \frac{\exp(-\sigma_j F_j)}{\exp(F_j) + \exp(-F_j)}. \tag{14.20}$$

Mesoscopic Domains

General Description

As with most nonequilibrium systems, such as lasers, chemical systems, fluids, and ecologic systems (Haken, 1983; van Kampen, 1981), a mesoscopic scale is needed to formulate the statistical mechanics of the microscopic system, from which the macroscopic scale can be developed (Haken, 1983). The neocortex is particularly interesting in this context because a clear scale for the mesoscopic system exists, both anatomically (structurally) and physiologically (functionally). "Minicolumns" of about $N \approx 110$ neurons (about 220 in the visual cortex) comprise modular units vertically oriented relative to the warped and convoluted neocortical surface throughout most, if not all, regions of the neocortex (Gilbert and Wiesel, 1983; Goldman and Nauta, 1977; Hubel and Wiesel, 1962; Imig and Reale, 1980; Jones et al, 1978; Mountcastle, 1978). Clusters of about 100 neurons are thought to be reasonably based on other considerations (Bullock, 1980). Because the short-ranged interactions between neurons occur within ~1 mm, which is the extent of a "macrocolumn" comprising $\sim 10^3$ minicolumns of $N^* \approx 10^5$ neurons, and because macrocolumns also exhibit rather specific information-processing features, this theory has retained the divergence-convergence of macrocolumn–minicolumn, efferent–afferent interactions by considering domains of minicolumns as having similar synaptic interactions within the extent of a macrocolumn. This macrocolumnar-averaged minicolumn is designated in this theory as a "mesocolumn."

Given this observed situation, $N \approx 10^2$ is just the right order of magnitude to permit a formal analysis using methods of mathematical physics just developed for statistical systems in the late 1970s (Graham, 1977a; Langouche et al, 1982). N is small enough to permit nearest-neighbor interactions to be formulated, such that interactions between mesocolumns are small enough to be considered gradient perturbations on otherwise independent mesocolumnar firing states. This is consistent with rather continuous spatial gradient interactions observed among columns (Dykes, 1983) and with the basic hypothesis that nonrandom differentiation of properties among broadly tuned individual neurons coexists with functional columnar averages representing superpositions of patterned information (Erickson, 1982). This is a definite mathematical convenience, because otherwise a macrocolumn of $\sim 10^3$ minicolumns must be described by a system of minicolumns with as many as 16th-order next-nearest neighbors. (Consider 1000 minicolumns spread in a two-dimensional grid of about 33 by 33 minicolumns, and focus attention on the center minicolumn.) Also N is large enough to permit the derived binomial distribution of afferent minicolumnar firing states to be well approximated by a Gaussian distribution, a luxury not afforded an "average" neuron, even in this otherwise similar physical context. Finally, mesocolumnar interactions occur through one to several relays of neuronal interactions, so their time scales are similarly $\tau \approx 5$ to 10 milliseconds.

Even after statistically shaping the microscopic system, the parameters of the mesoscopic system are still macrocolumnar-averaged synaptic parameters, that is reflecting the statistics of millions of synapses with regard to their chemical and electrical properties. Explicit laminar circuitry, and more complicated synaptic interactions, such as those that depend on all combinations of presynaptic and postsynaptic firings, can be included without loss of detailed analysis (Ingber, 1983a).

The mathematical development of mesocolumns establishes a mesoscopic Lagrangian $\underline{L}$, which may be considered as a "cost function" with variables M^G, $\dot{M}^G$, and ∇M^G, and with parameters defined by the macrocolumnar-averaged chemical–electrical entities developed below. (See Figure 14-2.)

The Einstein summation convention is used for compactness, whereby any index appearing more than once among factors in any term is assumed to be summed over, unless otherwise indicated by vertical bars ($|G|$). The mesoscopic probability distribution P is expressed by the product of microscopic probability distributions p_{σ_i}, constrained such that the aggregate mesoscopic excitatory firings $M^E = \Sigma_{j \in E} \sigma_j$, and the aggregate mesoscopic inhibitory firings $M^I = \Sigma_{j \in I} \sigma_j$

$$P = \prod_G P^G[M^G(r; t + \tau) | M^{\bar{G}}(r'; t)]$$

$$= \sum_{\sigma_j} \delta \left(\sum_{j \in E} \sigma_j - M^E(r; t + \tau) \right) \delta \left(\sum_{j \in I} \sigma_j - M^I(r; t + \tau) \right) \prod_j^N p_{\sigma_j} \qquad (14.21)$$

$$\approx \prod_G (2\pi\tau g^{GG})^{-1/2} \exp(-N\tau \underline{L}^G)$$

where the final form is derived using $N > 100$. $\bar{G}$ represents contributions from E and I sources. This defines the Lagrangian, in terms of its first-moment drifts g^G, its second-moment diffusion matrix $g^{GG'}$, and its potential $\underline{V}'$, which all depend sensitively on threshold factors F^G

$$
\begin{aligned}
P &\approx (2\pi\tau)^{-1/2} g^{1/2} \exp(-N\tau\underline{L}) \\
\underline{L} &= \underline{T} - \underline{V} \\
\underline{T} &= (2N)^{-1}(\dot{M}^G - g^G) g_{GG'} (\dot{M}^{G'} - g^{G'}) \\
\underline{V} &= \underline{V}' - M^G J_G/(2N\tau) \\
\underline{V}' &= \sum_G \underline{V}''^G_{G'} (\rho \nabla M^{G'})^2 \\
g^G &= -\tau^{-1}(M^G + N^G \tanh F^G) \\
g^{GG'} &= (g_{GG'})^{-1} = \delta^{G'}_G \tau^{-1} N^G \operatorname{sech}^2 F^G \\
g &= \det(g_{GG'}) \\
F^G &= \frac{(V^G - a^{|G|}_{G'} v^{|G|}_{G'} N^{G'} - \frac{1}{2} A^{|G|}_{G'} v^{|G|}_{G'} M^{G'})}{(\pi[(v^{|G|}_{G'})^2 + (\phi^{|G|}_{G'})^2](a^{|G|}_{G'} N^{G'} + \frac{1}{2} A^{|G|}_{G'} M^{G'}))^{1/2}} \\
a^G_{G'} &= \frac{1}{2} A^G_{G'} + B^G_{G'}
\end{aligned}
\tag{14.22}
$$

where $A^G_{G'}$ and $B^G_{G'}$ are macrocolumnar-averaged interneuronal synaptic efficacies, $v^G_{G'}$ and $\phi^G_{G'}$ are averaged means and variances of contributions to neuronal electric polarizations, and nearest-neighbor interactions $\overline{V}'$ are detailed in other SMNI articles (Ingber, 1982, 1984a). $M^{G'}$ and $N^{G'}$ in F^G are afferent macrocolumnar firings, scaled to efferent minicolumnar firings by $N/N^* \sim 10^{-3}$, where N^* is the number of neurons in a macrocolumn. Similarly, $A^{G}_{G}{}'$ and $B^{G}_{G}{}'$ have been scaled by $N^*/N \sim 10^3$ to keep F^G invariant. This scaling is for convenience only. This mathematical description defines the mesocolumn concept introduced previously.

At this stage, severe approximation in modeling typically is needed to proceed toward solutions. However, we can take advantage of experimentally observed columnar structure to try to scale the neuronal system analytically into mesoscopic domains that are still relatively microscopic compared with the macroscopic regions to be described (Fitzpatrick and Imig, 1980; Goldman and Nauta, 1977; Hubel and Wiesel, 1977; Jones et al, 1978; Mountcastle, 1978; Takeuchi and Amari, 1979). For macroscopic description, the minicolumnar structure effectively averages the neuronal interactions spatially within one to several firing periods.

The following development is proposed that (1) reasonably includes and averages over millions of synaptic interactions that exist between groups of hundreds of neurons, (2) analytically establishes the integrity of columnar domains and specifies

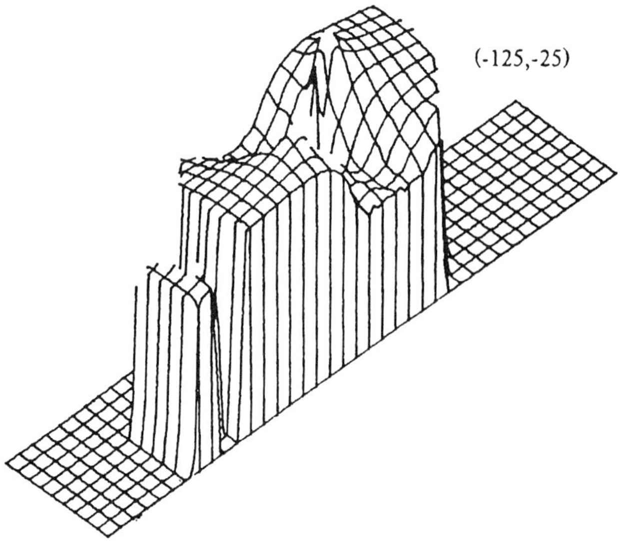

Figure 14-2. Examination of the minima structure of the spatially averaged and temporally averaged, nonlinear Lagrangian provides some quick intuitive details about the most probable states of the system. This is supported by further analysis detailing the actual spatial-temporal minima structure. Illustrated is the surface of the static (time-independent) mesoscopic neocortical Lagrangian $\bar{\underline{L}}$ over the excitatory-inhibitory firing plane ($\bar{M}^E - \bar{M}^I$), for a specific set of synaptic parameters. All points on the surface higher than $5 \times 10^{-3}/\tau$ were deleted to expose this fine structure.

their interactions, and (3) prepares the formulation of the first two factors to foresee their analytic inclusion into studies of macroscopic regions.

To describe anatomic or physiologic properties of neurons, it is incorrect to postulate an "average" neuron. However, with macroscopic brain function, when considering millions of neurons, we should respect the similar modular structure present in all regions of the neocortex (Gilbert and Wiesel, 1983; Goldman and Nauta, 1977; Hubel and Wiesel, 1962; Imig and Reale, 1980; Jones et al, 1978; Mountcastle, 1978), but still allow for the differentiation among the laminar structure of individual modules and among neurons active at different temporal and spatial scales.

In this context, the neocortex has about 5×10^{10} neurons distributed uniformly over approximately 5×10^8 minicolumns. (The visual cortex is twice as dense.) Within these minicolumns, a "vertical" structure is defined perpendicular to six convoluted laminae of total thickness $\approx 2.5 \times 10^3$ μm, principally by the efferent pyramidal cells. They show vertical apical bundling of their dendrites in the upper laminae, and some of their recurrent axonal collaterals also ascend to upper laminae. Several other fusiform, Martinotti, and stellate cells (granule cells in the sensory cortex and basket cells in the motor cortex) also contribute to this vertical organization. In general, laminae I to IV are afferent and laminae V and VI are efferent (Afifi and Bergman, 1978).

However, "horizontal" dendritic basal arborizations (tree-like structures) of the pyramidal cells (tangential to the laminae), horizontal axonal collaterals of the pyramidal cells, and horizontal processes of stellate, Martinotti, and neonatal horizontal cells all impart horizontal stratification to columnar interactions. Therefore, although the columnar concept has anatomic and physiologic support, the minicolumnar boundaries are not so clearly defined (Dykes, 1978). If this stratification and other long-range afferent input to groups of minicolumns are incorporated, future work may have to define a physiologic unit that encompasses a mesocolumn consisting of one to perhaps several minicolumns outputting to a macrocolumnar extent. This study formalizes these circumstances by defining a mesocolumn with extent greater than 10^2 μm, as an intermediate integral physiologic unit encompassing one minicolumn (Figure 14-1b). Dynamic nearest-neighbor interactions between mesocolumns are analytically defined by their overlapping neuronal interactions, in accordance with the observed horizontal columnar stratifications outlined previously (Figure 14-1b). This approach permits future analytic modifications, as differences between inter- and intraminicolumnar interactions and circuitries become experimentally clarified.

The resulting columnar interactions are relatively more simple than a mass of interacting neurons, but not so simple to be useless. A collection of average excitatory and inhibitory neuronal firings, as depicted in Figure 14-1a, define a continuum of mesocolumnar firings. A zero-order binomial distribution is easily intuited: Let G denote E or I firings. Using the magnetic analogy, consider E as a spin-up and I as a spin-down magnet. A column of N^G neurons can have a total firing of Nn^G, within time τ, where n^G is the fraction firing, ranging by 2s between $-N^G \leq Nn^G \leq N^G$. (Count firing as $+1$, nonfiring as -1.) For convenience, assume $Nn^G > 0$, which arises from Nn^G firings plus $\frac{1}{2}(N^G - Nn^G)$ cancelling pairs of firings and nonfirings. This yields a total of $\frac{1}{2}(N^G - Nn^G) + Nn^G = \frac{1}{2}(N^G + Nn^G)$ firings and $N^G - \frac{1}{2}(N^G + Nn^G)$ nonfirings. The degeneracy factor, as a function of the firing rate Nn^G, is the number of ways N^G neurons can produce a given firing pattern, that is, the binomial distribution. The binomial coefficient is unity for states of all firing or all nonfiring, and peaks as $N^G!/[(N^G/2)!]^2 \approx 2^{N^G+1/2}(\pi N^G)^{-1/2}$ for $Nn^G = 0$. In the range $Nn^G \approx 0$, there is maximal degeneracy of information encoded by mesocolumnar firings. This argument analytically articulates the meaning of "neuronal degeneracy" and also of the ubiquitous, often ambiguous "average neuron." However, reasonable properties of mesocolumns, not of average neurons, are developed here for macroscopic study.

The properly calculated distribution contains nearest-neighbor mesocolumnar interactions expressed as spatial-derivative correction terms. This verifies that in macroscopic activity, in which patterns of mesocolumnar firing vary smoothly over neighboring mesocolumns, it is consistent to approximate mesocolumnar interactions by including only second-order gradient correction terms. We calculate macroscopic states of mesocolumnar firings, which are subject to these constraints. Excitatory and inhibitory sensitivity to the neuronal parameters survive, similar to the sensitivity encountered by single neurons.

Nearest-neighbor interactions are "induced" between minicolumns in the following manner. Most short-range interactions engaging the neurons in a minicolumn do not occur within the minicolumn but rather within a spatial extent the size of a macrocolumn, comprising about 1000 minicolumns. If we consider the area of influence of a minicolumn as extending to a macrocolumn's reach, then the area of interactions engaged by nearest-neighbor minicolumns has an offset circle of influence (Ingber, 1984a) (Figure 14-3). Therefore, within one or two epochs spanning the refractory periods of a typical neuron, interactions engaged by a given minicolumn can be extended to areas of influence engaged by their nearest neighbors. This is physically calculated by a careful mathematical treatment of overlapping interactions. In this manner, microscopic degrees of freedom of many types of neurons (many are only crudely classified by these definitions), synapses, neurotransmitters, cellular architecture, and circuitries can be practically weighted and averaged for macroscopic considerations.

In these steps, the mesocolumnar conditional probability that a given mesocolumn will fire is calculated, given its direct interactions with other mesocolumns just previously fired. Thus a transition rate from one state of mesocolumnar firing to another state closely following the first state is obtained. A string or path of these conditional probabilities connects the mesocolumnar firings at one time to the firing at any subsequent time. Many paths may link the same initial and final state. In this way, the long-time conditional probability of all possible mesocolumnar firings at any given time is obtained. A Lagrangian is thus derived that explicitly describes the time evolution of the neocortical region in terms of its initial distribution of firings and is expressed in terms of its mesoscopic order parameters that retain a functional form derived from microscopic neuronal interactions. An important benefit of this formalism is a variational principle that allows us to develop extrema equations. This also allows us to draw analogies to the orienting field and temperature of other collective systems.

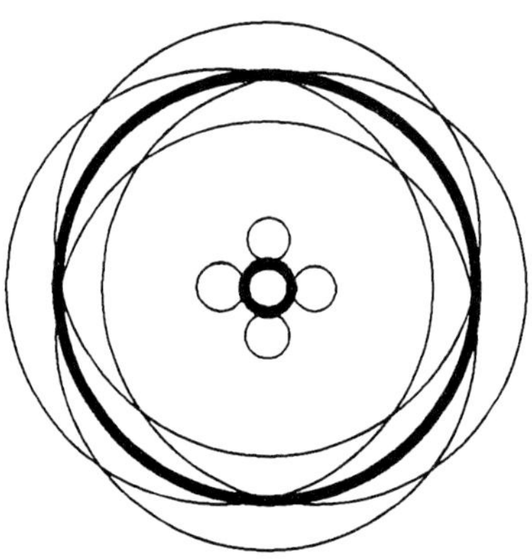

Figure 14-3. Nearest-neighbor interactions between mesocolumns. Afferent minicolumns of $\sim 10^2$ neurons are represented by the inner circles, and efferent macrocolumns of $\sim 10^5$ neurons are denoted by the outer circles. Illustrated are the nearest-neighbor interactions between a mesocolumn, represented by the thick circles, and its nearest neighbors, represented by thin circles. The area outside the outer thick circle represents the effective number of efferent macrocolumnar nearest-neighbor neurons. That is, these neurons outside the macrocolumnar area of influence of the central minicolumn are contacted through interactions with neurons in the central macrocolumn.

Further Development of a Mesocolumn Model

As noted in this derivation (Ingber, 1982, 1983a), this microscopic scale represents a high aggregation of submicroscopic scales, aggregating effects of tens of thousands of quanta of chemical transmitters as they influence the 5×10^{-3} μm scale of bimolecular leaflets of phospholipid molecules. This microscopic scale has been aggregated up to the mesoscopic scale, again using the general property of probability distributions—that the aggregated distribution P_q of variable q is calculated from the joint distribution $P_{q_1q_2}$ of underlying variables q_1 and q_2

$$P_q(q) = \int dq_1\, dq_2 P_{q_1q_2}(q_1, q_2)\delta(q - (q_1 + q_2)) \tag{14.23}$$

To summarize to this point, the mathematical development of mesocolumns establishes a mesoscopic Lagrangian $\underline{L}$, defining the short-time probability distribution of firings in a minicolumn, composed of $\sim 10^2$ neurons (Gilbert and Wiesel, 1983; Goldman and Nauta, 1977; Hubel and Wiesel, 1962; Imig and Reale, 1980; Jones et al, 1978; Mountcastle, 1978; Szentagothai, 1978), given its previous interactions with all other neurons in its macrocolumnar surround

$$\begin{aligned} P &= \prod_G P^G[M^G(r; t + \tau)|M^{\bar{G}}(r'; t)] \\ &= \sum_{\sigma_j} \delta\left(\sum_{jE} \sigma_j - M^E(r; t + \tau)\right) \delta\left(\sum_{jI} \sigma_j - M^I(r; t + \tau)\right) \prod_j^N p_{\sigma_j} \\ &\approx \prod_G (2\pi\tau g^{GG})^{-1/2} \exp(-N\tau \underline{L}^G) \\ P &\approx (2\pi\tau)^{-1/2} g^{1/2} \exp(-N\tau\underline{L}) \end{aligned} \tag{14.24}$$

where $\underline{L}$ is defined in terms of its drift, diffusion, and potential, all of which depend sensitively on the threshold factor F^G

$$F^G = \frac{V^G - a^{|G|}_{G'} v^{|G|}_{G'} N^{G'} - \frac{1}{2} A^{|G|}_{G'} M^{G'}}{\left\{\pi[(v^{|G|}_{G'})^2 + (\phi^{|G|}_{G'})^2]\left(a^{|G|}_{G'} N^{G'} + \frac{1}{2} A^{|G|}_{G'} M^{G'}\right)\right\}^{1/2}} \tag{14.25}$$

In the first SMNI articles, long-range interactions were included in $\underline{L}$ by adding potential terms simulating these constraints, that is, adding $J_G M^G$ to $\underline{L}$, where J_G was numerically adjusted to account for these interactions.

To include more properly long-range fibers (corticocortical axons, as discussed in Chapter 2) so interactions among macrocolumns may be included in the numeric EEG studies, the J_G terms are dropped and more realistically replaced by a modified threshold factor F^G

$$F^G = \frac{V^G - a_{G'}^{|G|} \nu_{G'}^{|G|} N^{G'} - \frac{1}{2} A_{G'}^{|G|} \nu_{G'}^{|G|} M^{G'} - a_{G'}^{\ddagger|G|} \nu_{G'}^{|G|} N^{\ddagger|G|'} - \frac{1}{2} A_{G'}^{\ddagger|G|} \nu_{G'}^{|G|} M^{\ddagger G'}}{(\pi[(\nu_{G'}^{|G|})^2 + (\phi_{G'}^{|G|})^2](a_{G'}^{|G|} N^{G'} + \frac{1}{2} A_{G'}^{|G|} M^{G'} + a_{G'}^{\ddagger|G|} N^{\ddagger G'} + \frac{1}{2} A_{G'}^{\ddagger|G|} M^{\ddagger G'}))^{1/2}}$$

$$A_E^{\ddagger I} = A_I^{\ddagger E} = A_I^{\ddagger I} = B_E^{\ddagger I} = B_I^{\ddagger E} = B_I^{\ddagger I} = 0$$

$$a_E^{\ddagger E} = \frac{1}{2} A_E^{\ddagger E} + B_E^{\ddagger E} \tag{14.26}$$

Afferent contributions from $N^{\ddagger E}$ long-range excitatory fibers, such as corticocortical neurons, have been added, where $N^{\ddagger E}$ might be about 10% of N^*: Nearly every pyramidal cell has an axon branch that makes a corticocortical connection; that is, the number of corticocortical fibers may be as high as 10^{10} (Braitenberg, 1978).

At this point, we draw attention to the similar algebraic structure of the threshold factors in (14.18 and 14.26), illustrating common forms of interactions between their entities, that is, neurons and columns of neurons, respectively. The nonlinear threshold factors are defined in terms of electrical-chemical synaptic and neuronal parameters lying within their experimentally observed ranges.

The net short-time probability distribution can be folded over and over (multiplied) in time increments Δt to yield a path-integral algorithm for calculating the long-time probability distribution (Langouche et al, 1982). This result depends on the use of the Markov property of our distribution, wherein the short-time evolution of the system at time $t + \tau$ depends only on the state of the system at time t. For example, in a very compacted notation, labeling u intermediate time epochs by s, that is, $t_s = t_0 + s\Delta t$ in the limits $u \rightarrow \infty$ and $\Delta t \rightarrow 0$ and assuming $M_{t_0} = M(t_0)$ and $M_t = M(t \equiv t_{u+1})$ are fixed

$$P[M_t|M_{t_0}] = \int \cdots \int dM_{t-\Delta t}\, dM_{t-2\Delta t} \cdots dM_{t_0+\Delta t} \times P[M_t|M_{t-\Delta t}]P[M_{t-\Delta t}|M_{t-2\Delta t}] \cdots P[M_{t_0+\Delta t}|M_{t_0}] \tag{14.27}$$

$$P[M_t|M_{t_0}] = \int \cdots \int \underline{D}M \exp\left(-\sum_{s=0}^{u} \Delta t \underline{L}_s\right)$$

$$\underline{D}M = (2\pi \hat{g}_0^2 \Delta t)^{-1/2} \prod_{s=1}^{u} (2\pi \hat{g}_s^2 \Delta t)^{-1/2}\, dM_s$$

Similarly, the short-time probability distribution P can be folded over and over at each point r, to give a field-theoretic Lagrangian, L(r, t). The above "prepoint-discretization" representation of $\underline{L}$ derived for the neocortex, such as $g_s^G = g^G[M^G(t_0 + s\Delta t)]$, disguises the Riemannian geometry induced by the nonconstant metric $g_{GG'}$, which is discussed further below.

Macroscopic Development

General Description

Inclusion of all these microscopic and mesoscopic features of neocortex permits a true nonphenomenologic Gaussian-Markovian formal development for macroscopic regions encompassing $\sim 5 \times 10^3$ macrocolumns of spatial extent $\sim 5 \times 10^9$ μm^2, albeit one that is still highly nonlinear and not in equilibrium. The development of mesocolumnar domains presents conditional probability distributions for mesocolumnar firings with spatially coupled nearest-neighbor interactions. The macroscopic spatial folding of these mesoscopic domains and their macroscopic temporal folding of tens to hundreds of τ, with a resolution of at least τ/N (Ingber, 1984a), yields a true path-integral formulation in terms of a macroscopic Lagrangian possessing a variational principle for most-probable firing states. At this point in formal development, no continuous-time approximation has been made; this is done, with clear justification, only for some applications discussed below. Much of this algebra is facilitated by, but does not require, Riemannian geometry to develop the nonlinear means, variances, and "potential" contributions to the Lagrangian (Langouche et al, 1982).

This formalism can also be recast in several other representations (Langouche et al, 1982), perhaps more familiar to other investigators, and sometimes more useful for particular calculations. For example, a Hamiltonian formulation can be obtained, one that does not permit simple energy-type conservation approximations, but does permit the usual circumstances of time evolution. The time-dependent differential macroscopic probability distribution, or "propagator," satisfies a true Fokker-Planck second-order partial-differential equation, expressing the rate of change of the distribution as the sum of contributions from nonlinear drifts and diffusion in the space of E and I firings. With respect to a reference stationary state, a well-defined information, or "entropy," can be formulated. Also a set of Langevin rate equations for E and I firings can be obtained, expressing the rate of change of firings as the sum of drifts and multiplicative noise. The most-probable firing states derived variationally from the path-integral Lagrangian as the Euler-Lagrange equations represent a reasonable average over the noise in the Langevin system; the noise cannot be indiscriminately neglected. Because of the presence of multiplicative noise, the Langevin system differs in its Itô (prepoint) and Stratonovich (midpoint) discretizations. Furthermore, a midpoint-discretized covariant description, in terms of the Feynman Lagrangian $\underline{L}_F$, is defined such that fluctuations occur in solutions to the Euler-Lagrange variational equations. In contrast, the usual Itô and corresponding Stratonovich discretizations are defined such that the path-integral reduces to the Fokker-Planck equation in the weak-noise limit.

Using the Lagrangian formulation, a systematic numeric procedure was developed for fitting parameters in such stochastic nonlinear systems to data using methods of ASA (Ingber, 1989, 1993c, 1993a), and then integrating the path-integral using a non-Monte Carlo technique especially suited for nonlinear systems

(Wehner and Wolfer, 1983a, 1983b, 1987). This numeric method has been applied with success to military modeling (Ingber et al, 1991; Ingber and Sworder, 1991) and to financial markets (Ingber, 1990; Ingber et al, 1991); as discussed below, we are using it now in this neocortical system to correlate EEG to behavioral states (Ingber, 1991a; Ingber and Nunez, 1990).

Riemannian Geometry

A series of articles recognized that a few of the most popular Riemannian-geometric transformation properties possessed by physics systems might be advantageous for a theory of cortical interactions, particularly in the cerebellum, and they have gone further to postulate this geometry as the essential component of their theory (Pellionisz and Llinás, 1979, 1980; Pellionisz, 1984).

As developed most notably by Einstein (Einstein et al, 1923), Riemannian geometry has been established firmly as a necessary component of the foundations of physics. There are still two viable camps of opinions, considering this geometry itself as a basic foundation (Misner et al, 1973), or considering the physical entities on which its transformations operate as the basic foundation (Weinberg, 1972). However, all agree that Riemannian geometry is an essential theoretical construct that explains some observed physical phenomena. Riemannian geometry also is a natural mathematical consequence of properties possessed by general stochastic systems, including those models of neural systems assumed or endorsed by most investigators (Arbib and Amari, 1985). These properties have been stressed in the SMNI article series.

We want to stress these general properties and make the short but important observation that mathematical support exists on which to conjecture possible neural mechanisms that might result from invariance under Riemannian-geometric transformations. This observation then leads us back to the spirit, if not the essence, of other neuroscience investigations. However, whereas they hypothesize a Riemannian metric between cortical regions, SMNI derives a Riemannian metric within each cortical region or within an aggregate set of interacting cortical regions, which is an important physical distinction.

Corresponding to the differential-operator ordering problem in the Fokker-Planck equation is the discretization problem in the path-integral and in the Langevin rate equations, which are both equivalent mathematical representations of the Fokker-Planck equation (Dekker, 1980; Grabert and Green, 1979; Graham, 1977a; Graham, 1977b; Langouche et al, 1982; Schulman, 1981). An overview of these equations is required to at least note where the Riemannian geometry applies. The appendix of an SMNI article provides a brief derivation (Ingber, 1991a).

The output need not be confined to complex algebraic forms or tables of numbers. Because $\underline{L}_F$ possesses a variational principle, sets of contour graphs, at different long-time epochs of the path-integral of P and integrated over all its variables at all intermediate times, provide a visually intuitive and accurate decision aid to view the dynamic evolution of the scenario. For example, this Lagrangian approach permits a quantitative assessment of concepts that are usually only loosely defined.

Concept	Lagrangian equivalent
Momentum	$\Pi^G = \dfrac{\partial \underline{L}_F}{\partial(\partial M^G/\partial t)}$
Mass	$g_{GG'} = \dfrac{\partial \underline{L}_F}{\partial(\partial M^G/\partial t)\partial(\partial M^{G'}/\partial t)}$
Force	$\dfrac{\partial \underline{L}_F}{\partial M^G}$
F = ma	$\delta \underline{L}_F = 0 = \dfrac{\partial \underline{L}_F}{\partial M^G} - \dfrac{\partial}{\partial t}\dfrac{\partial \underline{L}_F}{\partial(\partial M^G/\partial t)}$

(14.28)

These physical entities provide another form of intuitive, but quantitatively precise, analyses (Ingber, 1991b).

The key issue is that Riemannian geometry is not needed to derive the mathematics of multiplicative Gaussian-Markovian systems. More interestingly, based on this derivation, the space of random variables induces a Riemannian geometry, obtained explicitly by simply (in hindsight) reorganizing terms in their defining equations. Then the differential and path-integral representations can be rewritten only in terms of functions f(M) of random variables M that are tensor invariant under generally nonlinear point transformations, that is, $M' = M'(M)$.

The derived probability distribution also is invariant under an equivalence class of discretizations. This is not equivalent to incorporating bona fide physical delays, such as those that can yield EEG wave propagation in local circuits, as emphasized in SMNI, or in long-range circuits (Nunez, 1981a).

The possibility of rewriting any theory or model of neural systems, which can be described by multiplicative Gaussian-Markovian dynamics, into an algebraic form invariant under Riemannian-geometric transformations does not require that neural systems develop or elect mechanisms to take advantage of these transformations. However, the most obvious candidate for a physical consequence of invariance under such transformations is the information Υ, developed in SMNI, sometimes loosely called the "entropy" of the system. The invariance of Υ implies that, although different cortical regions may have different anatomic features and superficially appear to have different sets of firing states, they may indeed share, encode, or decode the same information using their own anatomic and physiologic features to develop their own sets of firing states related to each other by (nonlinear) transformations.

This possibility reflects the original spirit of other authors, who were attracted to Riemannian geometry to explain how information in sensory regions might be transmitted to motor regions although their neural properties differ in many respects. Statistical mechanics of neocortical interactions develop columnar interactions; we have been tempted to conjecture that local and global processing of columnar firing patterns is enhanced, if not primarily effected, by transmitting blocks of information that are invariant under nonlinear transformations of firing states.

Ultimately, these issues must be resolved by experiment. No evidence, pro or con, bears on the issue of the explicit Riemannian-geometric nature of information processing of neural firings. In principle, this could be accomplished by numerically fitting neuronal firing data to Lagrangians that describe regions behaviorally proved to process similar information, similar to fits to data proposed for other artificial intelligence systems (Ingber, 1985d).

INFORMATION, POTENTIAL, AND LONG-RANGE INTERACTIONS

Some investigators have tried to use information as an index of EEG activity (Gersch, 1987; Mars and Lopes da Silva, 1987). However, these attempts have focused on the concept of "mutual information" to find correlations of EEG activity under different electrodes. At the outset, the SMNI approach recognizes that, for most brain states of late latency, at least a subset of regions measured by several electrodes should be considered as one system, and their interactions should be explicated by mathematical or physical modeling of the underlying neuronal processes. Then it is not relevant to compare joint distributions over a set of electrodes with marginal distributions over individual electrodes. The concept of information, as expressed below, may yet prove to be a useful valid measure to compare different subjects within certain categories.

With reference to a steady-state $\bar{P}(\tilde{M})$, when it exists, an analytic definition of the information gain $\hat{Y}$ in state $\tilde{P}(\tilde{M})$ is defined by (Graham, 1978; Haken, 1983)

$$\hat{Y}[\tilde{P}] = \int \cdots \int \underline{D}\tilde{M}\tilde{P}\ \ln(\tilde{P}/\bar{P}) \qquad (14.29)$$

where again a path integral is defined such that all intermediate-time values of $\tilde{M}$ appearing in the folded short-time distributions $\tilde{P}$ are integrated over. This is general for any system that can be described as Gaussian-Markovian (Haken, 1988), even if only in the short-time limit, such as the SMNI theory. (As time evolves, the distribution probably no longer behaves in a Gaussian manner, and the apparent simplicity of the short-time distribution typically must be supplanted by numeric calculations.) Although $\hat{Y}$ is well defined and useful for discussing macroscopic neocortical activity, it may not be as useful for all applications. Many important local changes of information effected by the neocortical system are a function of the microscopic degrees of freedom already averaged for this study. However, the path-integral represents many spatial-temporal degrees of freedom of the mesoscopic system. For example, even neglecting specific coding of presynaptic and postsynaptic membranes, detailed neuronal circuitry, and the dynamics of temporal evolution, in a hypothetical region of 10^9 neurons with 10^{13} synapses and considering each synapse as only conducting or not conducting, there are $\approx \exp(7 \times 10^{12})$ possible synaptic combinations; considering only each neuron as firing or not firing, there are $\approx \exp(7 \times 10^{8})$ neuronal combinations;

considering only each mesocolumn as having integral firings between -100 and 100, there are $\approx \exp(5 \times 10^7)$ mesocolumnar combinations.

$\underline{T}$, defined as the "kinetic-energy" $\underline{V}$-independent part of $\underline{L}$ in (14.22), is scale independent of N. Therefore, the small scale of the neocortical system, about which the system fluctuates, is derived to be N^{-1}, the inverse of the number of neurons in a mesocolumn. This is interpreted as the effective "temperature" or inherent noise of the system. Thus STM defines a "hot" and volatile system, wherein the relevant activity occurs on the same order as N^{-1}. In contrast, some long-term memory calculations described below (Ingber, 1983a) are consistent with the interpretation that they occur at a much lower temperature and in a locally more stable environment.

Verification of SMNI

Because it is relevant to the use of the SMNI model to fit experimental data, we are justified in considering this approach a viable description of the real neocortex. As outlined below, the mesoscopic scale developed by SMNI was verified by calculations detailing some properties of short-term memory. (Of course, this does not mean that some other theories do not possess similar numeric verification.) The macroscopic scale developed by SMNI was verified by calculations detailing some properties of phenomena associated with EEG measurements. The aggregate calculations suggest mechanisms for long-term storage of memories through synaptic modifications.

Short-Term Memory

General Description

The most detailed and dramatic application of the theory outlined here is to predict stochastic bounds for human STM capacity during focused selective attention (Ingber, 1972, 1981b, 1984a, 1985b, 1985e), which occurs in tenths of a second to seconds and is limited to the retention of 7 ± 2 items (Miller, 1956). This is true even for apparently exceptional memory performers who, although they may encode and retrieve STM more efficiently, and although they may "chunk" larger patterns of information into single items, nevertheless they are limited to a STM capacity of 7 ± 2 items (Ericsson and Chase, 1982). This is verified for acoustical STM, but for visual or semantic STM, which typically require longer times for rehearsal in an hypothesized articulatory loop of individual items, STM capacity appears to be limited to two to four (Zhang and Simon, 1985). This STM capacity-limited chunking phenomenon also has been noted with items requiring varying depths and breadths of processing (Ingber, 1972, 1976, 1981b, 1981c, 1985e). Another interesting phenomenon of STM capacity explained by this theory is the primacy-versus-recency effect in STM serial processing, wherein first-learned items are recalled most error-free, with last-learned items still more error-free than those in the middle (Murdock, 1983).

The basic assumption being made is that a pattern of neuronal firing that persists for many τ cycles is a candidate to store the "memory" of activity that produced this pattern. If several firing patterns can exist simultaneously, then several memories can be stored. The short-time probability distribution derived for the neocortex is the primary tool to seek such firing patterns. Because this distribution is exponentially sensitive to (minus) the Lagrangian function $\underline{L}$, it is more convenient to address $\underline{L}$ directly, whereby its minima specify the most probable states that can be sustained at a given time. Then several important features of these patterned states can be investigated, as is done for other physical systems (Haken, 1983), such as the evolution of these states, the "time of first passage" to jump from one state to another state, hysteresis between states that have different depths (values of the Lagrangian at these local minima), the stability of each state under external forces, and so forth.

We define the "stationary" (sometimes called the "uniform") Lagrangian, $\bar{\underline{L}}$, by setting to zero all temporal and spatial derivatives of M^G, as in (14.22). Contour plots of the stationary Lagrangian, $\bar{\underline{L}}$, for typical synaptic parameters balanced between predominately inhibitory and predominately excitatory firing states are examined at many scales when the background synaptic noise is only modestly shifted to cause efferent and afferent mesocolumnar firing states to have a common most-probable firing, centered at $M^{*G} = M^G = 0$ (Ingber, 1984a). Within the range of synaptic parameters considered, for values of $\tau\bar{\underline{L}} \sim 10^{-2}$, this "centering" mechanism causes the appearance of from 5 to 10 or 11 extrema for values of $\tau\bar{\underline{L}}$ of about 10^{-2}. The centering mechanism is achieved by modestly shifting $B^G_{G'}$ to cause $(V^G - a^{|G|}_{G'}v^{|G|}_{G'}N^{G'})$ to become zero, thereby driving the threshold factor F^G to zero. (At $F^G = 0$, the mesoscopic derivation of Gaussian $\underline{L}$ breaks down, so we can only consider a finite region, heavily weighted by N, about this point.) In the absence of external constraints and this centering mechanism, no stable minima are found; that is, the system either shuts down, with no firings, or it becomes epileptic, with maximal firings at the upper limits of excitatory or of excitatory and inhibitory firings. The appearance of these extrema due to the centering mechanism clearly depends on the nonlinearities present in the derived Lagrangian, stressing competition and cooperation among excitatory and inhibitory interactions at columnar and neuronal scales (Figure 14-4).

These numbers of minima are determined when the resolution of the contours is commensurate with the resolution of columnar firings, that is, about 5 to 10 neuronal firings per columnar mesh point. If the resolution is forced to decrease to one neuronal firing per columnar mesh point, then typically only about one half of these minima are found. The coarser resolution, in fact, is the one appropriate for numeric solution of the derived time-dependent path-integral: Most important contributions to the probability distribution P come from ranges of the time slice θ and the "action" $N\underline{L}$, such that $\theta N\underline{L} \leq 1$. By considering the contributions to the first and second moments of ΔM^G for small time slices θ, conditions on the time and variable meshes can be derived (Wehner and Wolfer, 1983a).

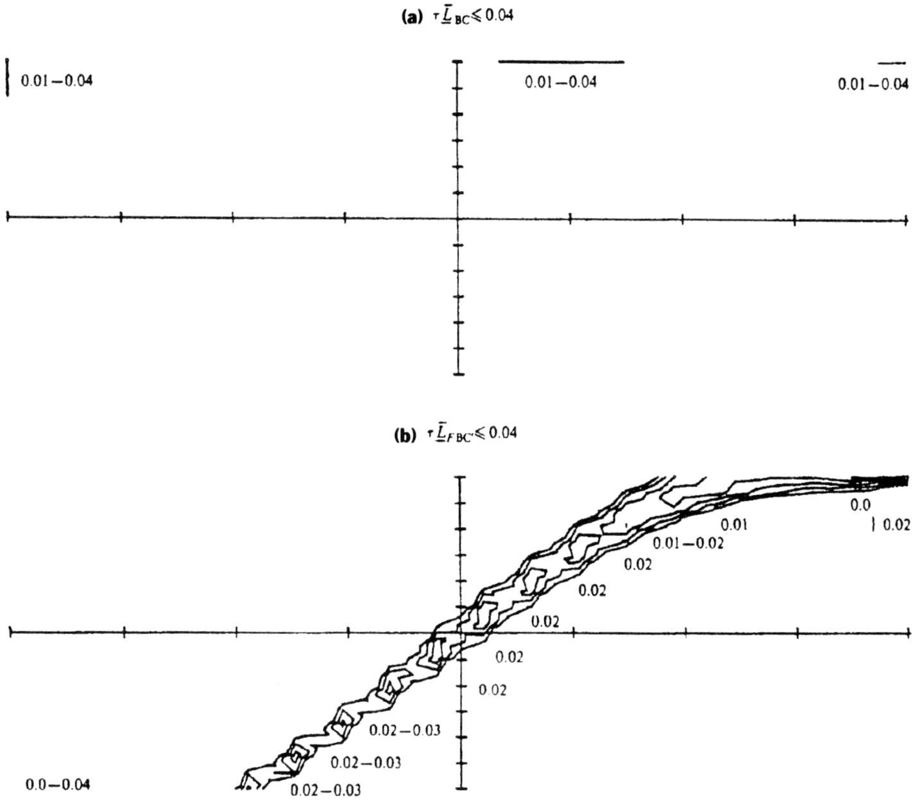

Figure 14-4. Contours of the Lagrangian illustrate "valleys" that trap firing states of mesocolumns. ($\tau\underline{\bar{L}}_{BC}$ can be as large as 10^3.) These valleys are candidates for short-term memories. Detailed calculations support the identification of the inner valleys with stable short-term memory states that have durations on the order of tenths of a second. (**a**) Contours for values less than 0.4 are drawn for $\tau\underline{\bar{L}}_{BC}$, where BC designates the balanced case of firing states at a moderate level of excitatory and inhibitory firings. The $\bar{M}^E$ axis increases to the right, from $-N^E = -80$ to $N^E = 80$. The $\bar{M}^I$ axis increases to the right, from $-N^I = -30$ to $N^I = 30$. In each cluster, the smaller values are closer to the center. There are no closed contours in the interior space. (**b**) Contours for values less than 0.04 are drawn for $\tau\underline{\bar{L}}_{FBC'}$, where BC′ denotes that the "centering mechanism" has been turned on, and F denotes that the full Feynman Lagrangian was used. A right brace } signifies enclosure of other nested closed contours above and to the left of this brace.

The variable mesh, a function of M^G, is optimally chosen such that ΔM^G is measured by the covariance $g^{GG'}$ (diagonal in the neocortex because of the independence of E and I chemical interactions) or $\Delta M^G \sim (g^{GG}\theta)^{1/2}$ in the notation of SMNI articles. For $N \sim 10^2$ and $\underline{\bar{L}} \sim 10^{-2}/\tau$, it is reasonable to pick $\theta \sim \tau$. Then it is calculated that optimal meshes are $\Delta M^E \sim 7$ and $\Delta M^I \sim 4$, which are essentially the resolutions used in the published SMNI coarse contour plots.

Because the extrema of the Lagrangian appear to lie fairly well along a line in the two-dimensional M^G space, and because coefficients of slowly varying dM^G/dt terms in the nonstationary $\bar{L}$ are small perturbations on $\bar{L}$ (Ingber, 1983a), a solution to the stationary probability distribution was hypothesized to be proportional to $\exp(-\Phi/D)$, where $\Phi = CN^2\bar{L}$, the diffusion $D = N/\tau$, and C is a constant. Surprisingly, at least until more recent research showed the generality of such results (Colet et al, 1990), along the line of the extrema, for $C \approx 1$, this is an accurate solution to the full two-dimensional Fokker-Planck equation (Ingber, 1985b). A weak-noise high-barrier regimen defined by $\Delta\Phi/D > 1$, where $\Delta\Phi$ is the difference in Φ from minima to maxima, can be assumed for further analyses (Shenoy and Agarwal, 1984). This is very useful, because a linear stability analysis shows that stability with respect to mesocolumnar fluctuations induced by several neurons changing their firings is determined by the second derivatives of $-\Phi$ (Agarwal and Shenoy, 1981); here this just measures the parabolic curvature of $\bar{L}$ at the extrema. Thus all the extrema of the stationary Lagrangian are determined to be stable minima of the time-dependent dynamic system. However, it is unlikely that a true potential exists over all M^G space (Graham et al, 1985; Graham and Tél, 1984).

This stationary solution is also useful for calculating the time of first passage, $t_{\nu p}$, to fluctuate out of a valley in one minimum over a peak to another minimum (Agarwal and Shenoy, 1981). The values of $\tau\bar{L} \sim 10^{-2}$ for which the minima exist are just right to give $t_{\nu p}$ at about tenths of a second for about nine of the minima when the maximum of 10 to 11 are present. The other minima give $t_{\nu p}$ of approximately many seconds, which is large enough to cause hysteresis to dominate single jumps between other minima (Ingber, 1984a). Thus 7 ± 2 is the capacity of STM, for memories or new patterns that can be accessed in any order during tenths of a second, all as observed experimentally (Ericsson and Chase, 1982). When the number of neurons per minicolumn is ~220, modeling the visual neocortex (Ingber, 1984a), then the minima become deeper and sharper, consistent with sharper depth of processing, but several minima become isolated from the main group. This effect might be responsible for the lowering of STM capacity for visual processing, as noted previously. The statistical time of passage between clusters becomes many hours, longer than STM, whereas the time between minima within a cluster, now with only 2 to 4 minima per cluster, is on the order of tenths of a second, as observed. This effect also illustrates that the "practical" number of emergent mesoscopic stable states does not necessarily increase with an increasing number of microscopic units (Figure 14-5).

This estimate of the number of minima involves a very sensitive calculation. That is, if N were a factor of 10 larger, or if $\tau\bar{L} \sim 0.1$ at the minima, then $t_{\nu p}$ is measured in hours rather than seconds, becoming unrealistic for STM durations. Alternatively, if $t_{\nu p}$ were much smaller, that is less than $\sim 5\tau$, this case would be inconsistent with observed time scales necessary for formation of any memory trace (Libet, 1982). In this context, the threshold factor of the probability distribution scales is $(N^*N)^{1/2}$, necessitating that both the macrocolumnar divergence

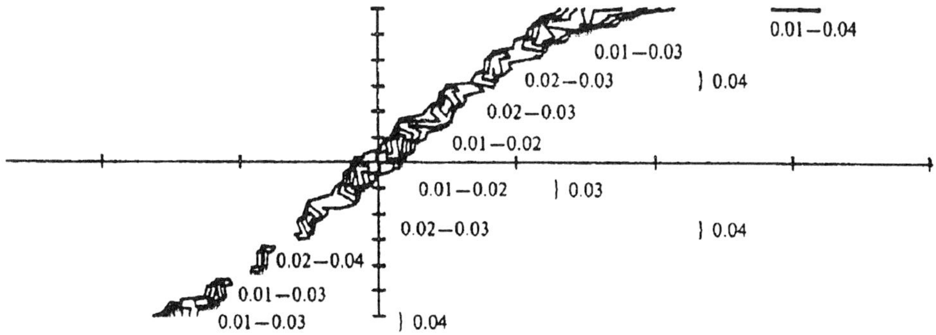

Figure 14-5. When N = 220, modeling the number of neurons per minicolumn in the visual neocortex, then only clusters containing 2 to 4 or as many as 5 to 6 minima are found, consistent with visual STM. These minima are more narrow, consistent with the sharpness required to store visual patterns.

and minicolumnar convergence of mesocolumnar firings be tested by these calculations.

These results pose serious problems for other models, such as "mean-field" theories or reductionist doctrines. The mean-field approach essentially sets N = 1, and N* is assumed, by some investigators, to be $\sim 10^5$, the size of a macrocolumn, but others even consider it to be as large as $\sim 10^{10}$, the total number of neurons in the neocortex. The reductionist doctrine claims that only circuitries among a few to several neurons are responsible for a specific pattern of neocortical function, and this effectively sets $N \approx N^*$, to about a few neurons. It is difficult to understand how both the capacity and duration of STM can be explained by these other models, even assuming they were or could be derived with realistic synaptic interactions and correct statistical dynamics.

The statistical nature of this storage and processing also explains the primacy-versus-recency effect: The deepest minima of the Lagrangian are more likely to be accessed than the others of this probability distribution, and these valleys are sharper than the others. That is, they are more readily accessed and sustain their patterns against fluctuations more accurately than do the relatively more shallow minima. The more recent memories or newer patterns may be presumed to be those having synaptic parameters that are more recently tuned, more actively rehearsed, or both. Thus both the nonlinearities and the statistical nature of this theory are tested by STM capacity. These insights have helped to correct the beliefs of some experimentalists who claimed they could not find this effect in the visual cortex: Their experimental paradigms were testing the visual cortex using rules of auditory capacity (that is, they were testing 7 ± 2 instead of 4 ± 2) and therefore they were canceling this effect.

These calculations give experimental support to the derivation of the mesoscopic probability distribution, yielding similar algebraic structures of the threshold factors in (14.18) and (14.26), illustrating common forms of interactions between their entities, that is, neurons and columns of neurons, respectively. The nonlinear threshold factors are defined in terms of electrical-chemical synaptic and neuronal parameters all lying within their experimentally observed ranges.

STM CALCULATION

Three cases of neuronal firings were considered (Ingber, 1984a). That reference is recommended for several figures that exhibit the minima structures algebraically described below. Because STM duration is still long relative to τ, stationary solutions of $\bar{\underline{L}}$, derived from $\underline{L}$ in (14.24), were investigated to determine how many stable minima, $\langle\langle \bar{M}^G \rangle\rangle$, may simultaneously exist within this duration. Also individual mesocolumns were studied, that is, taking the uniform limit of $\dot{M}^G = 0 = \nabla \bar{M}^G$. Although the $\dot{M}^G = 0$ limit should only be taken in the midpoint-discretized Lagrangian $\underline{L}_F$, this is a small difference here (Ingber, 1984a).

A model of dominant inhibition describes how minicolumnar firings are suppressed by their neighboring minicolumns. For example, this could be effected by developing nearest-neighbor mesocolumnar interactions (Ingber, 1983a), but here the averaged effect is established by inhibitory mesocolumns (IC) by setting $A^I_E = A_E = 2A^E_E = 0.01N^*/N$. Because there appears to be relatively little I − I connectivity, $A^I_I = 0.0001N^*/N$. The background synaptic noise is understood to be $B^E_I = B^I_E = 2B^E_E = 10B^I_I = 0.002N^*/N$. Because minicolumns are observed to have ~110 neurons (the visual cortex appears to have approximately twice this density) (Mountcastle, 1978), and because there is a predominance of E over I neurons (Nunez, 1981a), assume that here $N^E = 80$ and $N^I = 30$. Use $N^*/N = 10^3$, $J_G = 0$ (absence of long-range interactions), and V^G, $\nu^G_{G'}$, and $\phi^G_{G'}$ as estimated previously, that is, $V^G = 10$ mV, $|\nu^G_{G'}| = 0.1$ mV, $\phi^G_{G'} = 0.1$ mV. The "threshold factors" F^G_{IC} for this IC model are then

$$
\begin{aligned}
F^E_{IC} &= \frac{0.5\bar{M}^I - 0.25\bar{M}^E + 3.0}{\pi^{1/2}(0.1\bar{M}^I + 0.05\bar{M}^E + 9.80)^{1/2}} \\
F^I_{IC} &= \frac{0.005\bar{M}^I - 0.5\bar{M}^E - 45.8}{\pi^{1/2}(0.001\bar{M}^I + 0.1M^E + 11.2)^{1/2}}
\end{aligned}
\qquad (14.30)
$$

In the prepoint-discretized deterministic limit, the threshold factors determine when and how smoothly the "step functions" $\tanh F^G_{IC}$ in $g^G(t)$ change $M^G(t)$ to $M^G(t + \theta)$. F^I_{IC} will cause afferent $\bar{M}^I$ to fire for most of its values, because $\bar{M}^I \sim -N^I \tanh F^I_{IC}$ will be positive for most values of $\bar{M}^G$ in F^I_{IC}, which is already weighted heavily with a term −45.8. Looking at F^E_{IC}, the relatively high positive values of efferent $\bar{M}^I$ require at least moderate values of positive efferent $\bar{M}^E$ to cause firings of afferent $\bar{M}^E$.

The calculations presented here support the contention that the neocortex functions at multiple hierarchies. Although specific long-term memory (LTM) information is probably coded at the microscopic neuronal level, the mesoscopic scale probably provides the context for multiple most-probable firing patterns that process STM and that facilitate plastic synaptic encoding of LTM (Ingber, 1983a). For example, $\tau\bar{\underline{L}}$ can range from 0 to values greater than 10^3 (Ingber, 1982, 1983a). However, realistic constraints on STM duration dictate that only values of $\tau\bar{\underline{L}} \leq 0.04$ are of interest here. Detailed mesoscalar calculations show that only this range has sufficient nonlinear structure to support STM phenomena.

More minima of $\bar{\underline{L}}$ are created, or "restored," if the numerator of F^G contains terms only in $\bar{M}^G$, tending to center $\bar{\underline{L}}$ about $\bar{M}^G = 0$. Of course, any mechanism producing more and deeper minima is statistically favored. However, this particular "centering" mechanism has plausible support: $M^G(t + \tau) = 0$ is the state of afferent firing with highest statistical weight. That is, there are more combinations of neuronal firings, $\sigma_j = \pm 1$, yielding this state than any other $M^G(t + \tau)$; for example, $\sim 2^{N^G + 1/2}(\pi N^G)^{-1/2}$ relative to the states $M^G = \pm N^G$. Similarly, $M^{*G}(t)$ is the state of efferent firing with highest statistical weight. Therefore, it is natural to explore mechanisms that favor common highly weighted efferent and afferent firings in ranges consistent with favorable firing threshold factors $F^G \approx 0$.

Detailed calculations demonstrate that typically either $\bar{\underline{L}}^E$ or $\bar{\underline{L}}^I$ separately yield more multiple minima, $\approx$10, than permitted by their sum $\bar{\underline{L}}$ at this resolution. This "loss" of minima apparently is an interesting consequence of E − I competition at the mesoscopic scale. On one hand, because $\bar{\underline{L}}^G$ scales as N^G/N for relatively large $\bar{M}^G$, $\bar{\underline{L}}^E$ dominates because of the larger $\bar{M}^E$ in its mean g^E. On the other hand, for relatively small $\bar{M}^G$, g^G typically is small if there are several multiple minima in $\bar{\underline{L}}^G$, because most of the minima are found to cluster about the origin. Therefore, $\bar{\underline{L}}^G$ scales as $(N^G)^{-1}$ from the variances $(g^{GG})^{-1}$, and $\bar{\underline{L}}^I$ dominates for small $\bar{M}^G$.

The centering effect of the IC model of dominant inhibition, labeled here as the IC′ model, is easy for the neocortex to accommodate. For example, this can be accomplished simply by readjusting the synaptic background noise from B^G_E to B'^G_E

$$B'^G_E = \frac{V^G - \left(\frac{1}{2} A^G_I + B^G_I\right) \nu^G_I N^I - \frac{1}{2} A^G_E \nu^G_E N^E}{\nu^G_E N^G} \tag{14.31}$$

for G = E and G = I. This is easily modified when regional influences from $M^{\ddagger E}$ are included, as in (14.26). In general, B^G_E and B^G_I (and possibly A^G_E and A^G_I as a result of actions of neuromodulators, and J_G or $M^{\ddagger E}$ constraints from long-range fibers) are available to force the constant in the numerator to zero, giving an extra degree(s) of freedom to this mechanism. (If B'^G_E were negative, we would have unphysical results in the square-root denominator of F^G. Here, in all examples in which this occurs, we can instead find positive B'^G_I to appropriately shift the numerator of F^G.) In this context, we observe experimentally that the synaptic sensitivity of neurons engaged in selective attention is altered, presumably by the influence of chemical neuromodulators on postsynaptic neurons (Mountcastle et al, 1981).

By this centering mechanism, $B_E'^E = 1.38$ and $B_I'^I = 15.3$, and F_{IC}^G is transformed to $F_{IC'}^G$

$$
\begin{aligned}
F_{IC'}^E &= \frac{0.5\bar{M}^I - 0.25\bar{M}^E}{\pi^{1/2}(0.1\bar{M}^I + 0.05\bar{M}^E + 10.4)^{1/2}} \\
F_{IC'}^I &= \frac{0.005\bar{M}^I - 0.5\bar{M}^E}{\pi^{1/2}(0.001\bar{M}^I + 0.1\bar{M}^E + 20.4)^{1/2}}
\end{aligned}
\tag{14.32}
$$

Aside from enforced vanishing of the constant terms in the numerators of $F_{IC'}^G$, the only other change in $F_{IC'}^G$ relative to F_{IC}^G is to moderately affect the constant terms in the denominators. This increases the number of minima of $\tau\bar{\underline{L}}_{IC'}$ to four. The two minima clustered close to the origin cannot be discerned for $\tau\bar{\underline{L}}_{IC'} > 0.03$.

The other "extreme" of normal neocortical firings is a model of dominant excitation, produced by establishing excitatory mesocolumns (EC) by using the same parameters $\{B_{G'}^G, \nu_{G'}^G, \phi_{G'}^G, A_{I}^{I}\}$ as in the IC model, but setting $A_E^E = 2A_E^I = 2A_I^E = 0.01N^*/N$. This yields

$$
\begin{aligned}
F_{EC}^E &= \frac{0.25\bar{M}^I - 0.5\bar{M}^E - 24.5}{\pi^{1/2}(0.05\bar{M}^I + 0.10\bar{M}^E + 12.3)^{1/2}} \\
F_{EC}^I &= \frac{0.005\bar{M}^I - 0.25\bar{M}^E - 25.8}{\pi^{1/2}(0.001\bar{M}^I + 0.05\bar{M}^E + 7.24)^{1/2}}
\end{aligned}
\tag{14.33}
$$

The negative constant in the numerator of F_{EC}^I inhibits afferent $\bar{M}^I$ firings. Although there is also a negative constant in the numerator of F_{EC}^E, the increased coefficient of $\bar{M}^E$ (relative to its corresponding value in F_{IC}^E), and the fact that $\bar{M}^E$ can be as large as $N^E = 80$, readily permits excitatory firings throughout most of the range of $\bar{M}^E$. This permits three minima.

Applying the centering mechanism to EC, $B_I'^E = 10.2$ and $B_I'^I = 8.62$. The net effect in $F_{EC'}^G$, in addition to removing the constant terms in the numerators of F_{EC}^G, is to change the constant terms in the denominators: 12.3 in F_{EC}^E is changed to 17.2 in $F_{EC'}^E$, and 7.24 in F_{EC}^I is changed to 12.4 in $F_{EC'}^I$. Now six prominent minima are possible along a line through $\bar{M}^G = 0$, and two others are at $\bar{M}^G = \pm N^G$. Each pair of minima above and below the $\bar{M}^I = 0$ axis merge into single minima for $\tau\bar{\underline{L}}_{EC'} > 0.02$, and these lose resolution for $\tau\bar{\underline{L}}_{EC'} > 0.03$.

It is natural to examine a balanced case between IC and EC, labeled BC. This is accomplished by changing $A_E^E = A_E^I = A_I^E = 0.005N^*/N$. This yields

$$
\begin{aligned}
F_{BC}^E &= \frac{0.25\bar{M}^I - 0.25\bar{M}^E - 4.50}{\pi^{1/2}(0.050\bar{M}^E + 0.050\bar{M}^I + 8.30)^{1/2}} \\
F_{BC}^I &= \frac{0.005\bar{M}^I - 0.25\bar{M}^E - 25.8}{\pi^{1/2}(0.001\bar{M}^I + 0.050\bar{M}^E + 7.24)^{1/2}}
\end{aligned}
\tag{14.34}
$$

Three minima are possible, on the boundaries of $\bar{M}^G$ space.

Applying the centering mechanism to BC, $B_E'^E = 0.438$ and $B_I'^I = 8.62$. The net effect in $F_{BC'}^G$, in addition to removing the constant terms in the numerators of F^G_{BC}, is to change the constant terms in the denominators: 8.30 in F^E_{BC} is changed to 7.40 in $F^E_{BC'}$, and 7.24 in F^I_{BC} is changed to 12.4 in $F^I_{BC'}$. Now 10 minima are possible. The nine minima along the diagonal line lose resolution for $\tau \bar{\underline{L}}_{BC'} > 0.01$ above $\bar{M}^I = 0$ and for $\tau \bar{\underline{L}}_{BC'} > 0.02$ below $\bar{M}^I = 0$.

The effects of using the full Feynman Lagrangian $\bar{\underline{L}}_F$ were considered, including all the Riemannian and other nonlinear corrections, discussed above. The net effect is to raise slightly the threshold at which minima dissipate, to about $\tau \bar{\underline{L}}_{BC'} \geq 0.03$, which is relevant for the duration of STM, which is discussed subsequently. However, the minima structure is essentially the same (Figure 14-4).

To show that multiple minima are not an effect of nonlinearities induced by the denominators of F^G, the net effect in $\bar{\underline{L}}_{BC'}$ by dropping the $\bar{M}^G$ terms in the denominators of $F^G_{BC'}$, is such that the valleys of minima are only slightly increased. However, these denominators are still important contributions derived from synaptic interactions. For example, even with the $\bar{M}^G$ terms dropped, the denominators contribute factors of $\sim 1/5$ to $F^G_{BC'}$.

If N^* is scaled larger or smaller, this effectively scales $A^G_{G'} = A^{*G}_{G'} N^*/N$ and $B^G_{G'} = B^{*G}_{G'} N^*/N$, disturbing the relatively sensitive balance that permits a few percent of efferent firings to affect their afferents. Then the number of possible minima typically is reduced to one or two. If N is scaled larger or smaller, the number of minima is altered and the duration of STM is affected. However, for N still in the range of a few hundred, the number of possible minima is not severely reduced. The case $N = 220$, such as the visual cortex, was considered: For model BC′, the number of prominent minima found was 11, but they formed clusters, with higher peaks between clusters than betwen minima within a cluster. The larger N sharpens the minima and therefore the resolution of visual information processing (Figure 14-5).

The sharpness of the tanh F^G step-function contribution to the mean firing is sensitive to a factor of $N^{1/2}$ in F^G. In addition, the strength of coupling between mesocolumns scales as $N^{3/2}$. Thus the neuronal size of mesocolumns directly affects the breadth and depth of the information processing capability of the neocortex. The human visual cortex, which may be assumed to require the finest tuning in the neocortex, is unique in having twice the number of neurons per minicolumn than other regions of the neocortex (Mountcastle, 1978).

These results are unchanged qualitatively for modest changes of any neocortical parameters. However, we can reasonably conjecture that more drastic abnormal changes in the neocortical parameters might severely reduce the number of minima. This conjecture is based on calculations wherein F^G do not possess the relatively sensitive balances allowing a few percent of efferent neurons to control firings in their afferent neurons. In calculations using these unrealistic or abnormal parameters, only one or two minima survive.

STM Stability and Duration

The calculation of stability and time of duration in most probable states of firing starts by using the differential equation Hamiltonian formulation of the path-integral Lagrangian, called the Fokker-Planck equation. For future reference, when EEGs are discussed in the context of considering a given local minimum, the time-dependent differential macroscopic probability distribution $\tilde{P} = \Pi_r P$, or "propagator," satisfies a true Fokker-Planck equation but has nonlinear drifts and diffusions in the space of E and I firings. The Fokker-Planck equation for the region Ω is

$$\frac{\partial \tilde{P}}{\partial t} \approx \Omega^{-1} \int d^2r \left[\frac{1}{2} (g^{GG'}\tilde{P})_{,GG'} - (g^G\tilde{P})_{,G} + N\underline{V}'\tilde{P} \right]$$
$$(\cdots)_{,G} \equiv \partial(\cdots)/\partial M^G \tag{14.35}$$

The true Fokker-Planck equation is actually more general, for example when long-range spatial structures are included, in which the independent variables M^G are fields that may depend on space and time coordinates. The above equation is derived in the nearest-neighbor approximation from the general equation using functional derivatives (Ingber, 1984a)

$$\partial(\cdots)/\partial M^G \rightarrow \delta(\cdots)/\delta M^G$$
$$\delta(\cdots)/\delta M^G = (\cdots)_{,G} - \nabla_i(\cdots)_{,\nabla_i G} + \nabla_i^2(\cdots)_{,\nabla_i^2 G} \tag{14.36}$$

where we have used the compacted notation introduced previously (Ingber, 1984a).

An estimate of a stationary solution P_{stat} to the Fokker-Planck differential equation for the probability distribution P of M^G firings for an uncoupled mesocolumn, that is, $\underline{V}' = 0$, is denoted by the stationary limit of the short-time propagator

$$P_{stat} \approx N_{stat} g^{1/2} \exp(-CN\tau\bar{\underline{L}})$$
$$g = \det(g^{GG'})^{-1} \equiv \det(g_{GG'}) = g_{EE}g_{II} \tag{14.37}$$

where N_{stat} and C are constant factors. The approximation made is estimated by seeking values of constants C, such that the stationary Fokker-Planck equation is satisfied exactly. Contour plots of C versus $\bar{M}^G$ show that real positive C exists, that may only range from $\sim 10^{-1}$ to ~ 1, for which unbroken contours of C pass through or at least border the line of minima (Ingber, 1985b). At each point $\bar{M}^G$, this leaves a quadratic equation for C to be solved. Dropping the $g^{1/2}$ factor causes C not to be real throughout the domain of $\bar{M}^G$.

Thus we have defined a solution with potential $N^2\bar{\underline{L}} = \int A\, dM$, drift A, and diffusion N/τ. Stability of transient solutions, defined for $\underline{\delta M}^G$ about a stationary state by

$$\underline{\delta \dot{M}}^G \approx -A_{,G}\underline{\delta M}^G = -N^2\bar{\underline{L}}_{,GG}\underline{\delta M}^G \tag{14.38}$$

therefore is equivalent to $\langle\langle \bar{M} \rangle\rangle$ being a minimum of $\bar{\underline{L}}$.

Because the minima of the Lagrangian lie deep in a valley along a line, the time for first passage, $t_{\nu p}$, is estimated in analogy to a one-dimensional system as (Agarwal and Shenoy, 1981)

$$t_{\nu p} \approx \pi N^{-2}[|\bar{L}_{,GG'}(\langle\langle \bar{M} \rangle\rangle_p)|\bar{L}_{,GG'}(\langle\langle \bar{M} \rangle\rangle_\nu)]^{-1/2}$$
$$\times \exp\{CN\tau[\bar{L}(\langle\langle \bar{M} \rangle\rangle_p) - \bar{L}(\langle\langle \bar{M} \rangle\rangle_\nu)]\} \tag{14.39}$$

where $\langle\langle \bar{M} \rangle\rangle_\nu$ is the minimum at the valley of $\underline{\bar{L}}$ in question, and $\langle\langle \bar{M} \rangle\rangle_p$ is the maximum at a peak separating two minima. These equations are reasonable but crude estimates, and future numeric work is needed to prove the extent of their validity.

The exponential factor can be very large in some instances and very small in others. As noted previously (Ingber, 1983a), differences in $\underline{\bar{L}}$ from valleys to peaks are still large relative to the Riemannian correction terms and relative to differential spatial-temporal contributions, thereby permitting this simpler analysis. However, values of $\tau\underline{\bar{L}}$ at maxima separating the far minima may be greater than 1, thereby yielding a very large $t_{\nu p}$, typical of many physical systems undergoing hysteresis (Ingber, 1983a). Relaxation times t_r about this stationary state are estimated by $|g^G_{;G}|^{-1}$ (Agarwal and Shenoy, 1981), and are on the order of τ.

Hysteresis can be more probable than simple jump behavior to another firing state. This provides a mechanism whereby an extended temporal firing pattern of information can be processed beyond the time scale of relaxation periods, such as reverberation among several local minima. The effects of long-range influences on mesoscopic synaptic parameters, such as those calculated in previous SMNI articles (Ingber, 1983a), can create more complex examples of spatial-temporal hysteresis. These sustaining mechanisms permit other biochemical processes to store information for longer periods as stable synaptic modifications, such as LTM. As detailed previously (Ingber, 1983a), changes in synaptic parameters may duplicate the effects of long-range interactions, providing a mechanism whereby columnar firings encode long-range firing constraints. If this encoding of firing patterns can be established on short enough time scales, then columnar coding of long-range firings could be a precursor mechanism initiating the centering mechanism above, especially across large regions of the neocortex. Then a more uniform gradation of mechanism(s) would establish STM and LTM.

However, to address the issue of limited capacity of STM, we should require that within time spans of tenths of a second to tens of seconds, simple jumps among minima are more probable than hysteresis. This permits all minima to be accessed readily during STM duration, in any ordering (Ericsson and Chase, 1982), at least more so than if hysteresis were more probable. In accord with this empirical requirement, as detailed in previous studies, $\tau[\underline{\bar{L}}(\langle\langle \bar{M} \rangle\rangle_p) - \underline{\bar{L}}(\langle\langle \bar{M} \rangle\rangle_\nu)] \sim 0.01$ to 0.03 for these models using empirical values for synaptic parameters. Then for $|\tau\underline{\bar{L}}_{,CC'}| \sim 10^{-3}$, $t_{\nu p} \sim 10\tau$ to 100τ, on the order of several tenths of a second to a second. The full Feynman Lagrangian $\underline{\bar{L}}_F$ increases $t_{\nu p}$ slightly. For these relatively short $t_{\nu p}$, the second inequality above is violated, and simple jumps are more probable than hysteresis, as required for STM.

Under conditions of serial processing, the deeper valleys of $\underline{\bar{L}}$ representing the more probable firing states will be occupied first. In all cases considered here, some valleys are deeper than the others. This implies that the last several items in STM should be harder to encode (learn) and retain, with the possible exception of the last one or two items, which represent the most recent shifting of firing patterns $\bar{M}^G$ to these minima $\langle\langle \bar{M} \rangle\rangle_\nu$ of $\underline{\bar{L}}$. These conclusions are consistent with empirical observations and are obtained independent of any other rehearsal mechanisms that may exist.

Calculations in these models establish that the prefactor most often is $\sim\tau$. However, points close to the corners $\bar{M}^G = \pm(N^E, N^I)$ have more rapid variations. Therefore, minima at these corners, even when $\tau\underline{L}(\langle\langle\bar{M}\rangle\rangle_p) \sim 0.01$ to 0.03, because of their sharp peaks, typically have $t_{\nu p}$ of about tens of seconds to jump to minima clustered on the diagonal. This is within the range where hysteresis is more probable for these minima. Therefore, minima at the corners of $\bar{M}^G$ space probably do not contribute to STM, reducing the number of available minima to 7 ± 2, as empirically observed.

EEG Dispersion Relations

General Description

Linear expansions about specific extrema, specified by the Euler-Lagrange variational equations, permit the development of stability analyses and dispersion relations in frequency-wave number space (Ingber, 1982, 1983a, 1985a). Of course, such linear expansions are justified only after the nonlinear problem, such as that encountered for STM, is solved for locations of minima. In this regard, the corresponding wave propagation velocities pace interactions over several minicolumns, to be of magnitude sufficient to permit simultaneous information processing within $\sim 10^{-1}$ seconds with interactions mediated by long-range fibers possessing much greater propagation velocities of ~600 to 900 cm/second (Ingber, 1985a). For example, detailed auditory and visual processing can feed information to the association cortex, where it can be processed simultaneously, possibly giving feedback to the primary sensory regions. The propagation velocities calculated by SMNI, ~1 cm/second, also are consistent with observed movements of attention (Tsal, 1983) and of hallucinations (Cowan, 1982) across the visual field. This strongly suggests that nearest-neighbor mesocolumnar interactions, as developed here, are an important mechanism in these movements. These velocities scale strongly with the values of $\bar{M}^G$ minima, increasing with their distsance from $\bar{M}^G \sim 0$, the range of maximal firing combinations. This effect must be investigated further; the appropriate calculations should test the nearest-neighbor spatial dependence of the SMNI theory.

These mesoscopic dispersion relations also are consistent with global macroscopic dispersion relations derived and fitted to EEG data (Nunez, 1981a; see Chapters 11 and 12), yielding oscillatory solutions consistent with the alpha rhythm, that is, $\omega \approx 10^2$ second^{-1}, equivalent to $\nu = \omega/(2\pi) \approx 16$ cp (Hertz). This suggests that these complementary local and global theories may be confluent, considered as a joint set of dispersion relations evolving from the deterministic limit of a joint Lagrangian, similar to "equations of motion," but linearly simplified in neighborhoods of minima of the stationary Lagrangian.

Other researchers have developed different approaches to investigating macroscopic neocortical activity, for example stressing that systematics of rhythmic EEG (alpha rhythm, sleep delta, and so on) can be modeled by resonant modes of macroscopic dipole-layered firing patterns of the neocortex (Nunez, 1974, 1981a, 1981b, 1981c), as discussed in Chapter 11. These resonances, in linearized, coupled, excitatory-inhibitory spatial-temporal integral equations describing dipole-layered sources, yield a macroscopic dispersion relation relating firing frequencies to spatial wave vectors, consistent with experimental observations. Although many other investigators also accept dipole layers to model EEG activity, at least to the extent of recognizing activity perpendicular to laminae, they also show that there are respectable candidates for mechanisms that might be fundamentally responsible for macroscopic activity, other than those proposed here, that detail synaptic dynamics of mesocolumnar interactions (Amari, 1983; Anninos et al, 1983; Basar, 1980; Freeman, 1978; Klemm and Sherry, 1981; Steriade, 1981; Traub and Llinás, 1979). For example, given the present lack of experimental knowledge, we can formulate macroscopic neocortical activity in terms of statistics of either membrane or synaptic microscopic neuronal activities, although they obviously depend on each other (Dudek et al, 1980). Therefore, the results of this statistical theory derived earlier (Ingber, 1985a) might be interpreted as suggesting that mesocolumnar activity instigates macroscopic activity or as suggesting that mesocolumnar activity strongly interacts with ongoing macroscopic activity that is instigated or sustained by other mechanisms.

The two approaches outlined above, that is local mesocolumnar versus global nonmesocolumnar, give rise to important alternative conjectures. Other studies also have proposed that EEG may be due to a combination of short-range and long-range interactions that combine to form a single dispersion relation with multiple branches (Nunez, 1989), as discussed in Chapter 11.

Studies of the origin of rhythmic EEG might give direct insight into related mechanisms underlying evoked potentials. However, in contrast to the alpha rhythm and other gross EEG phenomena that gauge general alertness for processing information, the time-locked averaged evoked potentials appear to gauge more selective attention to information being processed. Therefore, to derive a plausible description of the nature of evoked potentials, probably more details of local interaction among columnar interactions should be included, such as those discussed below.

The first SMNI approach to scalp EEG assumed that the Euler-Lagrange variational limit of the stochastic Lagrangian was a suitable averaging procedure over masses of neurons contributing to this relatively coarse spatial phenomenon (Ingber, 1982).

At this point in the development of our "bottom-up" description, we have overlapped with our initial "top-down" description and thus have provided a relatively first-principles approach to better understand these issues. We also show that most probable trajectories of the mesoscopic probability distribution, representing averages over columnar domains, give a description of the systematics nature of macroscopic EEG in accordance with experimental observations.

EULER-LANGRANGE VARIATIONAL EQUATIONS

This calculation begins by considering the Lagrangian $\underline{L}_F$, the Feynman midpoint-discretized Lagrangian. The Euler-Langrange variational equation associated with $\underline{L}_F$ leads to a set of 12 coupled first-order differential equations, with coefficients nonlinear in M^G, in the 12 variables $\{M^G, \dot{M}^G, \ddot{M}^G, \nabla M^G, \nabla^2 M^G\}$ in (r; t) space. In the neighborhood of extrema $\langle\langle\bar{M}^G\rangle\rangle$, $\underline{L}_F$ can be expanded as a Ginzburg-Landau polynomial, that is, in powers of M^E and M^I. To investigate first-order linear oscillatory states, only powers up to 2 in each variable are retained, and from this the variational principle leads to a relatively simple set of coupled linear differential equations with constant coefficients

$$0 = \delta \underline{L}_F = \underline{L}_{F,\dot{G}:t} - \delta_G \underline{L}_F$$

$$\approx -\underline{f}_{|G|}\ddot{\underline{M}}^{|G|} + \underline{f}^1_G \dot{\underline{M}}^{G\neg} - \underline{g}_{|G|}\nabla^2 \underline{M}^{|G|} + \underline{b}_{|G|}\underline{M}^{|G|} + \underline{bM}^{G\neg},\ G\neg \neq G$$

$$(\cdots)_{,\dot{G}:t} = (\cdots)_{,\dot{G}G'}\dot{M}^{G'} + (\cdots)_{,\dot{G}\dot{G}'}\ddot{M}^{G'}$$

$$\underline{M}^G = M^G - \langle\langle\bar{M}^G\rangle\rangle,\ \underline{f}^1_E = -\underline{f}^1_I \equiv \underline{f} \tag{14.40}$$

These equations are Fourier transformed, and the resulting dispersion relation is examined to determine for which values of the synaptic parameters and of the normalized wave number $\underline{\xi}$, the conjugate variable to r, can oscillatory states $\omega(\underline{\xi})$ persist. For example, solutions are sought of the form

$$\underline{M}^G = \mathrm{Re}\ \underline{M}^G_{osc} \exp[-i(\underline{\xi}\cdot r - \omega t)]$$

$$\underline{M}^G_{osc}(r, t) = \int d^2\underline{\xi}\ d\omega \hat{\underline{M}}^G_{osc}(\underline{\xi}, \omega)\exp[i(\underline{\xi}\cdot r - \omega t)] \tag{14.41}$$

For instance, a typical example is specified by extrinsic sources $J_E = -2.63$ and $J_I = 4.94$, $N^E = 125$, $N^I = 25$, $V^G = 10$ mV, $A^G_E = 1.75$, $A^G_I = 1.25$, $B^G_{G'} = 0.25$, and $\nu^G_{G'} = \phi^G_{G'} = 0.1$ mV. The synaptic parameters are within observed ranges (Shepherd, 1979), and the J_G values are just those required to solve the Euler-Lagrange equations at the selected values of M^G. The global minimum is at $\bar{M}^E = 25$ and $\bar{M}^I = 5$. This set of conditions yields (dispersive) dispersion relations

$$\omega\tau = \pm\{-1.86 + 2.38(\xi\rho)^2;\ -1.25i + 1.51i(\xi\rho)^2\} \tag{14.42}$$

where $\xi = |\underline{\xi}|$. The propagation velocity defined by $d\omega/d\xi$ is ~1 cm/second, taking typical wave numbers ξ to correspond to macrocolumnar distances ~30ρ. Calculated frequencies ω are similar to EEG frequencies ~10^2 second^{-1}, equivalent to $\nu = \omega/(2\pi) = 16$ cp (Hz). These mesoscopic propagation velocities permit processing over several minicolumns ~10^{-1} cm, simultaneous with the processing of mesoscopic interactions over tens of centimeters through association fibers with propagation velocities ~600 to 900 cm/second. That is, both intraregional and inter-regional information processing can occur within ~10^{-1} second. This propagation velocity is not "slow": Visual selective attention moves at ~8 milliseconds/degree (Tsal, 1983), which is ~0.5 mm/second if a macrocolumn of an approximately square millimeter is assumed to span 180 degrees. This suggests that nearest-neighbor interactions play some part in disengaging and orienting selective attention.

Direct Fit of SMNI to EEG

Statistical mechanics of neocortical interactions can give an even more detailed description of EEG than can the Euler-Lagrange limit of the Lagrangian. The full SMNI probability distribution can be used to process raw stochastic EEG data. A pilot project described explicitly how this can be accomplished (Ingber, 1991a). We collected EEG spontaneous and averaged evoked potential data from a multielectrode array under a variety of conditions. We fit data collected under a project sponsored by the National Institute on Alcohol Abuse and Alcoholism (Holden, 1991; Porjesz and Begleiter, 1990).

Algebraic Development

We use (14.6) as the basic probability distribution to fit these data. We also take advantage of and extend the results gained for the STM analysis discussed previously, such as the nature of the parabolic well of the Lagrangian. Accordingly, we assume a linear relation (about minima to be fit to data) between the M^G firing states and the measured scalp potential Φ_ν, at a given electrode site ν representing a macroscopic region of neuronal activity

$$\Phi_\nu - \phi = aM^E + bM^I \tag{14.43}$$

where $\{\phi, a, b\}$ are constants determined for each electrode site. In the prepoint discretization, the postpoint $M^G(t + \Delta t)$ moments are expressed by

$$\begin{aligned} m &\equiv \langle \Phi_\nu - \phi \rangle = a\langle M^E \rangle + b\langle M^I \rangle = ag^E + bg^I \\ \sigma^2 &\equiv \int \langle (\Phi_v - \phi)^2 \rangle - \langle \Phi_v - \phi \rangle^2 = a^2 g^{EE} + b^2 g^{II} \end{aligned} \tag{14.44}$$

where the M^G-space drifts, g^G, and diffusions, $g^{GG'}$, have been derived above. The macroscopic drifts and diffusions of the Φ_v values are simply linearly related to the nonlinear mesoscopic drifts and diffusions of the M^G values. For the prepoint $M^G(t)$ firings, we assume the same linear relation in terms of $\{\phi, a, b\}$.

The data we fit are consistent with invoking the "centering" mechanism discussed previously. Therefore, for the prepoint $M^E(t)$ firings, we also take advantage of the parabolic trough derived for the STM Lagrangian, and use

$$M^I(t) = cM^E(t) \tag{14.45}$$

where the slope c is determined for each electrode site. This permits a complete transformation from M^G variables to Φ variables.

Similarly, as appearing in the modified threshold factor F^G given in (14.26), each regional influence from electrode site μ acting at electrode site ν, given by afferent firings $M^{\ddagger E}$, is expressed as

$$M^{\ddagger E}_{\mu \to \nu} = d_\nu M^{E}_{\mu}(t - T_{\mu \to \nu}) \tag{14.46}$$

where d_ν are constants to be fitted at each electrode site, and $T_{\mu \to \nu}$ is the delay time estimated for interelectrode signal propagation, based on current anatomic knowledge of the neocortex and of velocities of propagation of action potentials of long-range fibers that are typically one to several multiples of $\tau = 5$ milliseconds. Some terms in which d directly affects the shifts of synaptic parameters $B^{G}_{G'}$, when calculating the centering mechanism, also contain long-range efficacies (inverse conductivities) B^{*E}_{E}. Therefore, the latter were fixed with the other electrical-chemical synaptic parameters during these fits. In future fits, we will try using the T values as parameters.

This defines the conditional probability distribution for the measured scalp potential Φ_ν

$$\begin{aligned} P_\nu[\Phi_\nu(t + \Delta t) | \Phi_\nu(t)] &= \frac{1}{(2\pi\sigma^2 \Delta t)^{1/2}} \exp(-L_\nu \Delta t) \\ L_\nu &= \frac{1}{2\sigma^2} (\dot{\Phi}_\nu - m)^2 \end{aligned} \tag{14.47}$$

where m and σ have been derived just above. As noted previously in defining macroscopic regions, the probability distribution for all electrodes is the product of all these distributions

$$\begin{aligned} P &= \prod_\nu P_\nu \\ L &= \sum_\nu L_\nu \end{aligned} \tag{14.48}$$

We are also strongly invoking the current belief in the dipole or nonlinear string model. The model SMNI, derived for $P[M^G(t + \Delta t) | M^{\bar{G}}(t)]$, is for a macrocolumnar-averaged minicolumn, and thus we expect it to be a reasonable approximation of a macrocolumn, scaled to its contribution to Φ_ν. Therefore, we use L to represent this macroscopic regional Lagrangian, scaled from its mesoscopic mesocolumnar counterpart $\underline{L}$. However, the above expression for P_ν uses the dipole assumption to represent several to many macrocolumns present in a region under an electrode that is at a scale measured in centimeters: A macrocolumn has a spatial extent of about a millimeter. A scalp electrode, under very favorable experimental circumstances, has a resolution as small as perhaps one centimeter, directly competing with the spatial resolutions under similar circumstances attributed to magnetoencephalography (Cohen et al, 1990), but often most data collected under typical conditions represent a resolution that is more likely to be several centimeters and many macrocolumns. Still, investigators often argue that typically at least several tens of macrocolumns firing coherently account for the electric potentials measured by one scalp electrode (Nunez, 1990). This stage of the SMNI model tested the scaling paradigm up to a representative region of many macrocolumns, including subsets of tens of coherently firing macrocolumns. While these results seem to confirm this approach, further MNN development of SMNI discussed next will make it possible to model tens of macrocolumns with greater resolution.

Mesoscopic Neural Nets

As noted early in this development (Ingber, 1981a, 1985d), basing information processing at macroscopic scales on processes at mesoscopic scales leads to new kinds of computational algorithms, such as proposed here. This approach is consistent with the view that many complex nonlinear nonequilibrium systems develop mesoscopic intermediate structures, such as Gaussian-Markovian statistics to maximize the flow of information (Graham, 1978; Haken, 1983). By viewing the neocortex as the prototypical information processor, a mesoscopic-neural-network (MNN) algorithm can be developed to store and predict patterns of activity inherent in many such nonlinear stochastic multivariate systems.

SMNI–MNN

Although the development of nearest-neighbor interactions into a potential term V' was useful to explore EEG dispersion relations (Ingber, 1984a, 1985a), for our purposes this is not necessary and, as permitted in the development of SMNI, we simply incorporate nearest-neighbor minicolumnar interactions with firings $M^{\dagger G}$ by again redefining F^G in (14.26)

$$
\begin{aligned}
F^G &= \frac{V^G - \nu_{G'}^{|G|} T_{G'}^{|G|}}{(\pi[(\nu_{G'}^{|G|})^2 + (\phi_{G'}^{|G|})^2] T_{G'}^{|G|})^{1/2}} \\
T_{G'}^{|G|} &= a_{G'}^{|G|} N^{G'} + \frac{1}{2} A_{G'}^{|G|} M^{G'} + a_{G'}^{\dagger|G|} N^{\dagger G'} + \frac{1}{2} A_{G}^{\dagger|G|} M^{\dagger G'} \\
&\quad + a_{G'}^{\ddagger|G|} N^{\ddagger G'} + \frac{1}{2} A_{G'}^{\ddagger|G|} M^{\ddagger G'} \qquad (14.49) \\
a_{G'}^{\dagger G} &= \frac{1}{2} A_{G'}^{\dagger G} + B_{G'}^{\dagger G} \\
A_E^{\ddagger I} &= A_I^{\ddagger E} = A_I^{\ddagger I} = B_E^{\ddagger I} = B_I^{\ddagger E} = B_I^{\ddagger I} = 0,\ a_E^{\ddagger E} = \frac{1}{2} A_E^{\ddagger E} + B_E^{\ddagger E}
\end{aligned}
$$

This result presents an SMNI–MNN as a set of nodes, each described by a short-time probability distribution interacting with the other nodes. A set of 1000 such nodes is a macrocolumn, scaled to represent a "dipole" current source (Ingber, 1991a). A circuitry among patches of macrocolumns represents a typical circuit of activity correlated to specific behavioral states, as recorded by EEG under specific experimental or clinical conditions. We apply SMNI–MNN to identify patterns of a person's EEG and to predict possible future states of brain activities, anomalies, and so forth. The methods used are general and can be described generically.

Generic MNN

We can generalize this SMNI–MNN, generated from (14.22), to model other large-scale nonlinear stochastic multivarate systems, by considering general drifts and diffusions to model such systems, letting G represent an arbitrary number of variables. Ideally, these systems inherently will be of the Fokker-Planck type

$$\frac{\partial P}{\partial t} = \frac{\partial(-g^G P)}{\partial M^G} + \frac{1}{2}\frac{\partial^2(g^{GG'}P)}{\partial M^G \partial M^{G'}} \tag{14.50}$$

The topology, geometry, and connectivity of MNN of course can be generalized. For example, we need not be restricted to nearest-neighbor interactions, although this is simpler to implement, especially on parallel processors. Also we can include "hidden layers" to increase the complexity of MNN, although the inclusion of nonlinear structure in the drifts, g^G, and diffusions, $g^{GG'}$, may make this unnecessary for many systems. A detailed description for using "learning" and "prediction" of information has been reported for these systems (Ingber, 1992).

Conclusions

Extracting Signal from Noise

Several factors in the SMNI development support optimism for extracting more signal from noise than is now possible.

Logical and Testable Development Across Multiple Scales

In the course of a logical, nonlinear, stochastic development of aggregating neuronal and synaptic interactions to increasingly larger scales, techniques of mathematical physics can be used to overcome several technical hurdles. Paradigms and metaphors from other disciplines do not substitute for logical SMNI development.

Validity Across Multiple Scales

The SMNI theoretical model has independent validity in describing EEG dispersion relations, systematics of short-term memory, velocities of propagation of information across neocortical fields, recency-versus-primacy effects, and so on.

Fits of such models to data should do better to extract signal from noise than do ad hoc phenomenologic models.

Use of ASA and PATHINT on Nonlinear Stochastic Systems

Adaptive simulated annealing (ASA) enables the fitting of quite arbitrary nonlinear stochastic models to such data as presented by EEG systems (Ingber, 1993a). This means that functional dependences in the noise itself (the different matrix) and the functional dependences in the driving terms (the drift vector) can be fit directly. A new C-language code, PATHINT, has been developed to handle n-dimensional Fokker-Planck type of systems, using the algorithm noted previously (Ingber 1994b, 1994c). Once fit, PATHINT can evolve the system, testing long-time corelations between the model(s) and the data and it can predict events.

Inclusion of Short-Range and Long-Range Interactions

Statistical mechanics of neocortical interactions proposes that models to be fit to data include models of activity under each electrode, such as those due to short-range neuronal fibers, and models of activity across electrodes, such as those due to long-range fibers.

Riemannian Invariants

Yet to be explored are the consequences of using the derived (not hypothesized) Riemannian metric induced by multivariate Fokker-Planck type of systems (Ingber, 1982, 1983a, 1988a). This seems to form a natural invariant measure of information that could, or should, be used to explore the flow of information between neocortical regions.

Renormalization of Attenuated Frequencies

The SMNI approach shows how to "renormalize" the spatial activity to create a model that more closely matches the experimental situation of scalp measurement, wherein ranges of wave numbers are attenuated (Ingber and Nunez, 1990). Although SMNI is most logically tested using data collected from brain surface recordings, the necessity and utility of performing noninvasive EEG scalp recordings argues strongly that SMNI should be developed further to extract better signal out of noise from scalp recordings.

Importance of Modeling at Multiple Scales

To learn more about complex systems, inevitably we must form functional models to represent huge data sets. Indeed, modeling phenomenon is as much a cornerstone of 20th century science as is collection of empirical data (Jammer, 1974).

The ability to fit data to these particular SMNI functional forms goes beyond nonlinear statistical modeling of data. The plausibility of the SMNI model, as emphasized in this and previous SMNI papers, as spanning several important neuroscientific phenomena, suggests that the fitted functional forms may yet help to explicate some underlying biophysical mechanisms responsible for the normal and abnormal behavioral states being investigated, such as excitatory and inhibitory influences and background electromagnetic influences from nearby firing states (by using SMNI synaptic conductivity parameters in the fits).

Analyzing, understanding, and attempting to predict neocortical phenomena at the spatial scales encountered in EEG scalp recordings involves measuring firings from millions of neurons; in intracortical measurements, at least tens of thousands of neurons may be involved. Statistical mechanics of neocortical interactions approaches such scales as new systems with emergent phenomena. Just as physics and chemistry could not have progressed during this century if all theoretical and experimental research were inappropriately constrained to be understood at the level of quantum mechanics (or quarks or strings), so neuroscience must accept that all brain phenomena are not best understood or perhaps understood at all at the level of simple neuron–neuron interactions (or membrane dynamics or macrocmolecular interactions). Different scales present new complex systems that must be approached as such and often with different approaches.

For example, both artificial neural networks (ANN) and SMNI structures are represented in terms of units with algebraic properties that greatly simplify specific realistic neuronal components. Of course, there is a clear logical difference between considering a small ensemble of simple ANN units (each unit representing an "average" neuron) to study the properties of small ensembles of neurons, and considering distributions of interactions between model neurons to develop a large ensemble of units (each unit representing a column of neurons) developed by SMNI to study properties of large ensembles of columns; only the latter has a chance for any statistical justification. Unlike SMNI, ANN models may yield insights into specific mechanisms of learning, memory, retrieval, information processing among small ensembles of model neurons, and so forth. However, consider that there are several million neurons located under a square-centimeter area of neocortical surface. Current estimates are that one to several percent of coherent neuronal firings can account for the amplitudes of electric potential measured on the scalp. This translates into considering firings of hundreds of thousands of neurons as contributing to activity measured under a typical electrode. Even when EEG recordings are made directly on the brain surface, tens of thousands of neurons contribute to activity measured under electrodes. Artificial neural network models cannot approach the order of magnitude of neurons participating in phenomena at the scale of EEG, just as neither ANN nor SMNI can detail relatively smaller scale activity at the membrane or atomic levels. Attempts to do so probably would require statistical interpretations such as are made by SMNI; otherwise the output of the models would just replace the data collected from many neuronal firings—a regression from 20th century science to empiricism.

Although ANN models use simplified algebraic structures to represent real neurons, SMNI models develop the statistics of large numbers of realistic neurons representing even larger numbers of synaptic interactions—there are 10^4 to 10^5 synapses per neuron. Furthermore, unlike most ANN approaches, SMNI accepts constraints on all its macrocolumnar averaged parameters to be taken from experimentally determined ranges of synaptic and neuronal interactions; there are no unphysical parameters. The stochastic and nonlinear nature of SMNI development is derived directly from experimentally observed synaptic interactions and from the mathematical development of observed minicolumns and macrocolumns of neurons. Statistical mechanics of neocortical interactions has required the use of mathematical physics techniques first published in the late 1970s in the context of developing an approach to multivariate nonlinear nonequilibrium statistical mechanics.

Modeling EEG and SMNI

To detail such a model of EEG phenomena, "top-down" models are useful, such as the nonlinear string model representing nonlinear dipoles of neuronal columnar activity. To construct a more detailed "bottom-up" model that could give reasonable algebraic functions with physical parameters to be fit by data, we needed to compile a wealth of empirical data and modern techniques of mathematical physics across multiple scales of neocortical activity. At each of these scales, we had to derive and establish reasonable procedures and submodels for climbing the scales. Each of these submodels could then be tested against some experimental data to determine if we were on the right track. For example, at the mesoscopic scale, we checked the consistency of SMNI with known aspects of visual and auditory short-term memory; at the macroscopic scale, we checked consistency with known aspects of EEG and the propagation of information across the neocortex. Here we showed that the currently accepted dipole EEG model can be derived as the Euler-Langrange equations of an electric-potential Lagrangian.

The theoretical and experimental importance of specific scaling of interactions in the neocortex has been shown quantitatively: The explicit algebraic form of the probability distribution for mesoscopic columnar interactions is driven by a nonlinear threshold factor of the same form used to describe microscopic neuronal interactions, where electrical-chemical synaptic and neuronal parameters all lie within their experimentally observed ranges; these threshold factors largely determine the nature of the drifts and diffusions of the system. This mesoscopic probability distribution has successfully described STM phenomena and, when used as a basis to derive the most probable trajectories using the Euler-Lagrange variational equations, it also has described the systematics of EEG phenomena. More recently, we considered the mesoscopic form of the full probability distribution more seriously for macroscopic interactions, deriving macroscopic drifts and diffusions linearly related to sums of their (nonlinear) mesoscopic counterparts, scaling its variables to describe regional interactions correlated with observed electric activities measured by electrode recordings of scalp EEG, with apparent success. These results provide strong quantitative support for an accurate intuitive perspective, portraying neocortical interactions as having common algebraic or physics mechanisms that span disparate spatial scales and functional or behavioral phenomena, that is, those that describe interactions among neurons, columns of neurons, and regional masses of neurons.

The SMNI methods also define an algorithm to construct an MNN based on realistic neocortical processes and parameters, to record patterns of brain activity, and to compute the evolution of this system. At this scale, we can overlap with work being done using artificial neural networks. Furthermore, this new algorithm is generic and can be used to process information in other systems in a similar manner, especially, but not limited to, those amenable to modeling by mathematical physics techniques alternatively described by path-integral Lagrangians, Fokker-Planck equations, or Langevin rate equations. This methodology is made possible and practical by a confluence of techniques drawn from SMNI itself, modern methods of functional stochastic calculus defining nonlinear Lagrangians, adaptive simulated eannealing (ASA), and parallel-processing computation.

Work in Progress

Much more work needs to be done. We have not yet addressed the "renormalization" issues raised, which are based on the nature of EEG data collection and are amenable to this framework. Although the fitting of these distributions condenses the experimental data into a reasonable algebraic model, which is a prime task of most physical theory, even more data reduction must be performed to be useful to clinicians (and therefore to give more feedback to theory). We must experiment with path-integral calculations and some methods of "scientific visualization" to determine what minimal, or at least small, set of "signatures" might suffice, which would be faithful to the data yet useful to clinicians. We also must examine the gains that might be made by putting these codes onto a parallel processor, which might enable real-time diagnoses based on noninvasive EEG recordings.

We are conducting a parallelizing of ASA and PATHINT project (PAPP). Codes and papers can be accessed via the world wide web at http://alumni.caltech.edu/~ingber/.

We can reasonably speculate on the evolutionary desirability of developing Gaussian-Markovian statistics at the mesoscopic columnar scale from microscopic neuronal interactions and of maintaining this type of system to the macroscopic regional scale. That is, this permits maximal processing of information (Graham, 1978), an entity that can be codified as invariants in a Riemannian geometry induced by the stochastic system. This concept must be tested against experimental data. Although much work remains, we believe that modern methods of statistical mechanics have led the way to promising approaches.

References

Adey, W.R. Long-range electromagnetic field interactions at brain cell surfaces. In: *Magnetic Field Effect on Biological Systems.* New York: Plenum, 1978.

Afifi, A.K. and Bergman, R.A. *Basic Neuroscience.* Baltimore, MD: Urban & Schwarzenberg, 1978.

Agarwal, G.S. and Shenoy, S.R. Observability of hysteresis in first-order equilibrium and nonequilibrium phase transitions. *Phys. Rev. A.* 23:2719–2723, 1981.

Amari, S.-I. Field theory of self-organizing neural nets. *IEEE Transactions on Systems, Man, and Cybernetics.* 13:741–748, 1983.

Anninos, P., Zenone, S., and Elul, R. Artificial neural nets: Dependence of the EEG amplitude's probability distribution on statistical parameters. *J. Theor. Biol.* 103:339–348, 1983.

Arbib, M.A. and Amari, S.-I. Sensori-motor transformations in the brain (with a critique of the tensor theory of cerebellum). *J. Theor. Biol.* 112:123–155, 1985.

Babloyantz, A. and Kaczmarek, L.K. Self-organization in biological systems with multiple cellular contacts. *Bull. Math. Biol.* 41:193–201, 1979.

Basar, E. *EEG-Brain Dynamics.* Amsterdam: Elsevier, 1980.

Boyd, I.A. and Martin, A.R. The end-plate potential in mammalian muscle. *J. Physiol. (London).* 132:74–91, 1956.

Braitenberg, V. *Cortical Architectonics: General and Areal.* New York: Raven, 1978.

Bullock, T.H. Reassessment of neural connectivity and its specification. In: *Information Processing in the Nervous System.* (H.M. Pinsker and Willis, W.D., Jr., Eds.) New York: Raven Press, 1980.

Caillé, A., Pink, D., de Verteuil, F., and Zuckermann, M.J. Theoretical models for quasi-two-dimensional mesomorphic monolayers and membrane bilayers. *Can. J. Phys.* 58:1723–1726, 1980.

Cartling, B. From short-time molecular dynamics to long-time stochastic dynamics of proteins. *J. Chem. Phys.* 91:427–438, 1989.

Cohen, D., Cuffin, B.N., Yunokuchi, K., Maniewski, R., Purcell, C., Cosgrove, G.R., Ives, J., Kennedy, J., and Schomer, D. MEG versus EEG localization test using implanted sources in the human brain. *Ann. Neurol.* 28:811–817, 1990.

Colet, P., Wio, H.S., and San Miguel, M. Colored noise: A perspective from a path-integral formalism. *Phys. Rev. A.* 39:6094–6097, 1989.

Cowan, J.D. Spontaneous symmetry breaking in large scale nervous activity. *International Journal of Quantum Chemistry.* 22:1059–1082, 1982.

Cragg, B.G. and Temperley, H.N.V. The organization of neurons: A cooperative analogy. *Electroencephalogr. Clin. Neurophysiol.* 6:85–92, 1954.

Dekker, H. Quantization in curved spaces. In: *Functional Integration: Theory and Applications.* (J.P. Antoine and Tirapegui, E., Eds.) New York: Plenum, pp. 207–224, 1980.

DeWitt, B.S. Dynamical theory in curved spaces. I. A review of the classical and quantum action principles. *Rev. Mod. Phys.* 29:377–397, 1957.

Dismukes, R.K. New concepts of molecular communication among neurons. *Behavioral Brain Science.* 2:409–448, 1979.

Dudek, F.E., Hatton, G.I., and Macvicar, B.A. Intracellular recordings from the paraventricular nucleus in slices of rat hypothalamus. *J. Physiol.* 301:101–114, 1980.

Dykes, R.W. The anatomy and physiology of the somatic sensory cortical regions. *Prog. Neurobiol.* 10:33–88, 1978.

Dykes, R.W. Parallel processing of somatosensory information: A theory. *Brain Research Reviews.* 6:47–115, 1983.

Einstein, A., Lorentz, A., Minkowski, H., and Weyl, H. *The Principle of Relativity.* New York: Dover, 1923.

Erickson, R.P. The across-fiber pattern theory: An organizing principle for molar neural function. *Sensory Physiology.* 6:79–110, 1982.

Ericsson, K.A. and Chase, W.G. Exceptional memory. *American Scientist.* 70:607–615, 1982.

Feynman, R.P., Leighton, R.B., and Sands, M. *The Feynman Lectures on Physics.* Reading, MA: Addison-Wesley, 1963.

Fitzpatrick, K.A. and Imig, T.J. Auditory cortico-cortical connections in the owl monkey. *J. Comput. Neurol.* 192:589–601, 1980.

Freeman, W.J. *Mass Action in the Nervous System.* New York: Academic Press, 1975.

Freeman, W.J. Spatial properties of an EEG event in the olfactory bulb and cortex. *Electroencephalogr. Clin. Neurophysiol.* 44:586–605, 1978.

Gardiner, C.W. *Handbook of Stochastic Methods for Physics, Chemistry and the Natural Sciences.* Berlin: Springer-Verlag, 1983.

Gersch, W. Non-stationary multichannel time series analysis. In: *Methods of Brain Electrical and Magnetic Signals. EEG Handbook.* (A.S. Gevins and Remond, A., Eds.) New York: Elsevier, pp. 261–296, 1987.

Gilbert, C.D. and Wiesel, T.N. Functional organization of the visual cortex. *Prog. Brain Res.* 58:209–218, 1983.

Goel, N.S. and Richter-Dyn, N. *Stochastic Models in Biology.* New York: Academic Press, 1974.

Goldman, P.S. and Nauta, W.J.H. Columnar distribution of cortico-cortical fibers in the frontal association, limbic, and motor cortex of the developing rhesus monkey. *Brain Res.* 122:393–413, 1977.

Grabert, H. and Green, M.S. Fluctuations and nonlinear irreversible processes. *Phys. Rev. A.* 19:1747–1756, 1979.

Graham, R. Covariant formulation of non-equilibrium statistical thermodynamics. *Zeitschrift fur Physik.* B26:397–405, 1977a.

Graham, R. Lagrangian for diffusion in curved phase space. *Phys. Rev. Lett.* 38:51–53, 1977b.

Graham, R. Path-integral methods on nonequilibrium thermodynamics and statistics. In: *Stochastic Processes in Nonequilibrium Systems.* (L. Garrido, Seglar, P., and Shepherd, P.J., Eds.) New York: Springer, pp. 82–138, 1978.

Graham, R., Roekaerts, D., and Tél, T. Integrability of Hamiltonians asociated with Fokker-Planck equations. *Phys. Rev. A.* 31:3364–3375, 1985.

Graham, R. and Tél, T. Existence of a potential for dissipative dynamical systems. *Phys. Rev. Lett.* 52:9–12, 1984.

Griffith, J.S. *Mathematical Neurobiology.* New York: Academic Press, 1971.

Haken, H. *Information and Self-Organization: A Macroscopic Approach to Complex Systems.* Berlin: Springer, 1988.

Haken, H. *Synergetics.* Third ed. New York: Springer, 1983.

Hebb, D.O. *The Organisation of Behavior.* New York: Wiley, 1949.

Holden, C. Probing the complex genetics of alcoholism. *Science.* 251:163–164, 1991.

Hubel, D.H. and Wiesel, T.N. Functional architecture of Macaque monkey visual cortex. *Proc. R. Soc. London Ser. B.* 198:1–59, 1977.

Hubel, D.H. and Wiesel, T.N. Receptive fields, binocular interaction and functional architecture in the cat's visual cortex. *J. Physiol.* 160:106–154, 1962.

Imig, T.J. and Reale, R.A. Patterns of cortico-cortical connections related to tonotopic maps in cat auditory cortex. *J. Comp. Neurol.* 192:293–332, 1980.

Ingber, L. Editorial: Learning to learn. *Explore.* 7:5–8, 1972.

Ingber, L. *The Karate Instructor's Handbook.* Solana Beach, CA: Physical Studies Institute-Institute for the Study of Attention, 1976.

Ingber, L. Towards a unified brain theory. *J. Social Biol. Struct.* 4:211–224, 1981a.

Ingber, L. *Karate: Kinematics and Dynamics.* Hollywood, CA: Unique, 1981b.

Ingber, L. Attention, physics and teaching. *J. Social Biol. Struct.* 4:225–235, 1981c.

Ingber, L. Statistical mechanics of neocortical interactions. I. Basic formulation. *Physica D.* 5:83–107, 1982.

Ingber, L. Statistical mechanics of neocortical interactions. Dynamics of synaptic modification. *Phys. Rev. A.* 28:395–416, 1983a.

Ingber, L. Riemannian corrections to velocity-dependent nuclear forces. *Phys. Rev. C.* 28:2536–2539, 1983b.

Ingber, L. Statistical mechanics of neocortical interactions. Derivation of short-term-memory capacity. *Phys. Rev. A.* 29:3346–3358, 1984a.

Ingber, L. Path-integral Riemannian contributions to nuclear Schrödinger equation. *Phys. Rev. D.* 29:1171–1174, 1984b.

Ingber, L. Statistical mechanics of nonlinear nonequilibrium financial markets. *Mathematical Modelling.* 5:343–361, 1984c.

Ingber, L. Statistical mechanics of neocortical interactions. EEG dispersion relations. *IEEE Trans. Biomed. Eng.* 32:91–94, 1985a.

Ingber, L. Statistical mechanics of neocortical interactions: Stability and duration of the 7 ± 2 rule of short-term-memory capacity. *Phys. Rev. A.* 31:1183–1186, 1985b.

Ingber, L. Towards clinical applications of statistical mechanics of neocortical interactions. *Innov. Tech. Biol. Med.* 6:753–758, 1985c.

Ingber, L. Statistical mechanics algorithm for response to targets (SMART). In: *Workshop on Uncertainty and Probability in Artificial Intelligence: UC Los Angeles, 14–16 August 1985.* (P. Cheeseman; Ed.) Menlo Park, CA: American Association for Artificial Intelligence, pp. 258–264, 1985d.

Ingber, L. *Elements of Advanced Karate.* Burbank, CA: Ohara, 1985e.

Ingber, L. Statistical mechanics of neocortical interactions. *Bull. Am. Phys. Soc.* 31:868, 1986a.

Ingber, L. Riemannian contributions to short-ranged velocity-dependent nucleon-nucleon interactions. *Physical Review D.* 33:3781–3784, 1986b.

Ingber, L. Applications of biological intelligence to Command, Control and Communications. In: *Computer Simulation in Brain Science: Proceedings, University of Copenhagen, 20–22 August 1986.* R. Cotterill, Ed.) London: Cambridge University Press, pp. 513–533, 1988a.

Ingber, L. Statistical mechanics of mesoscales in neocortex and in command, control and communications (C^3). Proceedings, Sixth International Conference, St. Louis, Missouri, 4–7 August 1987. *Mathematical Computer Modelling.* 11:457–463, 1988b.

Ingber, L. Mesoscales in neocortex and in command, control and communications (C^3) systems. In: *Systems with Learning and Memoroy Abilities: Proceedings, University of Paris 15–19 June 1987*. (J. Delacour and Levy, J.C.S., Eds.) Amsterdam: Elsevier, pp. 387–409, 1988c.

Ingber, L. Very fast simulated re-annealing. *Mathematical Computer Modelling*. 12:967–973, 1989.

Ingber, L. Statistical mechanical aids to calculating term structure models. *Phys. Rev. A*. 42:7057–7064, 1990.

Ingber, L. Statistical mechanics of neocortical interactions: A Scaling paradigm applied to electroencephalography. *Phys. Rev. A*. 44:4017–4060, 1991a.

Ingber, L. Statistical mechanical measures of performance of combat. In: *Proceedings of the 1991 Summer Computer Simulation Conference 22–24 July 1991, Baltimore, MD*. (D. Pace, Ed.) San Diego, CA: Society for Computer Simulation, pp. 940–945, 1991b.

Ingber, L. Generic mesoscopic neural networks based on statistical mechanics of neocortical interactions. *Phys. Rev. A*. 45:R2183–R2186, 1992.

Ingber, L. *Adaptive Simulated Annealing (ASA)*. [ftp.alumni.caltech.edu:pub/ingber], McLean, VA: Lester Ingber Research, 1993a.

Ingber, L. Statistical mechanics of combat and extensions. In: *Toward a Science of Command, Control, and Communications*. (C.R. Jones, Ed.) Washington, DC: American Institute of Aeronautics and Astronautics, pp. 117–149, 1993b.

Ingber, L. Simulated annealing: Practice versus theory. *Mathematical Computer Modelling*. pp. 18, 29–57, 1993c.

Ingber, L. Multiple scales of EEG. In: *Frontier Science in EEG Symposium: Proceedings, New Orleans, 9 Oct 1993*. (R. Dasheiff and Major-Vincent, D., Eds.) Pittsburgh, PA: University of Pittsburgh, 1994a.

Ingber, L. Statistical mechanics of neocortical interactions: Path-integral evolution of short-term memory. *Phys. Rev. E*. 49:4652–4664, 1994b.

Ingber, L. Path-integral evolution of multivariate systems with moderate noise. *Phys. Rev. E*. (submitted), 1994c.

Ingber, L., Fujio, H., and Wehner, M.F. Mathematical comparison of combat computer models to exercise data. *Mathematical Computer Modelling*. 15:65–90, 1991.

Ingber, L. and Nunez, P.L. Multiple scales of statistical physics of neocortex: Application to electroencephalography. *Mathematical Computer Modelling*. 13:83–95, 1990.

Ingber, L. and Sworder, D.D. Statistical mechanics of combat with human factors. *Mathematical Computer Modelling*. 15:99–127, 1991.

Ingber, L., Wehner, M.F., Jabbour, G.M., and Barnhill, T.M. Application of statistical mechanics methodology to term-structure bond-pricing models. *Mathematical Computer Modelling*. 15:77–98, 1991.

Jammer, M. *The Philosophy of Quantum Mechanics*. New York: Wiley, 1974.

John, E.R. Switchboard versus statistical theories of learning and memory. *Science*. 177:850–864, 1972.

Jones, E.G., Coulter, J.D., and Hendry, S.H.C. Intracortical connectivity of architectonic fields in the somatic sensory, motor and parietal cortex of monkeys. *J. Comput. Neurol*. 181:291–348, 1978.

Kaczmarek, L.K. and Babloyantz, A. Spatiotemporal patterns in epileptic seizures. *Biol. Cybernetics*. 26:199–208, 1977.

Katchalsky, A.K., Rowland, V., and Blumenthal, R. Dynamic patterns of brain assemblies. *Neurosci. Res. Prog. Bull*. 12, 1–187, 1974.

Katz, B. *Nerve, Muscle, and Synapse*. New York: McGraw-Hill, 1966.

Klemm, W.R. and Sherry, C.J. Serial ordering in spike trains: What's it 'trying to tell us'? *Int. J. Neurosci*. 14:15–33, 1981.

Korn, H. and Mallet, A. Transformation of binomial input by the postsynaptic membrane at a central synapse. *Science.* 225:1157–1159, 1984.

Korn, H., Mallet, A., and Faber, D.S. Fluctuating responses at a central synapse: n of binomial fit predicts number of stained presynaptic boutons. *Science.* 213:898–900, 1981.

Kubo, R., Matsuo, K., and Kitahara, K. Fluctuation and relaxation of macrovariables. *J. Stat. Phys.* 9:51–96, 1973.

Landau, L.D., Lifshitz, E.M., and Pitaevskii, L.P. *Statistical Physics.* New York: Pergamon, 1980.

Langouche, F., Roekaerts, D., and Tirapegui, E. *Functional Integration and Semiclassical Expansions.* The Netherlands: Riedel, Dordrecht, 1982.

Libet, B. Brain stimulation in the study of neuronal functions for conscious sensory experience. *Human Neurobiology.* 1:235–242, 1982.

Little, W.A. The existence of persistent states in the brain. *Mathematical Biosciences.* 19:101–120, 1974.

Little, W.A. and Shaw, G.L. Analytic study of the memory storage capacity of a neural network. *Mathematical Bioscience.* 39:281–290, 1978.

Ma, S.-K. *Modern Theory of Critical Phenomena.* Reading, MA: Benjamin/Cummings, 1976.

Ma, S.-K. *Statistical Mechanics.* Philadelphia: World Scientific, 1985.

Mars, N.J.I. and Lopes da Silva, F.H. EEG analysis methods based on information theory. In: *Methods of Brain Electrical and Magnetic Signals. EEG Handbook.* (A.S. Gevins and Remond, A., Eds.) New York: Elsevier, pp. 297–307, 1987.

Mathews, J. and Walker, R.L. *Mathematical Methods of Physics.* Second ed. New York: Benjamin, 1970.

McCulloch, W.S. and Pitts, W. A logical calculus of the ideas immanent in nervous activity. *Bulletin Mathematical Biophysiology.* 12:207–219, 1943.

McGeer, P.C., Eccles, J.C., and McGeer, E.G. *Molecular Neurobiology of the Mammalian Brain.* New York: Plenum, 1978.

Miller, G.A. The magical number seven, plus or minus two. *Psychol. Rev.* 63:81–97, 1956.

Misner, C.W., Thorne, K.S., and Wheeler, J.A. *Gravitation.* San Francisco: Freeman, 1973.

Mountcastle, V.B. An organizing principle for cerebral function: The unit module and the distributed system. In: *The Mindful Brain.* (G.M. Edelman and Mountcastle, V.B., Eds.) Cambridge, MA: Massachusetts Institute of Technology, pp. 7–50, 1978.

Mountcastle, V.B., Andersen, R.A., and Motter, B.C. The influence of attentive fixation upon the excitability of the light-sensitive neurons of the posterior parietal cortex. *J. Neurosci.* 1:1218–1235, 1981.

Murdock, B.B., Jr. A distributed memory model for serial-order information. *Psychol. Rev.* 90:316–338, 1983.

Nicolis, G. and Prigogine, I. *Self-Organization in Nonequilibrium Systems.* New York: Wiley, 1973.

Nunez, P.L. The brain wave equation: A model for the EEG. *Math. Biosci.* 21:279–297, 1974.

Nunez, P.L. *Electric Fields of the Brain: The Neurophysics of EEG.* London: Oxford University Press, 1981a.

Nunez, P.L. A study of origins of the time dependencies of scalp EEG: I—Theoretical basis. *IEEE Trans. Biomed. Eng.* 28:271–280, 1981b.

Nunez, P.L. A study of origins of the time dependencies of scalp EEG: II—Experimental support of theory. *IEEE Trans. Biomed. Eng.* 28:281–288, 1981c.

Nunez, P.L. Generation of human EEG rhythms by a combination of long and short-range neocortical interactions. *Brain Topography.* 1:199–215, 1989.

Nunez, P.L. Localization of brain activity with electroencephalography. In: *Advances in Neurology. Vol. 54: Magnetoencephalography.* (S. Sato, Ed.) New York: Raven Press, pp. 39–65, 1990.

Pellionisz, A.J. Coordination: A vector-matrix description of transformations of overcomplete CNS coordinates and a tensorial solution using the Moore-Penrose generalized inverse. *J. Theor. Biol.* 110:353–375, 1984.

Pellionisz, A. and Llinás, R. Brain modeling by tensor network theory and computer simulation. The cerebellum: Distributed processor for predictive coordination. *Neuroscience.* 4:323–348, 1979.

Pellionisz, A. and Llinás, R. Tensorial approach to the geometry of brain function: Cerebellar coordination via a metric tensor. *Neuroscience.* 5:1125–1136, 1980.

Perkel, D.H. and Feldman, M.W. Neurotransmitter release statistics: Moment estimates for inhomogeneous Bernoulli trials. *J. Math. Biol.* 7:31–40, 1979.

Porjesz, B. and Begleiter, H. Event-related potentials individuals at risk for alcoholism. *Alcohol.* 7:465–469, 1990.

Rapp, P.E., Bashore, T.R., Martinerie, J.M., Albano, A.M., Zimmerman, I.D., and Mees, A.I. Dynamics of brain electrical activity. *Brain Topography.* 2:99–118, 1989.

Schmitt, F.O., Dev, P., and Smith, B.H. Electronic processing of information by brain cells. *Science.* 193:114–120, 1976.

Schulman, L.S. *Techniques and Applications of Path Integration.* New York: Wiley, 1981.

Scott, A.C. The electrophysics of a nerve fiber. *Rev. Mod. Phys.* 47:487–533, 1975.

Shaw, G.L. and Vasudevan, R. Persistent states of neural networks and the random nature of synaptic transmission. *Math. Biosci.* 21:207–218, 1974.

Shenoy, S.R. and Agarwal, G.S. First-passage times and hysteresis in multivariable stochastic processes: The two-mode ring laser. *Phys. Rev. A.* 29:1315–1325, 1984.

Shepherd, G.M. *The Synaptic Organization of the Brain.* Second ed. New York: Oxford University Press, 1979.

Sommerhoff, G. *Logic of the Living Brain.* New York: Wiley, 1974.

Steriade, M. Mechanisms underlying cortical activation: Neuronal organization and properties of the midbrain reticular core and intralaminar thalamic nuclei. In: *Brain Mechanisms and Perceptual Awareness.* (O. Pompeiano and Marsan, C.A., Eds.) New York: Raven, pp. 327–377, 1981.

Szentágothai, J. The 'module-concept' in cerebral cortex architecture. *Brain Res.* 95:475–496, 1975.

Szentagothai, J. The neural network of the cerebral cortex: A functional interpretation. *Proc. R. Soc. Lon.* 201:219–248, 1978.

Szentágothai, J. and Arbib, M.A. Conceptual models of neural organization. *Neuroscience Research Bulletin.* 12:307–510, 1974.

Takeuchi, A. and Amari, S. Formation of topographic maps and columnar microstructures in nerve fields. *Biol. Cybern.* 35:63–72, 1979.

Traub, R.D. and Llinás, R. Hippocampal pyramidal cells: Significance of dendritic ionic conductances for neuronal function and epileptogenesis. *J. Neurophysiol.* 42:476–496, 1979.

Tsal, Y. Movements of attention across the visual field. *J. Exp. Psychol.* 9:523–530, 1983.

van Kampen, N.G. Fluctuations in closed and open non-linear systems. In: *Statistical*

Physics. (L. Pál and Szépfalusy, P., Eds.) Amsterdam: North-Holland, pp. 29–48, 1976.

van Kampen, N.G. *Stochastic Processes in Physics and Chemistry*. Amsterdam: North-Holland, 1981.

von der Heydt, I., von der Heydt, N., and Obermair, G.M. Statistical model of current-coupled ion channels in nerve membranes. *Z. Physik*. 41:153–164, 1981.

von der Marlsburg, C. Development of ocularity domains and growth behavior of axon terminals. *Biol. Cybern*. 32:49–62, 1979.

Vu, E.T. and Krasne, F.B. Evidence for a computational distinction between proximal and distal neuronal inhibition. *Science*. 255:1710–1712, 1992.

Wehner, M.F. and Wolfer, W.G. Numerical evaluation of path-integral solutions to Fokker-Planck equations. I. *Phys. Rev. A*. 27:2663–2670, 1983a.

Wehner, M.F. and Wolfer, W.G. Numerical evaluation of path-integral solutions to Fokker-Planck equations. II. Restricted stochastic processes. *Phys. Rev. A*. 28:3003–3011, 1983b.

Wehner, M.F. and Wolfer, W.G. Numerical evaluation of path integral solutions to Fokker-Planck equations. III. Time and functionality dependent coefficients. *Phys. Rev. A*. 35:1795–1801, 1987.

Weidlich, W. and Haag, G. *Concepts and Models of a Quantitative Sociology*. Berlin: Springer, 1983.

Weinberg, S. *Gravitational Cosmology*. New York: Wiley, 1972.

Williamson, S.J., Kaufman, L., and Brenner, D. Evoked neuromagnetic fields of the human brain. *J. Appl. Phys*. 50:2418–2421, 1979.

Wilson, H.R. and Cowan, J.D. Excitatory and inhibitory interactions in localized populations of model neurons. *Biophys. J*. 12:1–23, 1972.

Wilson, H.R. and Cowan, J.D. A mathematical theory of the functional dynamics of cortical and thalamic nervous tissue. *Kybernetik*. 13:55–80, 1973.

Wilson, H.R. Hysteresis in binocular grating perception: Contrast effects. *Vision Res*. 17:843–851, 1977.

Wilson, K.G. and Kogurt, J. The renormalization group and the ε expansion. *Physics Reports C*. 12:75–200, 1974.

Wilson, K.G. Problems in physics with many scales of length. *Sci. Am*. 241:158–179, 1979.

Zhang, G. and Simon, H.A. STM capacity for Chinese words and idioms: Chunking and acoustical loop hypotheses. *Memory and Cognition*. 13:193–201, 1985.

APPENDIX

Solutions to the Equations for Global Neocortical Dynamics

PAUL L. NUNEZ

1. BASIC GLOBAL EQUATIONS

The basic equations relating the dependent variables $h_E(\mathbf{r},t)$, $h_I(\mathbf{r},t)$, and $g(\mathbf{r},t)$ over the cortical surface Ω_1 are

$$h_E(\mathbf{r},t) = u(\mathbf{r},t) + \int_0^\infty d\text{v} \int_{\Omega_1} R_E(\mathbf{r},\mathbf{r}_1,\text{v})g\left(\mathbf{r}_1,t - \frac{|\mathbf{r} - \mathbf{r}_1|}{\text{v}}\right)d\Omega_1 \quad (11.1)$$

$$h_I(\mathbf{r},t) = u_0 + \int_{\Omega_1} R_I(\mathbf{r},\mathbf{r}_1)g(\mathbf{r}_1,t)d\Omega_1 \quad (11.2)$$

The one-dimensional equations for waves in an infinite closed strip are obtained by assuming that corticocortical and intracortical connections are highly anisotropic such that

$$R_E(\mathbf{r},\mathbf{r}_1,\text{v}) = \delta(y_1)R_E(x,x_1,\text{v}) \quad (\text{A.1})$$

$$R_I(\mathbf{r},\mathbf{r}_1,\text{v}) = \delta(y_1)R_I(x,x_1) \quad (\text{A.2})$$

Here x and y are coordinates parallel and perpendicular to the cortical strip (in the anterior-posterior direction of one hemisphere, for example). The one-dimensional distribution functions for excitatory and inhibitory synaptic connections are given by

$$R_E(x,x_1,\text{v}) = \frac{1}{2}\sum_{n=1}^{N} \rho_n\lambda_n f_n(\text{v})e^{-\lambda_n|x-x_1|} \quad (11.7)$$

$$R_I(x,x_1) = \frac{1}{2}\rho_I\lambda_I e^{-\lambda_I|x-x_1|} \quad (11.8)$$

The sum in (11.7) is over N excitatory fiber systems, including the possibility of multiple corticocortical and intracortical systems with different decays of connection density determined by the $\lambda_n(\text{cm}^{-1})$ parameters. Define small modulations of the three dependent variables

$$H_E(x,t) \equiv \delta h_E(x,t) \tag{A.3}$$

$$H_I(x,t) \equiv \delta h_I(x,t) \tag{A.4}$$

$$G(x,t) \equiv \delta g(x,t) \tag{A.5}$$

2. INFINITE NEORCORTICAL STRIP

Define the Fourier transform of the excitatory modulation variable $H_E(x,t)$

$$H_E(k,\omega) = \int_{-\infty}^{+\infty} e^{-jkx}dx \int_{-\infty}^{+\infty} H_E(x,t)e^{-j\omega t}dt \tag{A.6}$$

with similar definitions for $H_I(k,\omega)$ and $G(k,\omega)$. Consider a modulation of (11.1), substitute (A.1) into (11.1), and integrate over the infinite strip as in (A.6). This procedure is valid only for waves in an infinite strip; however, it provides a good approximation for all but the lowest mode (as shown in Section 3 of the Appendix). The resulting equation for the Fourier transformed modulation of excitatory synaptic action due to input $U(k,\omega)$ is

$$H_E(k,\omega) = U(k,\omega) + \frac{1}{2}\sum_{n=1}^{N} \rho_n\lambda_n \int_0^{\infty} f_n(\text{v})d\text{v} \int_{-\infty}^{+\infty} G(x_1,\omega)e^{-jkx_1}dx_1 \cdot \int_{-\infty}^{+\infty} e^{-(j\omega/\text{v}+\lambda_n)|x-x_1|-jk(x-x_1)}dx \tag{A.7}$$

If wave damping is restricted to

$$Real\left(j\frac{\omega}{\text{v}} + \lambda_n\right) > 0 \qquad \text{or} \qquad \gamma > -\lambda_n \text{v}_{\min} \tag{A.8}$$

where $\text{v}_{\min}$ is the minimum velocity of action potential propagation allowed by the distribution functions, the inner integral over x in (A.7) is independent of x_1 and yields

$$\frac{2\left(\lambda_n + j\dfrac{\omega}{\text{v}}\right)}{\left(\lambda_n + j\dfrac{\omega}{\text{v}}\right)^2 + k^2} \tag{A.9}$$

Equation (A.7) then reduces to

$$H_E(k,\omega) = U(k,\omega) + \rho_E G(k,\omega)F(k,\omega) \tag{A.10}$$

where the following function is defined

$$F(k,\omega) \equiv \sum_{n=1}^{N} \frac{\rho_n}{\rho_E} \int_0^\infty \frac{\lambda_n^2 v^2 + j\omega\lambda_n v}{(\lambda_n v + j\omega)^2 + k^2 v^2} f_n(v)dv \qquad (11.26)$$

The Fourier transformed version of (11.2) yields a similar expression for the modulation of inhibitory synaptic action

$$H_I(k,\omega) = \frac{\rho_I G(k,\omega)}{1 + k^2/\lambda_I^2} \approx \rho_I G(k,\omega) \qquad (A.11)$$

This approximation is valid for all scalp-recorded waves since $\lambda_I > 100\ \text{cm}^{-1}$, that is inhibitory connection density between neurons decreases rapidly with separation distance.

3. LINEARIZED GLOBAL THEORY

The linear approximation for input/output in a neural mass with no local time delays is given by

$$\delta g = \frac{\partial g}{\partial h_E} H_E + \frac{\partial g}{\partial h_I} H_I \qquad (11.3)$$

where we have used the notation defined in (A.3) through (A.5). With the definitions (11.4), we obtain

$$G(k,\omega) = Q_E H_E(k,\omega) - Q_I H_I(k,\omega) \qquad (A.12)$$

where Q_E and Q_I are the partial derivatives in (11.3) at the fixed state $g = g_0$. Equations (A.10), (A.11), and (A.12) determine the three dependent variables $H_E(k,\omega)$, $H_I(k,\omega)$, and $G(k,\omega)$. Solving for $H_E(k,\omega)$ yields a global relation connecting cortical input $U(k,\omega)$ to output $H_E(k,\omega)$ given by

$$H_E(k,\omega) = \frac{U(k,\omega)}{D_G(k,\omega)} \qquad (11.9)$$

where $D_G(k,\omega)$ and $T_G(k,\omega) \equiv D_G^{-1}(k,\omega)$ are the global dispersion function and transfer function, respectively. The dispersion relation is given by

$$D_G(k,\omega) = 1 - \frac{Q_E}{Q_I} \sum_{n=1}^{N} \frac{\rho_n}{\rho_I} \int_0^\infty \frac{\lambda_n^2 v^2 + j\omega\lambda_n v}{(\lambda_n v + j\omega)^2 + k^2 v^2} f_n(v)\, dv = 0 \qquad (11.10)$$

If all fiber systems but one ($n = 1$ or $n \rightarrow E$) have effectively infinite propagation velocity (negligible global delays), (11.10) yields

$$1 - B(k) \int_0^\infty \frac{\lambda_E^2 v^2 + j\omega\lambda_E v}{(\lambda_E v + j\omega)^2 + k^2 v^2} f_E(v)dv = 0 \qquad (11.11)$$

The control function B(k) is only weakly dependent on wave number k for waves of relatively long wavelength, and may be considered a control parameter given by

$$B = \frac{\dfrac{Q_E \rho_E}{Q_I \rho_I}}{1 - \dfrac{Q_E}{Q_I} \sum\limits_{n \neq E} \dfrac{\rho_n}{\rho_I}} \tag{11.19}$$

Here the sum is over all excitatory systems (both inter- and intracortical) that have negligible delays due to action potential propagation.

4. SINGLE FIBER SYSTEM WITH PEAKED VELOCITY DISTRIBUTION

If the velocity distribution is sharply peaked such that $f_E(v) = \delta(v - v_E)$, the dispersion relation (11.11) reduces to

$$D_G(k,\omega) = 1 - \frac{B\left(1 + j\dfrac{\omega}{\lambda_E v_E}\right)}{\left(1 + j\dfrac{\omega}{\lambda_E v_E}\right)^2 + \left(\dfrac{k}{\lambda_E}\right)^2} = 0 \tag{A.13}$$

The solution to (A.13) with $\omega(k) = \omega_R(k) - j\gamma(k)$ is

$$\left(\frac{\omega_R}{\lambda_E v_E}\right)^2 = \left(\frac{k}{\lambda_E}\right)^2 - \frac{B^2}{4} \tag{11.14}$$

$$\frac{\gamma}{\lambda_E v_E} = \frac{B}{2} - 1 \tag{11.15}$$

Here $\gamma < 0$ indicates damping, and $\gamma > 0$ ($B > 2$) corresponds to unstable waves (or perhaps limit cycles in more accurate quasi-linear theories).

5. WAVES IN A FINITE ONE-DIMENSIONAL STRIP

Here we examine the approximation of a finite strip of cortex. Following Srinivasan (1994), (A.6) is replaced by

$$H_E(x,\omega) = \sum_{m=-\infty}^{+\infty} e^{-jk_m x} \int_{-\infty}^{+\infty} H_E(x,t) e^{-j\omega t}\, dt \tag{A.14}$$

Periodic boundary conditions in the strip of circumference L restrict the wave numbers such that $H_E(x,t)$ and $\frac{\partial H_E(x,t)}{\partial x}$ are continuous functions of x, that is

$$k_m = \frac{2\pi m}{L} \qquad m = \pm 1, \pm 2, \pm 3, \ldots \tag{11.6}$$

The derivation is similar to that for the infinite strip and yields a dispersion relation

$$D_G(k_m,\omega) = 1 - B \left[\frac{1 + j\dfrac{\omega}{\lambda_E v_E}}{\left(1 + j\dfrac{\omega}{\lambda_E v_E}\right)^2 + \left(\dfrac{k_m}{\lambda_E}\right)^2} \right] \cdot \left\{ \frac{1 + (-1)^{m+1} exp\left[-\left(1 + j\dfrac{\omega}{\lambda_E v_E}\right) \dfrac{\lambda_E L}{2} \right]}{1 - e^{-\lambda_E L/2}} \right\} = 0 \tag{A.15}$$

which reduces to the solution for an infinite loop (A.13) in the limit $\lambda_E L \gg 1$ for waves with damping $\gamma > -\lambda_E v_E$. The complex roots of (A.15) were obtained using IMSL program ZANLY. Real and imaginary parts analogous to the equivalent solution for the infinite strip given by (11.14) and (11.15) are plotted in Figure 11-22. These results can be compared directly with frequency and damping plots for waves in an infinite strip (Figure 11-30) and waves on a spherical surface (Figure 11-33). The main difference between solutions in the infinite and finite strips is the absence of a weakly damped mode m = 1 in the finite strip.

6. WAVES ON A SPHERICAL SURFACE

The solution to the brain wave equations (11.1) and (11.2) for a spherical surface using the linear approximation (11.3) was originally obtained by Katznelson (1981, 1982). Here we generalize his solution in order to make the presentation more consistent with the one-dimension derivation and to include multiple fiber systems. A small modulation of (11.1) yields

$$H_E(\mathbf{r},t) = U(\mathbf{r},t) + \int_0^\infty dv \int_{\Omega_1} R_E(\mathbf{r},\mathbf{r}_1,v)G\left(\mathbf{r}_1, t - \frac{|\mathbf{r} - \mathbf{r}_1|}{v}\right) d\Omega_1 \tag{A.16}$$

In the example of waves on a spherical surface, the vectors $\mathbf{r}$ and $\mathbf{r}_1$ locate the surface positions (θ,ϕ) and (θ_1, ϕ_1), respectively. Define the temporal Fourier transform

$$H_E(\theta,\phi,\omega) = \int_{-\infty}^{+\infty} H_E(\theta,\phi,t)e^{-j\omega t}dt \tag{A.17}$$

Take the temporal Fourier transform of (A.16) to obtain

$$H_E(\theta,\phi,\omega) = U(\theta,\phi,\omega) + \int_0^\infty dv \int_{\Omega_1} R_E(\theta,\phi,\theta_1,\phi_1,v)G(\theta_1,\phi_1,\omega)e^{-j\frac{\omega R}{v}\beta(\theta,\phi,\theta_1,\phi_1)}d\Omega_1 \tag{A.18}$$

where the distance between locations on the surface of a sphere of radius of R is $R\beta$ and the angle β is defined by

$$\cos\beta = \cos\theta\cos\theta_1 + \sin\theta\sin\theta_1\cos(\phi - \phi_1) \tag{A.19}$$

The distribution function for fiber connections on a spherical surface must (by definition) satisfy the condition

$$\int_0^\infty dv \int_0^{2\pi} d\phi_1 \int_0^\pi R_E(\theta,\phi,\theta_1,\phi_1,v)\sin\theta_1 d\theta_1 = \rho(\theta,\phi) = \sum_{n=1}^N \rho_n \tag{A.20}$$

where $\rho(\theta,\phi)$ is the number density of excitatory synapses per target neuron. If our model cortex has homogeneous, isotropic fiber connections, the appropriate generalization of the one-dimensional distribution function (11.7) is

$$R_E(\theta,\phi,\theta_1,\phi_1,v) = \frac{1}{2\pi}\sum_{n=1}^N \frac{\rho_n(1 + \lambda_n^2R^2)f_n(v)e^{-\lambda_n R\beta}}{1 + e^{-\pi\lambda_n R}} \tag{A.21}$$

Here ρ_n is the local number of the excitatory synapses per neuron associated with the *n*th fiber system, and the factor multiplying the velocity distribution function $f_n(v)$ is determined by the normalization (A.20).

We express the solution $H_E(\theta,\phi,\omega)$ for waves on the surface of a sphere in a manner analogous to (A.14). That is, expand the solution in a series of spherical harmonics $Y_{\ell m}(\theta,\phi)$

$$H_E(\theta,\phi,\omega) = \sum_{\ell=0}^\infty \sum_{m=-\ell}^{+\ell} H_{E\ell m}(\omega)Y_{\ell m}(\theta,\phi) \tag{A.22}$$

The spherical harmonics are orthogonal in the Hermitian sense on the sphere so that (A.22) yields

$$H_{E\ell m}(\omega) = \int_0^{2\pi} d\phi \int_0^\pi H_E(\theta,\phi,\omega)Y^*_{\ell m}(\theta,\phi)\sin\theta\, d\theta \tag{A.23}$$

Expansions similar to (A.22) definite $H_{I\ell m}(\omega)$ and $G_{\ell m}(\omega)$. In order to simplify the notation, we write double sums

$$\sum_{\ell=0}^{\infty} \sum_{m=-\ell}^{+\ell} = \sum_{\ell,m} \tag{A.24}$$

and surface integrals like (A.23) as

$$H_{E\ell m} = \int_{\Omega} H_E(\Omega) Y^*_{\ell m}(\Omega) d\Omega \tag{A.25}$$

with the functional dependence on ω made implicit and the surface element sinθ dθ dϕ replaced by dΩ. Substitute (A.21) into (A.18) to obtain

$$H_E(\Omega) = U(\Omega) + \int_{\Omega_1} F(\Omega,\Omega_1) G(\Omega_1) d\Omega_1 \tag{A.26}$$

where we define the function

$$F(\Omega,\Omega_1) \equiv \sum_{n=1}^{N} \rho_n \left(\frac{1 + \lambda_n^2 R^2}{1 + e^{-\pi\lambda_n R}} \right) \int_0^{\infty} f_n(\mathrm{v}) e^{-\left(j\frac{\omega}{\mathrm{v}} + \lambda_n\right) R\beta(\Omega,\Omega_1)} d\mathrm{v} \tag{A.27}$$

Expand the functions $H_E(\Omega)$, $U(\Omega)$, and $G(\Omega_1)$ in (A.26) as in (A.22)

$$\sum_{\ell,m} H_{E\ell m} Y_{\ell m}(\Omega) = \sum_{\ell,m} U_{\ell m} Y_{\ell m}(\Omega) + \frac{1}{2\pi} \sum_{\ell,m} \int_{\Omega_1} F[\beta(\Omega,\Omega_1)] Y_{\ell m}(\Omega_1) d\Omega_1 \tag{A.28}$$

If the function $F(\Omega, \Omega_1)$ is continuous on the sphere, the surface integral in (A.28) may be simplified using the Funk-Hecke theorem (Erdelyi, 1953)

$$\int_{\Omega_1} F[\beta(\Omega,\Omega_1)] Y_{\ell m}(\Omega_1) d\Omega_1 = 2\pi Y_{\ell m}(\Omega) \int_0^{\pi} F(\beta) P_\ell(\cos\beta) \sin\beta \, d\beta \tag{A.29}$$

where $P_\ell(\cos\beta)$ is the usual Lengendre polynomial and β is the angle between surface locations Ω and Ω_1. Thus each coefficient in the spherical harmonic expansion satisfies

$$H_{E\ell m}(\omega) = U_{\ell m}(\omega) + F_{E\ell} G_{\ell m}(\omega) \tag{A.30}$$

where

$$F_{E\ell}(\omega) \equiv \sum_{n=1}^{N} \rho_n \left(\frac{1 + \lambda_n^2 R^2}{1 + e^{-\pi\lambda_n R}} \right) \int_0^{\infty} f_n(\mathrm{v}) d\mathrm{v} \int_0^{\pi} e^{-\left(j\frac{\omega}{\mathrm{v}} + \lambda_n\right) R\beta} P_\ell(\cos\beta) \sin\beta \, d\beta \tag{A.31}$$

In a similar manner, we obtain the following relations between spherical harmonic coefficients from (11.2) and (A.12)

$$H_{I\ell m}(\omega) = F_{I\ell}G_{\ell m}(\omega) \tag{A.32}$$

$$G_{\ell m}(\omega) = Q_E H_{E\ell m}(\omega) - Q_I H_{I\ell m}(\omega) \tag{A.33}$$

Here the inhibitory version of (A.31) is

$$F_{I\ell} \equiv \rho_I\left(\frac{1 + \lambda_I^2 R^2}{1 + e^{-\pi\lambda_I R}}\right)\int_0^\pi e^{-\lambda_I R\beta}P_\ell(\cos\beta)\sin\beta\, d\beta \tag{A.34}$$

Since λ_I is greater than 100 cm^{-1} and R ~ 10 cm, $\lambda_I R >> 1$, and the integral may be easily evaluated as

$$\int_0^\pi e^{-\lambda_I R\beta}P_\ell(\cos\beta)\sin\beta\, d\beta \cong \int_0^\pi \beta e^{-\lambda_I R\beta}\, d\beta \cong \frac{1}{\lambda_I^2 R^2} \tag{A.35}$$

which yields

$$F_{I\ell} \cong \rho_I \tag{A.36}$$

consistent with (A.11).

Combine (A.30), (A.32), and (A.33) to obtain

$$H_{E\ell m}(\omega) = \frac{U_{\ell m}(\omega)}{D_\ell(\omega)} \tag{11.44}$$

where the dispersion relation $D_\ell(\omega) = 0$ determines normal mode frequencies ω_ℓ for $\ell = 0,1,2,3....$ The dispersion function is given by

$$D_\ell(\omega) = 1 - \frac{Q_E F_{E\ell}(\omega)}{Q_I \rho_I} \tag{A.37}$$

where the number of inhibitory synapses per neuron was assumed to be sufficiently large so that $\rho_I Q_I >> 1$.

In order to solve (A.37) for the normal mode frequencies ω_ℓ, we must evaluate $F_{E\ell}$ from (A.31). Define a new frequency variable

$$Z_n \equiv j\frac{\omega R}{v} + \lambda_n R \tag{A.38}$$

which is a generalization of (11.46) for multi-fiber systems. The inner integral in (A.31) is then

$$S_{n\ell} = \int_0^\pi e^{-Z_n\beta}P_\ell(\cos\beta)\sin(\beta)\, d\beta \tag{A.39}$$

These integrals were evaluated recursively by Katznelson (Appendix H of Nunez, 1981)

$$S_{n0} = \frac{1 + e^{-\pi Z_n}}{1 + Z_n^2} \tag{A.40}$$

$$S_{n1} = \frac{1 - e^{-\pi Z_n}}{4 + Z_n^2} \tag{A.41}$$

$$S_{n\ell} = \frac{(\ell - 2)^2 + Z_n^2}{(\ell + 1)^2 + Z_n^2} S_{n,\ell-2} \tag{A.42}$$

Consider the special case of a single corticocortical fiber system (n = 1 or n → E) with velocity distribution for action potential propagation

$$f_n(v) = \delta(v - v_E) \tag{11.13}$$

In this example, (A.31) simplifies to

$$F_{E\ell} = \rho_E\left(\frac{1 + \lambda_E^2 R^2}{1 + e^{-\pi\lambda_E R}}\right) S_{E\ell}(Z) \tag{A.43}$$

where

$$Z = j\frac{\omega R}{v_E} + \lambda_E R \tag{11.46}$$

The dispersion relation (A.37) reduces to

$$D_\ell(\omega) = 1 - B_{2D} S_{E\ell}(Z) = 0 \tag{A.44}$$

where the two-dimensional control parameter is

$$B_{2D} \equiv \left(\frac{1 + \lambda_E^2 R^2}{1 + e^{-\pi\lambda_E R}}\right) B \tag{11.48}$$

and B is the one-dimensional control parameter given by

$$B = \frac{Q_E \rho_E}{Q_I \rho_I} \tag{A.45}$$

which is a limiting case of (11.19) when only one excitatory fiber system is included. Multiple short-range fiber systems with $Real\left(\frac{\omega}{\lambda_n v_n}\right) << 1$ and $\lambda_n R >> 1$ for all systems n > 1 satisfy the dispersion relation (A.44) provided the definition of B in (A.45) is replaced by the modified version (11.19). This occurs as a consequence of approximating integrals in (A.31) for different excitatory fiber systems in an analogous manner to the approximation in (A.34) and (A.35).

The inclusion of multiple systems may be critical to comparisons of (A.44) with experimental data since representation of corticocortical connections by a single parameter λ_E may not be valid.

If λ_E is too large (fibers too short), no weakly damped waves are found as solutions to (A.44). By contrast, a single system with long fibers can produce weakly or negatively damped waves (limit cycle modes, for example). Numerical solutions to (A.44) were obtained by the author using IMSL program ZANLY. The complex roots Z_ℓ are related to complex frequency by means of

$$\omega_\ell = \omega_{R\ell} - j\gamma_\ell \tag{A.46}$$

where γ_ℓ is defined such that $\gamma_\ell < 0$ corresponds to positive damping, thus

$$\frac{\omega_{R\ell} R}{v_E} = Imag(Z_\ell) \tag{A.47}$$

$$\frac{\gamma_\ell R}{v_E} = Real(Z_\ell) - \lambda_E R \tag{A.48}$$

Normal mode frequencies and relative damping for waves on a sphere are plotted versus the one-dimensional control parameter B in Figure 11-31 ($\lambda_E R = 0.7$), Figure 11-32 ($\lambda_E R = 1.5$), and Figure 11-33 ($\lambda_E R = 1.0$). Direct comparison with the one-dimensional solution may be obtained using Figure 11-30 ($\lambda_E R = 1.0$).

7. MULTIPLE CORTICOCORTICAL FIBER SYSTEMS

Our approach to multiple excitatory fiber systems as described by (11.7) or (A.21) has been to separate these systems into two categories, depending on whether action propagation velocity can be considered infinite. If $f_n(v) = \delta(v - v_n)$, "infinite propagation velocity" means

$$\frac{\omega}{\lambda_n v_n} << 1 \tag{A.49}$$

If, for example, there are two corticocortical fiber systems in one direction that do not satisfy (A.49) and one intracortical excitatory system that does satisfy (A.49), (11.10) reduces to

$$D_G(k,\omega) = 1 - \frac{B_1\left(1 + j\dfrac{\omega}{\lambda_1 v_1}\right)}{\left(1 + j\dfrac{\omega}{\lambda_1 v_1}\right)^2 + k^2/\lambda_1^2} - \frac{B_2\left(1 + j\dfrac{\omega}{\lambda_2 v_2}\right)}{\left(1 + j\dfrac{\omega}{\lambda_2 v_2}\right)^2 + k^2/\lambda_2^2} = 0 \tag{A.50}$$

where the control parameters B_1 and B_2 are given by (11.30). Equation (A.50) yields a quartic algebraic equation in mode frequency ω. Example solutions are shown in Figures 11-15 and 11-16 for the two branches of the dispersion relation which occur when two fiber systems have different functional decreases in connection density with separation distance ($\lambda_1 \neq \lambda_2$).

If corticocortical fibers consist of a mixture of myelinated and nonmyelinated axons, (A.50) may also be used to simulate the resulting effect on mode frequencies. Figure 11-21 shows frequency and relative damping for an example in which 22% of corticocortical fibers are nonmyelinated, having propagation velocity $v_1 = 0.1v_2$. In this example, equal length constants ($\lambda_1 = \lambda_2$) is assumed.

8. DISTRIBUTED CORTICOCORTICAL PROPAGATION VELOCITIES

If a single corticocortical fiber system has distributed velocities, the dispersion relation is given by (11.11). Define the nondimensional velocity

$$u = \frac{v}{v_E} \tag{A.51}$$

and corresponding distribution

$$f(u) = f_E(uv_E)v_E \tag{A.52}$$

where v_E is some characteristic velocity appropriate for the distribution function $f_E(v)$. Define the nondimensional frequency Z by

$$Z = j\frac{\omega}{\lambda_E v_E} \tag{A.53}$$

With these definitions, (11.11) may be written

$$1 - B\int_0^\infty \frac{(u^2 + Zu)f(u)\,du}{(u + Z)^2 + (k/\lambda_E)^2u^2} = 0 \tag{A.54}$$

Three methods were used to find solutions Z to this integral equation for several velocity distributions $f(u)$ which were defined to be zero for $u < u_{min}$. A small cut-off velocity u_{min} is chosen to avoid poles on the real u axis. This is essentially condition (A.8).

1. Equation (A.54) was solved for the control parameter B for a large number of assumed values of Z. Physiologically realistic problems with small relative damping or small instability correspond to $|Real(Z)| << |Imag(Z)|$ and $Imag(B) = 0$.
2. IMSL program ZANLY was used to find roots to (A.54) for different values of the control parameter B and spatial mode k.
3. The symbolic manipulation program MACSYMA was used to obtain an analytic integral in (A.54) when $f(u)$ is the rectangular function (11.35) (Ko-

walski and Nunez, 1991). The NAG library root solving program was used to find roots to (A.54). This procedure was used to check roots obtained by method (*ii*). MACSYMA was not able to obtain an analytic integral when $f(\mathrm{u})$ is the exponential function (11.37). In this case, methods (*i*) and (*ii*) were used to find roots. Solutions are shown in Figures 11-23 through 11-25.

When $f(\mathrm{u})$ is a distributed function, the singularities in the function given by (11.9) are not necessarily poles so that a dispersion relation need not exist in the usual sense (Montgomery and Tidman 1964, Nunez 1971). However, we still expect neocortical spacial-temporal filtering such that the frequency ranges given by $D_G(k,\omega) \approx 0$ are dominant. We have not examined examples in which the integral in (A.54) includes a pole on the real u axis. This does not appear to be important in neocortex, although a similar mathematical issue occurs in hot plasma theory in connection with Landau damping (Montgomery and Tidman 1964).

9. INCLUSION OF LINEAR LOCAL CIRCUIT FEEDBACK MECHANISMS

The linearization about a fixed state (11.3) implies an instantaneous response of action potential modulation $G(\mathbf{r},t)$ to the modulation of excitatory $H_E(\mathbf{r},t)$ and inhibitory $H_I(\mathbf{r},t)$ input to each neural mass. Actually, local circuit effects may influence the response in a number of ways ranging from simple delays to very complex behavior based on multiple nonlinear feedback mechanisms. This range of possible behavior is believed to be effected by various neuromodulators that act to alter local control parameters as discussed in Chapter 13. We have not emphasized detailed theoretical development of local circuit dynamics because of the severe limitations to obtaining valid models at the local level. However, the following examples provide a rough idea of how local-global interactions may occur.

Consider a model system in which inhibitory synaptic input to each neural mass causes an immediate, linear reduction in action potential output as in (11.3), but excitatory synaptic input produces positive and negative feedback within the mass. If the modulation of these feedback mechanisms is approximately linear, we may replace (11.3) or (A.12) by

$$G(\mathbf{r},t) = Q_E \int_0^\infty d\tau \int_{\Omega_1} T_L(\mathbf{r}_1, \tau) H_E(|\mathbf{r} - \mathbf{r}_1|, t - \tau)\, d\Omega_1 - Q_I H_I(\mathbf{r},t) \tag{A.55}$$

Here Q_E is defined as the local gain and $T_L(\mathbf{r}_1, \tau)$ is the weighing function for the local circuit, defined in a manner similar to that of linear systems with no spatial extent as in (8.4). Equation (A.55) expresses the idea that the output $G(\mathbf{r},t)$ depends on the input $H_E(\mathbf{r},t)$ at earlier times and other locations with weighing given by $T_L(\mathbf{r}_1, \tau)$. Since the output at any time cannot respond to future inputs, we require

$$T_L(\mathbf{r}_1, \tau) = 0 \qquad \tau < 0 \tag{A.56}$$

Thus, the lower limit of the τ integral in (A.55) may be replaced by minus infinity. The use of (A.55) is based on a homogeneous, isotropic neocortex; however it is not difficult to consider examples in which this restriction is relaxed somewhat. This issue of intracortical connection properties is different than the issue of corticocortical isotropy and homogeneity. The Fourier transform of the local weighing function on a spherical surface is given by

$$T_{L\ell m}(\omega) = \int_{\Omega_1} Y^*_{\ell m}(\Omega_1)\, d\Omega_1 \int_{-\infty}^{+\infty} T_L(\Omega_1, \tau) e^{-j\omega\tau} d\tau \tag{A.57}$$

If neural mass is distributed over a spherical surface, (A.55) may be integrated over this surface and over time as in (A.57) to obtain

$$G_{\ell m}(\omega) = Q_E T_{L\ell m}(\omega) H_{E\ell m}(\omega) - Q_I H_{I\ell m}(\omega) \tag{A.58}$$

Equation (A.58) is (A.33) modified by the local transfer function. The local dispersion function is, by definition, the inverse of the local transfer function

$$D_{L\ell m}(\omega) = T^{-1}_{L\ell m}(\omega) \tag{A.59}$$

If neural tissue is distributed along an infinite strip, the one-dimensional version of (A.57) is

$$T_L(k,\omega) = \int_{-\infty}^{+\infty} e^{-jkx_1} dx_1 \int_{-\infty}^{+\infty} T_L(x_1, \tau) e^{-j\omega\tau} d\tau \tag{A.60}$$

Here, the wave number k replaces the two-dimensional indices associated with the spherical harmonic $Y^*_{lm}(\Omega_1)$ used in (A.57). The one-dimensional version of (A.58) is

$$G(k,\omega) = Q_E T_{\mathrm{L}}(k,\omega) H_E(k,\omega) - Q_I H_I(k,\omega) \tag{A.61}$$

Equation (A.61) reduces to (A.12) when local circuit feedback is neglected, that is

$$T_L(k,\omega) = 1 \tag{A.62}$$

or

$$T_L(x_1, \tau) = \delta(x_1)\delta(\tau) \tag{A.63}$$

10. INFLUENCE OF LOCAL FEEDBACK ON NEOCORTICAL MODES

The general influence of local feedback on neocortical EEG can be estimated by comparison of (A.61) with (A.12). The dispersion relation for waves in an infinite strip obtained in Section 4 of the Appendix is given by (A.13). Modification by local feedback yields a local-global dispersion relation.

$$1 - \frac{B\left(1 + j\dfrac{\omega}{\lambda_E v_E}\right) T_L(k,\omega)}{\left(1 + j\dfrac{\omega}{\lambda_E v_E}\right)^2 + (k/\lambda_E)^2} = 0 \qquad \text{(A.64)}$$

Equation (A.64) is a special case of (11.27) which occurs when corticocortical fibers consist of a single system with peaked action potential velocity at $v = v_E$. Equation (A.64) may be re-written based on the definition of the dispersion function (A.59), that is

$$D(k,\omega) = D_L(k,\omega) - \frac{B\left(1 + j\dfrac{\omega}{\lambda_E v_E}\right)}{\left(1 + j\dfrac{\omega}{\lambda_E v_E}\right)^2 + (k/\lambda_E)^2} = 0 \qquad \text{(A.65)}$$

which is essentially (11.27). If the local dispersion function (or transfer function) is a rational fraction, that is consisting of a ratio of polynomials in ω, (A.65) yields a dispersion relation for which each pair of roots corresponds to a different branch of the dispersion relation. For example, if the local transfer function is given by

$$T_L(k,\omega) = \frac{a_n\omega^n + a_{n-1}\omega^{n-1} + \cdots + a_0}{b_m\omega^m + b_{m-1}\omega^{m-1} + \cdots + b_0} \qquad \text{(A.66)}$$

with m > n, $T_L(k,\omega)$ is called a proper rational function. This condition ensures that

$$\lim_{Real(\omega)\to\infty} T_L(k,\omega) = 0 \qquad \text{(A.67)}$$

which is generally expected in neural tissue. Under these conditions, the local-global dispersion relation (A.65) yields a polynomial of degree m+2, corresponding to $\frac{m + 2}{2}$ branches of the dispersion relation. Such branches can be overdamped, underdamped or unstable; only the underdamped and unstable branches are observable. Unstable branches may become limit cycles as discussed in Section 12 of the Appendix.

The local circuit theory outlined in Chapters 5 and 8 (or any other linear, local theory) may be used to obtain $D_L(k,\omega)$. Examples of different branches of the resulting dispersion relation (A.65) are plotted in Figure 11-8. However, we can make several general observations about the influence of the local feedback circuits on global oscillatory behavior. Since global modes become more weakly damped for large values of the global control parameter B, introduction of the local transfer function in (A.64) is seen to result in an effective global control parameter which is largest when $T_L(k,\omega)$ is large. Thus, global mode frequencies close to local resonant frequencies are enhanced by local circuits. These global modes, in turn, can drive local circuits at their resonant frequencies, thereby producing a mechanism for strong coupling of local and global neocortical processes. Furthermore, local circuits are known to alter their properties in response to electrical stimulation (see Chapters 3, 5 and 13). Thus, one may speculate that global oscillations partly determined by global boundary conditions can alter local resonant frequencies because of neural plasticity.

11. LOCAL AND REGIONAL MODES

Regional circuits due to specific reciprocal corticocortical connections between neocortical locations are emphasized in Chapter 13. Such neural circuits are believed to continually reform in different neocortical locations during preparation and performance of cognitive tasks as discussed in Chapters 6 and 7. Regional circuits may be introduced into the basic one-dimensional theory by using a simple example in which local circuits cause a delay τ_L, and regional circuits cause a delay depending on a fixed distance x_R separating the two parts of the regional circuit, which are assumed to be connected by axons carrying action potentials with speed v_R. The local-regional weighing function is given by

$$T_{LR}(x_1, \tau) = A_L\delta(x_1)\delta(\tau - \tau_L) + A_R\delta(x_1 - x_R)\delta(\tau - x_R/v_R) \quad (A.68)$$

Here A_L and A_R depend on the strengths of the local and regional feedback, respectively.

The local-regional transfer function corresponding to (A.68) is

$$T_{LR}(k,\omega) = A_L e^{-j\tau_L\omega} + A_R e^{-j(x_R\omega/v_R + x_R k)} \quad (A.69)$$

The local-regional-global dispersion relation is then given by (A.64) with $T_L(k,\omega)$ replaced by $T_{LR}(k,\omega)$. Changes in purely global resonant frequencies due to local-regional modes depend on the magnitude of the local delay τ_L, the spatial separation of the (assumed) two parts of each regional circuit x_R, and the propagation velocity in regional circuits v_R. Modifications of global modes are minimal if

$$\tau_L\omega \sim 2\pi n \qquad n = 0, 1, 2, \ldots$$

or

$$\tau_L \sim \frac{n}{f} \qquad n = 0, 1, 2, \ldots \tag{A.70}$$

and

$$x_R\left(\frac{\omega}{v_R} + k\right) \sim 2\pi m \qquad m = 0, 1, 2, \ldots \tag{A.71}$$

For example, in the limit of infinite regional velocity, the phase of the global wavelength Λ may "match" the spatial extent of regional circuits in the sense

$$\Lambda \sim \frac{x_R}{m} \qquad m = 0, 1, 2, \ldots \tag{A.72}$$

Condition (A.70) is satisfied for $n=0$ if the global delay τ_L is very short. Condition (A.71) is satisfied for $m=0$ if the regional circuit extent x_R is small. However, there exist multiple ranges of these parameters for which modifications of global modes are small, and other local-regional parameter ranges which cause large modifications of global modes. Furthermore, local-regional modes may be driven by global modes for certain parameter ranges.

12. GLOBAL LIMIT CYCLES

We consider a quasi-linear solution to (11.1) and (11.2) when the control parameter B is greater than 2.0; that is, when unstable waves are predicted by the linear theory. The input-output curve shown in Figure 11-5a suggests that large magnitudes of the excitatory input $h_E(x,t)$ may result in a decrease in the local slope of this curve due perhaps to increased negative feedback, saturation effects in the neural mass, or both. Since the control parameter B is proportional to this slope and determines wave damping, we may reasonably postulate amplitude-dependent damping for large and perhaps even moderate magnitudes of $h_E(x,t)$.

A crude quasi-linear approximation of the neocortical dynamics of Sections 1–5 may be obtained from (A.10), (A.11), and the following modified version of (A.12)

$$G(k,\omega) = Q_E[H_E(k,\omega)]H_E(k,\omega) - Q_I[H_I(k,\omega)]H_I(k,\omega) \tag{11.38}$$

The simple relation between the Fourier transforms of midbrain synaptic input $U(k,\omega)$ and excitatory synaptic neocortical response $H_E(k,\omega)$ given by (11.9) is not valid for nonlinear systems. However, if the derivatives Q_E and Q_I remain close to their background magnitudes (as postulated for fixed brain states), we expect dynamic behavior to follow (A.13) approximately, but with the control parameter B replaced by

$$B_{k\omega}[H_E(k,\omega),\ H_I(k,\omega)] \tag{A.73}$$

which reflects small oscillations of Q_E and Q_I about their background states. We may invert the temporal Fourier transforms, for example

$$H_E(k,t) = \frac{1}{2\pi}\int_{-\infty}^{+\infty} H_E(k,\omega)e^{j\omega t}d\omega \tag{A.74}$$

to obtain

$$B_{k\omega} \rightarrow B_{kt}[H_E(k,t),\ H_I(k,t)] \tag{A.75}$$

The dynamics of our putative weakly nonlinear system (A.13) may evidently be approximated by the following differential equations for the spatial modes $H_E(k,t)$

$$\frac{d^2H_E}{dt^2} + \lambda_E v_E[2 - B_{kt}(H_E,\ H_I)]\frac{dH_E}{dt} + [(\lambda_E^2 + k^2)v_E^2 - \lambda_E^2 v_E^2 B_{kt}(H_E,\ H_I)]H_E = 0 \tag{11.39}$$

If B_{kt} are constant, temporal Fourier transform of (11.39) yields the dispersion relation (A.13). If B_{kt} are variable, Fourier transform of (11.39) involves nonlinear terms. However, if the B_{kt} undergo small oscillations about the background states B_{k0}, we may approximate

$$\int_{-\infty}^{+\infty} B_{kt}[H_E(k,t),\ H_I(k,t)]H_E(k,t)e^{-j\omega t}dt \cong B_{k0}H_E(k,\omega) \tag{A.76}$$

with a similar approximation for the term involving $\frac{dH_E}{dt}$. In this limiting case, (A.13) is again obtained, but with B replaced by B_{k0}.

Generally, the equations for excitatory synaptic action (11.39) are coupled to equations for inhibitatory synaptic action $H_I(k,t)$. For example, equations (A.10), (A.11), and (11.38) yield

$$H_I(k,\omega) = \frac{\rho_I}{\rho_E} B_{k\omega}[H_E(k,\omega),\ H_I(k,\omega)]H_E(k,\omega) \tag{A.77}$$

For illustrative purposes, we consider a simple example for which $Q_E = Q_E(H_E)$, but Q_I = constant. If we further restrict our solution to a single dominant excitatory system such that the sum in the denominator of (11.19) may be neglected, we obtain

$$B_{\mathrm{kt}}(H_E) = \frac{\rho_E Q_E(H_E)}{\rho_I Q_I} \qquad \text{(A.78)}$$

Expand the functions $B_{\mathrm{k}t}$ about their background states

$$B_{kt}(H_E) \cong B_{k0} + \left(\frac{\partial B_{kt}}{\partial H_E}\right)_0 H_E + \frac{1}{2}\left(\frac{\partial^2 B_{kt}}{\partial H_E^2}\right)_0 H_E^2 \qquad \text{(A.79)}$$

Consider an example in which each $B_{kt}(H_E)$ has an isolated maximum (point b of Figure A-1). This occurs, for example, if the functions $g(\mathrm{k},t) = \mathrm{g}[h_E(\mathrm{k},t)]$ are sigmoids. If the background state occurs at the points of maximum slopes of $g(\mathrm{k},t)$

$$\left(\frac{\partial B_{kt}}{\partial H_E}\right)_b = 0 \quad \text{and} \quad \left(\frac{\partial^2 B_{kt}}{\partial H_E^2}\right)_b < 0 \qquad \text{(A.80)}$$

Substitute (A.79) into (11.39) to obtain

$$\frac{d^2H}{dt^2} - 2\gamma(1 - H^2)\frac{dH}{dt} + [\omega_0^2 - 2\lambda_E^2 \mathrm{v}_\mathrm{E}^2 H^2]H = 0 \qquad \text{(A.81)}$$

Here the transformed dependent variable $H(\mathrm{k},t)$ and parameters ω_0 and γ are defined by

$$H(\mathrm{k},t) \equiv \left[\frac{-\left(\frac{\partial^2 B_{kt}}{\partial H_E^2}\right)_b}{2(B_{kb} - 2)}\right]^{1/2} H_E(\mathrm{k},t) \qquad \text{(A.82)}$$

where $B_{kb} > 2$, $\left(\frac{\partial^2 B_{kt}}{\partial H_E^2}\right)_b < 0$, and

$$\omega_0 = (\mathrm{k}^2 + \lambda_E^2)^{1/2}\mathrm{v}_\mathrm{E} \qquad \omega_0 > 0 \qquad \text{(A.83)}$$

$$\gamma = \lambda_E \mathrm{v}_E \left(\frac{B_{kb}}{2} - 1\right) \qquad \gamma > 0 \qquad \text{(A.84)}$$

Equation (A.81) is approximately the Van der Pol equation (10.8) if

$$\omega_0 >> \sqrt{2}\lambda_E \mathrm{v}_\mathrm{E}|H_{\max}| \qquad \text{(A.85)}$$

If, in addition

$$\frac{\gamma}{\omega_0} << 1 \qquad \text{(A.86)}$$

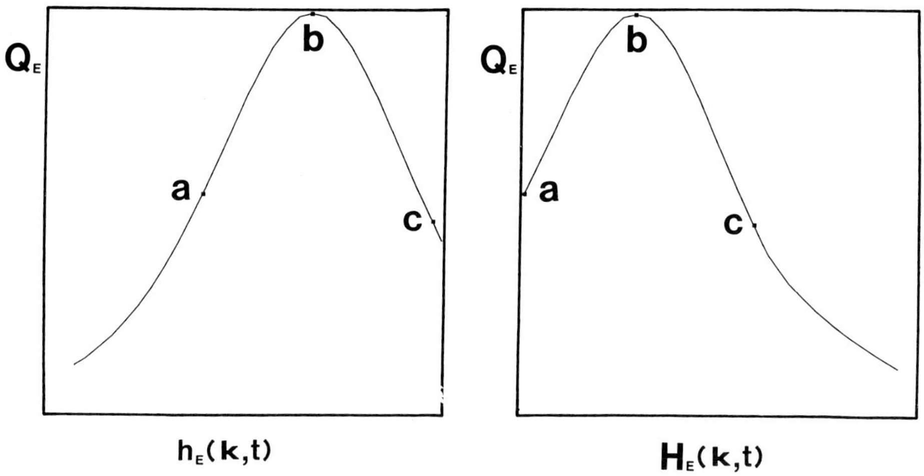

Figure A-1. **Left.** Symbolic representation of the assumed function $Q_E[h_E(k,t)]$ which is qualitatively consistent with the sigmoid function $g = g[h_E(\mathbf{r},t)]$ shown in Figure 11-5a. **Right.** The same function shifted to the left is $Q_E[H_E(k,t)]$. In this example, the background state h_{E0} is h_{Ea}. With condition (A.78), the control parameter B becomes a function of H_E (proportional to Q_E). When the background state is h_{Eb}, each spatial mode satisfies the van der Pol-like equation (A.81).

the Van der Pol equation has the approximate limit cycle solution

$$H \cong 2\cos(\omega_0 t) \tag{A.87}$$

Or in terms of the (Fourier transformed) modulation of excitatory synaptic action

$$H_E(\mathrm{k},t) \cong 2\left[\frac{2(B_{kb} - 2)}{-\left(\dfrac{\partial^2 B_{kt}}{\partial H_E^2}\right)_b}\right]^{1/2} \cos(\mathrm{k}\mathrm{v}_E t) \tag{11.40}$$

where conditions (A.85) and (A.86) require that $\mathrm{k} >> \lambda_E$.

More generally, we expect (A.81) to exhibit the following properties (see Figures 10-9 and 10-10):

(*i*) $B_{kb} > 2$ Limit cycle modes with amplitudes increasing and frequencies decreasing for increasing values of the parameters B_{kb}. We note that the correspondence of high amplitudes with low frequencies is a common EEG characteristic.
(*ii*) $B_{kb} < 2$ Point attractors that make much less contribution to observed EEG waveforms.

The quasi-linear approximations imply that the modulation of synaptic action may be approximated in a closed strip of length L by a linear combination of spatial modes

$$H_E(x,t) = \sum_{m=1}^{\infty} H_E(\mathrm{k}_m,t) \sin \mathrm{k}_m x \qquad \mathrm{k}_m = \frac{2m\pi}{L} \tag{11.41}$$

In the parlance of modern dynamic systems theory, the modes $H_E(\mathrm{k}_m,t)$ may be considered order parameters, a few of which may adequately describe the dynamics of a particular brain state. When the control parameters B_{kb} are changed (for example, by chemical changes in midbrain input), mode bifurcations may occur. For example, transition of one mode from point attractor to limit cycle, or from a limit cycle to chaotic motion (in more exact theories) may occur. In this manner, new order parameters (modes) characterize the new brain state.

Finally, we note the similarity of (11.39) or (A.81) to the nonlinear springs/linear string problem introduced in Chapter 2, in which the solution is expressed as a linear combination of spatial modes (2.8). We expect to observe only lower modes in scalp EEG recordings; however, these modes may be coupled to higher modes due, for example, to coupling of equations similar to (11.39) to nonlinear local circuit equations.

References

Erdelyi, A. *Higher Transcendentlal Functions, Vol.2*, New York: McGraw-Hill, 1953.

Katznelson, R.D. Normal modes of the brain: Neuroanatomical basis and a physiological theoretical model. In: *Electric Fields of the Brain: The Neurophysics of EEG*. (P.L. Nunez, Author) New York: Oxford University Press, 1981.

Katznelson, R.D. *Deterministic and Stochastic Field Theoretic Models in the Neurophysics of EEG*. Ph.D. Dissertation. LaJolla, CA: University of California at San Diego, 1982.

Kowalski, K. and Nunez, P.L. A mathematical study of a dispersion relation for brain waves using MACSYMA. Brain Physics Group Report, Tulane University, Jan. 15, 1991.

Montgomery, D.C. and Tidman, D.A. *Plasma Kinetic Theory*. New York: McGraw-Hill, pp. 51–63, 1964.

Nunez, P.L. Longitudinal wave propagation in plasma containing an external time dependent electric field. *Physics of Fluids*, 14: 633–639, 1971.

Srinivasan, R. *A Theoretical and Experimental Study of Neocortical Dynamics*. Ph.D. Dissertation. New Orleans, LA: Tulane University, 1994.

Index*

*"Thinking about thinking can make you crazy"; private communication from Richard Feynman to Lester Ingber (circa 1970).